ATLAS OF EMERGENCY MEDICINE

NOTICE

Medicine is an ever-changing science. As new research and clinical experience broaden our knowledge, changes in treatment and drug therapy are required. The editors and the publisher of this work have checked with sources believed to be reliable in their efforts to provide information that is complete and generally in accord with the standards accepted at the time of publication. However, in view of the possibility of human error or changes in medical sciences, neither the editors nor the publisher nor any other party who has been involved in the preparation or publication of this work warrants that the information contained herein is in every respect accurate or complete, and they are not responsible for any errors or omissions or for the results obtained from use of the information contained in this work. Readers are encouraged to confirm the information contained herein with other sources. For example and in particular, readers are advised to check the product information sheet included in the package of each drug they plan to administer to be certain that the information contained in this work is accurate and that changes have not been made in the recommended dose or in the contraindications for administration. This recommendation is of particular importance in connection with new or infrequently used drugs.

ATLAS OF EMERGENCY MEDICINE

Second Edition

Editors

Kevin J. Knoop, MD, MS

Program Director
Emergency Medicine Residency
Naval Medical Center
Portsmouth, Virginia

Lawrence B. Stack, MD

Associate Professor
Department of Emergency Medicine
Vanderbilt University Medical Center
Nashville, Tennessee

Alan B. Storrow, MD

Associate Professor of Emergency Medicine
Clinical Research Director, University of Cincinnati College of Medicine,
Cincinnati, Ohio

McGraw-Hill
MEDICAL PUBLISHING DIVISION

New York   Chicago   San Francisco   Lisbon   London   Madrid
Mexico City   Milan   New Delhi   San Juan   Seoul   Singapore   Sydney   Toronto

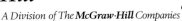

McGraw-Hill

A Division of The McGraw·Hill Companies

1234567890   IMPIMP   098765432

ISBN 0-07-135294-5

This book was set in Times Roman by TechBooks.
The editors were Andrea Seils, Kitty McCullough,
and Lester A. Sheinis.
The production supervisor was Richard C. Ruzycka.
The text and cover designer was Marsha Cohen/Parallelogram.
The indexer was Alexandra Nickerson.
Cayfosa-Quebecor, Barcelona, was printer and binder.

This book is printed on acid-free paper.

Library of Congress Cataloging-in-Publication Data

Atlas of emergency medicine / edited by Kevin J. Knoop,
    Lawrence B. Stack, Alan B. Storrow.—2nd ed.
    p.; cm.
  Includes bibliographical references and index.
  ISBN 0-07-135294-5
  1. Emergency medicine—Atlases.   I. Knoop, Kevin J.
II. Stack, Lawrence B.   III. Storrow, Alan B.
  [DNLM: 1. Emergency Medicine—methods—Atlases.
2. Critical Care—methods—Atlases.   3. Emergencies—Atlases.
WB 17 A8817 2002]
RC86.7.A85   2002
616.02´5—dc21   2002067849

To the outstanding Emergency Medicine residents of the Naval Medical Center, Portsmouth, Vanderbilt University Medical Center, and University of Cincinnati Medical Center, who teach us something new every day.

KJK

LBS

ABS

To Amelia and Stephen, you are my greatest teachers!
To Mary Jo, for your strength, support, love, and friendship.

KJK

To the patients who have allowed us to photograph their physical examination findings—may God bless you for allowing others to learn from your illness and injuries for the benefit of other patients.

LBS

To my patient, caring, and loving wife, Julia Ann.
To my children, Robert Leslie and Allison Marie. They bring me happiness every day.
Also in memory of my father, Hugh Alan Storrow, MD (1926–1996). He was a tenacious academician and a steadfast advocate for excellence in medical education.
His example is one I try to emulate daily.

ABS

CONTENTS

Part 1
REGIONAL ANATOMY   1

Chapter 1   HEAD AND FACIAL TRAUMA   3

David W. Munter
Timothy D. McGuirk

Chapter 2   OPHTHALMOLOGIC CONDITIONS   27

Frank Birinyi
Thomas F. Mauger

FUNDUSCOPIC FINDINGS   75   Chapter 3

David Effron
Beverly C. Forcier
Richard E. Wyszynski

OPHTHALMIC TRAUMA   97   Chapter 4

Dallas E. Peak
Carey D. Chisholm
Kevin J. Knoop

| Chapter 5 | EAR, NOSE, AND THROAT CONDITIONS | 117 |

Edward C. Jauch
Timothy Kaufman
Kevin J. Knoop

| Chapter 6 | MOUTH | 151 |

Edwin D. Turner
Edward C. Jauch

Oral Trauma   152

CHEST AND ABDOMEN   187   Chapter 7

Stephen Corbett
Lawrence B. Stack
Kevin J. Knoop

Chest and Abdominal Trauma   188

Chapter 8   UROLOGIC CONDITIONS   217

Jeffrey D. Bondesson

Chapter 9   SEXUALLY TRANSMITTED DISEASES AND ANORECTAL CONDITIONS 233

Diane M. Birnbaumer
Lynn K. Flowers

Sexually Transmitted Diseases   234

GYNECOLOGIC AND OBSTETRIC CONDITIONS 255 Chapter 10

Robert G. Buckley
Kevin J. Knoop

| Chapter 11 | EXTREMITY TRAUMA | 289 |

Deborah Gutman
Daniel L. Savitt
Alan B. Storrow

Upper Extremity 290

Pelvis and Hip 320

Lower Extremity 326

EXTREMITY CONDITIONS   347   Chapter 12

Selim Suner
Daniel L. Savitt

CUTANEOUS CONDITIONS   377   Chapter 13

Sean P. Collins

Part 2
SPECIALTY AREAS   431

PEDIATRIC CONDITIONS   433   Chapter 14

Javier A. Gonzalez del Rey
Richard M. Ruddy

| Chapter 15 | CHILD ABUSE | 479 |

Robert A. Shapiro
Charles J. Schubert

| Chapter 16 | ENVIRONMENTAL CONDITIONS | 513 |

Ken Zafren
R. Jason Thurman
Alan B. Storrow

FORENSIC MEDICINE   565   Chapter 17

William S. Smock
Lawrence B. Stack

Pattern Injuries of Domestic Violence, Assault, and Abuse   571

| Chapter 18 | WOUNDS AND SOFT TISSUE INJURIES | 577 |

Matthew D. Sztajnkrycer
Alexander T. Trott

| Chapter 19 | EMERGENCY ULTRASOUND | 609 |

Paul R. Sierzenski
Michael J. Lambert
Theodore J. Nielsen

| Chapter 20 | HIV CONDITIONS | 649 |

Shane Cline
Michael Krentz

MICROSCOPIC FINDINGS 675 Chapter 21

Diane M. Birnbaumer

Cerebrospinal Fluid Examination 688

CONTRIBUTORS

FRANK BIRINYI, MD, FACEP

Clinical Assistant Professor of Emergency Medicine
The Ohio State University
Attending Physician
Mount Carmel Medical Center
Mount Carmel East Hospital
Columbus, Ohio
Chapter 2

DIANE M. BIRNBAUMER, MD, FACEP

Associate Residency Director
Department of Emergency Medicine
Harbor–UCLA Medical Center
Torrence, California
Chapters 9, 21

JEFFREY D. BONDESSON, MD

Attending Physician
Kaiser Permanente Medical Center
San Diego, California
Chapter 8

ROBERT G. BUCKLEY, MD, FACEP, CDR, MC, USNR

Program Director
Emergency Medicine Residency
Naval Medical Center
San Diego, California
Chapter 10

CAREY D. CHISHOLM, MD, FACEP

Emergency Medicine Residency Director
Clinical Associate Professor of Emergency Medicine
Methodist-Indiana University
Indianapolis, Indiana
Chapter 4

SHANE CLINE, MD

Resident
Naval Medical Center
Portsmouth, Virginia
Chapter 20

SEAN P. COLLINS, MD

University of Cincinnati
Department of Emergency Medicine
Cincinnati, Ohio
Chapter 13

STEPHEN CORBETT, MD

Loma Linda University Medical Center
Department of Emergency Medicine
Loma Linda, California
Chapter 7

DAVID EFFRON, MD, FACEP

Department of Emergency Medicine
MetroHealth Medical Center
Cleveland, Ohio
Chapter 3

LYNN K. FLOWERS, MD, LCDR, MC, USNR

EMS Fellow
Charlotte Medical Center
Charlotte, North Carolina
Chapter 9

BEVERLY C. FORCIER, MD

Department of Emergency Medicine
MetroHealth Medical Center
Cleveland, Ohio
Chapter 3

JAVIER A. GONZALEZ DEL REY, MD, FAAP

Assistant Professor of Clinical Pediatrics and
Emergency Medicine
University of Cincinnati College of Medicine
Attending Physician, Division of Emergency Medicine
Children's Hospital Medical Center
Cincinnati, Ohio
Chapter 14

DEBORAH GUTMAN, MD

Department of Emergency Medicine
Rhode Island Hospital
Providence, Rhode Island
Chapter 11

EDWARD C. JAUCH, MD, MS

Assistant Professor
Department of Emergency Medicine
University of Cincinnati Medical Center
Cincinnati, Ohio
Chapters 5, 6

TIMOTHY KAUFMAN, MD

Resident
Department of Emergency Medicine
University of Cincinnati Medical Center
Cincinnati, Ohio
Chapter 5

KEVIN J. KNOOP, MD, MS, FACEP, CAPT, MC, USN

Program Director
Emergency Medicine Residency
Naval Medical Center
Portsmouth, Virginia
Chapters 4, 5, 7, 10

MICHAEL KRENTZ, MD, CAPT, MC, USN
Chairman, Emergency Medicine Department
Naval Medical Center
Portsmouth, Virginia
Chapter 20

MICHAEL J. LAMBERT, MD, RDMS
Fellowship Director, Emergency Ultrasound
Resurrection Medical Center
Chicago, Illinois
President, Windy City Ultrasound, Inc.
Darien, Illinois
Chapter 19

THOMAS F. MAUGER, MD
Associate Professor of Ophthalmology
Department of Ophthalmology
William H. Havener Eye Center
The Ohio State University
Columbus, Ohio
Chapter 2

**TIMOTHY D. McGUIRK, DO, FACEP,
CAPT, MC, USN**
Head, CIRD
Naval Medical Center
Portsmouth, Virginia
Chapter 1

**DAVID W. MUNTER, MD, FACEP,
CAPT, MC, USN**
Director, Medical Services
Naval Medical Center
Portsmouth, Virginia
Chapter 1

THEODORE J. NIELSEN, RT, RDMS
Vice President, Windy City Ultrasound, Inc.
Darien, Illinois
Chapter 19

DALLAS E. PEAK, MD
Attending Physician
Department of Emergency Medicine
Methodist-Indiana University
Indianapolis, Indiana
Chapter 4

RICHARD M. RUDDY, MD, FAAP
Professor of Clinical Pediatrics and Emergency
Medicine
University of Cincinnati College of Medicine
Director, Division of Emergency Medicine
Children's Hospital Medical Center
Cincinnati, Ohio
Chapter 14

DANIEL L. SAVITT, MD
Attending Physician and Residency Director
Department of Emergency Medicine
Rhode Island Hospital
Assistant Professor of Medicine
Brown University
Providence, Rhode Island
Chapters 11, 12

CHARLES J. SCHUBERT, MD, FAAP
Assistant Professor of Pediatrics
University of Cincinnati College of Medicine
Attending Physician, Division of Emergency Medicine
Children's Hospital Medical Center
Cincinnati, Ohio
Chapter 15

ROBERT A. SHAPIRO, MD
Medical Director, Mayerson Center for Safe &
Healthy Children
Children's Hospital Medical Center
Cincinnati, Ohio
Chapter 15

PAUL R. SIERZENSKI, MD, RDMS, FAAEM
Director, Emergency Medicine Ultrasound
Department of Emergency Medicine
Christiana Care Health System
Newark, Delaware
President, Emergency Ultrasound Consultants, LLC,
Bear, Delaware
Chapter 19

WILLIAM S. SMOCK, MD
Associate Professor and Director
Clinical Forensic Medicine Fellowship
Department of Emergency Medicine
University of Louisville School of Medicine
Louisville, Kentucky
Chapter 17

LAWRENCE B. STACK, MD, FACEP
Associate Professor
Department of Emergency Medicine
Vanderbilt University Medical Center
Nashville, Tennessee
Chapters 7, 17

ALAN B. STORROW, MD
Associate Professor of Emergency Medicine
Clinical Research Director
University of Cincinnati College of Medicine
Cincinnati, Ohio
Chapters 11, 16

SELIM SUNER, MD, MS
Assistant Professor of Surgery (Emergency Medicine)
Brown University School of Medicine
Department of Emergency Medicine
Rhode Island Hospital
Providence, Rhode Island
Chapter 12

MATTHEW D. SZTAJNKRYCER, MD, PhD
Assistant Professor of Emergency Medicine
University of Cincinnati College of Medicine
Cincinnati, Ohio
Chapter 18

R. JASON THURMAN, MD
Emergency Medicine Resident
University of Cincinnati College of Medicine
Cincinnati, Ohio
Chapter 16

ALEXANDER T. TROTT, MD
Professor of Emergency Medicine
University of Cincinnati College of Medicine
Cincinnati, Ohio
Chapter 18

EDWIN D. TURNER, MD
Attending Physician
Maplewood, Minnesota
Chapter 6

RICHARD E. WYSZYNSKI, MD
Department of Emergency Medicine
MetroHealth Medical Center
Cleveland, Ohio
Chapter 3

KEN ZAFREN, MD, FACEP
Providence Alaska Medical Center–Anchorage,
Alaska
Clinical Assistant Professor–Division of Emergency
Medicine
Stanford University Medical Center
Stanford, California
Medical Director, Denali National Park
Mountaineering Rangers and Lake Clark
National Park, Alaska
Associate Medical Director (USA), Himalayan
Rescue Association
Chapter 16

PHOTOGRAPHY CREDITS

BURT T. ACKERMAN, DO
Columbus, Georgia
American Academy of Ophthalmology
San Francisco, California

PAMELA AMBROZ, MD, LT, MC, USNR
Resident
Department of Obstetrics and Gynecology
Naval Medical Center
San Diego, California

American Academy of Pediatrics
Elk Grove Village, Illinois

American Society of Colon and Rectal Surgeons
Arlington Heights, Illinois

EDWARD S. AMRHEIN, DDS, CAPT, DC, USN
Head, Dental Department
Director, Oral & Maxillofacial Surgery Residency
Naval Medical Center
Portsmouth, Virginia

Armed Forces Institute of Pathology
Bethesda, Maryland

PAUL S. AUERBACH, MD, MS, FACEP
Chief Operating Officer
Sterling Health Care Group
Coral Gables, Florida
Formerly, Professor and Chief
Division of Emergency Medicine
Department of Surgery
Stanford University Medical Center
Stanford, California

MATTHEW BACKER JR., MD, RADM, MC, USNR (RET)
Attending Physician
Department of Obstetrics and Gynecology
Naval Medical Center
San Diego, California

JOHN D. BAKER, MD
Chief of Ophthalmology
Children's Hospital of Michigan
Clinical Professor of Ophthalmology
Wayne State University School of Medicine
Detroit, Michigan

RAYMOND C. BAKER, MD
Professor of Pediatrics
University of Cincinnati College of Medicine
Pediatrician, Division of Pediatrics
Children's Hospital Medical Center
Cincinnati, Ohio

WILLIAM S. BALL JR., MD
Professor of Radiology and Pediatrics
Chief, Section Neuroradiology and Staff Radiologist
Medical Director Imaging Research Center
Children's Hospital Medical Center
Cincinnati, Ohio

WILLIAM BARSAN, MD
Professor and Chair
Department of Emergency Medicine
University of Michigan
Ann Arbor, Michigan

KEITH F. BATTS, MD
Department Head
Emergency Medicine Department
Naval Hospital
Bremerton, Washington

JUDITH C. BAUSHER, MD
Associate Professor of Pediatrics and Emergency
Medicine
University of Cincinnati College of Medicine
Attending Physician, Division of Emergency
Medicine
Children's Hospital Medical Center
Cincinnati, Ohio

BILL BECK, CRA
Clinic Photographer, Florida Eye Clinic
Altamonte Springs, Florida

FRANK BIRINYI, MD, FACEP
Clinical Assistant Professor of Emergency Medicine
The Ohio State University
Attending Physician
Mount Carmel Medical Center
Mount Carmel East Hospital
Columbus, Ohio

DIANE M. BIRNBAUMER, MD, FACEP
Associate Residency Director
Department of Emergency Medicine
Harbor-UCLA Medical Center
Torrance, California

JEFFERY D. BONDESSON, MD
Attending Physician
Kaiser Permanente Medical Center
San Diego, California

JOHN BOYLE, MD, LT, MC, USNR
Resident
Department of Obstetrics and Gynecology
Naval Medical Center
San Diego, California

ALAN S. BRODY, MD
Staff Radiologist
Children's Hospital Medical Center
Cincinnati, Ohio

MICHAEL B. BROOKS, MD
Attending Physician
Joint Military Medical Centers Emergency Medicine
Residency
Brooke Army Medical Center
San Antonio, Texas

ROBERT G. BUCKLEY, MD, FACEP, CDR, MC, USNR
Program Director
Department of Emergency Medicine
Naval Medical Center
San Diego, California

SEAN P. BUSH, MD, FACEP
Staff Emergency Physician and Envenomation
Consultant
Associate Professor of Emergency Medicine
Loma Linda University Medical Center and School of
Medicine
Loma Linda, California

WILLIAM E. CAPPAERT, MD
Department of Emergency Medicine
MetroHealth Medical Center
2500 MetroHealth Drive
Cleveland, Ohio

CAREY D. CHISHOLM, MD, FACEP
Emergency Medicine Residency Director
Clinical Associate Professor of Emergency Medicine
Methodist-Indiana University
Indianapolis, Indiana

RICHARD A. CHOLE, MD, PhD
Lindburg Professor and Head
Department of Otolaryngology
Washington University School of Medicine
St. Louis, Missouri

JUDY CHRISTENSEN
Medical Illustrator
Graphics Division
Staff Education and Training
Naval Medical Center
San Diego, California

RICHARD A. CLINCHY III, PhD, NREMT-P
American College of Prehospital Medicine
Ft. Walton Beach, Florida

SHANE CLINE, MD
Staff Physician
Naval Hospital
Jacksonville, Florida

SEAN P. COLLINS, MD
Chief Resident
Department of Emergency Medicine
University of Cincinnati
Cincinnati, Ohio

MARCO COPOLLA, DO, FACEP
Program Director, Emergency Medicine Residency
Research Directory
Department of Emergency Medicine
Scott and White Memorial Hospital
Assistant Professor of Emergency Medicine
Texas A&M University Health Science Center
Temple, Texas

STEPHEN CORBETT, MD
Department of Emergency Medicine
Loma Linda University Medical Center
Loma Linda, California

ROBIN T. COTTON, MD
Professor
Department of Otolaryngology and Maxillofacial
Surgery
Children's Hospital Medical Center
Cincinnati, Ohio

BARBARA R. CRAIG, MD, CAPT, MC, USN
Medical Consultant for Child Abuse and Neglect
National Naval Medical Center
Bethesda, Maryland

Curatek Pharmaceuticals
Elk Grove Village, Illinois

TIMOTHY CURTIN, MD
Department of Dermatology
Naval Medical Center
Portsmouth, Virginia

Department of Dermatology
National Naval Medical Center
Bethesda, Maryland

Department of Dermatology
Naval Medical Center
Portsmouth, Virginia

Departments of Dermatology
Collective Files
Brooke Army Medical Center
Wilford Hall USAF Medical Center
San Antonio, Texas

Department of Ophthalmology
Naval Medical Center
Portsmouth, Virginia

Department of Otolaryngology
Children's Hospital Medical Center
Cincinnati, Ohio

HERBERT L. DUPONT, MD
Chief, Internal Medicine Service
St. Luke's Episcopal Hospital
Houston, Texas

LEE E. EDSTROM, MD
Surgeon in Chief
Division of Plastic Surgery
Rhode Island Hospital
Assistant Professor of Surgery
Brown University
Providence, Rhode Island

DAVID EFFRON, MD, FACEP
Department of Emergency Medicine
MetroHealth Medical Center
Cleveland, Ohio

MARK EICH, MD
Staff Physician
Naval Hospital
Jacksonville, Florida

ERIC EINFALT, MD, LCDR, MC, USNR
Staff Physician
Emergency Medicine Department
Naval Medical Center
Jacksonville, Florida

EDWARD M. EITZEN, JR., MD, MPH
Chief, Preventive Medicine Department
US Army Medical Research Institute of Infectious
Diseases
Fort Detrick, Maryland

JAMES P. ELROD, MD, PHD
Staff Hemopathologist
St. Thomas Hospital
Nashville, Tennessee

KIM MARIE FELDHAUS, MD
Emergency Medical Services
Denver General Hospital
Denver, Colorado

JOHN FILDES, MD, FACS
Attending Surgeon
Division of Trauma
Department of Surgery
Cook County Hospital
Chicago, Illinois

JEFFREY FINKELSTEIN, MD, FACEP
Chief, Division of Acute Care
Chairman, Department of Emergency Medicine
Wilford Hall Medical Center
Attending Physician
Joint Military Medical Centers
Emergency Medicine Residency
San Antonio, Texas

LYNN K. FLOWERS, MD, LCDR, MC, USNR
EMS Fellow
Charlotte Medical Center
Charlotte, North Carolina

BEVERLY C. FORCIER, MD
Department of Emergency Medicine
MetroHealth Medical Center
Cleveland, Ohio

SARA-JO GAHM, MD
Resident
Department of Emergency Medicine
Medical College of Pennsylvania
Philadelphia, Pennsylvania

Geisinger Medical Center
Department of Emergency Medicine
Danville, Pennsylvania

W. BRIAN GIBLER, MD
Professor and Chair
Department of Emergency Medicine
University of Cincinnati College of Medicine
Cincinnati, Ohio

JEFFREY S. GIBSON, MD, LCDR, MC, USNR
Staff Physician
Emergency Medicine Department
Naval Medical Center
Jacksonville, Florida

GLAXO-WELLCOME PHARMACEUTICALS

JAVIER A. GONZALEZ DEL REY, MD, FAAP
Assistant Professor of Clinical Pediatrics and
Emergency Medicine
University of Cincinnati College of Medicine
Attending Physician, Division of Emergency Medicine
Children's Hospital Medical Center
Cincinnati, Ohio

RALPH A. GRUPPO, MD
Professor of Pediatrics
University of Cincinnati College of Medicine
Director, Hemophilia Treatment Center
Children's Hospital Medical Center
Cincinnati, Ohio

DEBORAH GUTMAN, MD
Department of Emergency Medicine
Rhode Island Hospital
Providence, Rhode Island

PETER HACKETT, MD, FACEP
St. Mary's Hospital
Grand Junction, Colorado

H. HUNTER HANDSFIELD, MD
Professor of Medicine
University of Washington
Director, STD Control Program
Seattle-King County Department of Public Health
Seattle, Washington

BRIANA HILL, MD
Chairman
Department of Dermatology
Naval Medical Center
Portsmouth, Virginia

TIMOTHY HINMAN, MD, CDR, MC, USN
Head, Emergency Medicine Department
Naval Hospital
Okinawa, Japan

ROBERT S. HOFFMAN, MD, FACEP
Assistant Professor, Clinical Surgery and Emergency
Medicine
NYU School of Medicine
Director, NYC Poison Control Center
New York City, New York

KING K. HOLMES, MD, PhD
Director, University of Washington Center for AIDS
and STD
Professor of Medicine
University of Washington
Seattle, Washington

STEPHEN HOLT, MD
San Antonio, Texas

ROBERT B. HORTON, DDS
Professor of Clinical Surgery
Assistant Chief
Division of Oral and Maxillofacial Surgery
Department of Surgery
University of Cincinnati College of Medicine
Cincinnati, Ohio

CURTIS HUNTER, MD
Chief, Emergency Medical Services
General Leonard Wood Army Community Hospital
Fort Leonard Wood, Missouri

LIUDVIKAS JAGMINAS, MD
Attending Physician
Department of Emergency Medicine
Rhode Island Hospital
Assistant Professor of Medicine
Brown University
Providence, Rhode Island

JENNIFER JAGOE, MD, LT, MC, USNR
Resident
Department of Obstetrics and Gynecology
Naval Medical Center
San Diego, California

TIMOTHY JAHN, MD, LCDR, MC, USNR
Attending Physician
Department of Emergency Medicine
Naval Hospital
Great Lakes, Illinois

THEA JAMES, MD
Department of Emergency Medicine
Boston Medical Center
Boston University School of Medicine
Boston, Massachusetts

EDWARD C. JAUCH, MD, MS
Assistant Professor
Department of Emergency Medicine
University of Cincinnati Medical Center
Cincinnati, Ohio

IAN JONES, MD
Assistant Professor of Emergency Medicine
Director of Emergency Department Operations
Vanderbilt University
Nashville, Tennessee

ARTHUR M. KAHN, MD, FACS
Assistant Professor of Surgery
UCLA School of Medicine
Attending Surgeon
Cedars-Sinai Medical Center
Los Angeles, California

LEE KAPLAN, MD
Chief of Dermatology
VA Medical Center, San Diego, California
Associate Clinical Professor of Medicine and
Dermatology
University of California
San Diego, California

MARGARET J. KARNES, DO
Assistant Professor of Emergency Medicine
Texas A&M University Health Science Center
College Station, Texas
Senior Staff Physician
Department of Emergency Medicine
Scott and White Memorial Hospital and Clinic
Temple, Texas

TIMOTHY KAUFMAN, MD
Resident
Department of Emergency Medicine
University of Cincinnati Medical Center
Cincinnati, Ohio

KENNETH W. KIZER, MD
Distinguished Professor of Military and Emergency
Medicine
Uniformed Services University of the Health Sciences
Bethesda, Maryland
Former Undersecretary for Health
Department of Veteran Affairs
Washington, DC

**KEVIN J. KNOOP, MD, MS, FACEP, CAPT,
MC, USN**
Program Director
Emergency Medicine Residency
Naval Medical Center
Portsmouth, Virginia

PAUL J. KOVALCHIK, MD, FACS
Colorectal Surgeon
Chesapeake, Virginia

MICHAEL KRENTZ, MD, MPH, FACEP
Chairman, Emergency Medicine Department
Naval Medical Center
Portsmouth, Virginia

DAVID P. KRETZSCHMAR, DDS, MS
Chief, Department of Oral and Maxillofacial Surgery
2nd Medical Group
Barksdale AFB, Louisiana
Assistant Professor
Department of Surgery
Louisiana State University Medical Center
New Orleans, Louisiana

**JAMES L. KRETZSCHMAR, DDS, MS,
LTCOL, USAF**
OIC Flight Dental Clinic
Holloman AFB, New Mexico

JEFFERY KUHN, MD, CDR, MC, USNR
Department of Otolaryngology—Head and Neck
Surgery
Naval Medical Center
Portsmouth, Virginia

MICHAEL J. LAMBERT, MD, RDMS
Fellowship Director, Emergency Ultrasound
Resurrection Medical Center
Chicago, Illinois
President, Windy City Ultrasound, Inc.
Darien, Illinois

DOUGLAS R. LANDRY, MD
Staff Physician
Bayside Hospital
Virginia Beach, Virginia

PATRICK W. LAPPERT, MD, CAPT, MC, USN
Naval Medical Center, Portsmouth, Virginia
Clinical Assistant Professor, Department of Surgery
Uniformed Services University of the Health Sciences
Bethesda, Maryland

HILLARY J. LARKIN, PA-C
Director, Medical Sexual Assault Services
Department of Emergency Medicine
Alameda Sexual Assault Response Team
Highland General Hospital
Oakland, California

LORENZ F. LASSEN, MD, CAPT, MC, USN
Assistant Professor of Otolaryngology—Head and
Neck Surgery
Eastern Virginia Medical School
Service Line Leader
Reparative Services
Naval Medical Center
Portsmouth, Virginia

LOUIS LAVOPA, MD
Staff Physician
Emergency Medicine Department
Naval Hospital
Agana, Guam

WILLIAM LENINGER, MD, LT, MC, USNR
Resident
Department of Obstetrics and Gynecology
Naval Medical Center
San Diego, California

RICHARD C. LEVY, MD
Professor Emeritus of Emergency Medicine
Department of Emergency Medicine
University of Cincinnati
Cincinnati, Ohio

ANNE W. LUCKY, MD
Volunteer Professor of Dermatology and Pediatrics
University of Cincinnati College of Medicine
Director, Dermatology Clinic
Children's Hospital Medical Center
Cincinnati, Ohio

C. BRUCE MACDONALD, MD
Assistant Professor, Department of Otolaryngology
Boston University School of Medicine
Boston, Massachusetts

MARK L. MADENWALD, MD, LT, MC, USNR
Chief Resident
Emergency Medicine Department
Naval Medical Center
Portsmouth, Virginia

WILLIAM K. MALLON, MD, FACEP
Associate Director of Residency Training
Assistant Professor of Medicine
University of Southern California School of Medicine
Los Angeles, California

ROBIN MARSHALL, MD
Emergency Medicine Resident
Naval Medical Center
Portsmouth, Virginia

MASSIE RESEARCH LABORATORIES, INC.
Dublin, California

THOMAS F. MAUGER, MD
Associate Professor of Ophthalmology
Department of Ophthalmology
William H. Havener Eye Center
The Ohio State University
Columbus, Ohio

TIMOTHY D. MCGUIRK, DO, FACEP, CAPT, MC, USN
Department Head
Emergency Medicine Hospital
Okinawa, Japan

PATRICK H. MCKENNA, MD, FACS, FAAP
Assistant Clinical Professor of Urology and Pediatrics
University of Connecticut Health Center
Hartford, Connecticut

AURORA MENDEZ, RN
Sexual Assault Response Team Coordinator
Villavu Community Hospital
San Diego, California

JAMES MENSCHING, DO
Operational Medical Director
Emergency Medical Department
Naval Medical Center
Portsmouth, Virginia

SHERMAN MINTON, MD
Professor Emeritus
Department of Microbiology and Immunology
Indiana University School of Medicine
Indianapolis, Indiana

JOHN D. MITCHELL, MD
Program Director
Ophthalmology Residency
Washington National Eye Center
Washington Hospital Center
Washington, D.C.

MARGARET P. MUELLER, MD
Department of Emergency Medicine
Rhode Island Hospital and Brown University
Providence, Rhode Island

DAVID W. MUNTER, MD, FACEP, CAPT, MC, USN
Director, Medical Services
Naval Medical Center
Portsmouth, Virginia

GEORGE L. MURRELL, MD, LCDR, MC, USN
Department of Otolaryngology—Head and Neck Surgery
Naval Medical Center, Portsmouth, Virginia
Assistant Professor of Clinical Otolaryngology Head and Neck Surgery
Eastern Virginia Medical School
Norfolk, Virginia

THEODORE J. NIELSEN, RT, RDMS
Vice President, Windy City Ultrasound, Inc.
Darien, Illinois

DANIEL NOLTKAMPER, MD
Assistant Chairman
Department of Emergency Medicine
Naval Hospital
Camp Lejeune, North Carolina

JAMES NORDLUND, MD
Professor of Dermatology
Department of Dermatology
University of Cincinnati
Cincinnati, Ohio

MICHAEL J. NOWICKI, MD, CDR, MC, USN
Division of Pediatric Gastroenterology
Department of Pediatrics
Naval Medical Center
Portsmouth, Virginia

ALAN E. OESTREICH, MD
Professor of Radiology and Pediatrics
University of Cincinnati College of Medicine
Chief, Section of Diagnostic Radiology
Staff Radiologist
Children's Hospital Medical Center
Cincinnati, Ohio

EDWARD C. OLDFIELD, III, MD
Professor of Medicine
Director, Infectious Diseases Division
Eastern Virginia School of Medicine
Norfolk, Virginia

GERALD O'MALLEY, DO, LCDR, MC, USNR
Research Coordinator
Naval Medical Center
Portsmouth, Virginia

JAMES O'MALLEY, MD
Providence Alaska Regional Medical Center
Anchorage, Alaska

EDWARD J. OTTEN, MD
Professor of Emergency Medicine and Pediatrics
Director, Division of Toxicology
University of Cincinnati College of Medicine
Cincinnati, Ohio

JAMES PALOMBARO, MD, LCDR, MC, USNR
Attending Physician
Department of Obstetrics and Gynecology
Naval Medical Center
San Diego, California

LAURI PAOLINETTE, PA-C
Sexual Assault Examiner
Department of Emergency Medicine
Alameda Sexual Assault Response Team
Highland General Hospital
Oakland, California

DAVID O. PARRISH, MD
St. Petersburg, Florida

DALLAS E. PEAK, MD
Attending Physician
Department of Emergency Medicine
Methodist Hospital of Indiana
Indianapolis, Indiana

MICHAEL P. POIRIER, MD
Assistant Professor of Pediatrics
Eastern Virginia Medical School
Division of Pediatric Emergency Medicine
Children's Hospital of the King's Daughters
Norfolk, Virginia

MARK RALSTON, MD, MPH, CAPT, MC, USNR
Director
Children's Emergency Unit
Department of Emergency Medicine
Naval Medical Center
Portsmouth, Virginia

MICHAEL REDMAN, PA-C
Staff, Emergency Medicine
Fort Leonard Wood Army Community Hospital
Fort Leonard Wood, Missouri

SUE RIST, FNP, CAPT, NC, USN (RET)
Naval Training Center
San Diego, California

MICHAEL RITTER, MD
Laguna Beach, California

HAROLD RIVERA, HM1, USN
Optician
Department of Ophthalmology
Naval Medical Center
Portsmouth, Virginia

GREGORY K. ROBBINS, MD MPH
Instructor in Medicine
Massachusetts General Hospital
Partners AIDS Center
Harvard Medical School
Boston, Massachusetts

ROCHE LABORATORIES
Nutley, New Jersey

DONALD L. RUCKNAGEL, MD, PHD
Professor of Pediatrics and Internal Medicine
University of Cincinnati College of Medicine
Comprehensive Sickle Cell Center
Children's Hospital Medical Center
Cincinnati, Ohio

RICHARD M. RUDDY, MD, FAAP
Professor of Clinical Pediatrics and Emergency
Medicine
University of Cincinnati College of Medicine
Director, Division of Emergency Medicine
Children's Hospital Medical Center
Cincinnati, Ohio

WARREN K. RUSSELL, MD, LCDR, MC, USNR
Head, Emergency Medicine Department
Naval Hospital
Roosevelt Roads, Puerto Rico

SALLY SANTEN, MD
Assistant Professor
Department of Emergency Medicine
Vanderbilt University Medical Center
Nashville, Tennessee

KATRINA C. SANTOS, HM3, USN
Ocular Technician
Department of Ophthalmology
Naval Medical Center
Portsmouth, Virginia

ADAM R. SAPERSTON, MD, MS, CDR, MC, USN
Attending Physician
Emergency Medicine Residency
Naval Medical Center
Portsmouth, Virginia

CHRISTOPHER R. SARTORI, MD
Chief, Outpatient Dermatology
Wilford Hall Medical Center
San Antonio, Texas

DANIEL L. SAVITT, MD
Attending Physician and Residency Director
Department of Emergency Medicine
Rhode Island Hospital
Assistant Professor of Medicine
Brown University
Providence, Rhode Island

JOSEPH C. SCHMIDT, MD
Chief Resident
Joint Military Medical Centers Emergency Medicine
Residency
Wilford Hall Medical Center
San Antonio, Texas

ROBERT SCHNARRS, MD
Staff Physician
Department of Plastic Surgery
Sentara Norfolk General Hospital
Norfolk, Virginia

CHARLES J. SCHUBERT, MD
Assistant Professor of Pediatrics and Emergency
Medicine
University of Cincinnati College of Medicine
Attending Physician, Division of Emergency Medicine
Children's Hospital Medical Center
Cincinnati, Ohio

GARY SCHWARTZ, MD
Assistant Professor
Department of Emergency Medicine
Vanderbilt University Medical Center
Nashville, Tennessee

ROBERT A. SHAPIRO, MD
Medical Director, Mayerson Center for Safe and
Healthy Children
Children's Hospital Medical Center
Cincinnati, Ohio

VIRENDER K. SHARMA, MD
Fellow
Division of Digestive Disease and Nutrition
University of South Carolina School of Medicine
Columbia, South Carolina

REES W. SHEPPARD, MD, FACS
Assistant Director of Pediatric Ophthalmology
Children's Hospital Medical Center
Volunteer Associate Professor
University of Cincinnati College of Medicine
Cincinnati, Ohio

PAUL R. SIERZENSKI, MD, RDMS, FAAEM
Director of Emergency Medicine Ultrasound
Department of Emergency Medicine
Christiana Care Health System
Newark, Delaware
President, Emergency Ultrasound Consultants, LLC
Bear, Delaware

KENNETH SKAHAN, MD
Assistant Professor
Division of Infectious Diseases
University of Cincinnati
Cincinnati, Ohio

TIMOTHY L. SMITH, MD
Assistant Professor
Department of Otolaryngology—Head and Neck
Surgery
Vanderbilt University Medical Center
Nashville, Tennessee

WILLIAM S. SMOCK, MD
Associate Professor and Director
Clinical Forensic Medicine Fellowship
Department of Emergency Medicine
University of Louisville, School of Medicine
Louisville, Kentucky

SONOSITE, INC.
Bothell, Washington

D. J. SPALTON FRCS, MRCP
Consultant Ophthalmic Surgeon
Medical Eye Unit
St. Thomas's Hospital
London, United Kingdom

LAWRENCE B. STACK, MD, FACEP
Associate Professor
Department of Emergency Medicine
Vanderbilt University Medical Center
Nashville, Tennessee

WALTER STAMM, MD
Professor of Medicine
Head, Infectious Diseases Division
Harborview Medical Center
Seattle, Washington

JAMES F. STEINER, DDS
Professor of Pediatrics
University of Cincinnati College of Medicine
Pediatric Dentistry
Children's Hospital Medical Center
Cincinnati, Ohio

ALAN B. STORROW, MD, FACEP
Associate Professor of Emergency Medicine
Clinical Research Director
University of Cincinnati College of Medicine
Cincinnati, Ohio

RICHARD STRAIT, MD
Assistant Professor of Clinical Pediatrics
Children's Hospital Medical Center
University of Cincinnati
Cincinnati, Ohio

SELIM SUNER, MD, MS
Assistant Professor of Surgery (Emergency Medicine)
Brown University School of Medicine
Department of Emergency Medicine
Rhode Island Hospital
Providence, Rhode Island

MATTHEW D. SZTAJNKRYCER, MD
Assistant Professor of Emergency Medicine
University of Cincinnati College of Medicine
Cincinnati, Ohio

GARY TANNER, MD, CDR, MC, USN
Chairman, Department of Ophthalmology
Naval Medical Center
Portsmouth, Virginia

R. JASON THURMAN, MD
Emergency Medicine Resident
University of Cincinnati College of Medicine
Cincinnati, Ohio

ROBERT TRIEFF, MD (DECEASED)
Emergency Medicine Resident
Naval Medical Center
Portsmouth, Virginia

ALEXANDER T. TROTT, MD
Professor of Emergency Medicine
University of Cincinnati College of Medicine
Cincinnati, Ohio

GEORGE TURIANSKY, MD
Dermatology Service
Walter Reed Army Medical Center
Washington, D.C.

EDWIN D. TURNER, MD, FACEP
Attending Physician, Emergency Department
Unity Hospital
Fridley, Minnesota

JANICE E. UNDERWOOD, RDMS
Advanced Health Education Center, Inc.
Houston, Texas

US Government Printing Office
Washington, DC

LYNN UTECHT, MD
Chairman
Department of Dermatology
Naval Hospital
Rota, Spain

GERALD VAN HOUDT, MD, CDR, MC, USN
Resident
Department of Emergency Medicine
Naval Medical Center
San Diego

CATHLEEN M. VOSSLER, MD
Resident
Department of Emergency Medicine
Rhode Island Hospital and Brown University
Providence, Rhode Island

ARDEN H. WANDER, MD
Professor of Clinical Ophthalmology
University of Cincinnati
Cincinnati, Ohio

ERIC D. WILLIAMS, MD, CAPT, MC, USAF
Staff Emergency Physician
Eskan Clinic
Elemendorf Air Force Base, Alaska

ALEX WILSON
Nova Scotia Museum of Natural History
Halifax, Nova Scotia, Canada

Windy City Ultrasound, Inc.
Chicago, Illinois

RICHARD E. WYSZYNSKI, MD
Department of Emergency Medicine
MetroHealth Medical Center
Cleveland, Ohio

SCOTT W. ZACKOWSKI, MD
Director, Medical Services
Naval Hospital
Naples, Italy

KEN ZAFREN, MD, FACEP, FAAEM
Providence Alaska Medical Center
Anchorage, Alaska
Clinical Assistant Professor
Division of Emergency Medicine
Stanford University Medical Center
Stanford, California
Medical Director, Denali National Park
Mountaineering Rangers and
Lake Clark National Park, Alaska
Associate Medical Director (USA), Himalayan
Rescue Association

RICHARD ZIENOWICZ, MD
Attending Physician
Division of Plastic Surgery
Rhode Island Hospital
Assistant Professor of Surgery
Brown University
Providence, Rhode Island

FOREWORD

The second edition of the *Atlas of Emergency Medicine* is a rare book. Though it is an excellent stand-alone text, it is also perfectly suited to be a supplement to any other textbook in emergency medicine. The *Atlas* is a resource for all who study or practice emergency medicine. Medical students, nursing students, and others new to the Emergency Department, residents based in or rotating through emergency medicine, and, finally, clinicians and teachers will all find it invaluable.

The *Atlas of Emergency Medicine* is much more than simply an atlas with clear pictures, classic radiographs, microscopic reproductions, and instructive diagrams. It is also an easy-to-read textbook of emergency medicine told with innumerable clinical pearls and instructive teaching supplemented by pictures and illustrations. This second edition has four new chapters that reflect both emergency medicine's growth in the areas of ultrasound and forensic medicine and also the editors' desire to provide readers with in-depth pictorial expertise in wound care and AIDS. All of the other chapters have been updated, refined, and expanded where appropriate.

As has been said by many, the *Atlas of Emergency Medicine* can be used for many different purposes ranging from an introduction to acute care to a review text for board certification. It is one of the few texts that can be routinely utilized by students, practicing physicians, and experienced teachers.

Drs. Knoop, Stack and Storrow should be very proud of their work. They have improved upon an already classic text by adding appropriate new sections and expanding on existing chapters, yet they have succeeded in keeping their book concise, practical, and user-friendly.

Corey M. Slovis, MD

Scope

Text alone is simply not sufficient for assimilating the enormous amount of clinical knowledge necessary in today's practice of emergency medicine. Volumes of well-written text simply cannot replace what our eyes experience. The success of the first edition of *Atlas of Emergency Medicine* has born this out. The second edition significantly enlarges upon this theme by expanding the content and scope of the first edition.

We have incorporated the many changes suggested by the readership into this new edition. Feedback from journal reviews and abundant personal interactions has resulted in updates in every chapter with new items and photography. Another powerful source of the changes is the ever-evolving nature of our specialty. The addition of new chapters on Forensics, Wounds and Soft Tissue Injuries, Ultrasound, and HIV stems from our attempt to adjust to the ongoing transitions in emergency medicine. These areas are becoming prominent in our daily practice and deserve more dedicated attention.

Our goal is to continue to improve the *Atlas* with changes to future editions guided by reader feedback. All criticism is considered a "gift" and is accepted with gratitude and thanks. We hope this interchange with the readership will continue.

Purpose

Atlas of Emergency Medicine, second edition, continues to serve as the reference and teaching guide to the visual clues seen in emergency medicine. Despite the information explosion since the publication of the first edition, none of the many different atlases and color guides available today are comprehensive enough for use as a single reference in the Emergency Department or acute care clinic. The *Atlas* is not meant to be a comprehensive text nor a treatise on diagnosis. The images collected portray the scope and breadth of emergency practice and, as such, represent the most comprehensive collection of excellent emergency clinical images. Outside of the *Atlas,* such a book does not exist and we envision this text to continue to fill this void.

Intended Audience

The primary audience for this text is emergency medicine clinicians, educators, residents, and medical students who provide emergency care. We hope it will aid the clinician in making the diagnosis and help the teacher take the student "to the bedside." Many have found it useful as a review for the ABEM written examination. Other health care workers, such as internists, family physicians, and pediatricians will find the *Atlas* a useful guide in identifying and treating the many conditions for which visual cues significantly guide and expedite diagnosis and treatment. Physician extenders, such as nurse practitioners and physician assistants, may also appreciate the "clinical experience" this text can add to their training and practice. Finally, interested medical students can augment their clinical repertoire early in their training from the "visual discoveries" they will encounter in this text.

Organization

The organization of the *Atlas of Emergency Medicine,* second edition, is based on regional anatomy for Part 1, with Part 2 comprised of selected specialty areas. Part 2 has undergone a robust expansion with the addition of four new chapters mentioned above. The Contents shows the individual diagnoses displayed in each chapter. A brief text accompanies each diagnosis and, with the exception of the final chapter (Microscopic Findings), includes the following sections: Associated Clinical Features, Differential Diagnosis, Emergency Department Treatment and Disposition, and Clinical Pearls.

ATLAS OF EMERGENCY MEDICINE

PART 1

REGIONAL ANATOMY

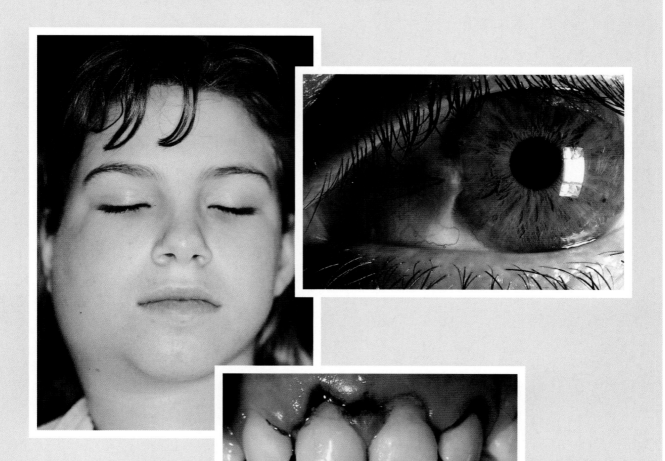

CHAPTER 1

HEAD AND FACIAL TRAUMA

David W. Munter
Timothy D. McGuirk

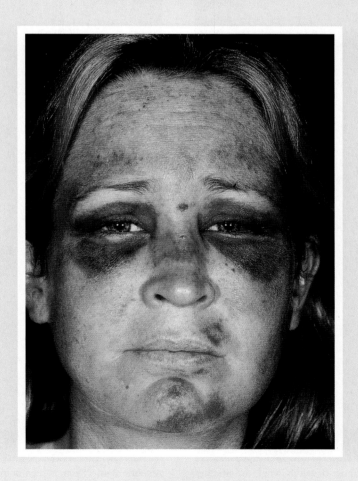

Associated Clinical Features

The skull base comprises the floors of the anterior, middle, and posterior cranial fossae. Trauma resulting in fractures to this basilar area typically does not have localizing symptoms. Plain skull radiographs are poor in identifying these fractures. Indirect signs of the injury may include visible evidence of bleeding from the fracture into surrounding soft tissue, such as a Battle's sign (Figs. 1.1, 1.2) or "raccoon eyes" (Fig. 1.3). Bleeding into other structures—including hemotympanum (Fig. 1.4) or blood in the sphenoid sinus seen as an air-fluid level—may also be seen. Cerebrospinal fluid (CSF) leaks may also be evident and noted as clear or pink rhinorrhea. If CSF is present, a dextrose stick test may be positive. The fluid can be placed on filter paper and a "halo" or double ring may be seen (Fig. 1.5).

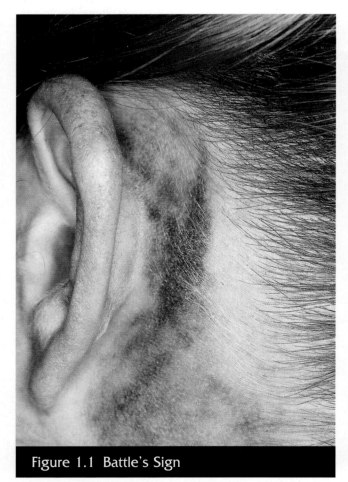

Figure 1.1 Battle's Sign

Ecchymosis in the postauricular area develops when the fracture line communicates with the mastoid air cells, resulting in blood accumulating in the cutaneous tissue. This patient had sustained injuries several days prior to presentation. (Courtesy of Frank Birinyi, MD.)

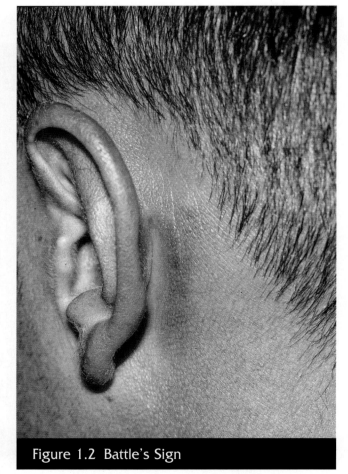

Figure 1.2 Battle's Sign

A subtle Battle's sign is seen in this patient with head trauma. This sign may take hours to develop fully. (Courtesy of Lawrence B. Stack, MD.)

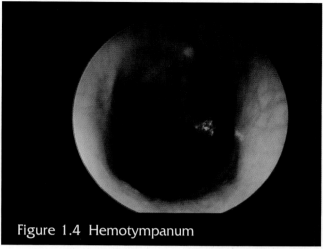

Figure 1.4 Hemotympanum

Seen in a basilar skull fracture when the fracture line communicates with the auditory canal, resulting in bleeding into the middle ear. Blood can be seen behind the tympanic membrane. (Courtesy of Richard A. Chole, MD, PhD.)

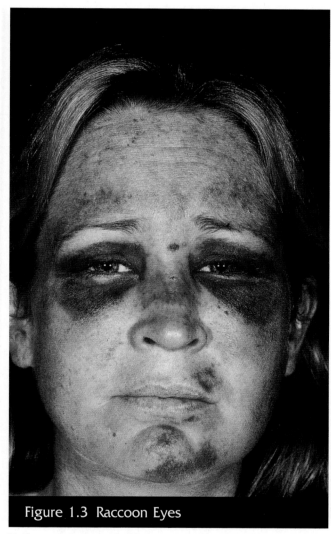

Figure 1.3 Raccoon Eyes

Ecchymosis in the periorbital area, resulting from bleeding from a fracture site in the anterior portion of the skull base. May also be caused by facial fractures. (Courtesy of Frank Birinyi, MD.)

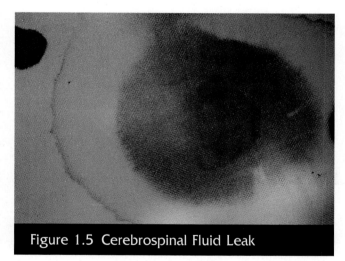

Figure 1.5 Cerebrospinal Fluid Leak

This example, from the nose, can be difficult to distinguish from blood or mucus. The distinctive double-ring sign, seen here, comprises blood (*inner ring*) and CSF (*outer ring*). The reliability of this test has been questioned. (Courtesy of David W. Munter, MD.)

Differential Diagnosis

Direct trauma without skull fracture can result in external ecchymosis. Barotrauma can cause hemotympanum. Facial injuries and fractures can cause facial ecchymosis.

Emergency Department Treatment and Disposition

The mainstay of therapy is to identify underlying brain injury, which is best accomplished by computed tomography (CT). CT is also the best diagnostic tool for identifying the fracture site, but fractures may not always be evident. Evidence of open communication, such as a CSF leak, mandates neurosurgical consultation and admission. Otherwise, the decision for admission is based on the patient's clinical condition, other associated injuries, and evidence of underlying brain injury as seen on CT. The use of antibiotics in the presence of a CSF leak is controversial because of the possibility of selecting resistant organisms.

Clinical Pearls

1. The clinical manifestations of basilar skull fracture may take several hours to fully develop.
2. Since plain films are unhelpful, there should be a low threshold for head CT in any patient with head trauma, loss of consciousness, obtundation, severe headache, visual changes, or nausea or vomiting.
3. The use of filter paper or a dextrose stick test to determine if CSF is present in rhinorrhea is not 100% reliable.

Associated Clinical Features

Depressed skull fractures typically occur when a large force is applied over a small area. They are classified as open if the skin above them is lacerated (Fig. 1.6) and closed if the overlying skin is intact. Abrasions, contusions, and hematomas may also be present over the fracture site. The patient's mental status can range from comatose to fully alert depending on the extent of the associated brain injury. Soft tissue bleeding and swelling may be present. Evidence of other injuries such as a basilar fracture or facial fractures may also be present.

Differential Diagnosis

Direct trauma can cause abrasions, contusions, hematomas, and lacerations without an underlying depressed skull fracture. Every laceration to the scalp should be explored and palpated to rule out depression of a fracture. Alterations in mental status may occur with or without fracture. Penetrating injuries to the skull and brain can produce a similar clinical picture.

Emergency Department Treatment and Disposition

Plain films have been suggested for suspected depressed skull fractures and if positive should be followed by CT, which will more accurately demonstrate the degree of depression as well as any underlying brain injury (Fig. 1.7). Others suggest that plain films offer little diagnostic utility and recommend CT with its more accurate bone windows for any suspected depressed skull fracture.

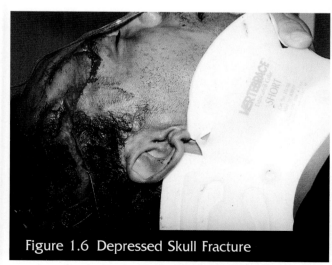

Figure 1.6 Depressed Skull Fracture

A scalp laceration overlying a depressed skull fracture. Wearing a sterile glove, the examiner should digitally explore all scalp lacerations for evidence of fracture or depression. (Courtesy of David W. Munter, MD.)

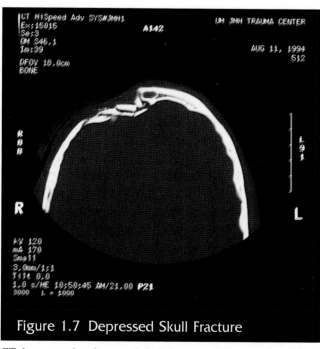

Figure 1.7 Depressed Skull Fracture

CT demonstrating depressed skull fracture. (Courtesy of David W. Munter, MD.)

When depressed skull fractures are noted on plain films or CT, immediate neurosurgical consultation is required. Open fractures also require antibiotics and tetanus prophylaxis as indicated. The decision to observe or operate immediately is made by the neurosurgeon. Children below 2 years of age with skull fractures can develop leptomeningeal cysts. These cysts, which are extrusion of CSF or brain through dural defects, are associated with skull fractures. For this reason, children below age 2 with skull fractures require follow-up or admission.

Clinical Pearls

1. Gently palpate all scalp injuries including lacerations for evidence of fractures or depression. When fragments are depressed more than 3 to 5 mm below the inner table, penetration of the dura and injury to the cortex are more likely.
2. Children with depressed skull fractures are more likely to develop epilepsy.
3. The index of suspicion for nonaccidental trauma should be raised for children below 2 years of age with depressed skull fractures.

Associated Clinical Features

Clinically significant nasal fractures are almost always evident on examination, with deformity, swelling, and ecchymosis present (Fig. 1.8). Injuries may occur to other surrounding bony structures, including fractures of the orbit, frontal sinus, or cribriform plate. A history of a mechanism with significant force, loss of consciousness, or findings of facial bone injury or CSF leak should alert the clinician to look for these associated injuries. Epistaxis may be due to a septal or turbinate laceration but can also be seen with fractures of surrounding bones, including the cribriform plate. Septal hematoma (Fig. 1.9) is a rare but important complication that, if untreated, may result in necrosis of the septal cartilage and a resultant "saddle-nose" deformity.

Differential Diagnosis

Nasal fractures may have associated facial injuries—such as orbital, frontal sinus, or cribriform plate fractures—and these more serious injuries must be ruled out. A simple nasal contusion may present identically to a simple nasal fracture with pain, swelling, and ecchymosis. A frontonasoethmoid fracture has nasal or frontal crepitus and may have associated telecanthus or obstruction of the nasolacrimal duct.

Emergency Department Treatment and Disposition

Look for more serious injuries first. Patients with associated facial bone deformity or tenderness may require radiographs to rule out facial fractures. Nasal fractures rarely require radiographs (Fig. 1.10). Obvious deformities are referred within 2 to 5 days for reduction, after the swelling has subsided. Nasal injuries without deformity need only conservative therapy with an analgesic and possibly a nasal decongestant. Septal hematomas must be immediately drained, with packing placed to prevent reaccumulation. In some cases, epistaxis may not be controlled by pressure alone and may require nasal packing. Lacerations overlying a simple nasal fracture should be vigorously irrigated and primarily closed with the patient placed on antibiotic coverage. Complex nasal lacerations with underlying fractures should be referred for closure. Nasal fractures with mild angulation

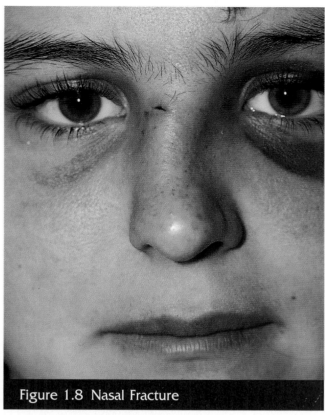

Figure 1.8 Nasal Fracture

Deformity is evident on examination. Note periocular ecchymosis indicating the possibility of other facial fractures (or injuries). The decision to obtain radiographs is based on clinical findings. A radiograph is not indicated for an isolated simple nasal fracture. (Courtesy of David W. Munter, MD.)

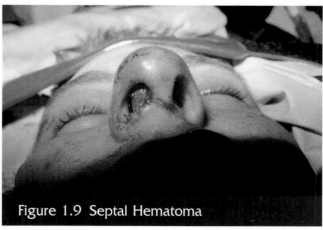

Figure 1.9 Septal Hematoma

A bluish, grapelike mass on the nasal septum. If untreated, this can result in septal necrosis and a saddle-nose deformity. An incision, drainage, and packing are indicated. (Courtesy of Lawrence B. Stack, MD.)

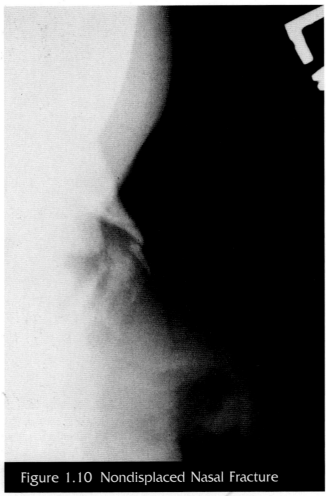

Figure 1.10 Nondisplaced Nasal Fracture

Radiograph of a fracture of the nasal spine, for which no treatment other than ice and analgesics is needed. This radiograph did not change the treatment or disposition of the patient. (Courtesy of Lorenz F. Lassen, MD.)

and without displacement may be reduced in the ED by manipulating the nose with the examiner's thumbs into the correct alignment.

Clinical Pearls

1. Rule out any life threats or serious associated injuries.
2. Control epistaxis to perform a good intranasal examination. If there is no epistaxis or deformity, treat the patient with ice and analgesics. If obvious deformity is present, including a new septal deviation or deformity, treat with ice and analgesics and provide ear/nose/throat (ENT) referral in 2 to 5 days for reduction.
3. Although the effectiveness of prophylactic antibiotics to prevent toxic shock syndrome is unproved, every patient discharged with nasal packing should be placed on antistaphylococcal antibiotics and referred to ENT in 2 to 3 days.
4. Consider cribriform plate fractures in patients with clear rhinorrhea after nasal injury, with the understanding that this finding may be delayed.
5. Check every patient for a septal hematoma.

Associated Clinical Features

The zygoma bone has two major components, the zygomatic arch and the body. The arch forms the inferior and lateral orbit, and the body forms the malar eminence of the face. Fractures to the zygoma are usually the result of blunt trauma. Direct blows to the arch can result in isolated arch fractures (Fig. 1.11). These present clinically with pain on opening the mouth secondary to the insertion of the temporalis muscle at the arch or impingement on the coronoid process. More extensive trauma can result in the "tripod fracture," which consists of fractures through three structures: the frontozygomatic suture; the maxillary process of the zygoma including the inferior orbital floor, inferior orbital rim, and lateral wall of the maxillary sinus; and the zygomatic arch (Figs. 1.12, 1.13). Clinically, patients present with a flattened malar eminence and edema and ecchymosis to the area, with a palpable step-off on examination. Injury to the infraorbital nerve may result in infraorbital paresthesia, and gaze disturbances may result from injury to orbital contents. Subcutaneous emphysema may be caused by a fracture of the antral wall at the zygomatic buttress.

Differential Diagnosis

Other facial fractures, including LeFort II and III fractures, may involve the zygoma bone or orbit. These fractures typ-

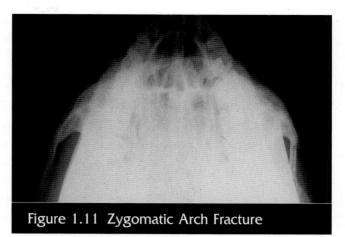

Figure 1.11 Zygomatic Arch Fracture

Jug-handle view of the zygomatic arch demonstrating a depressed fracture. In such a case, operative reduction can be delayed for several days. (Courtesy of Timothy D. McGuirk, DO.)

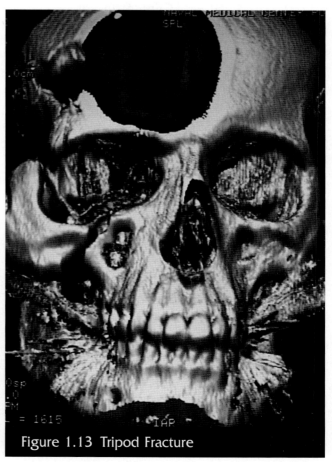

Figure 1.13 Tripod Fracture

The fracture lines involved in a tripod fracture are demonstrated in this three-dimensional CT reconstruction. The large defect in the frontal area is artifact from the reconstruction. (Courtesy of Patrick W. Lappert, MD.)

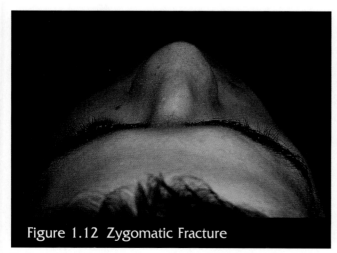

Figure 1.12 Zygomatic Fracture

Patient with blunt trauma to the zygoma. Flattening of the right malar eminence is evident. (Courtesy of Edward S. Amrhein, DDS.)

ically involve more extensive facial trauma. Orbital blowout fractures may present with entrapment and ocular injuries, but the malar eminence appears normal.

Emergency Department Treatment and Disposition

Plain films, including a Waters view and "jug-handle" view (a submental-vertex view of the zygomatic arches), demonstrate the fracture and evaluate the zygomaticomaxillary complex. In the case of a tripod fracture, facial CT will best show the involvement and degree of displacement. Since plain films often do not adequately demonstrate all elements of the fracture, patients with evidence of a tripod fracture should have CT on an urgent basis to help identify the extent of bony injuries. The CT results guide the need for urgent referral. Simple zygomatic arch or tripod fractures without eye injury can be treated with ice and analgesics and referred for delayed operative consideration in 5 to 7 days. More extensive tripod fractures or those with eye injuries should be referred more urgently. Decongestants and broad-spectrum antibiotics are generally recommended for tripod fractures, since the fracture crosses into the maxillary sinus.

Clinical Pearls

1. Tripod fractures are often associated with orbital and ocular trauma. Palpate the zygomatic arch and orbital rims carefully for a step-off deformity.
2. Examine for eye findings such as diplopia, hyphema, or retinal detachment. Check for infraorbital paresthesia indicating injury or impingement of the second division of cranial nerve V.
3. Visual inspection of the malar eminence from several angles (especially by viewing the area from over the head of the patient in the coronal plane, Fig. 1.12) allows detection of a subtle abnormality.
4. Insist on adequate radiographs of the zygomatic arches, which require good positioning of the patient.

Associated Clinical Features

All LeFort facial fractures involve the maxilla (Fig. 1.14). Clinically, the patient has facial injuries, swelling, and ecchymosis (Figs. 1.15, 1.16). LeFort I fractures are those involving an area under the nasal fossa. LeFort II fractures involve a pyramidal area including the maxilla, nasal bones, and medial orbits. LeFort III fractures, sometimes described as craniofacial dissociation, involve the maxilla, zygoma, nasal and ethmoid bones, and the bones of the base of the skull. Airway compromise may be associated with LeFort II and III fractures. Physical examination is sometimes helpful in distinguishing the three. The examiner places fingers on the bridge of the nose and tries to move the central maxillary incisors with the other hand. If only the maxilla moves, a LeFort I is present; movement of the upper jaw and nose indicates a LeFort II; and movement of the entire midface and zygoma indicates a LeFort III. Because of the extent of LeFort II and III fractures, they may be associated with cribriform plate fractures and CSF rhinorrhea. The force required to sustain a LeFort II or III fracture is considerable, and associated brain or cervical spine injuries are common.

Differential Diagnosis

LeFort II and III fractures can be difficult to distinguish, and combination LeFort fractures (e.g., LeFort II on one

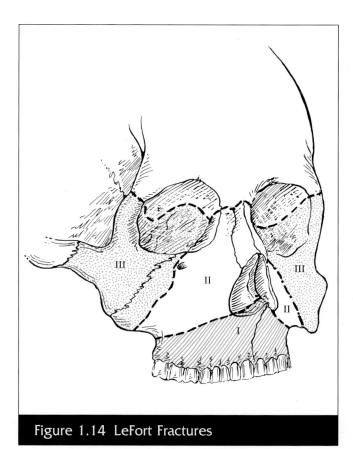

Figure 1.14 LeFort Fractures

Illustration of the fracture lines of LeFort I (alveolar), LeFort II (zygomatic maxillary complex), and LeFort III (cranial facial dysostosis) fractures.

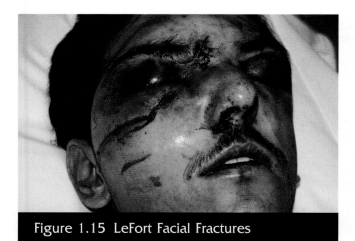

Figure 1.15 LeFort Facial Fractures

Clinical photograph of patient with blunt facial trauma. Note the ecchymosis and edema. This patient sustained a LeFort II/III fracture (a LeFort II fracture on one side and a LeFort III on the other), and associated intracranial hemorrhages. (Courtesy of Stephen Corbett, MD.)

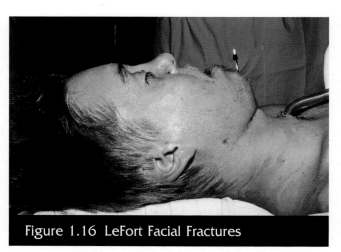

Figure 1.16 LeFort Facial Fractures

Clinical photograph of patient with blunt facial trauma. Patient demonstrates the classic "dish face" deformity (depressed midface) associated with bilateral LeFort III fractures. (Courtesy of Robert Schnarrs, MD.)

side and LeFort III on the other) are common. Tripod and frontonasoethmoid fractures may be present in blunt facial trauma as well.

Emergency Department Treatment and Disposition

Patients with associated facial bone deformity or tenderness may require radiographs to rule out facial fractures. Plain facial films will reveal the presence of facial fractures but are less helpful in determining the type or extent. Head and facial CT, including three-dimensional re-creations, offer much more useful information. Management of LeFort I fractures may involve only dental splinting and oral surgery referral, but management of LeFort II and III fractures normally requires admission because of associated injuries as well as definitive operative repair. Epistaxis may be difficult to control in LeFort II and III fractures, in rare cases requiring intraoperative arterial ligation.

Clinical Pearls

1. Attention should be focused on immediate airway management, since the massive edema associated with LeFort II and III fractures may quickly lead to airway compromise.
2. Nasotracheal intubation should be avoided because of the possibility of intracranial passage.
3. Any serious facial trauma may also be associated with cervical spine injuries.
4. Associated cranial injuries are common and are best evaluated by CT.
5. If not recognized, an occult CSF leak may result in significant morbidity. Suspected CSF leaks require neurosurgical consultation.
6. The best diagnostic modality for delineation of the extent of injuries is CT of the facial bones.

Associated Clinical Features

Blowout fractures occur when the globe sustains a direct blunt force. There are two mechanisms of injury. The first is a true blowout fracture, where all energy is transmitted to the globe. The spherical globe is stronger than the thin orbital floor, and the force is transmitted to the thin orbital floor or medially through the ethmoid bones, with the resultant fracture. The object causing the injury must be smaller than 5 to 6 cm, otherwise the globe is protected by the surrounding orbit. Fists or small balls are the typical causative agents. This mechanism of injury is more likely to cause entrapment and globe injury. The second mechanism of injury occurs when the energy from the blow is transmitted to the infraorbital rim, causing a buckling of the orbital floor. Entrapment and globe injury is less likely with this mechanism of injury. Patients with blowout fractures have periorbital ecchymosis and lid edema (Figs. 1.17, 1.18) but may sustain eye injuries as well, including chemosis, subconjunctival hemorrhage, or infraorbital numbness from injury to the infraorbital nerve. Other eye injuries should be sought and ruled out with a careful physical examination; they include corneal abrasion, hyphema, enophthalmos, proptosis, iridoplegia, dislocated lens, retinal tear, retinal detachment, and ruptured globe. If the inferior rectus muscle is extruded into the fracture, it may become entrapped; upward gaze is then limited, with resultant diplopia (Figs. 1.19, 1.20). Because of the communication with the maxillary sinus, subcutaneous emphysema is common.

Differential Diagnosis

Orbital contusions present with similar physical findings. Fractures of the orbital rim are clinically similar to orbital blowout fractures. Other facial fractures (zygoma, tripod, LeFort) may involve the orbital floor but are associated with more extensive injuries to the face outside of the orbit.

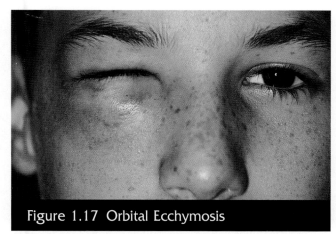

Figure 1.17 Orbital Ecchymosis

Sustained from blunt trauma to the globe, with some of the force directed to the inferior orbital rim. This patient presents with subtle signs only (ecchymosis and swelling with no entrapment or eye injury) yet has the classic signs on plain films (Figure 1.18). This patient demonstrates that orbital floor fractures can present with subtle physical findings. (Courtesy of Kevin J. Knoop, MD, MS.)

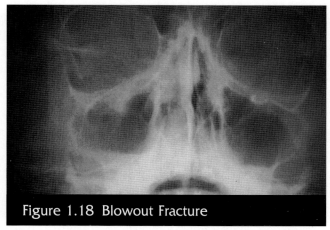

Figure 1.18 Blowout Fracture

Plain film demonstrating a fracture of the floor of the right orbit, with a teardrop sign due to extruded orbital contents. There is an associated air-fluid level in the maxillary sinus due to blood. Note the two lines seen at the inferior orbit: the infraorbital rim and inferior floor of the orbit. These are well visualized on the unaffected side but disrupted on the affected side. (Courtesy of Kevin J. Knoop, MD, MS.)

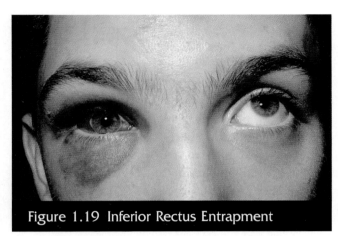

Figure 1.19 Inferior Rectus Entrapment

The inferior rectus muscle is entrapped within the blowout fracture. When the patient tries to look upward, the affected eye has limited upward gaze. The patient experiences diplopia with this maneuver. (Courtesy of Lawrence B. Stack, MD.)

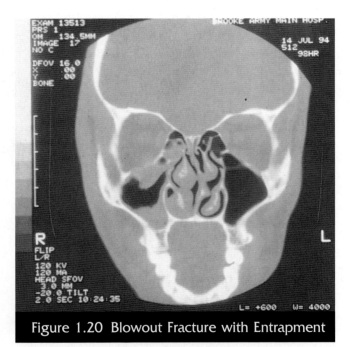

Figure 1.20 Blowout Fracture with Entrapment

CT of the patient in Fig. 1.19 demonstrating the entrapped muscle extruding into the maxillary sinus. (Courtesy of Lawrence B. Stack, MD.)

Emergency Department Treatment and Disposition

Plain radiography to include a Caldwell view (showing orbital rim and walls) and a Waters view (orbital floor and roof) demonstrates the fracture. Patients without eye injury or entrapment may be treated conservatively with ice and analgesics and referred for follow-up in 2 to 3 days. Patients with blood in the maxillary sinus are usually treated with antibiotics. Strongly consider an ophthalmology consultation in patients with a true blowout fracture (all energy transmitted to the globe), since up to 30% of these patients sustain a globe injury. Patients with entrapment should receive a CT of the orbits and be referred on a same-day basis. Most specialists will observe fractures with entrapment for 10 to 14 days to allow for resolution of edema prior to operative repair.

Clinical Pearls

1. Enophthalmos, limited upward gaze, diplopia with upward gaze, or infraorbital anesthesia from entrapment or injury to the infraorbital nerve should heighten suspicion of a blowout fracture.
2. Compare the pupillary level on the affected side with the unaffected side, since it may be lower from prolapse of the orbital contents into the maxillary sinus. Subtle abnormalities may be appreciated as an asymmetric corneal light reflex (Hirschberg's reflex).
3. Subcutaneous emphysema on clinical examination, a soft-tissue teardrop along the roof of the maxillary sinus on plain film, or an air-fluid level in the maxillary sinus on plain film should also be interpreted as evidence of a blowout fracture.
4. Some patients present with unusual complaints—for example, of an eye swelling up after the patient blows his or her nose (from subcutaneous emphysema) or air bubbles emanating from the tear duct.
5. Carefully examine the eye for visual acuity, hyphema, or retinal detachment. Remember to assess the nose for a septal hematoma.

Associated Clinical Features

A history of blunt trauma, mandibular pain, and possible malocclusion is normally seen with mandibular fractures. A step-off in the dental line (Fig. 1.21) or ecchymosis or hematoma to the floor of the mouth are often present. Mandibular fractures may be open to the oral cavity, as manifest by gum lacerations. Dental trauma may be associated. Other clinical features include inferior alveolar or mental nerve paresthesia, loose or missing teeth, dysphagia, trismus, or ecchymosis of the floor of the mouth (considered pathognomonic) (Figs. 1.22, 1.23). Multiple mandibular fractures are present in more than 50% of cases because of the ring-like structure of the mandible. Mandibular fractures are often classified as favorable or unfavorable, depending on the location and resultant displacement forces exerted by the associated musculature. Those frac-

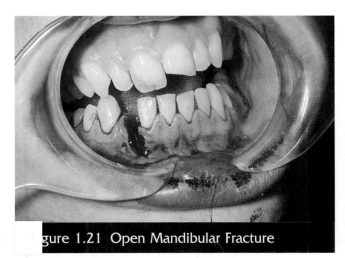

gure 1.21 Open Mandibular Fracture

The open fracture line is evident clinically. There is slight misalignment of the teeth. (Courtesy of Edward S. Amrhein, DDS.)

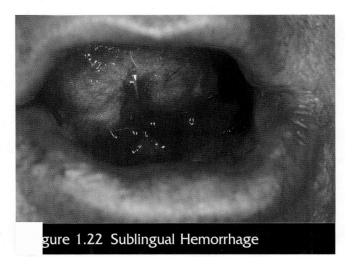

gure 1.22 Sublingual Hemorrhage

Hemorrhage or ecchymosis in the sublingual area is pathognomonic for mandibular fracture. (Courtesy of Lawrence B. Stack, MD.)

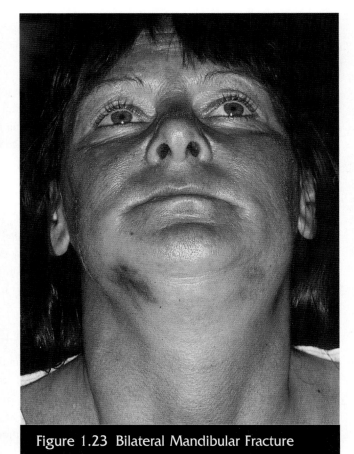

Figure 1.23 Bilateral Mandibular Fracture

The diagnosis is suggested by the bilateral ecchymosis seen in this patient. (Courtesy of Lawrence B. Stack, MD.)

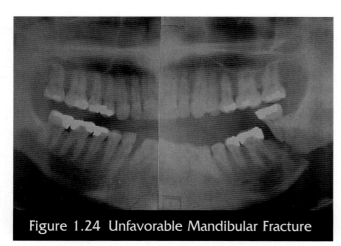

Figure 1.24 Unfavorable Mandibular Fracture

Dental panoramic view demonstrating a mandibular fracture with obvious misalignment due to the distracting forces of the masseter muscle. (Courtesy of Edward S. Amrhein, DDS.)

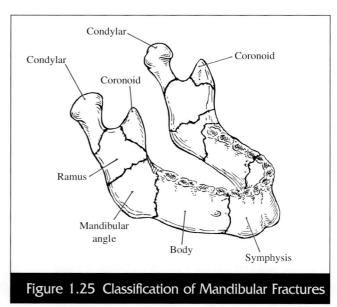

Figure 1.25 Classification of Mandibular Fractures

Classification based on anatomic location of the fracture.

tures displaced by the masseter muscle are unfavorable (Fig. 1.24) and inevitably require fixation, whereas fractures that are not displaced by traction are favorable and in some cases will not require fixation. Injuries creating unstable mandibular fractures may create airway obstruction because the support for the tongue is lost. Mandibular fractures are also classified based on the anatomic location of the fracture (Fig. 1.25).

Differential Diagnosis

Contusions have a similar presentation and can be differentiated only radiographically. Dislocation of the mandibular condyles may also result from blunt trauma and will always have associated malocclusion, typified by an inability to close the mouth. Isolated dental trauma may have a similar presentation, and underlying mandibular fracture should be ruled out.

Emergency Department Disposition and Treatment

The best view for evaluating mandibular trauma is a dental panoramic view, which should be obtained if available. Plain films should include anteroposterior (AP), bilateral oblique, and Townes views to evaluate the condyles. Nondisplaced fractures can be treated with analgesics, soft diet, and referral to oral surgery in 1 to 2 days. Displaced fractures, open fractures, and fractures with associated dental trauma need more urgent referral. All mandibular fractures should be treated with antibiotics effective against anaerobic oral flora (clindamycin, amoxicillin clavulanate) and tetanus prophylaxis given if needed. The Barton's bandage has been suggested to immobilize the jaw in the ED.

Clinical Pearls

1. The presence of disfiguring facial injuries can be distracting. The primary consideration in the evaluation of the patient with facial fractures is the assessment and treatment of life-threatening injuries.

2. Any patient with trauma and malocclusion should be considered to have a mandibular fracture.

3. The most sensitive sign of a mandibular fracture is malocclusion. The jaw will deviate toward the side of a unilateral condylar fracture on maximal opening of the mouth. A non-fractured mandible should be able to hold a tongue blade between the molars tightly enough to break it off. There should be no pain in attempting to rotate the tongue blade between the molars.

4. Bilateral parasymphyseal fractures may cause acute airway obstruction in the supine patient. This is relieved by pulling the subluxed mandible and soft tissue forward and, in patients in whom the cervical spine has been cleared, by elevating the patient to a sitting position.

Associated Clinical Features

Injuries to the external ear may be open or closed. Blunt external ear trauma may cause a hematoma (otohematoma) of the pinna (Fig. 1.26), which, if untreated, may result in cartilage necrosis and chronic scarring or further cartilage formation and permanent deformity ("cauliflower ear") (Fig. 1.27). Open injuries include lacerations (with and without cartilage exposure) and avulsions (Fig. 1.28).

Differential Diagnosis

These injuries are normally self-evident. Pinna hematomas and contusions can sometimes be difficult to distinguish, but flocculence is the hallmark of the hematoma.

Emergency Department Treatment and Disposition

Pinna hematomas must undergo incision and drainage or large needle aspiration using sterile technique, followed by a pressure dressing to prevent reaccumulation of the hematoma. This procedure may need to be repeated several times; hence, after ED drainage, the patient is treated

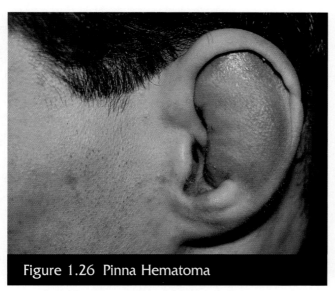

Figure 1.26 Pinna Hematoma

A hematoma has developed, characterized by swelling, discoloration, ecchymosis, and flocculence. Immediate incision and drainage or aspiration is indicated, followed by an ear compression dressing. (Courtesy of C. Bruce MacDonald, MD.)

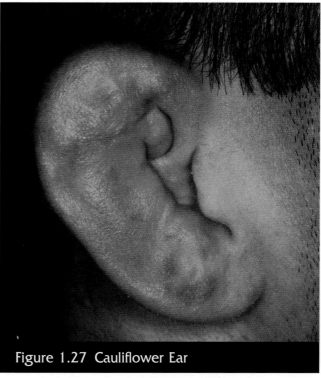

Figure 1.27 Cauliflower Ear

Repeated trauma to the pinna or undrained hematomas can result in cartilage necrosis and subsequent deforming scar formation. (Courtesy of Timothy D. McGuirk, DO.)

with antistaphylococcal antibiotics and referred to ENT or plastic surgery for follow-up in 24 h. Lacerations must be carefully examined for cartilage involvement; if this is present, copious irrigation, closure, and postrepair oral antibiotics covering skin flora are indicated. Simple skin lacerations may be repaired primarily with nonabsorbable 6-0 sutures. The dressing after laceration repair is just as important as the primary repair. If a compression dressing is not placed, hematoma formation can occur. Complex lacerations or avulsions normally require ENT or plastic surgery referral.

Clinical Pearls

1. Pinna hematomas may take hours to develop, so give patients with blunt ear trauma careful discharge instructions, with a follow-up in 12 to 24 h to check for hematoma development.

2. Failure to adequately drain a hematoma, reaccumulation of the hematoma owing to a faulty pressure dressing, or inadequate follow-up increases the risk of infection of the pinna (perichondritis) or of a disfiguring cauliflower ear.

3. Copiously irrigate injuries with lacerated cartilage, which can usually be managed by primary closure of the overlying skin. Direct closure of the cartilage is rarely necessary and is indicated only for proper alignment, which helps lessen later distortion. Use a minimal number of absorbable 5-0 or 6-0 sutures through the perichondrium.

4. Lacerations to the lateral aspect of the pinna should be minimally debrided because of the lack of tissue at this site to cover the exposed cartilage.

5. In the case of an avulsion injury, the avulsed part should be cleansed, wrapped in saline-moistened gauze, placed in a sterile container, then placed on ice to await reimplantation by ENT.

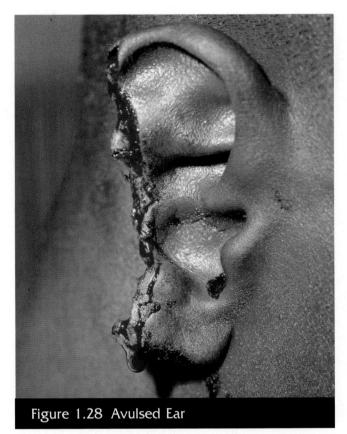

Figure 1.28 Avulsed Ear

This ear injury, sustained in a fight, resulted when the pinna was bitten off. Plastic repair is needed. The avulsed part was wrapped in sterile gauze soaked with saline and placed in a sterile container on ice. (Courtesy of David W. Munter, MD.)

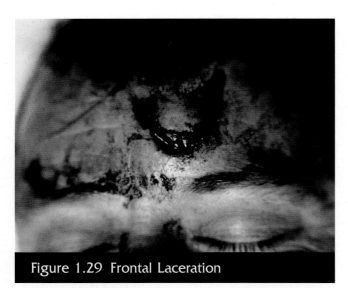

Figure 1.29 Frontal Laceration

Any laceration over the frontal sinuses should be explored to rule out a fracture. This laceration was found to have an associated frontal fracture. (Courtesy of David W. Munter, MD.)

Associated Clinical Features

Blunt trauma to the frontal area may result in a depressed frontal sinus fracture. Often, there is an associated laceration (Fig. 1.29). Isolated frontal fractures (Figs. 1.30, 1.31) normally do not have the associated features of massive blunt facial trauma such as seen in LeFort II and III fractures. Careful nasal speculum examination may reveal blood or CSF leak high in the nasal cavity. Posterior table involvement can lead to mucopyocoele or epidural empyema as late sequelae. Involvement of the posterior wall of the frontal sinus may occur and result in cranial injury or dural tear.

Differential Diagnosis

Simple lacerations or contusions of the frontal area may not involve fractures. Frontal fractures may be part of a complex of facial fractures, as seen in frontonasoethmoid fractures, but generally more extensive facial trauma is required.

Emergency Department Treatment and Disposition

Frontal sinus fractures revealed on plain films of the frontal bones, including posteroanterior (PA), lateral, and Waters views, may be quite subtle. The extent of the frontal injury,

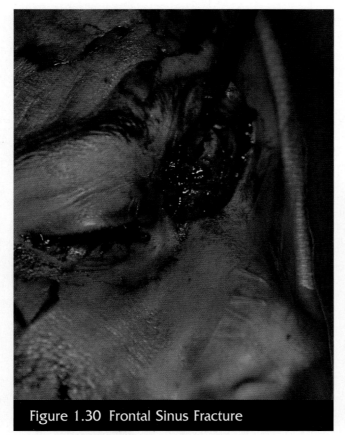

Figure 1.30 Frontal Sinus Fracture

Fracture defect seen at the base of a laceration over the frontal sinus. (Courtesy of Jeffrey Kuhn, MD.)

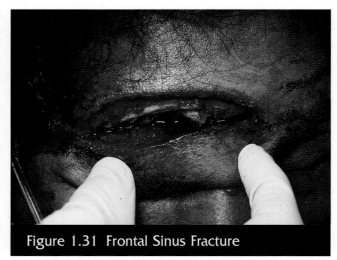

Figure 1.31 Frontal Sinus Fracture

Fracture of the outer table of the frontal sinus is seen under this forehead laceration. (Courtesy of Lawrence B. Stack, MD.)

especially posterior table involvement, is best investigated with bone windows on CT (Fig. 1.32). Fractures involving only the anterior table of the frontal sinus can be treated conservatively with referral to ENT or plastic surgery in 1 to 2 days. Fractures involving the posterior table require urgent neurosurgical referral. Frontal sinus fractures are usually covered with high-dose antibiotics against both skin and sinus flora (second- or third-generation cephalosporins). ED management also includes control of epistaxis, application of ice packs, and analgesia.

Clinical Pearls

1. Explore every frontal laceration digitally before repair. Digital palpation is sensitive for identifying frontal fractures, although false positives from lacerations extending through the periosteum can occur.
2. Communication of irrigating solutions with the nose or mouth indicates a breach in the frontal sinus.
3. For serious injuries, a CT scan is mandatory to assess the posterior aspect of the sinus and for possible intracranial injury.

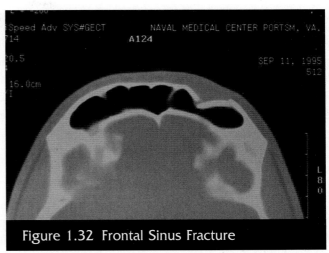

Figure 1.32 Frontal Sinus Fracture

CT of the patient in Figure 1.29 demonstrating a fracture of the anterior table of the frontal sinus. (Courtesy of David W. Munter, MD.)

Associated Clinical Features

Normally the result of blunt orbital trauma, the exophthalmos develops as a retrobulbar hematoma pushes the globe outward. Patients present with periorbital edema, ecchymosis (Fig. 1.33), a marked decrease in visual acuity, and an afferent pupillary defect in the involved eye. The exophthalmos, which may be obscured by periorbital edema, can be better appreciated from a superior view (Fig. 1.34). Visual acuity may be affected by the direct trauma to the eye, compression of the retinal artery, or, more rarely, neuropraxia of the optic nerve.

Differential Diagnosis

Periorbital ecchymosis and edema can result from blunt trauma without a retrobulbar hematoma. Traumatic chemosis can present with exophthalmos. Visual impairment can result from retinal detachment, hyphema, globe rupture, or any number of nontraumatic conditions. Nontraumatic exophthalmos can be caused by cavernous sinus thrombosis, a complication of frontal sinusitis, or endocrine (thyrotoxicosis) disorders.

Emergency Department Treatment and Disposition

CT is the best modality to determine the presence and extent of a retrobulbar hematoma and associated facial or orbital fractures (Fig. 1.35). Referral to ENT and ophthalmology is indicated on an urgent basis. An emergent lateral canthotomy decompresses the orbit and can be performed in the ED. Emergency treatment can be sight-saving.

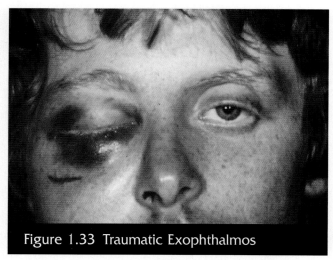

Figure 1.33 Traumatic Exophthalmos

Blunt trauma resulting in periorbital edema and ecchymosis, which obscures the exophthalmos in this patient. The exophthalmos is not obvious in the AP view and can therefore be initially unappreciated. Figure 1.34 shows the same patient viewed in the coronal plane from over the forehead. (Courtesy of Frank Birinyi, MD.)

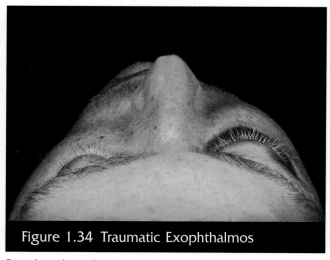

Figure 1.34 Traumatic Exophthalmos

Superior view, demonstrating the right-sided exophthalmos. (Courtesy of Frank Birinyi, MD.)

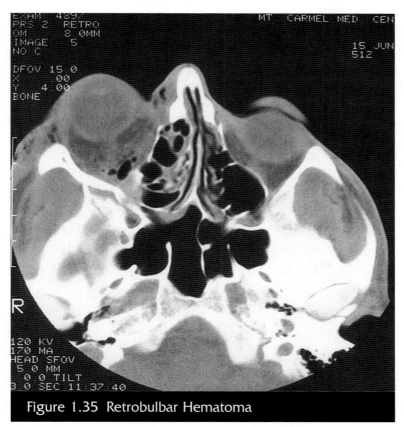

Figure 1.35 Retrobulbar Hematoma

CT of the patient in Figs. 1.33 and 1.34 with right retrobulbar hematoma and traumatic exophthalmos. (Courtesy of Frank Birinyi, MD.)

Clinical Pearls

1. The retrobulbar hematoma and resultant exophthalmos may not develop for hours. Give careful discharge instructions to any patient with periorbital trauma.

2. Perform a careful ophthalmic examination including visual acuity, since associated conditions such as hyphema or retinal detachment are common.

3. A subtle exophthalmos may be detected by looking down over the head of the patient and viewing the eye from the coronal plane.

4. Lateral canthotomy is indicated for emergent treatment of patients with traumatic exophthalmos who demonstrate profound ischemic signs and symptoms of an afferent pupillary defect and decreased vision.

5. An afferent pupillary defect in a patient with blunt trauma to the face or eye with normal visual acuity may be pharmacologically induced.

EYE

CHAPTER 2
OPHTHALMOLOGIC CONDITIONS

Frank Birinyi
Thomas F. Mauger

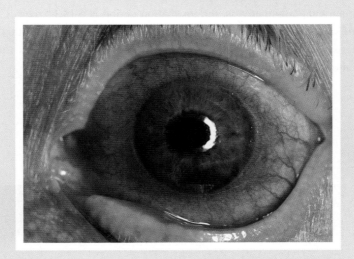

NEONATAL CONJUNCTIVITIS (OPHTHALMIA NEONATORUM)

Associated Clinical Features

Neonatal conjunctivitis is acquired either during birth with passage through the mother's cervix and vagina or from cross infection in the neonatal period. Microbiologic etiologies include *Chlamydia trachomatis,* viruses (herpes simplex), and bacteria (*Neisseria gonorrhoeae, Staphylococcus aureus, Streptococcus pneumoniae,* groups A and B streptococci, *Haemophilus* species, *Pseudomonas aeruginosa,* and *Escherichia coli*). Of these, *S. aureus* is the most frequent and *N. gonorrhoeae* the most important. Clinical findings in neonatal conjunctivitis include drainage, conjunctival hyperemia, chemosis, and lid edema.

Neisseria gonorrhoeae presents as a hyperacute bilateral conjunctivitis. Distinctive findings include a copious purulent drainage (Fig. 2.1) and preauricular adenopathy. The incubation period, like that for sexually transmitted *N. gonorrhoeae,* is 3 to 5 days, although the onset may vary. In chlamydial conjunctivitis, the incubation period is 5 to 12 days. Clinical features of chlamydial conjunctivitis include unilateral conjunctivitis and concomitant otitis media or pneumonia. Herpes simplex conjunctivitis generally begins 2 to 14 days after birth; fluorescein staining demonstrates epithelial dendrites.

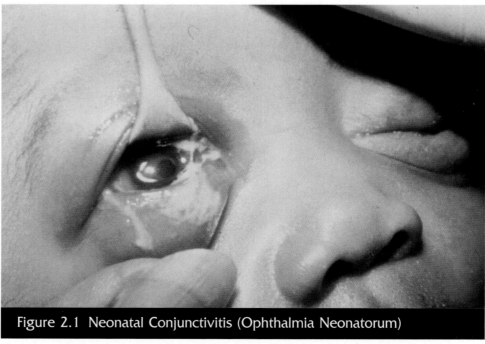

Figure 2.1 Neonatal Conjunctivitis (Ophthalmia Neonatorum)

Copious purulent drainage in a newborn with neonatal gonococcal conjunctivitis. (Reprinted with permission of the American Academy of Ophthalmology, *Eye Trauma and Emergencies: A Slide-Script Program.* San Francisco, 1985.)

Differential Diagnosis

Dacryocystitis, corneal abrasions, foreign body, and an obstructed nasolacrimal duct present with redness and tearing. Neonatal glaucoma may also be mistaken for conjunctivitis; findings include eye pain, photophobia, corneal haze, corneal enlargement, and excessive tearing.

Emergency Department Treatment and Disposition

The neonate with conjunctivitis must be evaluated carefully for systemic involvement. With any form of neonatal conjunctivitis, smears and cultures are mandatory and therapy should begin immediately thereafter. Scrapings of the palpebral conjunctiva for cultures and Gram stain are more revealing than examination of the discharge itself. Topical therapy for a neonate whose Gram stain demonstrates gram-negative diplococci includes aqueous penicillin (10,000 to 20,000 U/mL one drop every hour for 6 to 12 h, followed by one drop every 2 to 3 h until resolution). Saline irrigation of the conjunctival cul-de-sac prior to antibiotic instillation may be helpful. Systemic therapy involves intravenous penicillin G (50,000 U/kg/day in two or three doses for 7 days). Pediatric consultation is advised.

Chlamydial conjunctivitis is treated with oral erythromycin estolate. Neonatal bacterial conjunctivitis that is neither gonococcal nor chlamydial may be treated with antibiotic ointment (erythromycin, tetracycline, or gentamicin four to six times a day for 2 weeks) and should be reevaluated in 24 h. Herpes simplex conjunctivitis is treated with intravenous acyclovir and topical trifluorothymidine.

Evaluation of the newborn's parents should be undertaken in neonatal conjunctivitis due to *N. gonorrhoeae, Chlamydia,* or herpes simplex virus.

Clinical Pearls

1. Neonatal conjunctivitis may be caused by chemical, chlamydial, viral, and bacterial agents.
2. The "rule of fives" is fairly accurate in predicting the most likely bacterial etiology.

0 to 5 days:	*N. gonorrhoeae*
5 days to 5 weeks:	*Chlamydia*
5 weeks to 5 years:	*Streptococcus* or *Haemophilus influenzae*

3. The cornea should be examined for involvement. Corneal ulcers, perforation, permanent scarring, and blindness can quickly result from gonococcal eye infection in the neonate. It is one of the few urgent conjunctival infections.
4. A detailed maternal history may help with the diagnosis of neonatal conjunctivitis secondary to *N. gonorrhoeae, Chlamydia,* or herpes.

Associated Clinical Features

Bacterial conjunctivitis is characterized by the acute onset of conjunctival injection and muco-purulent drainage. *Staphylococcus aureus* is the most common causative bacterium. *Streptococcus pneumoniae* and *Haemophilus influenzae* occur more frequently in children. The purulent drainage (Fig. 2.2) commonly leads the eyelids to be stuck together on awakening. Lid edema and erythema, chemosis, and superficial punctate keratitis may also be present.

The most severe form of acute purulent conjunctivitis is associated with *Neisseria gonor-rhoeae*. Infection can be seen in children of any age, including the newborn. Clinical symptoms are hyperacute in onset and include a discharge that is prominent, thick, copious, and purulent. Other findings include marked eyelid swelling, along with tenderness, marked conjunctival hy-peremia, pain, chemosis, and preauricular adenopathy. The condition may progress to involve the cornea, because *Neisseria* species are capable of invading an intact corneal epithelium. Corneal findings include a diffuse epithelial haze, epithelial defects, marginal infiltrates, and peripheral ulcerative keratitis, which can rapidly progress to perforation.

Neonatal conjunctivitis is discussed separately.

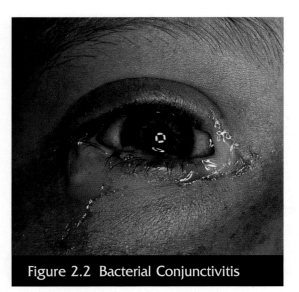

Figure 2.2 Bacterial Conjunctivitis

Mucopurulent discharge, conjunctival injection, and lid swelling in a 10-year-old with *Haemophilus influenzae* conjunctivitis. (Courtesy of Frank Birinyi, MD.)

Differential Diagnosis

Other etiologies of conjunctivitis (viral, allergic) as well as iritis, glaucoma, scleritis, and foreign body also present as a red eye.

Emergency Department Treatment and Disposition

Treatment involves local hygiene with warm, moist compresses and frequent hand washing, along with broad-spectrum antibiotic drops (10% sulfacetamide, gentamicin, ofloxacin, ciprofloxacin, or trimethoprim/polymyxin B). One drop every 3 h for 7 to 10 days usually results in rapid resolution. If there is no response, cultures and ophthalmologic consultation should be sought.

The treatment of gonococcal conjunctivitis is both systemic (ceftri-axone 25 to 50 mg/kg/day, not to exceed 4 g/day, given in one dose IM for 7 days) and topical (penicillin G 100,000 U/mL one drop every 2 h or bacitracin ophthalmic ointment 500 U/g every 2 h, tapering over 48 h to five times a day). Patients with corneal involvement should receive additional intravenous ceftriaxone (1 g every 12 h). Sexual partners should be advised and evaluated.

Clinical Pearls

1. Worsening symptoms during topical treatment with any antibiotic, particularly Neosporin or a sulfonamide (Sodium Sulamyd), may represent a contact allergic reaction.
2. Conjunctivitis due to *N. gonorrhoeae* must be considered in the sexually active adult with a prominent, thick, copious, and purulent eye discharge.
3. *Neisseria* species are capable of invading an intact corneal epithelium.
4. In early or mild cases of bacterial conjunctivitis, symptoms may be limited to mild con-junctival injection without frankly purulent drainage that is evident to the physician. Thus, empiric antibiotic therapy is warranted in most cases of conjunctivitis.

Associated Clinical Features

Viral conjunctivitis is an infection caused most commonly by adenoviruses. Clinical features range in severity but usually are mild and typically include burning or irritation, conjunctival injection, lid edema, chemosis, and a thin, watery discharge. The infection usually begins in one eye, but both eyes generally become involved because of autoinoculation (Fig. 2.3). The palpebral conjunctiva may demonstrate hyperemia and follicles, which are hyperplastic lymphoid tissue appearing as gray or white lobular elevations. The palpebral conjunctiva also may demonstrate papillae. Papillae are seen in many acute inflammatory diseases, secondary to a hyperplastic conunctival epithelium being thrown into numerous folds and projections. Clinically, papillae give the palpebral conjunctiva a velvety appearance. Preauricular adenopathy may be present. Severe cases may demonstrate focal or diffuse subconjunctival hemorrhages as well as pseudomembranes. A punctate keratitis may appear several days after the onset of symptoms, followed several weeks later by subepithelial infiltrates. The visual acuity and pupillary reactivity are normal.

Pharyngoconjunctival fever, usually caused by adenovirus type 3, is highly infectious and should be considered if there is fever, upper respiratory tract infection (cold, flu, or sore throat), and preauricular adenopathy. It is seen predominantly in the young and institutionalized, with epidemics occurring in families, schools, and military camps.

Epidemic keratoconjunctivitis is discussed separately.

Differential Diagnosis

Similar symptoms are seen in allergic and bacterial conjunctivitis and other causes of a red eye, such as scleritis, glaucoma, and iritis. Less common diagnoses include preseptal cellulitis and dacryoadenitis.

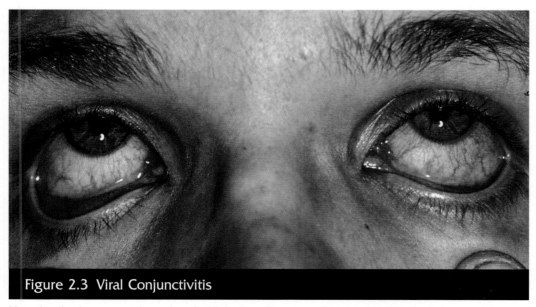

Figure 2.3 Viral Conjunctivitis

Note the classic asymmetric conjunctival injection. Symptoms first developed in the left eye, with symptoms spreading to the other eye a few days later. A thin watery discharge is also seen. (Courtesy of Kevin J. Knoop, MD, MS.)

Emergency Department Treatment and Disposition

Many cases are self-limited and mild. Cool compresses are helpful. Meticulous hygiene (hand washing by the family and instrument cleaning by medical personnel) is necessary to prevent spread. Because the signs and symptoms of viral conjunctivitis do not always suffice to distinguish it from bacterial conjunctivitis, antibacterial eye drops are usually prescribed. Antivirals are ineffective against adenovirus. Topical steroids should be avoided. Symptoms may persist for several weeks; follow-up is indicated if symptoms have not begun to resolve within 4 to 7 days.

Clinical Pearls

1. Adenoviruses are the most common cause of acute conjunctivitis. However, a complete eye examination is necessary to rule out other more serious causes of a red eye before the diagnosis of viral conjunctivitis is made.
2. Adenovirus most commonly demonstrates a follicular conjunctivitis. Papillae may also be seen on the palpebral conjunctiva.
3. Pharyngoconjunctival fever should be considered in the setting of fever, upper respiratory tract infection, and conjunctivitis.

Associated Clinical Features

Epidemic keratoconjunctivitis (EKC) is a severe and highly contagious adenovirus infection involving the conjunctiva and cornea. Viral transmission usually occurs through direct or indirect contact with the ocular secretions of infected individuals. The incubation period after exposure is about 8 days. Initial symptoms include watery or mucopurulent discharge, foreign-body sensation, and mild photophobia. Clinical findings include edema of the eyelids, chemosis, marked diffuse conjunctival hyperemia, subconjunctival hemorrhage, and a follicular and papillary conjunctival reaction (Fig. 2.4). Pseudomembranes overlying the palpebral conjunctiva and tender preauricular nodes may be present. A painful keratitis, typically involving the central cornea, develops in about 80% of patients, usually around the eighth day. The keratitis initially appears as fine punctate epithelial lesions that stain with fluorescein (Figs. 2.5, 2.6). These lesions coalesce

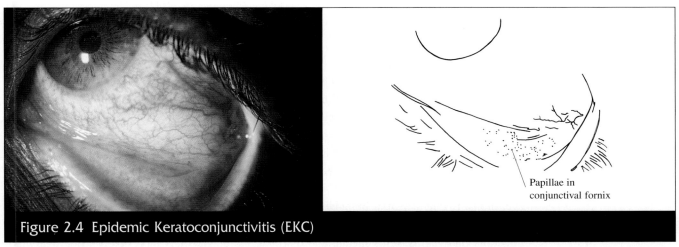

Papillae in
conjunctival fornix

Figure 2.4 Epidemic Keratoconjunctivitis (EKC)

Diffuse injection of the bulbar conjunctiva is seen in addition to a papillary reaction of the palpebral conjunctiva—a classic finding in EKC. (Courtesy of Katrina C. Santos.)

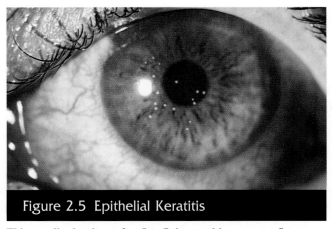

Figure 2.5 Epithelial Keratitis

This usually develops after 5 to 7 days and is seen as a fine punctate abrasion pattern over the cornea. (Courtesy of Katrina C. Santos.)

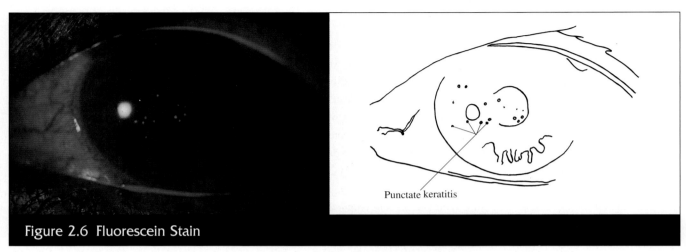

Figure 2.6 Fluorescein Stain

Punctate keratitis

This demonstrates epithelial keratitis from the prior photo. (Courtesy of Katrina C. Santos.)

and continue to stain with fluorescein. By the end of the second week, the keratitis is replaced by white macular, subepithelial infiltrates located in the central cornea. These lesions no longer stain with fluorescein. They may cause a significant decrease in vision and photophobia for months and even years, but they eventually resolve spontaneously. These subepithelial infiltrates are believed to result from a host immune response rather than from active viral replication.

Symptoms usually begin unilaterally in young adults during the fall and winter months. Bilateral involvement may develop 4 to 5 days later, with less severe symptoms in the second eye, probably due to partial immune protection of the host. There are few to no systemic complaints. Thus, in patients with systemic complaints and associated fever, upper respiratory tract infection, pharyngitis, otitis media, and diarrhea, the diagnosis is more likely to be pharyngo-conjunctival fever, which is also caused by an adenovirus. Pharyngoconjunctival fever is seen predominately in the young, with epidemics occurring in families and schools.

Differential Diagnosis

Other viruses and causes of red eye (bacterial conjunctivitis, iritis, scleritis, glaucoma, herpetic infection) need be considered.

Emergency Department Treatment and Disposition

Although EKC may be severe, the condition is self-limited and therapy is mainly palliative. Cool compresses, topical vasoconstrictors (Vasocon), and dark sunglasses provide symptomatic relief. Antibiotics and antivirals are ineffective. However, topical broad-spectrum antibiotic drops are usually prescribed, since it is difficult to distinguish viral from bacterial conjunctivitis. In the presence of pseudomembrane formation, topical broad-spectrum antibiotic ointments may be prescribed to lubricate and protect the cornea. The use of topical corticosteroids is controversial. They may have a role in patients with marked symptoms such as severe conjunctival pseudomembrane formation, severe foreign-body sensation, or reduced visual acuity secondary to epithelial or subepithelial keratitis. Although topical steroids do provide effective symptomatic relief, they have no beneficial therapeutic effect on the ultimate clinical outcome. Patients with EKC should limit their exposure to others for 2 weeks after the onset of the disease and use separate linens.

Clinical Pearls

1. A nonspecific adenoviral conjunctivitis will resolve in 10 to 14 days; a virulent adenovirus causing EKC will peak in 5 to 7 days and may last 3 to 4 weeks.
2. Frequent hand washing and the use of separate linens is advised for patients and family members to reduce exposure.
3. Pharyngoconjunctival fever should be considered if there is an associated fever and upper respiratory tract infection.
4. EKC may be nosocomially transmitted by tonometry (the footplate of the Schiøtz tonometer, the prism of the applanation tonometer), contaminated solutions (topical anesthetics), and the physician's fingers. Regular hand washing by the physician and patient and careful cleaning (using alcohol or Dakin's solution followed by rinsing) and sterilization of instruments are therefore important. Adenovirus can be recovered for extended periods of time from these surfaces.

Associated Clinical Features

Allergic conjunctivitis is a recurrent condition whereby airborne allergens precipitate hypersensitivity reactions in the conjunctiva. Potential allergens include pollens (ragweed, grasses, trees, weeds), animal dander, mold, and dust. Itching is the hallmark symptom. Allergic conjunctivitis is usually transient and self-limited and is seasonal if it is due to pollens. However, it can present as a single acute episode if the allergen is animal dander, mold, or dust. There may be a personal or family history of atopy, eczema, asthma, and allergic rhinitis (hay fever). Ocular allergic conditions are more common in males and tend to commence in the first or second decade of life.

In addition to the hallmark symptom of itching, associated clinical features include conjunctival injection and edema, burning, discharge (clear, white, or mucopurulent), and chemosis (swelling of the bulbar conjunctiva). Chemosis may be marked and may actually balloon beyond the lids. Small to medium-sized papillae (hyperplastic conjunctival epithelium thrown into numerous folds and projections) appear as small elevations on the palpebral conjunctiva (Fig. 2.7) and give the tissue a velvety appearance. Pallor of the palpebral conjunctiva may be present due to edema. The eyelids may be red and swollen.

Vernal conjunctivitis is an infrequent but serious form of allergic conjunctivitis that mainly affects young males (4 to 16 years of age) during the warm months or in tropical climates. Again, a family or personal history of atopy is common. In addition to a hereditary predisposition, exogenous factors play a role in the severity and likelihood of this disease. The Middle East and North Africa, with arid areas and wind and dust storms, have the highest incidence of vernal conjunctivitis. Symptoms of vernal conjunctivitis are similar to those of allergic conjunctivitis but greater in degree. Itching is intense, and a vigorous knuckle rubbing is a typical observation. Giant, raised, pleomorphic papillae ("cobblestones") are seen over the upper tarsal plate (but rarely over the lower tarsal plate) and are pathognomonic for the disease (Fig. 2.8). The drainage of vernal conjunctivitis is also pathognomonic and is characteristically tenacious, copious, thick, and ropy. Corneal findings include a sterile ulcer (well delineated with an oval or shield shape

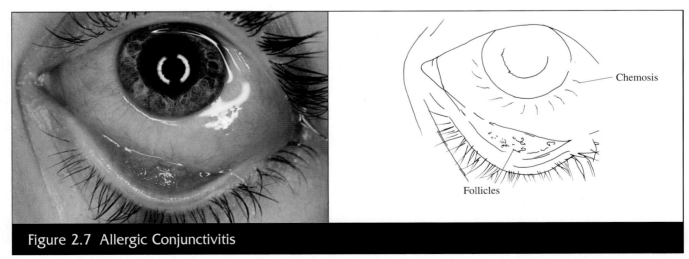

Figure 2.7 Allergic Conjunctivitis

Conjunctival injection, chemosis, and a follicular response in the inferior palpebral conjunctiva in this patient with allergic conjunctivitis secondary to cat fur. (Courtesy of Timothy D. McGuirk, DO.)

and no surrounding haze or iritis), Horner-Trantas dots (raised white limbal infiltrates), and superficial punctate keratopathy.

Differential Diagnosis

Other etiologies of a red eye (scleritis, iritis, glaucoma, bacterial conjunctivitis) should be considered.

Emergency Department Treatment and Disposition

The severity of the allergic condition is directly proportional to the level and duration of the allergen exposure. Therefore, initial therapy is primarily aimed at identification and elimination of the allergen. Avoiding animal dander, using air conditioners with appropriate filters, limiting time outdoors (to avoid pollen-bearing wind), or the use of goggles or glasses outdoors will improve the condition.

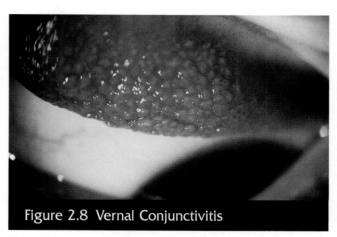

Figure 2.8 Vernal Conjunctivitis

The tarsal conjunctiva demonstrates giant papillae and a cobblestone appearance pathognomonic for vernal conjunctivitis. (Courtesy of William Beck.)

Topical tear substitutes (four to eight times a day) are effective in diluting or washing away the allergen. For mild allergic conjunctivitis, H_1 antihistamine-vasoconstrictor combinations successfully alleviate itching, redness, and swelling. Vasocon-A (one to two drops every 3 to 4 h) is effective and contains an antihistamine (0.5% antazoline) and a vasoconstrictor (0.05% naphazoline). Olopatadine (0.1%, one to two drops bid) is an antihistamine with mast cell–stabilizing properties that also relieves the itching and redness effectively. Mild topical steroids are an option after consultation with an ophthalmologist for those cases where all other modalities have been explored. A short course of prednisolone (0.12%) two to three times a day is unlikely to result in any ocular complications.

Additional therapeutic agents for vernal conjunctivitis include cromolyn sodium solution 4% (one to two drops every 4 to 6 h), aspirin (650 mg four times a day orally), and cold compresses. Topical cyclosporine (0.5%) may be useful in resistant cases of vernal conjunctivitis.

Clinical Pearls

1. Itching is the hallmark symptom of ocular allergy.
2. Removal of the offending allergen, if possible, is the first step in the treatment of allergic conjunctivitis. The patient is usually the best source for identifying the allergen to which he or she is sensitive.
3. Vasocon-A and olopatadine are effective in treating allergic conjunctivitis.
4. Topical corticosteroids may be used in severe cases but should be prescribed only with ED ophthalmology consultation. Complications include glaucoma, cataract formation, secondary infection, and corneal perforation.
5. Vernal conjunctivitis affects mainly children and adolescents; it peaks in the warmer months.
6. Evert the upper lid to appreciate the giant conjunctival papillae in vernal conjunctivitis. Their cobblestone appearance is pathognomonic.

Associated Clinical Features

A hordeolum is an acute purulent infection and a localized abscess involving the meibomian glands, the glands of Zeis, or the glands of Moll (Fig. 2.9). *Staphylococcus aureus* is the most frequent isolate. An external hordeolum (stye) involves an eyelash follicle and the adjacent glands of Zeis or Moll (Fig. 2.10). An internal hordeolum involves the meibomian glands within the tarsal plate. A chalazion is a chronic localized lipogranulomatous inflammation that results from the obstruction of the meibomian glands. A chalazion may evolve from a hordeolum but usually arises spontaneously secondary to blockage or obstruction of the gland. The impacted secretions of the gland are then extruded into the surrounding tissues, producing a foreign-body reaction to sebum and a lipogranulomatous inflammation. Chalazia are commonly seen in the ED (Fig. 2.11).

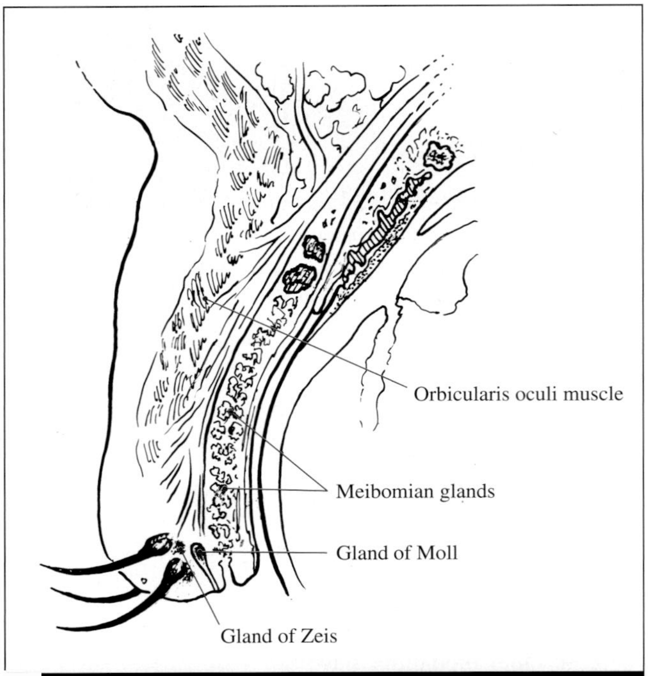

Common signs and symptoms include pain, focal swelling, edema, erythema, and tenderness. In the case of an external hordeolum (stye), an abscess localizes around the root of an eyelash, followed by necrosis of the skin and spontaneous evacuation of the abscess at the lid margin. An internal hordeolum, produced by obstruction of the meibomian duct with associated bacterial infection, demonstrates a localized inflammation of the tarsal plate. In the case of a chalazion, focal inflammation may cause pointing of the lesion either anteriorly (toward the skin of the eyelid) or posteriorly (toward the tarsal conjunctiva) (Figs. 2.12, 2.13). A chalazion may become sufficiently large as to press on the globe and cause astigmatism (corneal distortion that prevents focus). A chronic chalazion may appear as focal lid swelling without associated signs of inflammation.

There may be associated marginal blepharitis (Fig. 2.14) (a chronic low-grade inflammation of the lid margins with crusts around the lashes) or acne rosacea (a dermatologic condition with facial hyperemia, acneiform lesions, hypertrophy of sebaceous glands, and rhinophyma).

Figure 2.9 Eyelid Anatomy

Orbicularis oculi muscle

Meibomian glands

Gland of Moll

Gland of Zeis

Anatomic structures related to eyelid pathology.

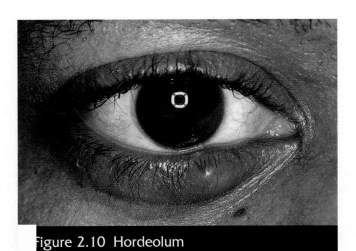

Figure 2.10 Hordeolum

Focal swelling and erythema at the lid margin are seen in this hordeolum. (Courtesy of Frank Birinyi, MD.)

Differential Diagnosis

Sebaceous cell or squamous cell carcinoma should be suspected in older patients with recurrent or persistent lesions. Preseptal cellulitis should be considered if the entire lid is erythematous and edematous. Pyogenic granuloma has a similar appearance but includes hypertrophic tissue as well as a vascular core, and it bleeds easily. Dacryocystitis should be considered if the lesion involves the medial aspect of the lower lid.

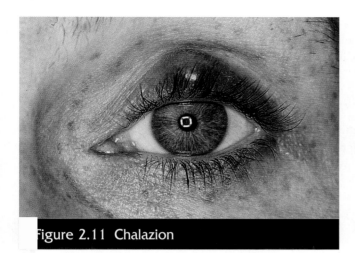

Figure 2.11 Chalazion

This chalazion shows nodular focal swelling and erythema. (Courtesy of Frank Birinyi, MD.)

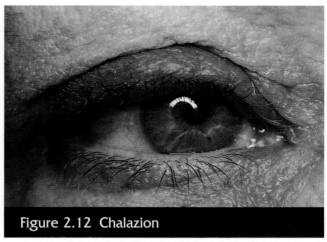

Figure 2.12 Chalazion

This chalazion is in an early stage. Lid swelling is evident, with pointing of the chalazion to the inner tarsal conjunctiva. (Courtesy of Kevin J. Knoop, MD, MS.)

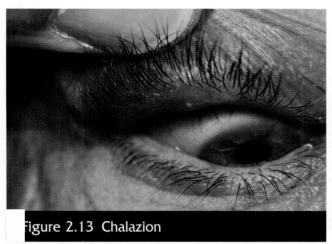

Figure 2.13 Chalazion

Pointing of the chalazion to the tarsal conjunctiva is more evident with slight lid eversion. (Courtesy of Kevin J. Knoop, MD, MS.)

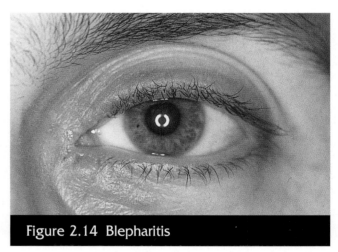

Figure 2.14 Blepharitis

Inflamed, erythematous eyelid margins consistent with blepharitis. (Courtesy of Kevin J. Knoop, MD, MS.)

Emergency Department Treatment and Disposition

The clinical course of a hordeolum may be self-limited, with spontaneous drainage of the abscess and resolution within 5 to 7 days. Treatment for both hordeola and chalazia includes warm compresses 2 to 4 times a day for 15 min. Warm compresses help to localize the infection and inflammation and may expedite spontaneous drainage. Systemic antibiotics are unnecessary unless there is a significant cellulitis. Topical antibiotic ointment cannot directly affect the inflammation inside the gland but is an adjunctive therapy to decrease the local bacterial flora. The application of a broad-spectrum antibiotic ointment, such as bacitracin or erythromycin, every 3 h to the conjunctival sac is effective. If the mass persists beyond 3 to 4 weeks or if the lesion is sufficiently large to distort vision, referral to the ophthalmologist should be made for incision and curettage or intralesional corticosteroid injection. Gentle scrubbing of the eyelids and lashes may be indicated if marginal blepharitis is noted.

Clinical Pearls

1. Chalazia are often found in patients with marginal blepharitis, probably because the orifices of the meibomian gland are blocked by the blepharitis infection.
2. Excisional biopsy is indicated for recurrent chalazia to exclude malignancy.

Associated Clinical Features

Dacryocystitis, an inflammation of the lacrimal sac, is usually secondary to obstruction of the nasolacrimal duct. Hallmark findings are tearing (epiphora) and discharge. Acute dacryocystitis is associated with pain, swelling over the lacrimal sac (Fig. 2.15), erythema, and tenderness. Mucopurulent discharge may be expressed from the punctum when pressure is applied over the lacrimal sac. In adults, acute infection is due to *Staphylococcus aureus* or occasionally beta-hemolytic streptococci.

In the newborn, 4 to 7% have a closed nasolacrimal passage. In these cases the duct usually opens spontaneously within the first month. Dacryocystitis is uncommon but may nevertheless develop, and aggressive treatment is required to avoid orbital cellulitis. *Haemophilus influenzae* is the most common organism isolated. Organisms usually seen in chronic dacryocystitis include *Streptococcus pneumoniae* or, rarely, *Candida albicans*.

Dacryocystitis is uncommon in the intermediate age groups unless it follows chronic sinusitis, facial trauma, or (rarely) neoplasm.

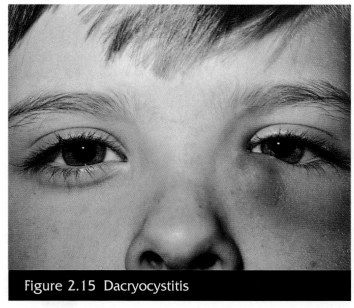

Figure 2.15 Dacryocystitis

Swelling and erythema over the medial lid and lacrimal sac developed in this 10-year-old patient with streptococcal pharyngitis. (Courtesy of Kevin J. Knoop, MD, MS.)

Differential Diagnosis

Chalazion, facial and orbital cellulitis, canaliculitis, canalicular stenosis, sinus tumors, ethmoid sinusitis, and mucoceles have similar features.

Emergency Department Treatment and Disposition

Acute dacryocystitis usually responds to oral antibiotics (amoxicillin-clavulanate), warm compresses, and gentle massage. Topical antibiotics may be used in chronic cases. Nonurgent ophthalmology or otolaryngology referral is required for definitive treatment—relief of the obstruction by dacryocystorhinostomy. In febrile and ill-appearing patients with acute dacryocystitis, hospitalization for intravenous antibiotics (cefuroxime) is indicated.

In infants with chronic dacryocystitis, both topical and oral antibiotics may be used. Referral is indicated if signs do not regress by 6 to 9 months of age or if acute dacryocystitis develops.

Clinical Pearls

1. The swelling is localized to the extreme nasal aspect of the lower lid and is usually unilateral.
2. The diagnosis of acute dacryocystitis may be confirmed by pressure on the lacrimal sac and the expression of purulent material from the punctum. The lacrimal sac and lacrimal fossa are situated in the inferior medial aspect of the orbit, not on the side of the nose.
3. The incidence follows a bimodal distribution. Dacryocystitis usually occurs in infants or persons over 40 years of age.

Associated Clinical Features

Dacryoadenitis is an uncommon condition involving inflammation of the lacrimal gland. Most acute cases are associated with systemic infection, although this may not be readily apparent. Findings are localized to the outer one-third of the upper eyelid and include fullness or swelling, conjunctival chemosis, and injection laterally (Fig. 2.16), erythema, and tenderness. A characteristic "S"-shaped deformity with mechanical ptosis of the upper lid is seen. The lacrimal gland may be palpable. Painful ophthalmoparesis and diplopia may be present secondary to involvement of the adjacent lateral rectus muscle.

Conditions associated with dacryoadenitis include sarcoidosis and Sjögren's syndrome. Infectious causes are more frequent; they include gonorrhea and mumps. Lacrimal gland masses, including lymphoma and epithelial tumors, may be neoplastic.

Differential Diagnosis

Chalazion, conjunctivitis, preseptal cellulitis, orbital cellulitis, and lacrimal gland tumor are other conditions to consider.

Emergency Department Treatment and Disposition

In the setting of acute bacterial infection, oral antibiotics (amoxicillin-clavulanate) are given for mild to moderate cases. In moderate to severe infections, intravenous antibiotics (ticarcillin-clavulanate) may be necessary. Viral dacryoadenitis (mumps) is treated with cool compresses and analgesics (acetaminophen); it resolves spontaneously without sequelae. Nonemergent ophthalmology follow-up is appropriate. Patients should be instructed to return to the ED urgently for symptoms suggestive of orbital cellulitis (decreased ocular motility or proptosis).

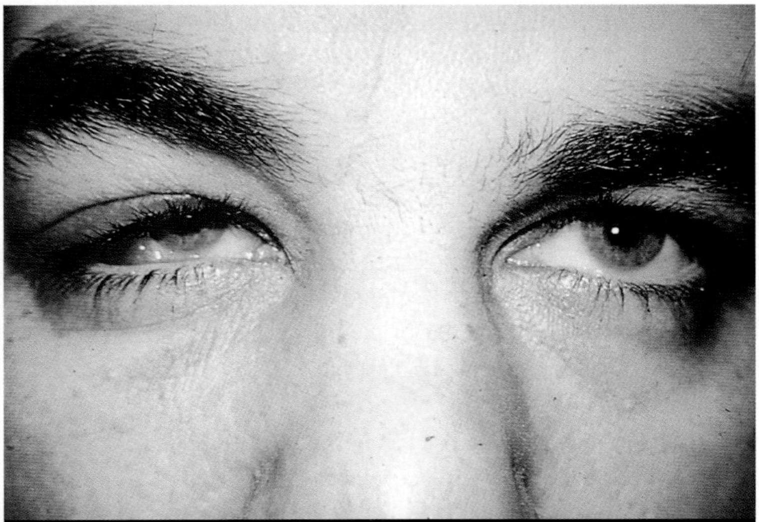

Figure 2.16 Dacryoadenitis

Unilateral localized swelling and chemosis are present laterally secondary to inflammation of the lacrimal gland. (Used with permission from the American Academy of Ophthalmology: *External Disease and Cornea: A Multimedia Collection.* San Francisco, 1994.)

Clinical Pearls

1. The swelling is usually unilateral and localized over the lateral one-third of the upper lid. It imparts an "S"-shaped curve to the lid margin.
2. In children, acute dacryoadenitis is most often seen as a complication of mumps with accompanying bilateral parotid swelling.
3. Approximately half of lacrimal gland masses are inflammatory; the other half are neoplastic.

Associated Clinical Features

A pinguecula (Latin: *pinguecula* meaning fatty) is a common degenerative lesion of the bulbar conjunctiva. It appears as a light brown or yellow-white amorphous conjunctival tissue adjacent to the limbus, usually nasally (Fig. 2.17). A pinguecula is usually asymptomatic and generally does not require treatment. It may become episodically inflamed, gradually enlarge over time, or become a pterygium.

A pterygium (Greek: *pterygion* meaning a wing-like thing) is a benign proliferation of fibrovascular tissue. It originates within the bulbar conjunctiva and extends onto the peripheral cornea. Early in its course a pterygium may be indistinguishable from a pinguecula. It may then enlarge to progressively encroach onto the cornea and visual axis. Typically a pterygium assumes a triangular configuration, with the apex of the lesion directed toward the pupil (Fig. 2.18). Growth occurs from this apex. Risk factors include exposure to ultraviolet light (sunlight), wind, and dust. Pterygia and pingueculae are generally seen in older individuals living in warmer areas with high levels of sunlight. Like pingueculae, pterygia are more likely to involve the nasal portion of the bulbar conjunctiva. Pterygia may be asymptomatic or become inflamed, giving rise to mild symptoms of irritation and foreign-body sensation. Decreased visual acuity may develop if the visual axis is involved or if the lesion induces astigmatism (irregular corneal curvature resulting in refractive error).

Differential Diagnosis

A pseudopterygium may have a similar appearance. A pseudopterygium is a fibrovascular scar arising in the bulbar conjunctiva and extending onto the cornea. It is the result of previous ocular inflammation (e.g., chemical burns, trauma, and infection). Episcleritis, corneal ulcer, and conjunctival neoplasm should be considered in the differential diagnosis.

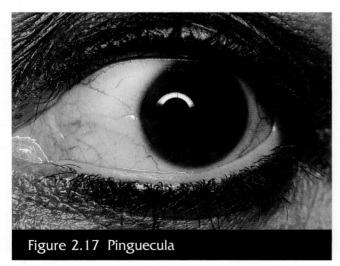

Figure 2.17 Pinguecula

A small area of yellowish "heaped up" conjunctival tissue is seen adjacent to the limbus on the nasal aspect. (Courtesy of Kevin J. Knoop, MD, MS.)

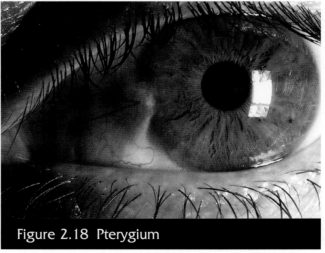

Figure 2.18 Pterygium

This pterygium appears as a raised vascular triangular area of bulbar conjunctiva that encroaches on the cornea. (Courtesy of the Department of Ophthalmology, Naval Medical Center, Portsmouth, VA.)

Emergency Department Treatment and Disposition

A patient with mild disease can be treated with artifical tears or a topical vasoconstrictor (Vasocon). In more severe cases, topical steroids may be prescribed after consultation. Nonemergent referral to an ophthalmologist is appropriate. Excision of a pinguecula (or pterygium) is indicated if the lesion interferes with contact lens wear, becomes chronically inflamed, or constitutes a cosmetic problem. Pterygia are excised if they cause persistent discomfort, encroach significantly on the cornea to involve the visual axis, or restrict the movement of extraocular muscles.

Clinical Pearls

1. Pterygia and pingueculae are usually found on the nasal conjunctiva, adjacent to the limbus, in the horizontal meridian.
2. Pterygia are a particular problem in sunny, hot, dusty regions. Eye protection (goggles, sunglasses) helps to reduce the irritation.

Associated Clinical Features

Scleritis is a destructive and serious inflammation involving the sclera. The sclera is the tough, flexible white outer covering of the eye, composed of collagen and elastic fibers. The onset of scleritis is gradual. Pain, tearing, and photophobia are prominent features. The pain, frequently severe, may awaken the patient at night. It may radiate to the forehead, temple, brow, or jaw. Ocular movement is usually painful.

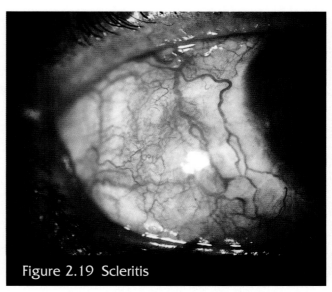

Figure 2.19 Scleritis

A prominent generalized vascular injection is present. These vessels do not move when the overlying conjunctiva is moved with a cotton-tipped applicator. (Courtesy of Thomas F. Mauger, MD.)

Patients with scleritis have an intensely red eye with a violaceous or purple hue, secondary to engorgement of the deep vessels of the episclera (Fig. 2.19). The blood vessels of the conjunctiva and superficial episclera are also commonly involved. Sectorial (versus diffuse) scleritis may mimic episcleritis. However, in scleritis, the globe is tender to palpation and the deep episcleral vessels do not move when the overlying tissues are moved with a cotton-tipped applicator, nor do they blanch with topical phenylephrine (2.5%). The normal radial vascular pattern of the episcleral vessels is lost. Scleral edema may be seen with slit-lamp biomicroscopy. (After the topical application of phenylephrine, the slit-lamp light beam appears to bow forward as the beam makes its excursion across the scleral surface.) Corneal involvement, iritis (with cells and flare in the anterior chamber) and decreased visual acuity frequently accompany scleritis. In patients with a previous history of scleritis, the uveal layer may be visible ("uveal show") in areas where scleral tissue has been lost.

Scleritis is associated with a number of autoimmune and infectious conditions; rheumatoid arthritis is the most common. Scleritis occurs more frequently in women and in the fourth to sixth decades of life.

Differential Diagnosis

Other causes of a red eye (conjunctivitis, iritis, episcleritis, trauma, glaucoma) should be considered. Scleritis may be confused with an inflamed pinguecula, pterygium, foreign body, or tumor.

Emergency Department Treatment and Disposition

Ophthalmology consultation and systemic therapy are required. Oral nonsteroidal anti-inflammatory drugs (NSAIDs) are recommended. Systemic steroids are added if oral NSAIDs are ineffective or for severe scleritis. Topical steroids and NSAIDs are occasionally effective. Immunosuppressive therapy (cyclophosphamide, methotrexate, azathioprine) is sometimes required, especially for progressive cases. Appropriate treatment of associated systemic autoimmune disease is also important. The intraocular pressure should be measured, since secondary glaucoma is associated with scleritis.

Clinical Pearls

1. Scleritis—unlike episcleritis, which may be self-limited—is destructive and threatens the patient's vision.
2. The eye is usually exquisitely tender, and patients frequently complain of severe pain. Episcleritis, on the other hand, is rarely associated with significant pain or tenderness.
3. Scleritis may be the presenting sign of a systemic disease. Rheumatoid arthritis is the most common.

Associated Clinical Features

Episcleritis is a common, benign, and frequently recurring inflammatory disease of the episclera; it typically affects young adults. The episclera is a thin layer of vascular elastic tissue overlying the primarily avascular sclera and is partly responsible for scleral nutrition. Tenon's capsule, a superficial layer within the episclera, acts as a synovial membrane for smooth movement of the eye. Episcleral vessels are large, run in a radial direction, and can be seen beneath the conjunctiva. Two separate vascular plexuses are found within the episclera. The superficial episcleral plexus is inflamed in episcleritis. These vessels blanch with the use of topical 2.5% phenylephrine drops. Vessels in the deep episcleral plexus, on the other hand, are associated with scleritis and remain dilated after the use of such drops.

Patients may complain of mild pain, foreign-body sensation, mild tenderness, irritation, photophobia, and excessive lacrimation. The affected eye appears normal except for nodular (or, rarely, diffuse) pink or bright red conjunctival and episcleral inflammation from dilation of the vessels in the superficial episcleral vascular plexus (Fig. 2.20). Visual acuity is normal. There is no history of trauma or purulent discharge.

Episcleritis is usually an isolated condition and the etiology is unknown. It has been associated with gout, systemic lupus erythematosus, rheumatoid arthritis, inflammatory bowel disease, and herpes zoster.

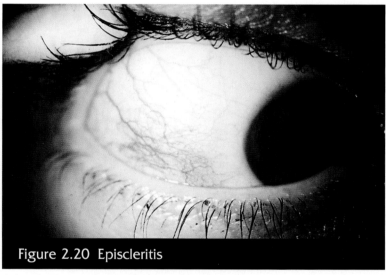

Figure 2.20 Episcleritis

A localized area of hyperemia consistent with episcleritis is seen in the lower lateral quadrant of the eye. (Courtesy of Thomas F. Mauger, MD.)

Differential Diagnosis

Other considerations include conjunctivitis and other causes of a red eye, such as iritis, acute glaucoma, trauma, corneal ulcer, scleritis, pinguecula, and phlyctenule (similar to episcleritis except that a nodule is present in the center of the lesion).

Emergency Department Treatment and Disposition

In mild cases, the condition is self-limited and may resolve spontaneously after 1 to 2 weeks. Artificial tears and topical vasoconstrictors (Naphcon) may be used. In those cases associated with rheumatoid arthritis or systemic lupus erythematosus, oral NSAIDs are recommended. Topical NSAIDS have not been shown to be effective. Ophthalmology referral is appropriate for confirmation and treatment.

Clinical Pearls

1. It is important to distinguish between episcleritis and scleritis, because the latter is an extremely serious problem that threatens the patient's vision.

2. While other causes of a red eye demonstrate a generalized redness, episcleritis is usually localized.

3. Dilated vessels in the superficial episcleral plexus will blanch with topical 2.5% phenylephrine. This test helps to distinguish between episcleritis and scleritis.

4. Episcleritis is unilateral two-thirds of the time and is seen in young and middle-aged adults. The gender incidence is equal.

5. Topical corticosteroids are not indicated in episcleritis. Although they may be effective temporarily, their use prolongs the natural history of resolution.

Associated Clinical Features

Glaucoma comprises a heterogeneous group of disorders causing optic nerve damage, usually in association with elevated intraocular pressure (IOP). It is a major and preventable cause of blindness. In angle closure glaucoma (ACG), the elevated IOP is due to an outflow obstruction of aqueous humor from the anterior chamber. Aqueous humor is initially produced by the ciliary body and first enters the posterior chamber. It then passes between the posterior surface of the iris and the anterior surface of the lens to enter the anterior chamber. After circulating within the anterior chamber, the aqueous humor leaves through the trabecular meshwork of the anterior chamber angle to enter Schlemm's canal. In ACG, the peripheral iris covers this trabecular meshwork, the angle is "closed," and aqueous outflow is blocked. Normal IOP is 10 to 21 mmHg; it rises to 50 to 100 mmHg in ACG.

There are several anatomic and physiologic factors that play a role in ACG. In the most common type of ACG, a major role is played by relative pupillary block. As the lens slowly enlarges due to normal development and aging, more of the lens's anterior surface makes contact with the iris's posterior surface. This increases the relative block of aqueous humor flow from the posterior chamber through the pupil to the anterior chamber. As a result, an increased pressure differential develops. The increased pressure in the posterior chamber causes the iris to bulge anteriorly ("iris bombé"). This bulging of the iris is maximal when the pupil is in the middilated position, generally 3 to 6 mm in diameter. The major factor that seems to predispose to an acute attack of ACG is prolonged, stationary middilation of the pupil. This sustained middilation can be seen with prolonged awake exposure to dim light or darkness with relaxation of the sphincter muscle, topical or systemic pharmacologic therapy that dilates the pupil, or prolonged severe emotional stress with secondary dilation due to adrenergic stimulation of the dilator muscle.

ACG presents as an acutely inflamed eye. Eye pain or headache varies in severity. Nausea and vomiting are common and may be the presenting complaints. As the IOP reaches the range of 50 to 60 mmHg, fluid is forced into the normal cornea, resulting in corneal edema. Because of this, patients may report blurred vision and rainbow-colored halos around lights. Clinical findings on examination include tearing, conjunctival injection with a perilimbal ("ciliary") flush, a cloudy ("steamy") cornea (Fig. 2.21), a nonreactive and middilated pupil (Fig. 2.22), mild anterior cham-

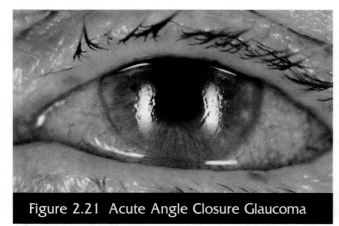

Figure 2.21 Acute Angle Closure Glaucoma

The cornea is edematous, manifest by the indistinctness of the iris markings and the irregular corneal light reflex. Conjunctival hyperemia is also present. (Courtesy of Kevin J. Knoop, MD, MS.)

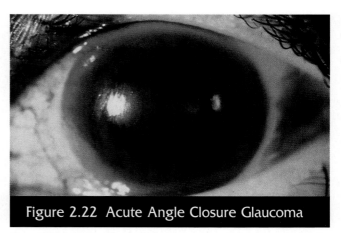

Figure 2.22 Acute Angle Closure Glaucoma

Note the cloudy or "steamy" appearance of the cornea and the midposition pupil. Conjunctival hyperemia is not as evident. (Courtesy of Gary Tanner, MD.)

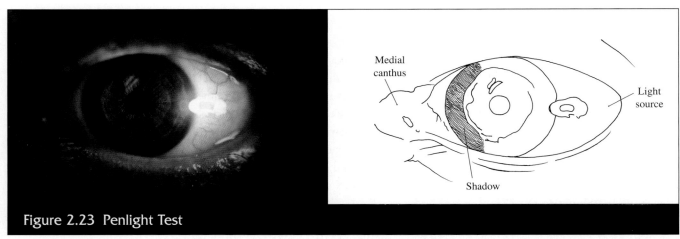

Figure 2.23 Penlight Test

A penlight, held laterally and directed nasally, projects a shadow on the nasal side of an iris with a shallow anterior chamber. This patient presented with acute angle closure glaucoma. (Courtesy of Alan B. Storrow, MD.)

ber inflammation, and increased intraocular pressure. Also, the anterior chamber is shallow. This is demonstrated by a penlight held laterally and directed nasally (Fig. 2.23). In an eye with a normal anterior chamber, the entire iris will be illuminated by the penlight. In an eye with a narrow angle or shallow anterior chamber, a shadow is cast on the nasal side of the iris secondary to the forward bowing of the iris. Alternatively, slit-lamp biomicroscopy may also be used to assess the anterior chamber's depth. Funduscopic examination demonstrates optic cupping only if there is preexisting glaucoma.

Tonometers available in the ED for measurement of IOP include the air-puff noncontact tonometer, the Schiøtz tonometer, the Tono-Pen, and the applanation tonometer. Tactile tonometry, using the examiner's fingers to ballot the globe, can easily detect ACG in patients with markedly elevated IOP.

Differential Diagnosis

Similar conditions include temporal arteritis, acute iritis, ulcer, and other causes of a red eye (conjunctivitis, trauma, scleritis, keratitis, foreign body).

Emergency Department Treatment and Disposition

ACG requires emergent ophthalmology consultation. Treatment is directed at reducing the IOP. Aqueous outflow is increased by the use of topical miotics (pilocarpine 1 or 2%, one drop every 5 min × 2. If the pupil does not respond, one drop every hour × 4 should be administered.) Topical miotics such as pilocarpine stimulate miosis to pull the peripheral iris taut, away from the trabecular meshwork. If the pupil does not respond within 5 to 10 min (or if it is not expected to respond because the IOP is greater than 50 to 60 mmHg or the attack is many hours old), other medications with a different mechanism of action to decrease the IOP should be administered. Decreased production of aqueous is accomplished with the use of a topical beta blocker (timolol maleate, 0.5%, one drop every 12 h) or an alpha-adrenergic agonist (apraclonidine, 1%, one drop every 12 h). Acetazolamide, a carbonic anhydrase inhibitor, can also be given (500 mg PO or 500 mg IV if the patient is nauseated or vomiting). The goal of these medicines, which decrease the production of aqueous, is to rapidly lower the IOP to less than 40 to 50 mmHg so as to allow for reperfusion of the pupillary sphincter, thereby permitting the muscle to respond to pilocarpine. Osmotic agents may also be used. Oral agents are tried first; if they are unsuccessful or if the patient is nauseous, systemic intravenous agents may then be used. Oral agents include glycerol (1.0 to 1.5 g/kg in a 50% solution). In diabetics, since glycerol can cause hyperglycemia, oral isosorbide can be substituted (1.5 to 2.0 g/kg). Intravenous agents include mannitol (20% solution, 2 g/kg given over 30 min). Hyperosmotics realize their maximal reduction within 45 to 60 min. A final agent to consider for use in ACG is the prostaglandin derivative latanoprost (0.005%, one drop once daily in the evening). Its mechanism of action is increased uveal-scleral outflow, acting to increase aqueous outflow through nontrabecular meshwork pathways.

Corneal indentation may be used in situations where the IOP is 50 mmHg or greater and topical miotics are ineffective secondary to ischemia of the iris constrictor. Indentation of the cornea displaces the aqueous to the peripheral anterior chamber, temporarily opening the angle. Corneal indentation is performed with topical anesthetics and any smooth instrument such as the Goldmann applanation prism. The prism is held with the fingers and firm pressure is applied for 30 s. This may successfully decrease the IOP and abort the attack; if the IOP has been of long standing, however, it is more likely to be unsuccessful.

The definitive treatment of ACG is laser peripheral iridectomy, usually done after the IOP normalizes.

Clinical Pearls

1. ACG may be inadvertently precipitated in the ED patient treated for corneal abrasion with a cycloplegic (cyclopentolate). Therefore the depth of the anterior chamber should always be evaluated in ED patients receiving cycloplegics.
2. In light of the associated severe headache and vomiting, patients with ACG may easily be misdiagnosed as having a migraine headache or a central nervous system (CNS) catastrophe.
3. The unaffected eye will also have a narrow anterior chamber. The presence of a shallow anterior chamber in only one eye casts doubt on the diagnosis of ACG, since ACG is the result of an anatomic configuration that is almost always bilateral.
4. Patients with ACG may be able to recall a previous (milder) attack that they felt was a migraine or some other type of headache.
5. The elevated IOP in acute ACG can be reduced pharmacologically by three mechanisms: first, by opening the closed angle with miotics; second, by reducing aqueous formation with beta blockers, alpha agonists, and carbonic anhydrase inhibitors; and third, by reducing the aqueous volume within the eye using osmotic agents.

Associated Clinical Features

The uvea is the middle layer of the eye and is composed of the iris, ciliary body, and choroid. *Uveitis* refers to inflammation within the uvea, and anterior uveitis localizes the inflammation to the anterior chamber, iris, ciliary body, and anterior vitreous.

In many cases of anterior uveitis, no definitive diagnosis can be made. A significant number, however, are associated with medically treatable systemic diseases. The list is extensive and includes inflammatory disorders (juvenile rheumatoid arthritis, rheumatoid arthritis, sarcoidosis, Behçet's disease, Sjögren's syndrome), conditions associated with HLA-B27, (ankylosing spondylitis, inflammatory bowel disease, Reiter's syndrome), and infectious diseases (tuberculosis, toxoplasmosis, herpes simplex, herpes zoster, cytomegalovirus, syphilis, AIDS). Finally, lymphoma and Kawasaki's disease may also manifest as an anterior uveitis. Therefore aggressive attempts to determine the underlying cause of the uveitis are warranted.

Clinical features of anterior uveitis include conjunctival hyperemia, hyperemic perilimbal vessels ("ciliary flush") (Fig. 2.24), decreased visual acuity, photophobia, miosis, pupillary irregularities (secondary to the formation of anterior or posterior synechiae), iris nodules, tearing (particularly when exposed to bright lights), and pain. A hypopyon (a layer of white blood cells in the dependent portion of the anterior chamber) may be seen (Fig. 2.25). The slit-lamp examination may demonstrate cells and flare. *Cells* refers to the finding of inflammatory cells seen in the anterior chamber, having the appearance of dust in a sunbeam (Fig. 2.26); *flare* is light scatter secondary to inflammatory cells and proteins circulating within the aqueous and anterior chamber and has the appearance of a headlight in fog (Fig. 2.27). Other significant slit-lamp findings in anterior uveitis include keratic precipitates, which are agglutinated inflammatory cells adherent to the posterior corneal endothelium (Fig. 2.28). Keratic precipitates appear either as fine gray-white deposits or as large, flat, confluent areas with a greasy surface ("mutton fat"). The intraocular pressure (IOP) may be elevated secondary to inflammatory debris within the trabecu-

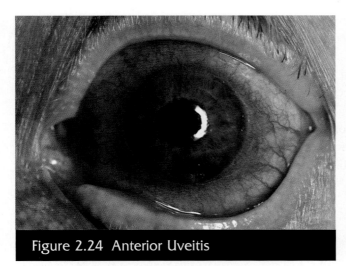

Figure 2.24 Anterior Uveitis

Marked conjunctival injection and perilimbal hyperemia ("ciliary flush") are seen in this patient with recurrent iritis. (Courtesy of Kevin J. Knoop, MD, MS.)

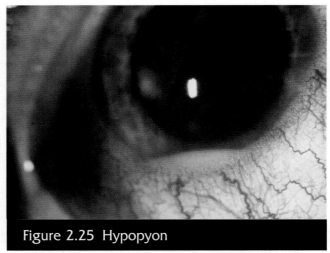

Figure 2.25 Hypopyon

A thin layering of white blood cells is present in the inferior anterior chamber. (Used with permission from Spalton DJ, Hitchings RA, Hunter PA (eds): *Atlas of Clinical Ophthalmology,* 2d ed. Mosby-Wolfe Limited, London, UK, 1994.)

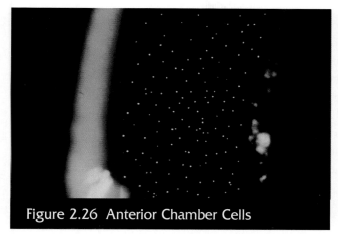

Figure 2.26 Anterior Chamber Cells

Cells in the anterior chamber are a sign of inflammation or bleeding and appear similar to particles of dust in a sunbeam. They are best seen with a narrow slit-lamp beam directed obliquely across the anterior chamber. (Used with permission from Spalton DJ, Hitchings RA, Hunter PA (eds): *Atlas of Clinical Ophthalmology,* 2nd ed. Mosby-Wolfe Limited, London, UK, 1994.)

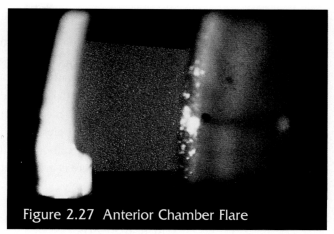

Figure 2.27 Anterior Chamber Flare

Flare in the anterior chamber represents an elevated concentration of plasma proteins from inflamed, leaking intraocular blood vessels. Flare seen in a slit-lamp beam appears similar to a car headlight cutting through the fog. (Used with permission from Spalton DJ, Hitchings RA, Hunter PA (eds). *Atlas of Clinical Ophthalmology.* Mosby-Wolfe Limited, London, UK, 1984.)

lae, obstructing outflow, or the IOP may be decreased secondary to decreased production of aqueous humor by the inflamed ciliary body.

Differential Diagnosis

Other conditions presenting with a red eye include glaucoma, conjunctivitis (bacterial, viral, allergic), scleritis, episcleritis, keratitis, and corneal ulcer. A hypopyon can also be seen with severe corneal ulcerations and penetrating trauma to the anterior chamber.

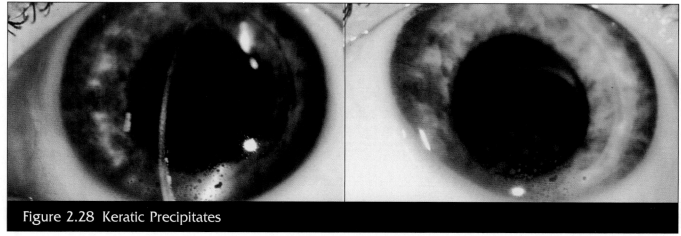

Figure 2.28 Keratic Precipitates

Deposits of cells on the *endothelial* layer of the cornea are seen in these photographs. (Used with permission from Spalton DJ, Hitchings RA, Hunter PA (eds): *Atlas of Clinical Ophthalmology,* 2nd ed. Mosby-Wolfe Limited, London, UK, 1994.)

Emergency Department Treatment and Disposition

In light of the common association of anterior uveitis with systemic disease, the evaluation of a uveitis patient in the ED is a systemic evaluation. The history should focus on rheumatic illness, dermatologic problems, bowel disease, infectious exposures, and sexual history. This history forms the basis for the subsequent physical examination and laboratory testing.

Treatment of the anterior uveitis itself is nonspecific. Topical cycloplegics (atropine) and corticosteroids may be prescribed in conjunction with the ophthalmologist. Although nonspecific, this therapy will greatly reduce the amount of scarring. Antibiotics are not usually prescribed or helpful unless there is a bacterial origin. Prompt ophthalmology follow-up is important if steroids are prescribed.

Clinical Pearls

1. Key diagnostic features of anterior uveitis are a miotic pupil, ciliary flush, and the finding of cells and flare in the anterior chamber.
2. When cells and flare are visualized in the anterior chamber using the slit lamp, the cells look like dust particles in a sunbeam, and the flare (the slit-lamp beam) looks like a headlight cutting through fog.
3. Inflammation of the anterior uveal tract (iris or ciliary body) produces the clinical symptom of photophobia.
4. The presence of anterior uveitis requires a search for associated systemic illness.
5. Topical analgesics (tetracaine, proparacaine) do not significantly ameliorate the pain of anterior uveitis, unlike the case with many of the common conditions seen in the ED, such as corneal abrasions.
6. The discharge associated with anterior uveitis is watery or nonexistent. A purulent discharge suggests an infectious condition such as conjunctivitis or keratitis.

Associated Clinical Features

Herpes zoster ophthalmicus develops secondary to activation of latent varicella zoster virus within the trigeminal ganglion. Neuronal spread of the virus through the ophthalmic division of the trigeminal nerve results in crops of grouped vesicles in a dermatomal distribution (Fig. 2.29).

Almost any ophthalmic abnormality in both the anterior and posterior segments of the eye may be seen with herpes zoster ophthalmicus. The most common corneal lesion is punctate epithelial keratitis, in which the cornea has a ground-glass appearance because of stromal edema. Pseudodendrites are also very common. Pseudodendrites form from the deposition of mucus, are usually peripherally located and stain moderately to poorly with fluorescein. Pseudodendrites may be differentiated from the dendrites of herpes simplex infection in that the pseudodendrites lack the rounded terminal bulbs at the end of the branches and are broader and more plaque-like. When they are wiped from the cornea, a layer of intact epithelium may remain, unlike the full-thickness epithelial defect seen with herpes simplex. The third most common corneal lesion—after punctate epithelial keratitis and pseudodendrites—is that of anterior stromal infiltrates. These are seen between the second and third weeks after the acute disease and are felt to be an immune response to viral antigen diffusing into the anterior stroma. They may be single or multiple.

Corneal anesthesia or hypoesthesia is a frequent complication of herpes zoster keratitis. Some 60% of patients will recover essentially normal sensitivity within 2 to 3 months. In about 25%, however, the anesthesia is permanent.

The anterior uvea is commonly involved in herpes zoster ophthalmicus and is second only to the cornea in frequency of involvement. Anterior uveitis may develop early or years after the acute disease—and independent of corneal pathology. Clinical findings range in severity and include ciliary flush, miosis, pain, cells and flare in the anterior chamber, photophobia, visual decrease, keratic precipitates (agglutinated inflammatory cells adherent to the posterior corneal endothelium), and anterior and posterior synechiae (adhesions from the iris to the cornea anteriorly or to the lens posteriorly).

Conjunctivitis is also extremely common; it is characterized by a watery discharge. Follicles (hyperplastic lymphoid tissue that appears as gray or white lobular elevations, particularly in the inferior cul-de-sac) and regional adenopathy may or may not be present.

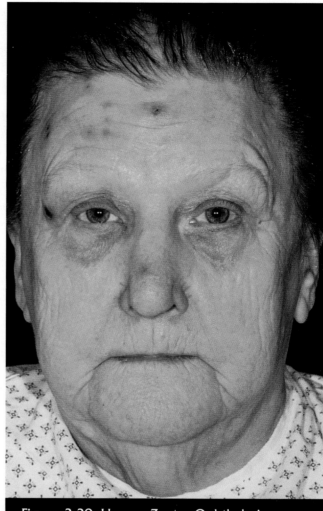

Figure 2.29 Herpes Zoster Ophthalmicus

A healing vesicular rash in the distribution of the ophthalmic division (V1) of the trigeminal nerve is present in this 72-year-old diabetic patient. The presence of the lesion on the tip of the nose (Hutchinson's sign) increases the risk of ocular involvement. (Courtesy of Frank Birinyi, MD.)

Differential Diagnosis

Keratitis secondary to herpes simplex may also present with rash, red eye, and dendriform corneal lesions. Ocular complications of herpes zoster ophthalmicus may follow the rash by many months to years; they have a highly variable presentation that can mimic almost any ophthalmic disease.

Emergency Department Treatment and Disposition

In patients with epithelial defects, topical broad-spectrum antibiotics should be administered bid to prevent secondary infection. Oral valacyclovir (1 g three times a day for 7 days), famciclovir (500 mg three times a day for 7 days), or acyclovir (800 mg five times a day for 10 days) is beneficial, particularly if given within 72 h of onset. Topical antivirals are clinically ineffective. Cycloplegics (cyclopentolate) are used if an iritis is present. Artificial tears and ointment may be recommended to the patient as necessary. Nonnarcotic and narcotic analgesics may be prescribed. An ophthalmology consult is appropriate.

Steroids in the past (before acyclovir) were among the mainstays of treatment. However, steroids have proved less successful than systemic acyclovir, famciclovir, and valacyclovir. Also arguing against steroid use is the risk of systemic dissemination of the herpes zoster virus should the zoster be an early presenting sign of immunosuppression. Therefore systemic steroids are largely out of favor.

Clinical Pearls

1. Nearly two-thirds of patients with herpes zoster ophthalmicus develop ocular lesions; thus careful eye examination with corneal staining should be performed to rule out corneal involvement.
2. Patients with skin lesions on the tip of the nose (Hutchinson's sign) are at higher risk for ocular involvement with herpes zoster. The sensory innervation to both the eye and the tip of the nose is supplied by the nasociliary branch of the ophthalmic division of cranial nerve V. This sign, however, is highly variable in its reliability. The eye may be involved without nasal involvement.
3. Corneal hypoesthesia and the appearance of dendrites with fluorescein staining are seen in both herpes zoster ophthalmicus and herpes simplex keratitis.
4. The severity of the cutaneous disease does not necessarily correlate with the severity of the ocular disease.
5. The prognosis is good, and recurrences—unlike those for herpes simplex keratitis—are rare.

Associated Clinical Features

Ocular herpetic disease may be neonatal, primary, or recurrent. Neonatal ocular herpes develops secondary to passage through an infected birth canal. Usually (80%) is herpes simplex virus (HSV) type 2. Most frequently the infection is a conjunctivitis, often associated with a keratitis. Fetal monitoring with a scalp electrode is associated with an increased risk for neonatal HSV infection.

Primary ocular herpes is an acute first HSV infection of a nonimmune host. It may present as blepharitis (vesicles on an erythematous base), conjunctivitis, or keratoconjunctivitis. Clinical disease may be seen 3 to 9 days after exposure. Patients with keratoconjunctivitis commonly have significant periorbital skin involvement. They note pain, irritation, foreign-body sensation, redness, photophobia, tearing, and occasionally decreased visual acuity. Follicles and preauricular adenopathy may be seen. Initially the keratitis is diffuse and punctate. After 24 h, fluorescein stain appears as either serpiginous ulcers without clear-cut branching or multiple diffuse microdendritic epithelial defects. True dendritic ulcers are rarely seen in primary disease.

The most likely clinical scenario facing the ED physician in cases of ocular herpes simplex is that of recurrent disease. Recurrences may be triggered by immunosuppression, fever, ultraviolet light exposure, trauma, systemic illness, stress, or menstruation. In recurrent disease, keratoconjunctivitis (Fig. 2.30), blepharitis, or iritis is seen, and the cornea is more likely to be involved (Fig. 2.31). With blepharitis and recurrent HSV disease, vesicles are grouped in focal clusters, with significantly less skin involvement than that seen in primary herpes. In those patients with recurrent HSV and keratoconjunctivitis, signs and symptoms include a watery discharge, conjunctival injection, irritation, blurred vision, and preauricular lymph node involvement. Corneal involvement initially may appear punctate but evolves into

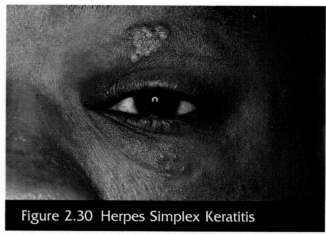

Figure 2.30 Herpes Simplex Keratitis

This 23-year-old has a history of ocular herpes infections since childhood. Grouped vesicles on an erythematous base with mild lid swelling are seen. The conjunctiva is mildly hyperemic. (Secondary impetigo may be present.) (Courtesy of Frank Birinyi, MD.)

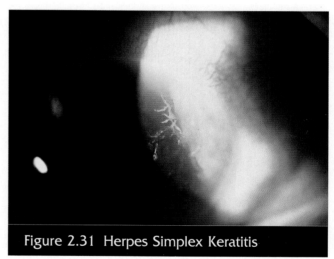

Figure 2.31 Herpes Simplex Keratitis

A slit-lamp view of unstained dendritic lesions. (Courtesy of Lawrence B. Stack, MD.)

a characteristic dendritic keratitis (Figs. 2.32, 2.33). Dendritic ulcers may be single or multiple. Their linear branches classically end in bead-like extensions called terminal bulbs. These are best seen with rose Bengal stain, which stains the epithelial defect as well as the infected cells surrounding the defect (Fig. 2.34). Fluorescein dye demonstrates primarily the corneal defect; punctate staining may be appreciated over the surrounding damaged epithelium. In addition to the dendritic pattern, fluorescein staining may instead take on a geographic appearance. This is particularly true when topical steroids have been (incorrectly) prescribed. Most patients (80%) with herpes simplex keratitis have decreased or absent corneal sensation in the area of the dendrite or geographic ulceration. Uninvolved areas of the cornea may retain normal sensation.

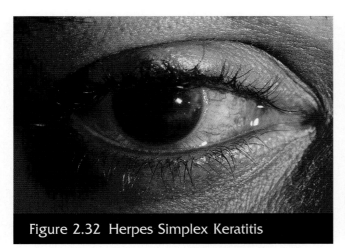

Figure 2.32 Herpes Simplex Keratitis

A large dendritic lesion after fluorescein staining. The patient had been diagnosed with "pink eye" in a prior visit. (Courtesy of Kevin J. Knoop, MD, MS.)

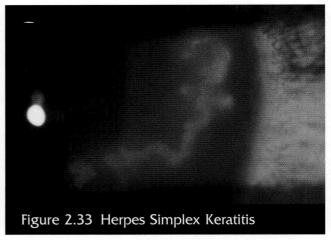

Figure 2.33 Herpes Simplex Keratitis

A magnified view via slit-lamp biomicroscopy shows the classic terminal bulbs pathognomonic for ocular HSV infection. (Courtesy of Department of Ophthalmology, Naval Medical Center, Portsmouth, VA.)

Following protracted and repeated episodes of HSV keratitis, corneal lesions occasionally scar, and a permanently decreased visual acuity can result. In some patients, melting and perforation of the cornea ensue secondary to structural damage.

Differential Diagnosis

Other causes of red eye (scleritis, iritis, glaucoma, conjunctivitis) should be considered. A similar fluorescein appearance may be seen with herpes zoster virus, recurrent corneal erosions, or a healing corneal abrasion.

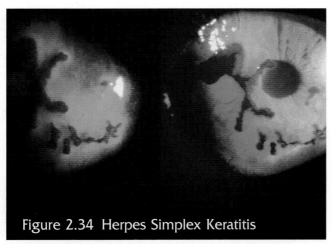

Figure 2.34 Herpes Simplex Keratitis

Fluorescein (*left*) and rose Bengal (*right*) stains demonstrate characteristic dendritic patterns. Whereas fluorescein staining is used to detect epithelial defects, rose Bengal staining additionally demonstrates degenerating or dead epithelial cells and is particularly good for demonstrating the club-shaped terminal bulbs at the end of each branch. (Used with permission from the American Academy of Ophthalmology: *External Disease and Cornea: A Multimedia Collection*, San Francisco, 1994.)

Emergency Department Treatment and Disposition

In neonatal ocular herpes infections, an emergency pediatric or infectious disease consultation is initiated. There is a high association between ocular neonatal HSV infection and potentially lethal systemic or neurologic infection. Therefore acyclovir is given intravenously. The ocular disease itself may be treated with topical antivirals (idoxuridine, vidarabine, trifluorothymidine).

Treatment of patients (beyond the neonatal period) with primary ocular herpes is usually successful and generally results in healing without scarring. For those with blepharitis or periocular dermatitis, warm wet soaks bid and general good hygiene is recommended. A prophylactic topical antiviral (trifluorothymidine drops five times a day, idoxuridine ointment tid or idoxuridine drops eight times a day) is administered to the adjacent eye until the skin lesions scab and dry. Patients with corneal involvement require a 2- to 3-week course of antiviral ointment or drops (trifluorothymidine 1% nine times a day, or idoxuridine 0.1% either q 1 h by day, q 2 h at night, or 1 drop q 5 min $\times$ 5 five times daily). Topical antibiotics bid are also recommended for those with corneal lesions to prevent secondary bacterial infection.

In patients with recurrent disease limited to HSV blepharitis, the lesions are superficial and heal without scarring. The goal of therapy in these patients is to protect the globe with prophylactic antiviral ointment tid or drops five to six times a day until the lesions have scabbed. No clinical trials have demonstrated oral acyclovir to prevent herpetic blepharitis. Nevertheless initiating acyclovir 400 mg PO five times a day for 5 days within 1 h of the first sign of recurrence is recommended and may alleviate some symptoms.

For most patients with recurrent HSV disease and corneal involvement, topical antivirals alone are effective. Trifluorothymidine (1% nine times a day for 14 to 21 days) is recommended. Topical antibiotics are administered bid while a corneal defect is present. Ophthalmology consultation is required.

Clinical Pearls

1. The diagnosis of acute neonatal ocular HSV should be entertained in any infant with non-purulent conjunctivitis or keratitis.
2. HSV is the most common cause of corneal ulceration and the most common infectious cause of corneal blindness in the western hemisphere.
3. HSV dendrites, when stained with fluorescein, appear as branching lesions with club-shaped or bead-like extensions called terminal bulbs at the end of each branch. In primary HSV disease, however, dendrites are rare. Terminal bulbs are not seen in herpes zoster dendrites.
4. Other patterns of fluorescein staining in HSV infection include a superficial punctate keratitis. This is seen particularly in primary disease and early in the course of recurrent disease.
5. With recurrent attacks, corneal pain may be diminished owing to increasing corneal hypoesthesia.

Associated Clinical Features

The term *corneal ulcer* denotes an inflammatory and ulcerative condition. Similar terms include *infectious keratitis, bacterial keratitis,* and *ulcerative keratitis.* Etiologies include bacteria (most commonly *Staphylococcus, Streptococcus,* and *Pseudomonas*) and viruses (herpes simplex). (Keratitis secondary to herpes simplex is discussed separately.) Bacterial corneal ulcers are commonly associated with extended-wear soft contact lenses and contaminated lens care solutions (Fig. 2.35), whereby minor corneal abrasion or chemical damage permits bacteria to penetrate the cornea. Fungal infection, although rare, should be suspected in cases of ocular trauma involving vegetable matter (a tree branch), chronic corneal disease (herpes keratitis), or cases involving steroid use. *Acanthamoeba* keratitis is associated with contaminated contact lens solutions.

Symptoms associated with corneal ulcer include pain, photophobia, decreased vision, discharge, and a foreign-body sensation. The ulcer appears as a corneal stromal infiltrate associated with conjunctival hyperemia (Fig. 2.36), a miotic pupil, and chemosis along with lid edema and erythema. Slit-lamp biomicroscopy demonstrates an epithelial defect with fluorescein uptake. Findings in the anterior chamber include cells (inflammatory cells that look like dust in a sunbeam) and flare (light scatter seen secondary to cells and proteins), keratic precipitates (inflammatory cells that have coalesced and adhered to the cornea), and hypopyon (a layer of white blood cells in the inferior or dependent portion of the anterior chamber).

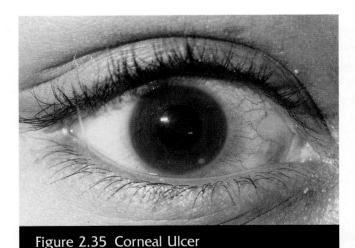

Figure 2.35 Corneal Ulcer

An elliptical ulcer at 5 o'clock near the periphery is seen. This location is atypical for a bacterial ulcer. The patient presented with painful red eyes and normal uncorrected vision, but was a new wearer of soft contact lenses (for cosmesis). Bilateral corneal ulcers were diagnosed, which cleared after treatment with topical cipro-floxacin. The impressive ciliary flush is pathognomonic for corneal (versus conjunctival) pathology. (Courtesy of Kevin J. Knoop, MD, MS.)

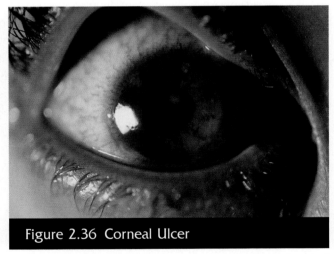

Figure 2.36 Corneal Ulcer

A circular corneal infiltrate is seen at 12 o'clock; conjunctival hyperemia is present. (A rectangular flash reflection is seen at 9 o'clock.) A mild limbal flush is noted superiorly. (Courtesy of Lawrence B. Stack, MD.)

Differential Diagnosis

Other possibilities include a residual corneal foreign body, a rust ring, and a sterile corneal infiltrate (secondary to an immune reaction to contact lens solution or *Staphylococcus*). Other causes of a red eye (conjunctivitis, glaucoma, scleritis) should also be considered.

Emergency Department Treatment and Disposition

Corneal ulcers should be treated as an ophthalmologic emergency and assumed to be bacterial until proven otherwise. An emergent ophthalmology consult is indicated, and stains and cultures should be obtained as expeditiously as possible before antibiotic treatment has commenced. Intensive topical treatment is the most effective way to treat corneal infections. Fortified (concentrated) cephalosporins or vancomycin combined with an aminoglycoside may be used every 30 to 60 min. A fluoroquinolone may be used as a single agent for mild cases of infectious keratitis. Clinical improvement is usually noted after 2 to 3 days of therapy; the frequency of antibiotic instillation can then be tapered. Subconjunctival injections of antibiotics every 12 to 24 h are used in severe cases. Systemic antibiotics are not usually used except in cases where the organism may have extended to the sclera (*Pseudomonas*) or if there is a high risk of concurrent systemic disease (*Neisseria, Haemophilus*). Cycloplegics (atropine) are usually recommended if there is an accompanying iritis. Epithelial debridement may be beneficial. Steroids and an eye patch are contraindicated in the initial management. A contact lens wearer must discontinue contact lens wear.

Clinical Pearls

1. A bacterial corneal infection must be treated as an ophthalmologic emergency.
2. Corneal injury, including recent contact lens procedures, is a risk factor for the development of a corneal ulcer.
3. *Pseudomonas aeruginosa* is capable of destroying the cornea within 6 to 12 h. It should be suspected by its aggressive course, thick yellow-green or blue-green tenacious, mucopurulent exudate, and ground-glass edema surrounding the ulcer.
4. *Acanthamoeba,* a ubiquitous protozoan, should be suspected in contact lens wearers with contaminated lens solutions or who swim wearing their contact lenses. These patients characteristically have pain out of proportion to their clinical findings.
5. Infectious ulcers tend to develop centrally, away from the vascular supply and immune system of the limbus, but they can also be peripheral.

Associated Clinical Features

Anisocoria is unequal pupil size. In room lighting, the normal diameter of pupils is 3 to 5 mm. Pupil size is larger in childhood and smaller with age. Anisocoria of 1 to 2 mm may be a normal finding, and is found in 5 to 20% of normal individuals. With normal (physiologic) anisocoria, the disparity in pupil size is the same in light as in dark. In addition, the pupils react normally to light and accommodation; they are perfectly round, extraocular movements are intact, and no ptosis or conjunctival injection is present.

Differential Diagnosis

Pupillary inequality is indicative of damage to one of the four iris muscles or their innervation. In order to establish which is the abnormal pupil, pupil sizes in light and dark should be compared. Anisocoria increases in the direction of action of the paretic iris muscle. If the iris sphincter muscle is paretic, its weakness will be accentuated in bright light, since reflex constriction is impaired. Conversely, if the iris dilator muscle is paretic, the anisocoria will be accentuated in darkness.

The most serious causes of anisocoria are neurogenic. In the setting of trauma, severe headache, or following intracranial surgery, anisocoria and a third-nerve palsy with ptosis, extraocular muscle palsies, and a nonreactive pupil are early signs of an aneurysm or an expanding supratentorial mass with tentorial herniation.

Other causes of anisocoria with an abnormally large pupil include an acute Adie's pupil, eye drops (atropine, phenylephrine, naphazoline), inadvertent contamination from a scopolamine patch, and ocular trauma with damage to the iris sphincter (Fig. 2.37). A patient with an Adie's pupil may note that he or she cannot focus with one eye, although the appearance of a dilated

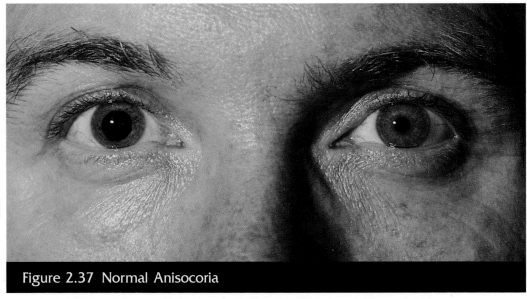

Figure 2.37 Normal Anisocoria

Marked chronic anisocoria secondary to prior trauma. (Courtesy of Kevin J. Knoop, MD, MS.)

pupil is more likely to prompt the ED visit. An Adie's pupil is dilated secondary to impairment in the postganglionic nerve supply to the iris sphincter. Causes include orbital trauma, infection, herpes zoster, diabetes, autonomic neuropathies, and Guillain-Barré syndrome, but in most instances the cause is unknown. Although an Adie's pupil is initially dilated, it may become miotic over time. A dilated pupil that is secondary to atropine eye drops does not react to light. Sympathomimetics eye drops such as phenylephrine, on the other hand, dilate the pupil, but the pupil still has some response to light. In addition, the conjunctiva may be blanched and the lid retracted. The slit-lamp examination helps to differentiate drug-induced dilation from dilation secondary to Adie's pupil. When dilation is drug-induced, the entire sphincter muscle is affected, whereas in Adie's, a segmental palsy is seen. (Segmental palsy is best appreciated with slit-lamp biomicroscopy. The curvature of the pupillary margin in those sections of the iris with palsy appears flatter. In addition, active pupil constriction is not radially symmetric.) The patient with ocular trauma and damage to the iris sphincter may show, on slit-lamp examination, evidence of a torn iris, an irregularly shaped pupil, hyphema, or lens dislocation.

An abnormally small pupil may be secondary to Horner's syndrome (see Fig. 2.38), chronic Adie's pupil (8 weeks or more after the event), iritis, and eye drops (pilocarpine). Associated clinical findings in Horner's syndrome include mild to moderate ptosis. The patient with iritis usually demonstrates conjunctival injection with a ciliary flush. Unilateral miosis may be transiently observed after ocular injury, followed by the development of mydriasis. Miosis in the setting of ocular trauma is secondary to spasm of the pupillary sphincter muscle.

Emergency Department Treatment and Disposition

The evaluation of anisocoria in the ED is dependent on the clinical presentation. A patient with acute onset of a third-nerve palsy and associated headache or trauma should be aggressively evaluated and treated as a neurosurgical emergency.

Pilocarpine may be helpful to differentiate pharmacologic pupil dilation from other causes of an abnormally dilated pupil, such as Adie's pupil and third-nerve palsy. With low concentrations of pilocarpine (0.125%), an Adie's pupil will constrict significantly more than the unaffected pupil because of denervation supersensitivity. With higher concentrations (1%), a pupil will constrict even if there is a third-nerve palsy. A pupil that fails to constrict with 1% pilocarpine localizes the etiology to the iris sphincter muscle itself. In this situation, the most likely diagnosis is the use of topical anticholinergic mydriatics such as scopolamine, atropine, or cyclopentolate. Other problems within the iris sphincter muscle that prevent constriction to 1% pilocarpine include synechiae (causing a mechanically immobile iris) and trauma to the iris muscle.

Clinical Pearls

1. The patient who presents with a dilated pupil should undergo a careful examination for ptosis and abnormal extraocular muscle movements, since their presence suggests compressive damage to the intracranial third nerve by an aneurysm or mass.
2. Pupil sizes in light and dark should be compared. In physiologic or normal anisocoria, the disparity in pupil size is the same in light as in dark. Anisocoria that is greater in the dark

suggests that the smaller pupil is abnormal due to paresis of its iris dilator muscle; anisocoria greater in the light suggests that the larger pupil is abnormal due to paresis of its iris sphincter muscle.

3. An old photograph or driver's license viewed with an ophthalmoscope may be helpful to document the prior existence of anisocoria.

4. Some brands of eye makeup contain belladonna alkaloids, which can cause mydriasis.

5. Adie's pupil initially is dilated but may become miotic over time. It is a benign condition that affects young adults, women more often than men.

Associated Clinical Features

Horner's syndrome consists of loss of ocular sympathetic innervation secondary to a lesion within the sympathetic pathway. This pathway can be interrupted in any location, from the hypothalamus down through the brainstem to the cervical cord, in the apex of the chest, along the carotid sheath, or in the cavernous sinus or orbit. Clinical features include unilateral miosis, along with mild to moderate unilateral ptosis (Fig. 2.38). Slight elevation of the lower lid may also be noted. Light and near reactions are intact. Acutely, conjunctival injection may be present on the affected side, and the intraocular pressure may be reduced. Anhidrosis of the ipsilateral face may be present, and the ipsilateral face may be warm and hyperemic. However, these findings are not present if the interruption of the sympathetic nerve supply occurs in a distal location, such as along the internal carotid artery. This is because vasoconstrictor fibers to the face, along with innervation to sweat glands, travel with branches of the external carotid artery.

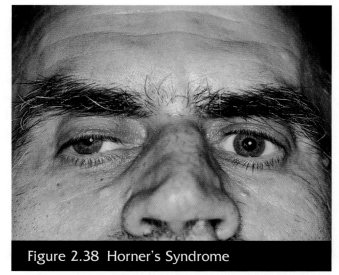

Figure 2.38 Horner's Syndrome

Unilateral miosis and ptosis are seen in this patient with Horner's syndrome and sarcoma metastatic to the spine. (Courtesy of Frank Birinyi, MD.)

A pupillary finding that is specific to Horner's syndrome is dilation lag. Normal pupil dilation is a combination of sphincter relaxation and dilator contraction, which produces a prompt dilation. A patient with Horner's syndrome, however, has a weak dilator muscle in one iris; as a result, that pupil dilates more slowly than the normal pupil. This anisocoria is maximal after 4 to 5 s. After 10 to 20 s, the anisocoria lessens, owing to the continued relaxation of the iris sphincter. Dilation lag is best seen if the patient is examined in a room where the lights can be turned off and a hand-held light illuminates the eyes from below.

Associated clinical findings are secondary to the neurologic lesion and its location. The causes of Horner's syndrome may involve first-order neurons (stroke or tumor in the hypothalamus and brainstem), second-order neurons (cervical spinal trauma, syringomyelia, cervical chain involvement by a Pancoast tumor, cervical rib, or tumor) or third-order neurons (internal carotid artery dissection, craniofacial or orbital trauma). Second-order neuron involvement may also occur during inadvertent injury from the placement of a central venous line or chest tube.

Horner's syndrome secondary to involvement of third-order neurons is often idiopathic.

Differential Diagnosis

Ptosis is seen in third-nerve palsies. Miosis may be due to eye drops (pilocarpine), iritis, an Argyll-Robertson pupil (a syphilitic pupil that accommodates but does not react), and long-standing Adie's pupil.

Pupillary inequality may be due to physiologic anisocoria.

Emergency Department Treatment and Disposition

Horner's syndrome is often caused by vascular disease, trauma, or tumor. The ED physician should attempt to elucidate associated signs and symptoms that help to localize the lesion. A patient with Horner's syndrome and cranial nerve abnormalities likely has brainstem or intracavernous pathology. Therefore an associated ipsilateral abducens palsy suggests a cavernous sinus lesion, since ocular sympathetics travel with the abducens nerve within the cavernous sinus. Wallenberg's syndrome, infarction of the lateral medulla, should be considered in a patient with numbness in the ipsilateral face and contralateral extremities. These types of patients should undergo computed tomography (CT) or magnetic resonance imaging (MRI).

In the setting of cervical spine trauma, neck immobilization and appropriate imaging studies are instituted. A patient with lung or breast malignancy, risk factors, or local or radicular shoulder pain should initially undergo a chest x-ray to evaluate for chest tumor. A Pancoast tumor is usually caused by bronchogenic carcinoma and may present, as its first sign, as a Horner's syndrome.

Neck pain in association with Horner's syndrome raises the possibility of carotid artery dissection. Third-order neuronal lesions should also be suspected in those who have had neck surgery, such as carotid endarterectomy.

Clinical Pearls

1. Patients with Horner's syndrome demonstrate a narrowed palpebral fissure secondary to a combined upper eyelid ptosis and higher than normal lower eyelid position ("reverse ptosis"). This is due to loss of sympathetic innervation to both Müller's muscle of the upper eyelid and as well as to the inferior tarsal muscle of the lower eyelid.
2. The ptosis of Horner's syndrome is moderate and never complete.
3. Carotid artery dissection should be entertained in the patient with neck pain and an ipsilateral Horner's syndrome.
4. Cluster headaches, with autonomic sympathetic system dysfunction, are capable of producing an ipsilateral Horner's syndrome.

Associated Clinical Features

Pupil size, controlled centrally by the Edinger-Westphal nucleus in the midbrain, is primarily based on the afferent light stimulus transmitted via the anterior visual pathway (Fig. 2.39). These afferents synapse both ipsilaterally and contralaterally within the midbrain, and pupillomotor fibers within the oculomotor nerves exit the midbrain to supply the direct and consensual responses. Even with a unilateral light stimulus, efferents travel to both pupils and, as a result, pupil size is symmetric. Efferents and pupil size are thus dependent upon the anterior visual structures, including the retina, optic nerve, chiasm, optic tract, and midbrain pathways. A defect anywhere along this pathway modulates the strength of the afferent light stimulus. An eye with, for example, retinal or optic nerve disease generates a diminished afferent response because less light is "perceived"; pupil contraction is decreased as a result. However, when the contralateral healthy eye is stimulated with light, the abnormal pupil's consensual response is normal, since the afferent light stimulus is normal. In this situation the diseased eye is said to demonstrate an afferent pupillary defect (APD), also called a Marcus Gunn pupil.

A Marcus Gunn pupil is best appreciated by the swinging flashlight test, which discloses differences in afferent stimuli between the two eyes. To perform this, a flashlight is directed onto one pupil and then the other. The normal pupillary response to the flashlight is a prompt constriction. (Generally this is followed by a slight "release" dilation.) Normally the brief interval

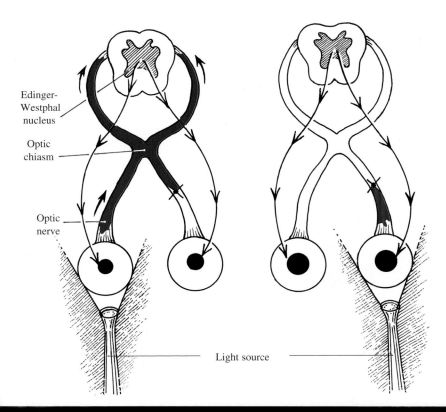

Edinger-
Westphal
nucleus

Optic
chiasm

Optic
nerve

Light source

Figure 2.39 Afferent Pupillary Defect

Schematic representation of an afferent pupillary defect (APD) due to neurologic lesion in the anterior visual pathway.

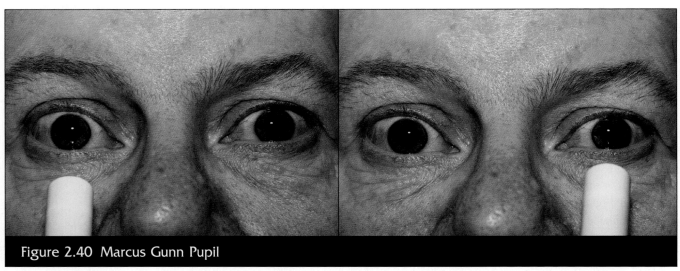

Figure 2.40 Marcus Gunn Pupil

These photographs demonstrate an afferent pupillary defect of the left pupil. When the light shines in the affected left eye, the pupils are less constricted than when the light shines in the right eye. Thus, when the light is swung from the right pupil to the left, the pupils appear to dilate. The anisocoria here is subtle. (Courtesy of Frank Birinyi, MD.)

required to move the light from one eye to the other permits the pupils to begin to dilate. Thus, under normal circumstances, when the light reaches the second eye, constriction can again be observed. In the abnormal situation with a diseased second eye, however, the pupils dilate instead of constrict (Fig. 2.40). This is because this second eye perceives less light than the first, and the midbrain therefore sets pupil size to be larger.

The swinging flashlight test is an extremely useful screening technique and one of the most important assessments for evaluation of optic nerve dysfunction. Although sensitive, the swinging flashlight test is not specific, since the pathology may be anywhere in the visual pathway from the retina to the midbrain. Within the globe, limited pathology such as a cataract or occlusion of a branch retinal vein or branch retinal artery is unlikely to produce a clinically detectable APD. However a detectable APD may be seen in cases of occlusion of the central retinal vein or artery, retinal detachment, or a dense hemorrhage in the anterior chamber or vitreous. An APD in the absence of gross ocular disease indicates pathology elsewhere in the anterior visual pathway, such as a compressive lesion involving the optic chiasm or tract. Typically, however, a positive finding is indicative of optic nerve disease. A Marcus Gunn pupil is best seen in conditions involving the optic nerve, such as ischemic optic neuropathy, optic neuritis (including that seen with multiple sclerosis), retrobulbar optic neuritis, and glaucoma.

In patients with an APD, associated findings may include decreased visual acuity and decreased visual fields. Funduscopic findings may demonstrate the basis for the APD; they include occlusion of a central retinal vein or artery, optic nerve pallor, optic nerve cupping, or severe vitreal hemorrhage.

Differential Diagnosis

An Adie's pupil, more common in young women, shows a diminished or absent reaction to light. It occurs with both direct and consensual response. Acutely, the Adie's pupil is dilated; chronically, it may be constricted. An Argyll-Robertson pupil, seen in neurosyphilis, is usually bilateral and miotic, it does not respond to light stimulation, but it does accommodate.

Emergency Department Treatment and Disposition

The finding of a Marcus Gunn pupil is nonspecific. A funduscopic examination may provide the basis for the APD, and ophthalmic consultation is indicated. If the funduscopic examination is normal, a neurologic evaluation (history, physical examination, and CT scan) is important to assess for treatable conditions. In the absence of gross ocular or neurologic disease, a clinically stable patient may be discharged from the ED with ophthalmology follow-up.

Clinical Pearls

1. Afferent pupillary defects do not cause anisocoria because any change in light input results in a bilaterally symmetric output from the midbrain.
2. Dim room illumination may be helpful in performing the swinging flashlight test. The patient should focus on an object 15 ft away to avoid the pupillary constriction normally seen with accommodation.
3. The normal pupillary response to bright light is an initial constriction followed by a small amount of dilation. In performing the swinging flashlight test, it is important to assess the initial reaction. In the Marcus Gunn pupil, this initial reaction is dilation.
4. A "subjective" APD (as can be seen in mild cases of optic neuritis) is demonstrated when no objective APD is seen but the patient perceives less light in the affected eye and has mildly decreased visual acuity.
5. If an eye is damaged or paralyzed or anisocoria is present, an APD can still be assessed by observing the response of the *normal* pupil with light that is shined alternately in each eye. As the light shines in the abnormal eye, the *normal* eye dilates if the abnormal eye "perceives" less light.

Associated Clinical Features

The third cranial nerve controls all extraocular muscles (except the lateral rectus and superior oblique) as well as the levator palpebrae muscle. It also supplies parasympathetic input to the pupillary constrictor and ciliary muscles. Thus symptoms of third-nerve palsy include double vision, droopy lid, an enlarged pupil, and blurred vision at near range. If the ptosis is complete, diplopia may not be recognized. The clinical examination demonstrates a dilated and unreactive pupil, limited extraocular movements, and ptosis (Fig. 2.41). The affected pupil faces laterally (exotropia) secondary to the unopposed action of the lateral rectus.

A third-nerve palsy can result from a lesion anywhere along its anatomic path, which begins in the brainstem nucleus, continues within the subarachnoid space, traverses the cavernous sinus, and terminates within the orbit. Associated signs and symptoms help to delineate a more precise location. An oculomotor palsy with contralateral hemiplegia suggests brainstem involvement. Infarction of the midbrain, involving the third nerve and corticospinal tracts (with contralateral hemiplegia), comprises Weber's syndrome.

In cases of isolated oculomotor palsy, the subarachnoid space is the most likely site of pathology. On leaving the brainstem, the nerve enters the subarachnoid space and travels alongside the posterior communicating artery. A common and extremely important cause for a third-nerve palsy with pupillary involvement is a posterior communicating artery aneurysm at the junction of the posterior communicating and internal carotid arteries. Because of the dorsal and medial location of the parasympathetic fibers (controlling pupillary constriction) within the oculomotor nerve bundle, these fibers are particularly susceptible to compressive lesions, and pupillary involvement often precedes ophthalmoparesis. With uncal herniation, enlarging lesions or edema in the middle fossa or temporal lobe push the medial edge of the uncus toward the midline and over the edge of the tentorium, compressing the underlying third nerve. Other causes of oculomotor dysfunction within the subarachnoid space include compressive neoplasms, inflammatory lesions, and trauma. Typically the trauma is severe enough to cause a skull fracture and loss of consciousness. An oculomotor palsy after minor trauma suggests an underlying mass lesion or aneurysm.

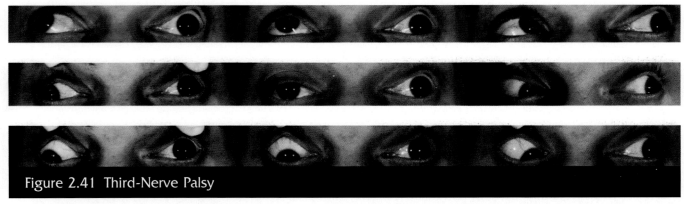

Figure 2.41 Third-Nerve Palsy

This composite shows the classic defects of a third cranial nerve palsy in all fields of gaze. The pupil is dilated. Conjugate eye movement is present in only one position, when the affected eye gazes laterally to the affected side (intact lateral rectus). When gaze is directly ahead, exotropia is seen secondary to the unopposed lateral rectus muscle of the affected side. (Courtesy of Frank Birinyi, MD.)

An oculomotor palsy secondary to pathology within the cavernous sinus may be inferred by associated involvement of the other structures within the cavernous sinus itself. These include the trochlear and abducens nerves, the first division of the trigeminal nerve, sympathetics to the eye, and the venous drainage of the eye and orbit. Causes for a third-nerve palsy within the cavernous sinus include neoplasms (pituitary, meningioma, craniopharyngioma, nasopharyngeal, metastatic), compression by carotid artery aneurysm, cavernous sinus thrombosis, and carotid-cavernous fistula. A carotid-cavernous fistula can present abruptly and dramatically as a result of reversal of blood flow in the orbital and ocular venous systems. These patients may complain of a bruit and pain. Clinical findings include pulsatile exophthalmos, elevated intraocular pressure, and chemosis. Vascular findings may be diffuse or localized. Conjunctival vessels are dilated and have a corkscrew appearance. A bruit may be audible by placing the bell of the stethoscope over the closed eyelid. Cavernous sinus thrombosis presents similarly to carotid-cavernous fistula, and the patients commonly have manifestations of sepsis. Within the anterior aspect of the cavernous sinus, the third nerve divides in two. The superior division innervates the levator palpebrae superioris and superior rectus muscles, while the inferior division innervates the medial rectus, inferior rectus, and inferior oblique muscles as well as the parasympathetics (preganglionic to the ciliary ganglion). Therefore third-nerve palsies due to cavernous sinus and orbital lesions are frequently partial, and the pupillomotor fibers may be spared.

Orbital lesions causing third-nerve palsies may be due to inflammation, trauma, neoplasms, and mucoceles. Associated clinical findings include proptosis, visual loss, and sixth-nerve involvement. As noted, an oculomotor palsy secondary to orbital pathology may be partial. In cases of trauma, the slit-lamp examination may demonstrate a tear in the iris sphincter.

An isolated third-nerve palsy is common with diabetic or hypertensive disease. The cause is felt to be microvascular ischemia. In this situation, the palsy rarely affects the pupil ("pupil sparing"). Microvascular third-nerve palsies, especially in diabetics, may be exquisitely painful.

Differential Diagnosis

Unilateral pupil dilation is also seen with minor eye trauma, eye drops (either alpha-adrenergic agents or anticholinergics such as atropine), inadvertent contamination from a scopolamine patch, and an acute Adie's pupil (a dilated and minimally reactive or nonreactive pupil, seen unilaterally and most often in young women). Myasthenia gravis, thyroid disease, temporal arteritis, and orbital inflammatory pseudotumor have similar features. Ptosis is seen in Horner's syndrome.

Emergency Department Treatment and Disposition

The evaluation of a patient with a third-nerve palsy is dependent upon the associated signs and symptoms that help to localize the pathology. In patients with involvement of the brainstem, CT or MRI is indicated. Associated fever, headache, depressed level of consciousness, neck stiffness, or other cranial nerve involvement should prompt consideration for CT scanning and subsequent spinal tap. If cavernous sinus involvement is suspected, MRI with gadolinium is preferred. For orbital pathology, CT scanning with contrast and thin coronal and axial views is recommended.

Of particular concern is the sudden onset of a third-nerve palsy accompanied by "thunderclap" headache, stiff neck, and a depressed level of consciousness. Even those with pupil sparing should be treated as neurosurgical emergencies and require immediate evaluation for an aneurysm or uncal herniation. The workup includes emergent CT or MRI. If subarachnoid hemorrhage is not found and suspicion of aneurysmal leakage remains high, a lumbar puncture should be performed. Options include CT with contrast and magnetic resonance angiography. However, the "gold standard" remains angiography, since small aneurysms can be missed, and even small aneurysms can rupture.

In the setting of head trauma, a patient with third-nerve palsy should undergo measures to reduce the intracranial pressure. These include elevation of the head of the bed, mannitol, and burr holes.

Patients under 50 years of age with isolated third-nerve palsy of any extent should undergo a full neurologic evaluation, including cerebral angiography. For patients older than 50 with vasculopathic risk factors who present with isolated pupil-sparing third-nerve palsies felt to be secondary to an ischemic neuropathy, the minimum ED evaluation should include measurement of the blood pressure and glucose. Such patients may be discharged from the ED provided that they can be observed closely for a week for evidence of pupillary involvement. Microvascular third-nerve palsies can be exquisitely painful and thus may require analgesics for 1 to 2 weeks. The majority of microvascular third-nerve palsies resolve within 3 months.

Clinical Pearls

1. A third-nerve palsy can result from pathology anywhere along its anatomic pathway, beginning with the brainstem, continuing within the subarachnoid space, traversing the cavernous sinus, and terminating within the orbit itself.
2. Patients with the abrupt onset of a "thunderclap" headache and third-nerve palsy require immediate neurosurgical evaluation for an aneurysm. (Posterior communicating artery is a common cause.)
3. In patients over 50 years of age with pupil-sparing third-nerve palsies, the etiology is usually hypertensive or diabetic vascular disease.
4. In the patient who presents with diplopia and possible third-nerve palsy, the ED physician should confirm the binocularity of the diplopia by monocular occlusion. Monocular diplopia is optical in origin.
5. A carotid-cavernous fistula most often (80%) results from trauma. It may be manifest at the time of injury or delayed for days or weeks. The trauma may be trivial in some patients.

Associated Clinical Features

The abducens nerve innervates the lateral rectus muscle and is the most common single-muscle palsy. Paralysis produces loss of abduction (Fig. 2.42) and horizontal diplopia. The diplopia is accentuated with gaze toward the affected side. Patients tend to turn their faces toward the affected eye to limit their diplopia. Other eye movements are normal; the lid and pupil are not affected.

Other associated findings are dependent upon the location of the lesion causing the sixth-nerve palsy. Within the pons, involvement of adjacent structures such as the corticospinal tract results in contralateral hemiparesis. Wernicke's encephalopathy affects the abducens nucleus and manifests as ipsilateral conjugate gaze palsy—i.e., paresis of the ipsilateral lateral rectus and contralateral medial rectus. This occurs because the abducens nucleus comprises two populations of neurons. One group forms the sixth nerve. The other group sends fibers to join the contralateral medial longitudinal fasciculus, with projection to the medial rectus subnucleus.

As the nerve emerges from the pons, the abducens ascends the clivus and is vulnerable to compression by downward or forward movement of the brainstem. In fact, the abducens nerve has the longest intracranial course of any nerve; it is therefore vulnerable to "stretching," resulting in sixth-nerve palsies, unilateral or bilateral, due to elevated intracranial pressure, trauma, neurosurgical manipulation, and cervical traction. Aneurysmal compression is much less common than is seen with third-nerve palsy. Any meningeal process (infectious, inflammatory, or neoplastic) is capable of affecting this portion of the sixth nerve.

Prior to entering the cavernous sinus, the abducens nerve crosses the petrous portion of the temporal bone. Trauma with temporal bone fracture can result in a combination of sixth- and seventh-nerve palsies, including bilateral palsies. Additional clinical findings of a basilar skull fracture include hemotympanum, Battle's sign, and leakage of CSF or blood from the external ear canal.

Pathology within the cavernous sinus can affect, in addition to the abducens nerve, the internal carotid artery, the

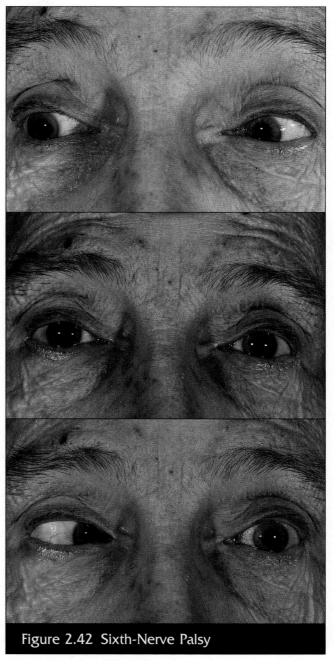

Figure 2.42 Sixth-Nerve Palsy

Loss of abduction of the left eye is seen in lateral gaze, demonstrating an isolated sixth-nerve palsy. (Courtesy of Frank Birinyi, MD.)

venous drainage of the eye and orbit, trochlear and oculomotor nerves, the first division of the trigeminal nerve, and the ocular sympathetics. The abducens tends to be particularly involved with vascular lesions within the cavernous sinus because of its adjacent position inferolateral to the carotid. A carotid-cavernous fistula can present abruptly and dramatically as a result of reversal of blood flow in the orbital and ocular venous systems. These patients may complain of a bruit and pain. Clinical findings include pulsatile exophthalmos, elevated intraocular pressure, and chemosis. Vascular findings may be diffuse or localized. Conjunctival vessels are dilated and have a corkscrew appearance. A bruit may be audible when the bell of the stethoscope is placed over the closed eyelid.

Within the orbit itself, isolated involvement of the sixth nerve is rare because of its short course prior to innervating the lateral rectus muscle.

The abducens nerve may be infarcted by microvascular changes secondary to diabetes, hypertension, giant cell arteritis, or arteriosclerosis. In children, a transient sixth-nerve palsy may follow a virus infection.

Differential Diagnosis

Thyroid eye disease, orbital inflammatory pseudotumor, myasthenia gravis, Duane's syndrome (congenital absence of the sixth-nerve nucleus), Parinaud's syndrome (dorsal midbrain syndrome), and medial rectus entrapment secondary to an ethmoid fracture have similar findings.

Emergency Department Treatment and Disposition

The ED evaluation is guided by the associated signs and symptoms. With involvement of the brainstem or cavernous sinus, CT or MRI is indicated. Pathology localized to the subarachnoid space should prompt consideration for CT scanning and subsequent spinal tap.

Children with antecedent viral illness and normal CT scan may be discharged provided that close follow-up is arranged. Children usually recover completely within 4 months. In the elderly, an isolated sixth-nerve palsy is likely ischemic, transient, and not indicative of underlying neurologic disease. In these cases, a glucose and an erythrocyte sedimentation rate (for evidence of giant cell arteritis) are appropriate. Although the palsy generally resolves in 3 to 4 months, these patients should be followed up carefully for the onset of additional neurologic abnormalities.

There is no treatment for the palsy itself except for patching the affected eye if diplopia is bothersome.

Clinical Pearls

1. Isolated sixth-nerve palsy is commonly due to microvascular disease, not an aneurysm.
2. An isolated lateral rectus palsy should not be considered nuclear in origin.
3. A deficit involving a sixth-nerve palsy with an ipsilateral Horner's syndrome is usually localized to the cavernous sinus, since sympathetic fibers, as they traverse from the internal carotid artery to the oculomotor nerve, may briefly accompany the abducens nerve.
4. Basilar skull fractures of the temporal bone are capable of producing a traumatic sixth-nerve palsy, since the nerve passes from the posterior fossa to the cavernous sinus via the petrous ridge.

EYE

CHAPTER 3

FUNDUSCOPIC FINDINGS

David Effron
Beverly C. Forcier
Richard E. Wyszynski

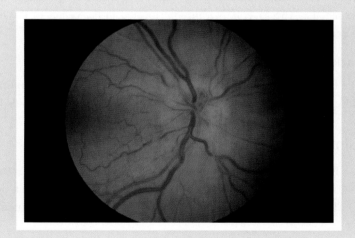

Associated Clinical Features

Disk

The disk is pale pink, approximately 1.5 mm in diameter, with sharp, flat margins (Fig. 3.1). The physiologic cup is located within the disk and usually measures less than six-tenths the disk diameter. The cups should be approximately equal in both eyes.

Vessels

The central retinal artery and central retinal vein travel within the optic nerve, branching near the surface into the inferior and superior branches of arterioles and venules, respectively. Normally the walls of the vessels are not visible; the column of blood within the walls is visualized. The venules are seen as branching, dark red lines. The arterioles are seen as bright red branching lines, approximately two-thirds or three-fourths the diameter of the venules.

Macula

This is an area of the retina located temporal to the disk; it is void of capillaries. The fovea is an area of depression approximately 1.5 mm in diameter (similar to the optic disk) in the center of the macula. The foveola is a tiny pit located in the center of the fovea. These areas correspond to central vision.

Background

The background fundus is red; there is some variation in the color, depending on the amount of individual pigmentation and the visibility of the choroidal vessels beneath the retina.

Clinical Pearls

1. Fundal examination should be an integral part of any eye examination.
2. The cup/disk ratio is slightly larger in the African-American population.
3. The normal fundus should be void of any hemorrhages, exudates, or tortuous vasculature.

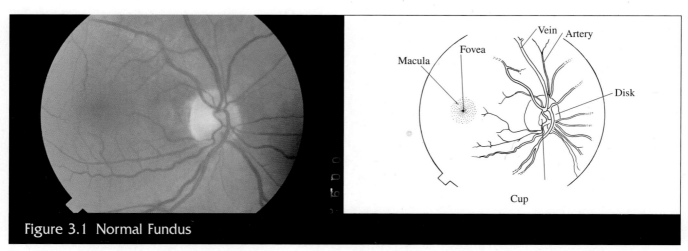

Figure 3.1 Normal Fundus

The disk has sharp margins and is normal in color, with a small central cup. Arterioles and venules have normal color, sheen, and course. Background is in normal color. The macula is enclosed by arching temporal vessels. The fovea is located by a central pit. (Courtesy of Beverly C. Forcier, MD.)

Associated Clinical Features

Age-related macular degeneration, the leading cause of blindness in the elderly, increases in incidence with each decade over 50. Degeneration of the macula may be evidenced by accumulation of either drusen (small, discrete, round, punctate nodules), or soft drusen (larger, pale yellow or gray, without discrete margins that may be confluent) (Fig. 3.2A and B). Most patients with drusen have good vision, although there may be decreased visual acuity and distortion of vision. There may be associated pigmentary changes and atrophy of the retina. Vision may slowly deteriorate if atrophy occurs.

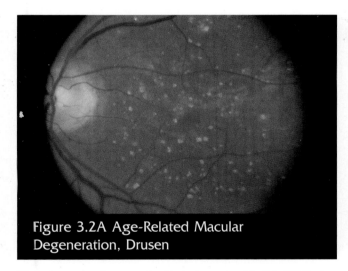

Figure 3.2A Age-Related Macular Degeneration, Drusen

Typical macular drusen and retinal pigment epithelial (RPE) atrophy (scalloped pigment loss) in age-related macular degeneration. (Courtesy of Richard E. Wyszynski, MD.)

Figure 3.2B Age-Related Macular Degeneration, Drusen

Drusen are clustered in the center of the macula. (Courtesy of Richard E. Wyszynski, MD.)

Patients with early or late degenerative changes of the macula are at risk of developing subretinal neovascularization (SRNV), which is associated with distortion of vision, blind spots, and decreased visual acuity. Macular appearance may show dirty gray lesions, hemorrhage, retinal elevation, and exudation (Fig. 3.3).

Differential Diagnosis

Hereditary macular degenerations, other acquired macular disorders including toxicities, and retinal exudation may present similarly.

Hemorrhages and exudates can present from vascular disease, ocular disorders such as inflammations or infections, tumors, trauma, and hereditary disorders.

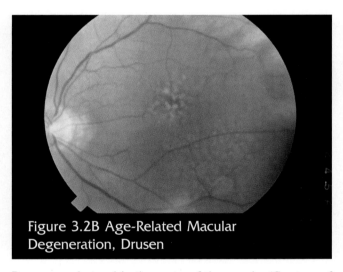

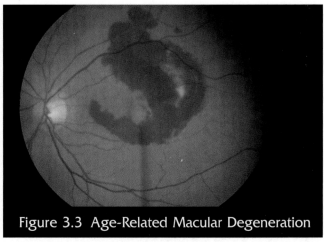

Figure 3.3 Age-Related Macular Degeneration

Hemorrhage seen beneath the retina in association with subretinal neovascularization. (Courtesy of Richard E. Wyszynski, MD.)

Emergency Department Treatment and Disposition

Patients with drusen need ophthalmologic evaluation every 6 to 12 months or sooner if visual distortion or decreasing visual acuity develops. If a patient complains of deterioration of visual acuity or image distortion, prompt ophthalmic evaluation is warranted, probably including fluorescein angiography. If SRNV is present, laser treatment may be indicated.

Clinical Pearls

1. Age-related macular degeneration is the leading cause of blindness in the United States in patients above 65 years of age.
2. Patient may have normal peripheral vision.
3. Untreated SRNV can lead to visual loss within a few days.
4. Patients frequently complain of distortion with SRNV.

Associated Clinical Features

Hard exudates (Figure 3.4A) are refractile, yellowish deposits with sharp margins composed of fat-laden macrophages and serum lipids. Occasionally the lipid deposits form a partial or complete ring (called a circinate ring) around the leaking area of pathology. If the lipid leakage is located near the fovea, a spoke, or star-type distribution of the hard exudates is seen.

Cotton wool spots, or soft "exudates," are actually microinfarctions of the retinal nerve-fiber layer, and appear white with soft or fuzzy edges (Fig. 3.4B).

Inflammatory exudates are secondary to retinal or chorioretinal inflammation.

Differential Diagnosis

Hard exudation and cotton wool spots are associated with vascular diseases such as diabetes mellitus, hypertension, and collagen vascular diseases but can be seen with papilledema and other ocular conditions. Inflammatory exudates are seen in patients with such diseases as sarcoidosis and toxoplasmosis.

Emergency Department Treatment and Disposition

Routine referral for ophthalmologic and medical workup is appropriate.

Clinical Pearl

1. Hard exudates that are intraretinal may easily be confused with drusen occurring near Bruch's membrane, which separates the retina from the choroid.

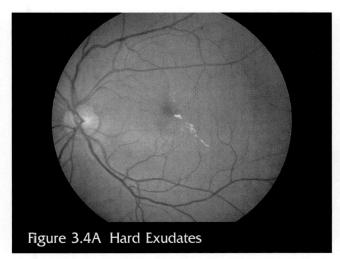

Figure 3.4A Hard Exudates

Linear collection of yellow lipid deposits with sharp margins in macula. (Courtesy of Beverly C. Forcier, MD.)

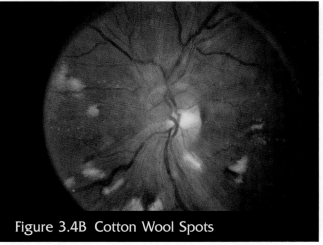

Figure 3.4B Cotton Wool Spots

White lesions with fuzzy margins, seen here approximately one-fifth to one-fourth disk diameter in size. Orientation of cotton wool spots generally follows the curvilinear arrangement of the nerve fiber layer. Intraretinal hemorrhages and intraretinal vascular abnormalities are also present. (Courtesy of Richard E. Wyszynski, MD.)

Associated Clinical Features

Roth's spots are retinal hemorrhages with a white or yellow center (Fig. 3.5). They are seen in patients with a host of diseases such as anemia, leukemia, multiple myeloma, diabetes mellitus, collagen vascular disease, other vascular disease, intracranial hemorrhage in infants, septic retinitis, and lung carcinoma.

Differential Diagnosis

Flamed-shaped or splinter hemorrhages or dot-blot hemorrhages may resemble Roth's spots.

Emergency Department Treatment and Disposition

Routine referral for general medical evaluation is appropriate.

Clinical Pearls

1. Roth's spots are not pathognomonic for any particular disease process and can represent a variety of clinical conditions.
2. These lesions represent red blood cells surrounding inflammatory cells.

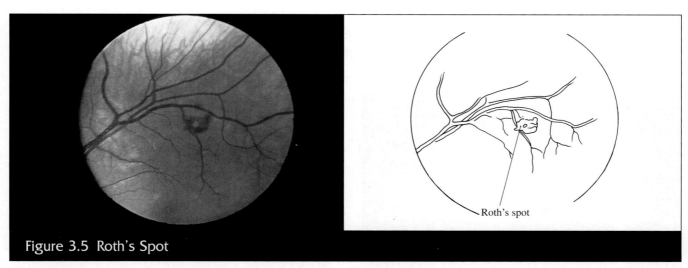

Figure 3.5 Roth's Spot

Retinal hemorrhage with pale center. (Courtesy of William E. Cappaert, MD.)

Associated Clinical Features

Plaques, if present, are often found at arteriolar bifurcations (Fig. 3.6). Patients may have signs and symptoms of vascular disease including a "source" of emboli such as carotid bruits or stenosis, aortic stenosis, aneurysms, or atrial fibrillation. Amaurosis fugax, a transient loss of vision often described as a curtain of darkness obscuring vision with sight restoration within a few minutes, may be present in the history.

Differential Diagnosis

Cholesterol emboli (Hollenhorst plaques), associated with generalized atherosclerosis often from carotid atheroma, are bright, highly refractile plaques; platelet emboli (carotid artery or cardiac thrombus) are white and very difficult to visualize; and calcific emboli (cardiac valvular disease) are irregular and white or dull gray and much less refractile.

Emergency Department Treatment and Disposition

Referral for routine general medical evaluation is appropriate unless the patient presents with signs or symptoms consistent with showering of emboli, transient ischemic attack, or cerebrovascular accident, in which case referral for admission is indicated.

Clinical Pearls

1. Retinal emboli may produce a loss of vision, either transient or permanent in nature.
2. Arteriolar occlusion may occur either in a central or peripheral branch location.

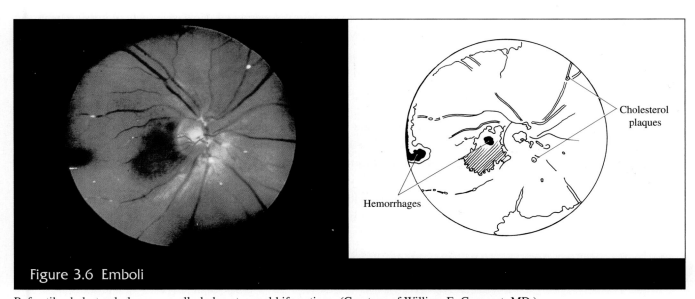

Figure 3.6 Emboli

Refractile cholesterol plaques usually lodge at vessel bifurcations. (Courtesy of William E. Cappaert, MD.)

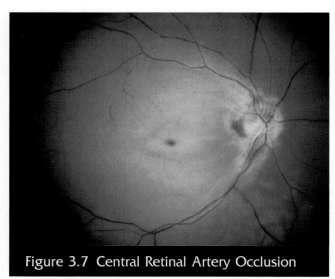

Figure 3.7 Central Retinal Artery Occlusion

The retinal pallor due to retinal edema is well demonstrated, contrasting with the "cherry red spot" of the nonedematous fovea. Note the vascular narrowing and the "boxcar" appearance of the venules. (Courtesy of Richard E. Wyszynski, MD.)

Associated Clinical Features

The typical patient experiences a sudden, painless monocular loss of vision, either segmental or complete. Visual acuity may range from finger counting or light perception to complete blindness. Fundal findings include: fundal paleness due to retinal edema; the fovea does not have the edema and thus appears as a cherry-red spot; the retinal arterioles are narrow and irregular; and the retinal venules have a "boxcar" appearance (Fig. 3.7).

Differential Diagnosis

Arteriosclerosis, arterial hypertension, carotid artery disease, diabetes mellitus, and valvular heart disease are the most common systemic disorders associated with central retinal artery occlusion (CRAO). Other associated disorders include vascular disorders, trauma, and coagulopathies. Temporal arteritis may present with similar visual complaints.

Emergency Department Treatment and Disposition

Attempts to restore retinal blood flow may be beneficial if performed in a very narrow time window after the acute event. This may be accomplished by (1) decreasing intraocular pressure with topical beta-blocker eye drops or intravenous acetazolamide; (2) ocular massage, applied with cyclic pressure on the globe for 10 s, followed by release and then repeated. Urgent consultation with an ophthalmologist if the CRAO is less than a few hours old is indicated to determine if more aggressive acute therapy (paracentesis) is warranted. However, such aggressive treatment rarely alters the poor prognosis. Medical evaluation and treatment of associated findings may be warranted.

Clinical Pearls

1. History should focus on how long ago the episode occurred. If the loss of vision occurred recently, then the patient should be triaged and examined quickly so as to consult an ophthalmologist within the treatment window.
2. Sudden, painless monocular vision loss is typical.
3. CRAO may be associated with temporal arteritis. This diagnosis should be strongly considered in all patients presenting with signs and symptoms of CRAO who are older than 55 years.

Associated Clinical Features

Patients are usually older individuals and complain of sudden, painless visual loss in one eye. The vision loss is usually not as severe as CRAO and may vary from normal to hand motion. Funduscopy in a classic, ischemic central retinal vein occlusion (CRVO) shows a "blood and thunder" fundus: hemorrhages (including flame, dot or blot, preretinal, and vitreous) and dilation and tortuosity of the venous system. The arterial system often shows narrowing. The disk margin may be blurred. Cotton wool spots and edema may be seen (Fig. 3.8).

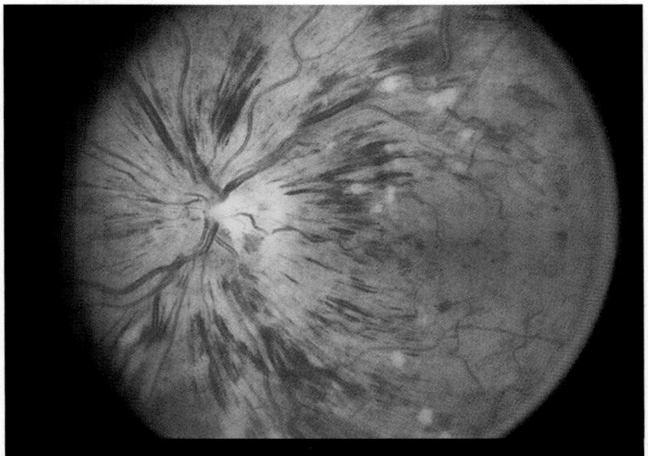

Differential Diagnosis

Retinal detachment, papilledema, and central retinal artery occlusion can have a similar appearance.

Emergency Department Treatment and Disposition

Figure 3.8 Central Retinal Vein Occlusion

The amount of hemorrhage is the most striking feature in this photograph. Also note the blurred disk margin, the dilation and tortuosity of the venules, and the cotton wool spots. Retinal edema is suggested by blurring of the retinal details. (Courtesy of Department of Ophthalmology, Naval Medical Center, Portsmouth, VA.)

Treatment is rarely effective in preventing or reversing the damage done by the occlusion and is directed toward systemic evaluation to identify and treat contributing factors, hopefully decreasing the chance of contralateral CRVO. Ophthalmologic evaluation is necessary to confirm the diagnosis, estimate the amount of ischemia, and follow the patient so as to minimize sequelae of possible complications such as neovascularization and neovascular glaucoma.

Clinical Pearls

1. Sudden, painless visual loss in one eye should be evaluated promptly to determine its etiology.
2. Look for the classic "blood and thunder" funduscopic findings.
3. Consider the differential diagnosis of acute *painful* (glaucoma, retrobulbar neuritis) versus *painless* vision loss (CRAO, anterior ischemic optic neuropathy, retinal detachment, subretinal neovascularization, and vitreous hemorrhage).

Associated Clinical Features

Fundus changes that may be seen with hypertension include generalized and focal narrowing of arterioles, generalized arteriolar sclerosis (resembling copper or silver wiring), arteriovenous crossing changes, hemorrhages (usually flame-shaped), retinal edema and exudation, cotton wool spots, microaneurysms, and disk edema (Fig. 3.9).

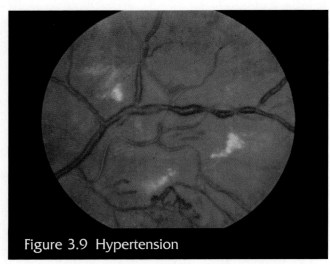

Figure 3.9 Hypertension

Chronic, severe systemic hypertensive changes are demonstrated by hard exudates, increased vessel light reflexes, and sausage-shaped veins. (Courtesy of Richard E. Wyszynski, MD.)

Differential Diagnosis

Diabetic retinopathy, many hemopoietic and vascular diseases, traumas, localized ocular pathology, and papilledema should all be considered.

Emergency Department Treatment and Disposition

Medical treatment of hypertension.

Clinical Pearls

1. Hypertensive arteriolar findings may be reversible if organic changes have not occurred in the vessel walls.
2. Always consider hypertensive retinopathy in the differential diagnosis of papilledema.

Associated Clinical Features

The early ocular manifestations of diabetes mellitus are referred to as background diabetic retinopathy (BDR). Fundus findings include flame or splinter hemorrhages (located in the superficial nerve fiber layer) or dot and blot hemorrhages (located deeper in the retina), hard exudates, retinal edema, and microaneurysms (Fig. 3.10A and B). If these signs are located in the macula, the patient's visual acuity may be decreased or at risk of becoming compromised, requiring laser treatment. Preproliferative diabetic retinopathy can show BDR changes plus cotton wool spots, intraretinal microvascular abnormalities, and venous beading. Proliferative diabetic retinopathy is demonstrated by neovascularization at the disk (NVD) or elsewhere (NVE) (Fig. 3.10C). These require laser therapy owing to risk of severe visual loss from sequelae: vitreous hemorrhage, tractional retinal detachment, severe glaucoma.

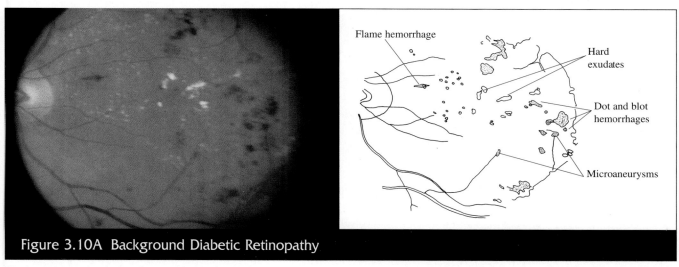

Figure 3.10A Background Diabetic Retinopathy

Hard exudates, dot hemorrhages, blot hemorrhages, flame hemorrhages, and microaneurysms are present. Because these changes are located within the macula, this is classified as diabetic maculopathy. (Courtesy of Richard E. Wyszynski, MD.)

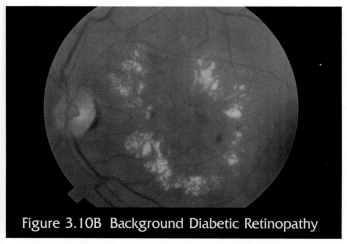

Figure 3.10B Background Diabetic Retinopathy

An example of diabetic maculopathy with a typical circinate lipid ring. (Courtesy of Richard E. Wyszynski, MD.)

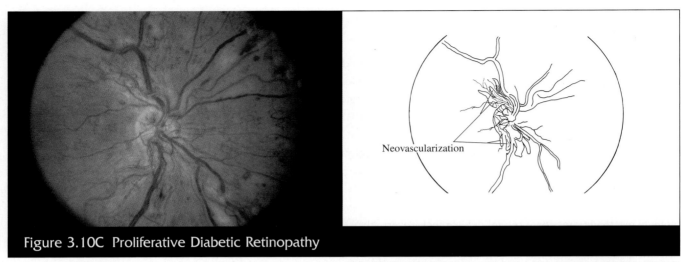

Neovascularization

Figure 3.10C Proliferative Diabetic Retinopathy

In addition to the signs seen in background and preproliferative diabetic retinopathy, neovascularization is seen here coming off the disk. (Courtesy of Richard E. Wyszynski, MD.)

Differential Diagnosis

Many vascular and hemopoietic diseases—such as collagen vascular disease, sickle cell trait, hypertension, hypotension, anemia, leukemia, inflammatory and infectious states—and ocular conditions can be associated with some of or all the above signs.

Emergency Department Treatment and Disposition

Routine ophthalmologic referral for laser or surgical treatment is indicated.

Clinical Pearls

1. Periodic ophthalmologic evaluations are recommended.
2. Microaneurysms typically appear 10 years after the initial onset of diabetes, although they may appear earlier in patients with juvenile diabetes.
3. Control of blood sugar alone does not prevent the development of vasculopathy.
4. Blurred vision can also occur from acute increases in serum glucose, causing lens swelling and a refractive shift even in the absence of retinopathy.

Associated Clinical Features

Patients may complain of sudden loss or deterioration of vision in the affected eye, although bilateral hemorrhage can occur. The red reflex is diminished or absent, and the retina is obscured because of the bleeding. Large sheets or three-dimensional collections of red to red-black blood may be detected (Fig. 3.11A and B).

Differential Diagnosis

Multiple underlying etiologies include proliferative diabetic retinopathy, retinal or vitreous detachments, hematologic diseases, trauma (ocular or shaken impact syndrome), subarachnoid hemorrhage, collagen vascular disease, infections, macular degeneration, and tumors.

Emergency Department Treatment and Disposition

Refer to an ophthalmologist and an appropriate physician for associated conditions. Ophthalmic observation, photocoagulation, and surgery are all therapeutic options. Bed rest may help to increase visualization of the fundus.

Clinical Pearl

1. The patient's vision may improve somewhat after a period of sitting or standing as the blood layers out.

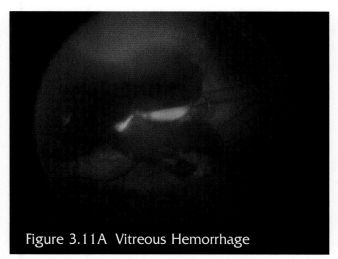

Figure 3.11A Vitreous Hemorrhage

Large amount of vitreous hemorrhage associated with metallic intraocular foreign body. The large quantity of blood obscures visualization of retinal details. (Courtesy of Richard E. Wyszynski, MD.)

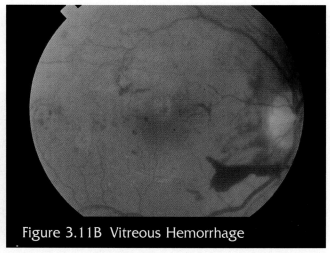

Figure 3.11B Vitreous Hemorrhage

A smaller amount of vitreous hemorrhage is more easily photographed. Gravitational effect on the vitreous blood creates the appearance of a flat meniscus (keel-shaped blood) in this patient with vitreous hemorrhage associated with proliferative diabetic retinopathy. (Courtesy of Richard E. Wyszynski, MD.)

Associated Clinical Features

Patients often complain of monocular decreased visual function and may describe a shadow or curtain descending over the eye. Other complaints include cloudy or smoky vision, floaters, or flashes of light. Central visual acuity is diminished with macular involvement. Fundal examination may reveal a billowing or tentlike elevation of retina compared with adjacent areas. The elevated retina often appears gray. Retinal holes and tears may be seen, but often the holes, tears, and retinal detachment cannot be seen without indirect ophthalmoscopy (Fig. 3.12).

Differential Diagnosis

Retinal detachments due to retinal tears or holes can be associated with trauma, previous ocular surgery, nearsightedness, family history of retinal detachment, and Marfan's disease. Retinal detachments due to traction on the retina by an intraocular process can be due to systemic influences in the eye, such as diabetes mellitus or sickle cell trait. Occasionally retinal detachments are due to tumors or exudative processes that elevate the retina. Symptoms of "light flashes" may occur with vitreous changes in the absence of retinal pathology. Patients may note flashes of light occurring only in a darkened environment because of the mechanical stimulation of the retina from the extraocular muscles, usually in a nearsighted individual.

Emergency Department Treatment and Disposition

Urgent ophthalmologic evaluation and treatment are warranted.

Clinical Pearls

1. Often patients have had sensation of flashes of light that occur in a certain area of a visual field in one eye, corresponding to the pathologic pulling on the corresponding retina.
2. Visual loss may be gradual or sudden.

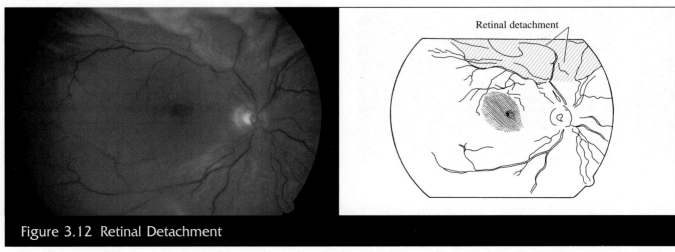

Figure 3.12 Retinal Detachment

A red, flat, well-focused macula is contrasted with the pale, undulating, out-of-focus, elevated retina surrounding the macula. (Courtesy of Richard E. Wyszynski, MD.)

Associated Clinical Features

Patients may complain of the gradual onset of the following visual sensations: floaters, scintillating scotomas (quivering blind spots), decreased peripheral visual field, and metamorphopsia (wavy distortion of vision). Cytomegalovirus (CMV) infiltrates appear as focal, small white lesions in the retina that look like cotton wool spots. CMV is a necrotizing virus that is spread hematogenously, so that damage is concentrated in the retina adjacent to the major vessels and the optic disk. Often hemorrhage is involved with significant retinal necrosis (dirty white with a granular appearance), giving the "pizza pie" or "cheese and ketchup" appearance (Fig. 3.13). Optic nerve involvement and retinal detachments can be present.

Differential Diagnosis

The differential includes other infections such as toxoplasmosis, other herpesviruses, syphilis, and occasionally other opportunistic infections.

Emergency Department Treatment and Disposition

Reversal, if possible, of immunosuppression. Ganciclovir and foscarnet have been used with some effectiveness.

Clinical Pearls

1. HIV retinopathy consists of scattered retinal hemorrhages and scattered, multiple cotton wool spots that resolve over time, whereas CMV lesions will typically progress.
2. Although exposure to the CMV virus is widespread, the virus rarely produces a clinically recognized disease in nonimmunosuppressed individuals.

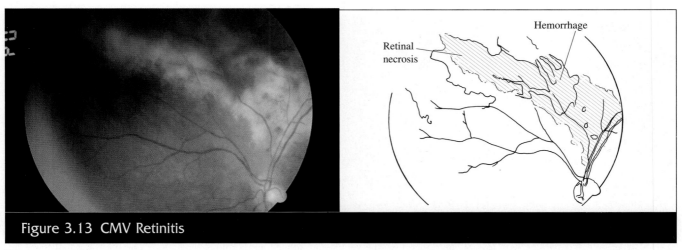

Figure 3.13 CMV Retinitis

"Pizza pie" or "cheese and ketchup" appearance is demonstrated by hemorrhages and the dirty, white, granular-appearing retinal necrosis adjacent to major vessels. (Courtesy of Richard E. Wyszynski, MD.)

Associated Clinical Features

Papilledema involves swelling of the optic nerve head, usually in association with elevated intracranial pressure. The optic disks are hyperemic with blurred disk margins; the venules are dilated and tortuous. The optic cup may be obscured by the swollen disk. There may be flame hemorrhages and infarctions (white, indistinct cotton wool spots) in the nerve fiber layer and edema in the surrounding retina (Fig. 3.14).

Differential Diagnosis

Ocular inflammation (e.g., papillitis), tumors or trauma, central retinal artery or vein occlusion, optic nerve drusen, and marked hyperopia may present with similar findings.

Emergency Department Treatment and Disposition

Expeditious ophthalmologic and medical evaluation is warranted.

Clinical Pearls

1. The top of a swollen disk and the surrounding unaffected retina will not both be in focus on the same setting on direct ophthalmoscopy.
2. Papilledema is a bilateral process, though it may be slightly asymmetric. A unilateral swollen disk suggests a localized ocular or orbital process.
3. Vision is usually normal acutely, though the patient may complain of transient visual changes. The blind spot is usually enlarged.
4. Diplopia from a sixth cranial nerve palsy can be associated with increased intracranial pressure and papilledema.

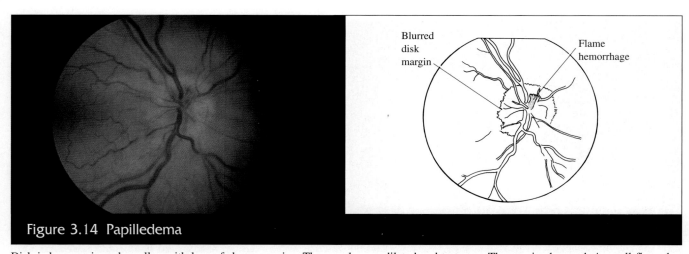

Figure 3.14 Papilledema

Disk is hyperemic and swollen with loss of sharp margins. The venules are dilated and tortuous. The cup is obscured. A small flame hemorrhage is seen at 12 to 1 o'clock on the disk margin. (Courtesy of Department of Ophthalmology, Naval Medical Center, Portsmouth, VA.)

Associated Clinical Features

Most cases of optic neuritis are retrobulbar and involve no changes in the fundus, or optic disk, during the acute episode. With time, variable optic disk pallor may develop (Fig. 3.15). Typical retrobulbar optic neuritis presents with sudden or rapidly progressing monocular vision loss in patients younger than 50 years. There is a central visual field defect that may extend to the blind spot. There is pain on movement of the globe. The pupillary light response is diminished in the affected eye. Over time the vision improves partially or completely; minimal or severe optic atrophy may develop. Papillitis, inflammation of the intraocular portion of the optic nerve, will accompany disk swelling, with a few flame hemorrhages and possible cells in the vitreous.

Differential Diagnosis

Optic neuritis must be differentiated from papilledema (bilateral disk swelling, typically with no acute visual loss with the exception of transient visual changes), ischemic neuropathy (pale, swollen disk in an older individual with sudden monocular vision loss), tumors, metabolic or endocrine disorders. Most cases of optic neuritis are of unknown etiology. Some known causes of optic neuritis include demyelinating disease, infections (including viral, syphilis, tuberculosis, sarcoidosis), or inflammations from contiguous structures (sinuses, meninges, orbit).

Emergency Department Treatment and Disposition

Treatment is controversial; often none is recommended. Oral steroids may worsen prognosis in certain cases. Intravenous steroids may be considered after consultation with an ophthalmologist.

Clinical Pearls

1. Monocular vision loss with pain on palpation of the globe or with eye movement are clinical clues to the diagnosis.
2. Sudden or rapidly progressing central vision loss is characteristic.
3. Most cases of acute optic neuritis are retrobulbar. Thus ophthalmoscopy shows a normal fundus.

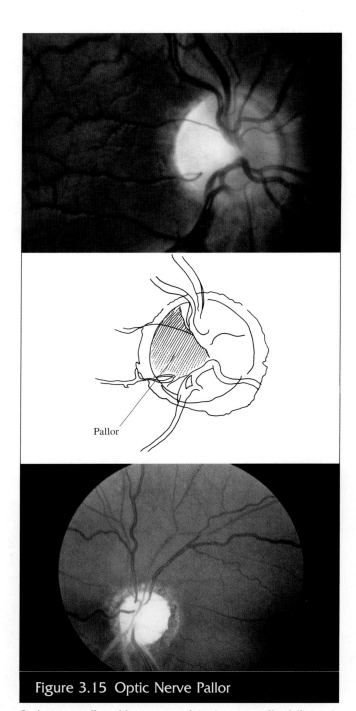

Figure 3.15 Optic Nerve Pallor

Optic nerve pallor, either segmental (*top*) or generalized (*bottom*), is a nonspecific change that may be associated with a previous episode of optic neuritis or other insults to the optic nerve. (Courtesy of Richard E. Wyszynski, MD.)

91

Associated Clinical Features

Anterior ischemic optic neuropathy (AION) presents with a sudden loss of visual field (often altitudinal), usually involving fixation, in an older individual. The loss is usually stable after onset, with no improvement, and only occasionally, progressive over several days to weeks. Pale disk swelling is present involving a sector or the full disk, with accompanying flame hemorrhages (Fig. 3.16).

Differential Diagnosis

The common, nonarteritic causes of AION (probably arteriosclerosis) need to be differentiated from arteritic ones, such as giant cell arteritis. If untreated, the latter will involve the other eye in 75% of cases, often in a few days to weeks. These elderly individuals often have weight loss, masseter claudication, weakness, myalgias, elevated sedimentation rate, and painful scalp, temples, or forehead.

Emergency Department Treatment and Disposition

Routine ophthalmologic and medical evaluation is appropriate.

Clinical Pearls

1. Consider AION in an elderly patient with sudden, usually painless visual field loss.
2. Rule out giant cell arteritis. These patients tend to be older (age > 55) and may have associated CRAO or cranial nerve palsies (III, IV, or VI) with diplopia.

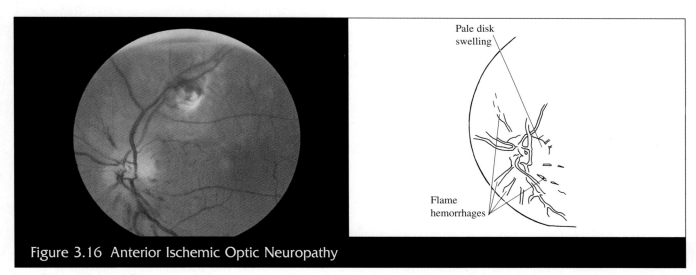

Figure 3.16 Anterior Ischemic Optic Neuropathy

Pale disk swelling and flame hemorrhages are present. This patient also has an unrelated retinal scar due to toxoplasmosis. (Courtesy of William E. Cappaert, MD.)

Associated Clinical Features

Narrow or closed-angle glaucoma results from a physical appositional impedance of aqueous humor outflow. Symptoms range from complaints of colored halos around lights and blurred vision to severe pain (may be described as a headache or brow ache) associated with nausea and vomiting. Intraocular pressures are markedly elevated. Perilimbal vessels are injected, the pupil is middilated and poorly reactive to light, and the cornea may be hazy and edematous (see also Chap. 2 for external ocular images).

Two-thirds of glaucoma patients have open-angle glaucoma due to an abnormality of primary tissues responsible for the outflow of fluid out of the eye. Often they are asymptomatic. They may have a family history of glaucoma. Funduscopy may show asymmetric cupping of the optic nerves (Fig. 3.17). The optic nerve may show notching, local thinning of tissue, or disk hemorrhage. Optic cups enlarge, especially vertically, with progressive damage. Tissue loss is associated with visual field abnormalities, usually in arcuate patterns. The intraocular pressure is often but not always greater than 21 mmHg.

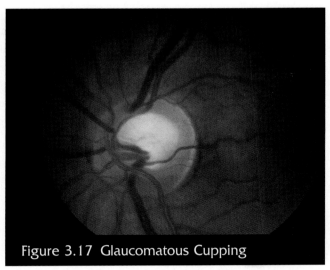

Figure 3.17 Glaucomatous Cupping

The cup is not central; it is elongated toward the rim superotemporally. (Courtesy of Department of Ophthalmology, Naval Medical Center, Portsmouth, VA.)

Differential Diagnosis

Acute Glaucoma

Painful visual loss (retrobulbar optic neuritis, iritis, endophthalmitis), referred pain from nonophthalmic source.

Chronic Glaucoma

Normal variants, ocular conditions like disk drusen or optic neuropathy.

Emergency Department Treatment and Disposition

Acute Narrow-Angle Glaucoma

Emergent ophthalmologic consultation and administration of medications to decrease intraocular pressure. Beta-blocker drops (timolol), carbonic anhydrase inhibitors (acetazolamide), cholinergic stimulating drops (pilocarpine), hyperosmotic agents (osmoglyn), and alpha-adrenergic agonists (apraclonidine) may be employed prior to laser or surgical iridotomy (see also Chap. 2).

Open-Angle Glaucoma

Long-term ophthalmic evaluation and treatment with medications and laser or surgery.

Clinical Pearls

1. A high index of suspicion must be maintained, since associated complaints such as nausea, vomiting, and headache may obscure the diagnosis.
2. Open-angle glaucoma usually causes no symptoms other than gradual loss of vision.
3. Congenital glaucoma is rare. However, because of prognosis if diagnosis is delayed, consider congenital glaucoma in infants and children with any of the following: tearing, photophobia, enlarged eyes, cloudy corneas.
4. Asymmetric cupping, enlarged cups, and elevated intraocular pressure are hallmarks of open-angle glaucoma.

SUBHYALOID HEMORRHAGE IN SUBARACHNOID HEMORRHAGE (SAH)

Associated Clinical Features

Subhyaloid hemorrhage appears as extravasated blood beneath the retinal layer (Fig. 3.18). These are often described as "boat-shaped" hemorrhages to distinguish them from the "flame-shaped" hemorrhages on the superficial retina. They may occur as a result of blunt trauma but are perhaps best known as a marker for subarachnoid hemorrhage (SAH). In SAH, the hemorrhages appear as a "puff" of blood emanating from the central disk.

Differential Diagnosis

SAH, shaken impact syndrome, hypertensive retinopathy, and retinal hemorrhage should all be considered and aggressively evaluated.

Emergency Department Treatment and Disposition

No specific treatment is required for subhyaloid hemorrhage. Treatment is dependent on the underlying etiology. Appropriate specialty referral should be made in all cases.

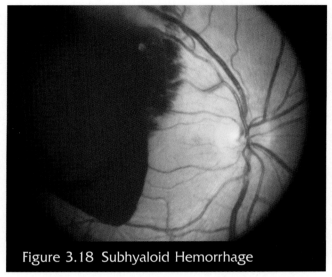

Figure 3.18 Subhyaloid Hemorrhage

Subhyaloid hemorrhage seen on funduscopic examination in a patient with subarachnoid hemorrhage. (From Edlow and Caplan: Primary care: Avoiding pitfalls in the diagnosis of subarachnoid hemorrhage. *N Engl J Med* 2000; 342:29–36, with permission.)

Clinical Pearl

1. A funduscopic examination looking for subhyaloid hemorrhage should be included in all patients with severe headache, unresponsive pediatric patients, or those with altered mental status.

EYE

CHAPTER 4

OPHTHALMIC TRAUMA

Dallas E. Peak
Carey D. Chisholm
Kevin J. Knoop

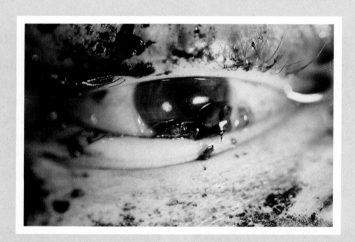

Associated Clinical Features

Corneal abrasions are heralded by the acute onset of eye discomfort accompanied by tearing and a foreign-body sensation. Conjunctival injection may also be noted. If the area of abrasion is large or central, visual acuity may be affected. Large abrasions or delays in seeking care may be accompanied by photophobia and headache from ciliary muscle spasm. Associated findings or complications include traumatic iritis, hypopyon, or a corneal ulcer (described in Chap. 2). Examination before and after instillation of fluorescein, preferably with a slit lamp, usually reveals the defect (Figs. 4.1 and 4.2). Fluorescein pools and stains the area where corneal epithelium has been denuded.

Differential Diagnosis

Corneal foreign body, conjunctivitis, conjunctival foreign body, iritis, and corneal ulcer can present with similar complaints.

Emergency Department Treatment and Disposition

Instillation of topical anesthetic drops permits a better examination and relieves pain. A short-acting cycloplegic (e.g., cyclopentolate 0.5%, homatropine 5%) may reduce ciliary spasm and pain and should be considered in patients with larger abrasions or in those who complain of headache or photophobia. Topical antibiotic drops or ointment—preferably broad-spectrum agents such as gentamicin, sulfacetamide, or erythromycin—are used to prevent secondary bacterial infection. A soft double-layer patch may also be applied. Neither treatment with topical antibiotics nor patching has been scientifically validated, and routine use of these practices has been called into question. Follow-up is required for any patient who is still symptomatic after 12 h.

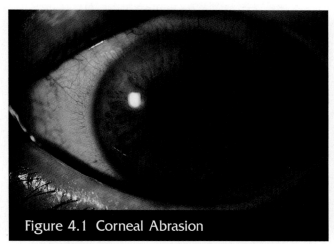

Figure 4.1 Corneal Abrasion

Seen under magnification from the slit lamp, corneal abrasion can sometimes be appreciated without fluorescein staining. This abrasion is seen without using the cobalt blue light. (Courtesy of Harold Rivera.)

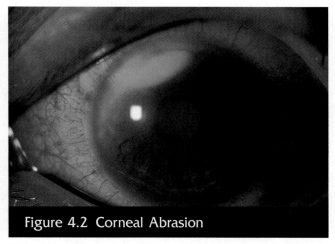

Figure 4.2 Corneal Abrasion

The same abrasion as Fig. 4.1 is seen under magnification from the slit lamp with fluorescein stain using the cobalt blue light. (Courtesy of Harold Rivera.)

Clinical Pearls

1. Only sterile fluorescein strips should be used, since the corneal epithelium, the primary barrier to infection, has been potentially disrupted.

2. Mucus may simulate the fluorescein uptake, but its position changes with blinking.

3. Multiple linear corneal abrasions, the "ice-rink sign," may result from the adherence of a foreign body to the conjunctiva under the lid (Fig. 4.3). The lid should always be everted to rule out a retained foreign body.

4. A high index of suspicion of a perforating injury should be maintained for any abrasion that occurs as a result of grinding or striking metal on metal.

5. Fluorescein streaming away from an "abrasion" (Seidel's test) may be an indication of a corneal perforation.

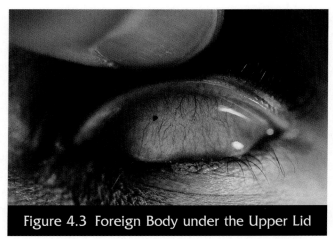

Figure 4.3 Foreign Body under the Upper Lid

Lid eversion is an essential part of the eye examination. (Courtesy of Kevin J. Knoop, MD, MS.)

Associated Clinical Features

Patients typically give a history of something in the eye or complain of foreign-body sensation. If the foreign body overlies the cornea, the patient's vision may be affected. There may be tearing, conjunctival injection, and ciliary flush (Fig. 4.4). If several hours have elapsed since the occurrence of the injury, there may be headache and photophobia in addition to the above signs and symptoms.

Differential Diagnosis

The most important consideration in the differential is the possibility of a penetrating injury to the globe. A meticulous history about the mechanism of injury (grinding or metal on metal) must be elicited. Conjunctival foreign body, corneal abrasion, intraocular foreign body, conjunctivitis, iritis, and glaucoma should also be considered.

Emergency Department Treatment and Disposition

If superficial, removal of the foreign body with a moist cotton-tipped applicator may be attempted; if unsuccessful, an eye spud or small (25-gauge) needle may be used. After removal, if a residual corneal abrasion is present, instill an antibiotic solution or ointment. A "short-acting" cycloplegic (e.g., cyclopentolate 0.5%) should be considered in patients with complaints of headache or photophobia. Metallic foreign bodies are often accompanied by a "rust ring" discoloration of the surrounding corneal epithelium (Fig. 4.5). Removal of the rust ring can be attempted, either with a needle or preferably with a small burr drill device available commercially. Alternatively, the patient may be referred to an ophthalmologist the following day.

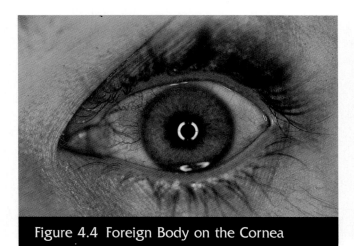

Figure 4.4 Foreign Body on the Cornea

A foreign body is lodged at 10 o'clock on the cornea. Note the localized ciliary flush in the surrounding conjunctiva at the limbus. (Courtesy of Kevin J. Knoop, MD, MS.)

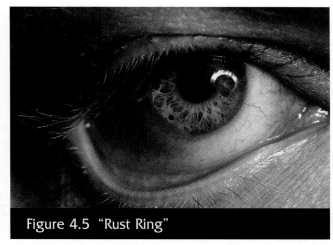

Figure 4.5 "Rust Ring"

A rust ring has formed from a foreign body (likely metallic) in this patient. A burr drill can be used for attempted removal, which, if unsuccessful, can be reattempted in 24 h. (Courtesy of Kevin J. Knoop, MD, MS.)

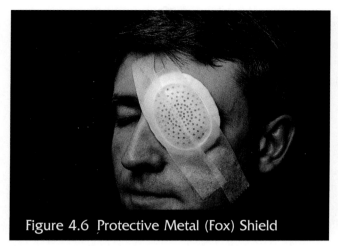

Figure 4.6 Protective Metal (Fox) Shield

A protective shield is used in the setting of a suspected or confirmed perforating injury. (Courtesy of Kevin J. Knoop, MD, MS.)

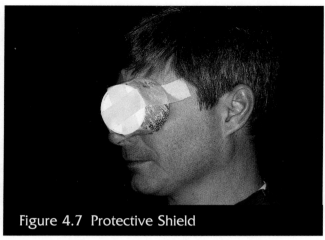

Figure 4.7 Protective Shield

A protective shield is readily fashioned from a paper cup if a metal shield is not available. (Courtesy of Kevin J. Knoop, MD, MS.)

Clinical Pearls

1. Treatment of a suspected penetrating injury to the globe includes immediate referral, eye rest, protective patching (Figs. 4.6, 4.7), and elevation of the head of the bed.

2. If history of ocular penetration is present, a diligent search for a foreign body is indicated. X-ray may identify the foreign body (Fig. 4.8), but computed tomography (CT) is the diagnostic study of choice.

3. Be sure to evert the upper lid and search carefully for a foreign body. A foreign body adherent to the upper lid abrades the cornea, producing the "ice-rink" sign, caused from multiple linear abrasions.

4. If a rust ring is present from a metallic foreign body, its removal can be attempted, or the patient may await ophthalmology follow-up in 24 h.

5. Multiple small corneal foreign bodies (e.g., glass or sand) may be removed by irrigating with normal saline or tap water. The instillation of a topical anesthetic facilitates the irrigation process.

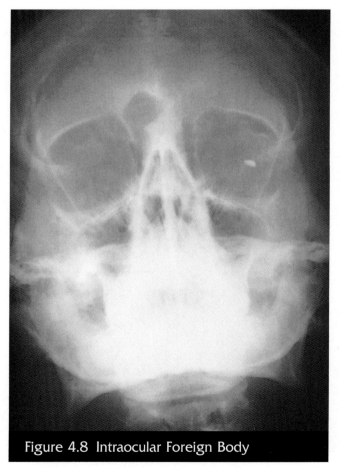

Figure 4.8 Intraocular Foreign Body

A metallic foreign body is seen on a plain radiograph and—with comparison with a lateral film—indicates the presence of an intraocular foreign body. (Courtesy of Department of Ophthalmology, Naval Medical Center, Portsmouth, VA.)

Associated Clinical Features

Eyelid lacerations should always prompt a thorough search for associated injury to the globe, penetration of the orbit, or involvement of surrounding structures (e.g., lacrimal glands, ducts, puncta) (Fig. 4.9). Depending on the mechanism of injury, a careful exclusion of foreign body may be indicated.

Differential Diagnosis

Laceration of the levator palpebrae musculature or tendinous attachments, laceration of the canthal ligamentous support, division of the lacrimal duct or puncta, and penetration of the periorbital septum should all be considered.

Emergency Department Treatment and Disposition

Eyelid lacerations involving superficial skin can be repaired with 6-0 nonabsorbable interrupted sutures, which should remain in place for 3 days. Lacerations through an anatomic structure called the gray line (see Fig. 4.9), situated on the palpebral edge, require diligent reapproximation and should be referred. Other injuries that require specialty consultation for repair include:

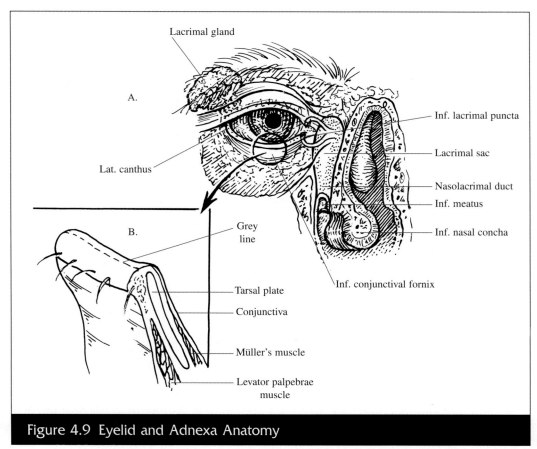

Figure 4.9 Eyelid and Adnexa Anatomy

Ocular trauma should prompt examination of surrounding anatomic structures for associated injuries.

—Lacerations through the lid margins: these require exact realignment to avoid entropion or extropion.

—Deep lacerations through the upper lid that divide the levator palpebrae muscles or their tendinous attachments: these must be repaired with fine absorbable suture to avoid ptosis.

—Lacrimal duct injuries: these are repaired by stenting of the duct, otherwise excessive spilling of tears (epiphora) will result.

—Medial canthal ligaments: these must be repaired to avoid drooping of the lids.

The most important objectives are to rule out injury to the globe and to search diligently for foreign bodies.

Clinical Pearls

1. Lacerations of the medial one-third of the lid (Fig. 4.10) should always raise suspicion for injury to the lacrimal ducts or puncta as well as the medial canthal ligament.

2. A small amount of adipose tissue seen within a laceration is a sign that perforation of the orbital septum has occurred (since there is no subcutaneous fat in the lids themselves).

3. Injuries involving the orbital septum carry a higher than normal risk of globe injury and intraorbital foreign body as well as a higher risk for orbital cellulitis. A CT scan and specialty consultation should be considered.

4. Any injury to the lids involving tissue loss or avulsion should be referred for specialty consultation.

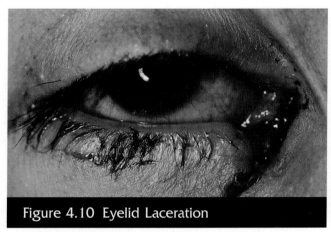

Figure 4.10 Eyelid Laceration

This laceration involving the medial third of the lid clearly violates the canalicular structures. The patient was struck by a person wearing a ring. (Courtesy of Kevin J. Knoop, MD, MS.)

Associated Clinical Features

Injury to the anterior chamber that disrupts the vasculature supporting the iris or ciliary body results in a hyphema. The blood tends to layer and because of gravity forms a meniscus (Fig. 4.11). Symptoms can include pain, photophobia, and possibly blurred vision secondary to obstructing blood cells. Nausea and vomiting may signal a rise in intraocular pressure (glaucoma) caused by blockage of the trabecular meshwork by blood cells or clot.

Differential Diagnosis

Hypopyon (pus within the anterior chamber), vitreous hemorrhage, iridodialysis, penetrating injury to the globe, and intraocular foreign body should be considered.

Emergency Department Treatment and Disposition

Prevention of further hemorrhage is the first goal. The patient should be kept at rest in the supine position with the head elevated slightly. A hard eye shield should be used to prevent further trauma from manipulation. Oral or parenteral pain medication and sedatives are appropriate, but avoid agents with antiplatelet activity such as nonsteroidal anti-inflammatory drugs (NSAIDs). Antiemetics should be used if the patient has nausea. Further treatment is at the discretion of specialty consultants but may include topical and oral steroids, antifibrinolytics such as aminocaproic acid, or surgery. Intraocular pressure (IOP) should be measured in all patients unless there is a suspicion of penetrating injury to the globe. If elevated, IOP should be treated with appropriate agents including topical beta blockers, pilocarpine, and, if needed, osmotic agents (mannitol, sorbitol) and acetazolamide. The need for admission for small hyphemas is variable, since some centers admit all whereas others individualize treatment. Ophthalmologic consultation is warranted to determine local practices.

Clinical Pearls

1. The patient should be told specifically not to read or watch television, as these activities result in greater than usual ocular activity.
2. Depending on the severity of the initial hyphema, rebleeding may occur in 10 to 25% of patients, commonly in 2 to 5 days as the original clot retracts and loosens.
3. Blood that is not absorbed from the anterior chamber may infiltrate and stain the cornea, leaving a brown discoloration.
4. An "eightball" or total hyphema occurs when blood fills the entire anterior chamber. These lesions require surgical evacuation.
5. Patients with sickle cell and other hemoglobinopathies are at risk for sickling of blood inside the anterior chamber (Fig. 4.12). This can cause a rise in IOP from physical obstruction of the trabecular meshwork.

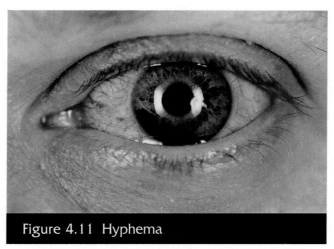

Figure 4.11 Hyphema

This hyphema has almost completely layered while the patient's head was tilted. Note the hazy greenish area at 6 o'clock in contrast to the remainder of the blue iris. This represents blood circulating in the anterior chamber that has not yet layered. (Courtesy of Kevin J. Knoop, MD, MS.)

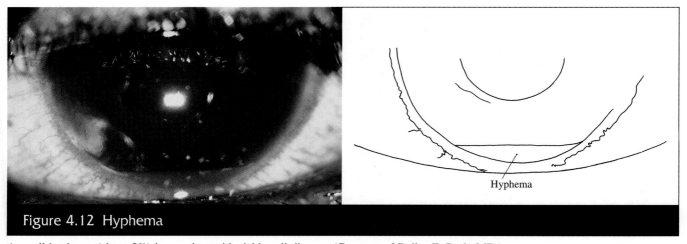

Figure 4.12 Hyphema

A small hyphema (about 5%) in a patient with sickle cell disease. (Courtesy of Dallas E. Peak, MD.)

Associated Clinical Features

Traumatic iridodialysis is the result of an injury, typically blunt trauma, that pulls the iris away from the ciliary body. The resulting deformity appears as a lens-shaped defect at the outer margin of the iris (Fig. 4.13). Patients may present complaining of a "second pupil." As the iris pulls away from the ciliary body, a small amount of bleeding may result. Look closely for associated traumatic hyphema.

Differential Diagnosis

Traumatic hyphema, penetrating injury to the globe, scleral rupture, intraocular foreign body, and lens dislocation causing billowing of the iris should all be considered.

Emergency Department Treatment and Disposition

A remote traumatic iridodialysis requires no specific treatment in the ED. Recent history of ocular trauma should prompt a diligent slit-lamp examination for associated hyphema or lens discoloration. If hyphema is present, it should be treated as discussed (see "Hyphema", above). Pure cases of iridodialysis may be referred for specialty consultation to exclude other injuries; if the defect is large enough to result in monocular diplopia, surgical repair may be necessary.

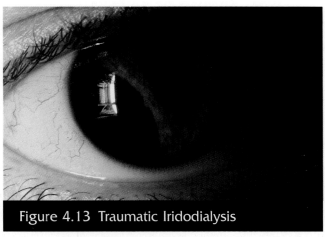

Figure 4.13 Traumatic Iridodialysis

The iris has pulled away from the ciliary body as a result of blunt trauma. (Courtesy of Department of Ophthalmology, Naval Medical Center, Portsmouth, VA.)

Clinical Pearls

1. The examination should carefully exclude posterior chamber pathology and hyphema.
2. A careful review of the history to exclude penetrating trauma should be made. If the history is unclear, CT scan may be used to exclude the presence of intraocular foreign body.
3. A careful examination includes searching for associated lens dislocation.

Associated Clinical Features

Lens dislocation may result from a sudden blow to the globe with resultant stretching of the zonule fibers that hold the lens in place (Fig. 4.14). The patient may experience symptoms of monocular diplopia or gross blurring of images, depending on the severity of the injury. The edge of the subluxed lens may be visible when the pupil is dilated (Fig. 4.15). If all the zonule fibers tear and the lens is dislocated, it may lodge in the anterior chamber or the vitreous.

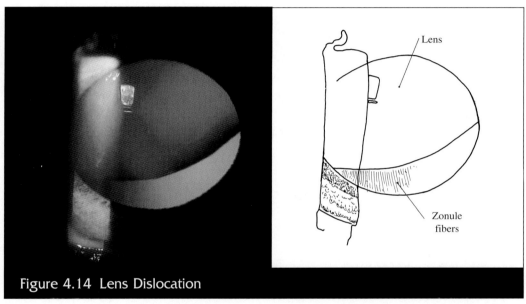

Figure 4.14 Lens Dislocation

Lens dislocation revealed during slit-lamp examination. Note the zonule fibers, which normally hold the lens in place. (Courtesy of Department of Ophthalmology, Naval Medical Center, Portsmouth, VA.)

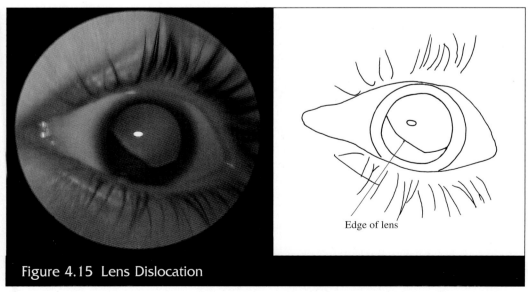

Figure 4.15 Lens Dislocation

The edge of this dislocated lens is visible with the pupil dilated as an altered red reflex. (Courtesy of Department of Ophthalmology, Naval Medical Center, Portsmouth, VA.)

Differential Diagnosis

Marfan's syndrome, tertiary syphilis, and homocystinuria may be present and should be considered in patients presenting with lens dislocation.

Emergency Department Treatment and Disposition

Almost all cases require surgery if the lens is totally dislocated; partial subluxations may require only a change in refraction.

Clinical Pearls

1. Patients may experience lens dislocation with seemingly trivial trauma if they have an underlying coloboma of the lens (see Fig. 4.20), Marfan's syndrome, homocystinuria, or syphilis.
2. Iridodonesis is a trembling movement of the iris noted after rapid eye movements and is a sign of occult posterior lens dislocation.

Associated Clinical Features

Open globe injuries resulting from penetrating trauma can be subtle and easily overlooked. All are serious injuries. Signs to look for are loss of anterior chamber depth caused by leakage of aqueous humor, a teardrop-shaped pupil, or prolapse of choroid through the wound (Fig. 4.16).

Differential Diagnosis

Iridodialysis, corneal foreign body, and scleral rupture may have similar presentations.

Emergency Department Treatment and Disposition

All open globe injuries require specialty consultation. A Fox (metal) eye shield should be placed over the affected eye. No attempts to examine, measure pressures, or manipulate the eye should be made. Intravenous antibiotics to cover gram-positive organisms are appropriate. Sedation and aggressive pain management are crucial and should be used liberally to prevent or decrease expulsion of intraocular contents due to crying, activity, or vomiting. Antiemetics should be given if nausea is present. Tetanus immunization should be updated. Many open globe injuries are associated with other significant blunt trauma injuries.

Clinical Pearls

1. When a large foreign body such as a pencil or nail protrudes from the globe, resist the temptation to remove it. Such objects should be left in place until definitively treated in the operating room.
2. Control of pain, activity, and nausea may be sight-saving and requires proactive use of appropriate medications.
3. Use of lid hooks, retractors (Fig. 4.17), or even retractors fashioned from paper clips (Fig. 4.18) is preferred to open the eyelids of trauma victims with blepharospasm or massive swelling. Attempts to do this with fingers can inadvertently increase the pressure on the globe.
4. Penetrating globe injuries are a relative contraindication to the sole use of depolarizing neuromuscular blockade (e.g., succinylcholine). Pretreatment with a small dose of a nondepolarizing agent should be given to abolish the fasciculations and resultant increased intraocular pressure.

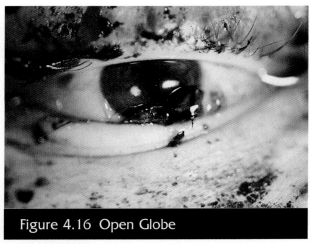

Figure 4.16 Open Globe

This injury is not subtle; extruded ocular contents (vitreous) can be seen; a teardrop pupil is also present. (Courtesy of Alan B. Storrow, MD.)

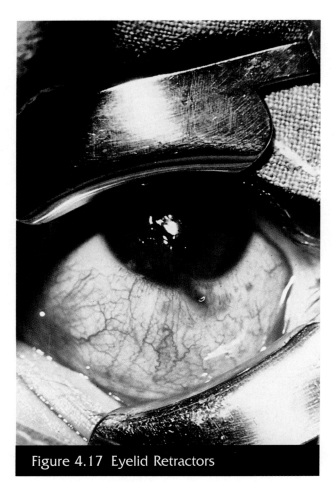

Figure 4.17 Eyelid Retractors

Retractors are used to gain exposure without applying pressure to the globe. (Courtesy of Dallas E. Peak, MD.)

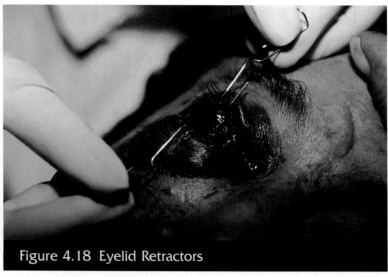

Figure 4.18 Eyelid Retractors

Retractors fashioned from paper clips can safely be used when standard retractors are not available. (Courtesy of Kevin J. Knoop, MD, MS.)

Associated Clinical Features

A forceful blow to the eye may result in a scleral rupture. The diagnosis is obvious when orbital contents are seen spilling from the globe itself. The diagnosis may be more occult in situations where only a tiny rent in the sclera has occurred. When rupture occurs at the limbus, a small amount of iris may herniate, resulting in an irregularly shaped pupil called a teardrop pupil (Fig. 4.19). A teardrop pupil may also be the result of a penetrating foreign body. Mechanism is the key to distinguishing these two causes. Another associated finding is bloody chemosis of the bulbar conjunctiva over the area of scleral rupture. This may be distinguished from a simple subconjunctival hematoma by bulging of the conjunctiva.

Differential Diagnosis

Subconjunctival hematoma, nontraumatic bloody chemosis, corneal-scleral laceration, intraocular foreign body, iridodialysis, and traumatic lens dislocation may have a similar presentation. A coloboma of the iris (Fig. 4.20) may appear similar to a teardrop pupil.

Emergency Department Treatment and Disposition

Urgent specialty consultation and operative management are mandatory. The eye should be protected by a Fox metal eye shield, and all further examination and manipulation of the eye should be discouraged to prevent prolapse or worsening prolapse of choriouveal structures. Tetanus status should be addressed. Intravenous antibiotics to cover suspected organisms are appropriate. Adequate sedation and use of parenteral analgesics is encouraged. Antiemetics should be given proactively, since vomiting may result in further prolapse of intraocular contents. CT scanning should be considered if the presence of a foreign body is suspected.

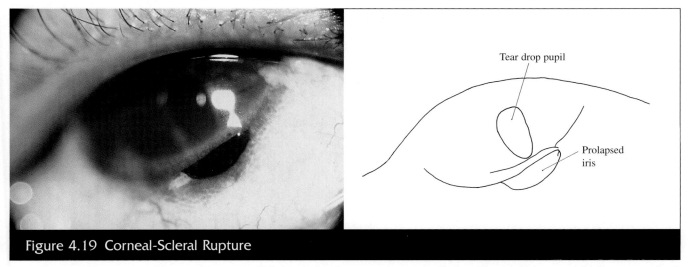

Figure 4.19 Corneal-Scleral Rupture

A teardrop pupil is present, with a small amount of iris herniating from a rupture at the limbus. These injuries may initially go unnoticed. (Courtesy of Dallas E. Peak, MD.)

Clinical Pearls

1. The eyeball may appear deflated or the anterior chamber excessively deep. Intraocular pressure will likely be decreased, but measurement should be avoided, since this may worsen herniation of intraocular contents.
2. Rupture usually occurs where the sclera is the thinnest, at the point of attachment of extraocular muscles and at the limbus.
3. Bloody chemosis from scleral rupture is distinguished from subconjunctival hematoma by bulging of the conjunctiva. A subconjunctival hematoma is flat in appearance (see Fig. 4.22).
4. A teardrop pupil may easily be overlooked in the triage process or in the setting of multiple traumatic injuries.
5. Seidel's test (instillation of fluorescein and observing for fluorescein streaming away from the injury) may be used to diagnose subtle perforation (Fig. 4.21).

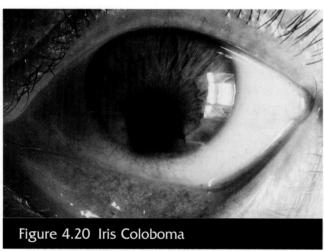

Figure 4.20 Iris Coloboma

Iris coloboma is a congenital finding resulting from incomplete closure of the fetal ocular cleft. It appears as a teardrop pupil and may be mistaken for a sign of scleral rupture. (Courtesy of Department of Ophthalmology, Naval Medical Center, Portsmouth, VA.)

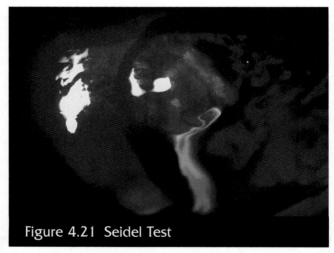

Figure 4.21 Seidel Test

A positive Seidel test shows aqueous leaking through a corneal perforation while being observed with the slit lamp. (Courtesy of John D. Mitchell, MD. Used with permission from Tintinalli JE et al: *Emergency Medicine: A Comprehensive Study Guide,* 5th ed. New York: McGraw-Hill; 2000.)

Associated Clinical Features

A subconjunctival hemorrhage or hematoma occurs with often trivial events such as a cough, sneeze, Valsalva maneuver, or minor blunt trauma. The patient may present with some degree of duress secondary to the appearance of the bloody eye. The blood is usually bright red and appears flat (Fig. 4.22). It is limited to the bulbar conjunctiva and stops abruptly at the limbus. This appearance is important to differentiate the lesion from bloody chemosis, which can occur with scleral rupture. Aside from appearance, this condition does not cause the patient any pain or diminution in visual acuity.

Differential Diagnosis

Scleral rupture, nontraumatic bloody chemosis (Fig. 4.23), conjunctivitis, iritis, corneal-scleral laceration, severe hypertension, and coagulopathy may have a similar appearance or presentation.

Emergency Department Treatment and Disposition

No treatment is required. The patient should be told to expect the blood to be resorbed in 2 to 3 weeks.

Clinical Pearls

1. Subconjunctival hematoma may be differentiated from bloody chemosis by the flat appearance of the conjunctival membranes.
2. A subconjunctival hematoma involving the extreme lateral globe after blunt trauma is very suspicious for zygomatic arch fracture.
3. Patients with nontraumatic bloody chemosis should be evaluated for an underlying metabolic (coagulopathy) or structural (cavernous sinus thrombosis) disorder.

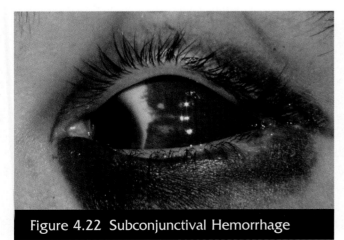

Figure 4.22 Subconjunctival Hemorrhage

Subconjunctival hemorrhage in a patient with blunt trauma. The flat appearance of the hemorrhage indicates its benign nature. (Courtesy of Dallas E. Peak, MD.)

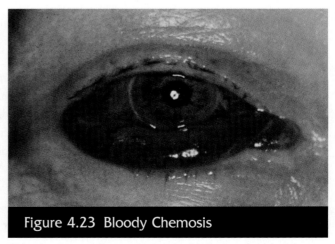

Figure 4.23 Bloody Chemosis

"Bloody chemosis" was confused with "subconjunctival hemorrhage" in this patient with no history of trauma and positive cranial nerve palsies. Cavernous sinus thrombosis was diagnosed. (Courtesy of Eric Einfalt, MD.)

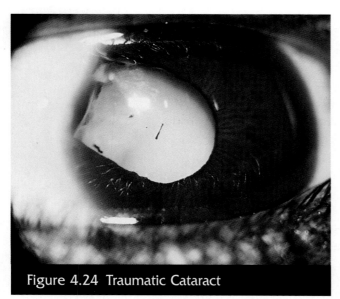

Figure 4.24 Traumatic Cataract

This traumatic cataract is seen as a large lens opacity overlying the visual axis. A traumatic iridodialysis is also present. (Courtesy of Dallas E. Peak, MD.)

Associated Clinical Features

Any trauma to the eye that disrupts the normal architecture of the lens may result in the development of a traumatic cataract—a lens opacity (Fig. 4.24). The mechanism behind cataract formation involves fluid infiltration into the normally avascular and acellular lens stroma. The lens may be observed to swell with fluid and become cloudy and opacified. The time course is usually weeks to months following the original insult. Cataracts that are large enough may be observed by the naked eye. Those that are within the central visual field may cause blurring of vision or distortion of light around objects (e.g., halos).

Differential Diagnosis

Lens dislocation, intraocular foreign body, hypopyon, corneal abrasion, and hyphema can present with similar complaints. History and physical examination are helpful in discriminating most of these conditions from traumatic cataract.

Emergency Department Treatment and Disposition

No specific treatment is rendered in the ED for cases of delayed traumatic cataract. Routine ophthalmologic referral is indicated for most cases.

Clinical Pearls

1. Traumatic cataracts are frequent sequelae of lightning injury. All lightning-strike victims should be warned of this possibility.
2. Cataracts may also occur as a result of electric current injury to the vicinity of the cranial vault.
3. Cataracts can be easily examined using the +10-diopter setting on an ophthalmoscope or in more detail with a slit lamp.
4. Leukocoria results from a dense cataract, which causes loss of the red reflex.
5. If a cataract develops sufficient size and "swells" the lens, the trabecular meshwork may become blocked, producing glaucoma.

Associated Clinical Features

Most symptomatic ocular exposures involve either immediate or delayed onset of eye discomfort accompanied by one or more of the following: itching, tearing, redness, photophobia, blurred vision, and/or foreign-body sensation. Conjunctival injection or chemosis may be noted on examination. Abrupt onset of more severe symptoms may indicate exposure to caustic alkaline or acidic substances and should be regarded as a true ocular emergency. Exposure to defensive sprays or riot-control agents (e.g., Mace or tear gas) causes immediate onset of severe ocular burning, intense tearing, blepharospasm, and irritation of the mucous membranes of the nose and oropharynx. Chemical conjunctivitis in the newborn may stem from the use of silver nitrate drops at delivery for prophylaxis against *Neisseria gonorrhoeae.* Many hospitals now favor erythromycin-based ointments.

Differential Diagnosis

Alkali or acid exposure, corneal foreign body, corneal abrasion, infectious conjunctivitis, and conjunctival foreign body should be considered.

Emergency Department Treatment and Disposition

Treatment should begin in the prehospital arena with immediate and copious irrigation. The patient who presents acutely with possible caustic exposure should be triaged to immediate treatment. An attempt should be made to determine the pH of the conjunctival sac with a broad-range pH paper, though this determination should not delay the initiation of treatment. Instillation of topical anesthetic drops will permit a better examination. The conjunctiva should be closely examined for concretions or foreign body, with eversion of the upper lid. Any debris should be removed with a moistened cotton-tipped applicator. If pH determination demonstrates acid or alkali exposure, irrigation with warmed normal saline (NS) or lactated ringers (LS) (preferred) solution should begin, using 1-L bags connected through standard intravenous tubing to a Morgan lens. A minimum of 2-L should be instilled, followed by a recheck of the pH or reassessment for continued symptoms. If a normal tear film pH of 7.4 has not been achieved, irrigation should be continued. Alkali exposures may cause severe injury due to liquification necrosis, which penetrates the deeper tissues (Fig. 4.25). Acids produce a coagulative necrosis, which creates a barrier to further penetration.

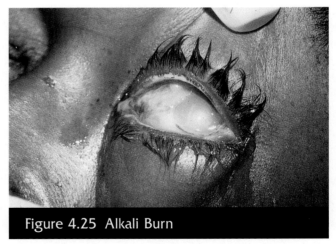

Figure 4.25 Alkali Burn

Diffuse opacification of the cornea occurred from a "lye" burn to the face. (Courtesy of Stephen Corbett, MD.)

Irrigation should be strongly considered after chemical exposure to a non–acid or alkali source. Many chemicals merely cause irritative symptoms; however, some may also denude the corneal epithelium and inflame the anterior chamber. All patients should undergo slit-lamp examination to document corneal injuries (e.g., abrasions, punctate erosions, opacities) or anterior chamber inflammation. Antibiotic drops may be indicated, particularly if corneal injury is noted. Cycloplegics may be of benefit as well to reduce ciliary spasm and pain in these cases.

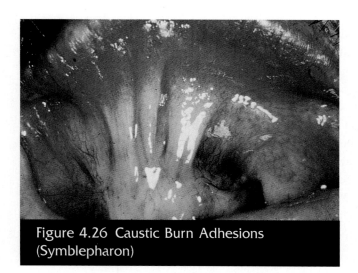

Figure 4.26 Caustic Burn Adhesions (Symblepharon)

Scarring of both palpebral and bulbar conjunctivae results in severe adhesions between the lids and the globe. (Courtesy of Arden H. Wander, MD.)

Clinical Pearls

1. Immediate onset of severe symptoms calls for immediate treatment and should prompt consideration of alkali or acid exposure.
2. Determination of ocular pH should be made in all cases of chemical exposure.
3. Prolonged (up to 24 h) irrigation may be needed for alkaline exposures.
4. Concretions from the exposure agent may form deep in the conjunctival fornices and must be removed to prevent further injury (Fig. 4.26).
5. Corneal abrasions or punctate erosions may be a direct result of the chemical agent or from treatment with irrigation or placement of the Morgan lens.

EAR, NOSE, AND THROAT

CHAPTER 5

EAR, NOSE, AND THROAT CONDITIONS

Edward C. Jauch
Timothy Kaufman
Kevin J. Knoop

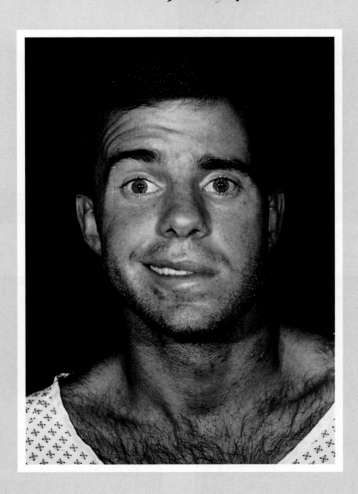

Associated Clinical Features

Children between the ages of 6 months and 2 years are at highest risk of developing acute otitis media (AOM). Males, North American Eskimos, non-breast-fed infants, and children with craniofacial anomalies have the highest incidence of AOM. Additionally, children who contract their first episode prior to their first birthday, have a sibling with a history of recurrent AOM, are in day care, or have parents who smoke are at increased risk of recurrent AOM.

In its most basic form, AOM is defined as an acute inflammation and effusion of the middle ear. Otoscopy of the middle ear should focus on color, position, translucency, and mobility. Compared with the tympanic membrane of a normal ear (Fig. 5.1), AOM causes the tympanic membrane to appear dull, erythematous or injected, bulging, and less mobile (Figs. 5.2 and 5.3).

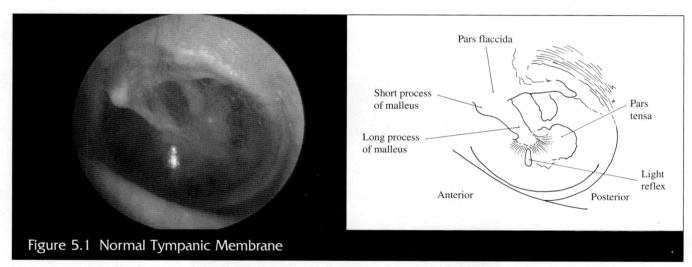

Figure 5.1 Normal Tympanic Membrane

Normal tympanic membrane anatomy and landmarks. (Courtesy of Richard A. Chole, MD, PhD.)

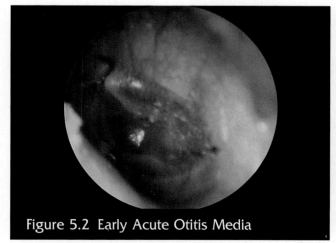

Figure 5.2 Early Acute Otitis Media

A mildly erythematous tympanic membrane is seen with a small purulent effusion in the middle ear. (Courtesy of C. Bruce MacDonald, MD.)

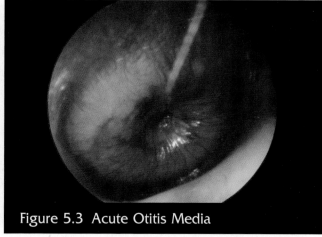

Figure 5.3 Acute Otitis Media

The middle ear is filled with purulent material behind an erythematous, bulging tympanic membrane. (Courtesy of Richard A. Chole, MD, PhD.)

Pneumatic otoscopy and tympanometry enhance accuracy in diagnosing AOM. The light reflex, normal tympanic membrane landmarks, and malleus become obscured.

There are many classifications and hence presentations of AOM based on symptom duration and clinical presentation. Regardless of classification, the common pathogenesis of AOM is eustachian tube dysfunction, allowing retention of secretions (serous otitis) (Figs. 5.4 and 5.5) and seeding of bacteria.

AOM is caused by a wide variety of viral, bacterial, and fungal pathogens. The most common bacterial isolates are *Streptococcus pneumoniae, Haemophilus influenzae, Moraxella catarrhalis,* and *Streptococcus pyogenes.* Approximately 20% of middle ear effusion aspirations are sterile. The prevalence of β-lactamase–producing strains of *H. influenzae* and *M. catarrhalis* is variable but increasing.

Patient presentations and complaints vary with age. Infants with AOM have vague, nonspecific symptoms such as irritability, lethargy, and decreased oral intake. Young children can be irritable, often febrile, and frequently pull at their ears, but they may also be completely asymptomatic. Older children and adults note ear pain, decreased auditory acuity, and occasionally otorrhea.

Differential Diagnosis

Myringitis, otitis externa, perforations of the tympanic membrane, and herpes zoster can mimic otitis media. Less common causes of ear pain include temporomandibular joint disorders, odontogenic infections, and sinusitis. Erythema of the tympanic membrane can appear in an otherwise healthy ear when a child cries.

Emergency Department Treatment and Disposition

Although AOM generally resolves spontaneously, most patients are treated with antibiotics and analgesics. Steroids, decongestants, and antihistamines do not alter the course in AOM but may improve upper respiratory tract symptoms. Rarely, myringotomy may be needed for pain relief.

Antibiotic selection is widely variable. Amoxicillin, in the dose range of 80 to 90 mg/kg/day divided tid, is a suitable first choice for an AOM. Alternatives for initial therapy include trimethoprimsulfamethoxazole, erythromycin-sulfisoxazole, and second-generation cephalosporins. If the patient remains symptomatic 48 to 72 h after beginning antibiotics, amoxicillin with clavulanate, cefixime, or the newer macrolides may provide broader coverage.

Patients should be instructed to follow up in 10 to 14 days or return if symptoms persist or worsen after 48 h. Patients who have significant hearing loss, failed two complete courses of out-

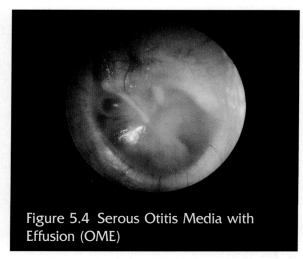

Figure 5.4 Serous Otitis Media with Effusion (OME)

Copious purulent drainage in a newborn with neonatal gonococcal conjunctivitis. (Reprinted with permission of the American Academy of Ophthalmology, *Eye Trauma and Emergencies: A Slide-Script Program.* San Francisco, 1985.)

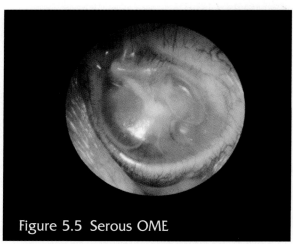

Figure 5.5 Serous OME

A clear, amber-colored effusion with multiple air-fluid levels is seen in the middle ear behind a normal tympanic membrane. (Courtesy of C. Bruce MacDonald, MD.)

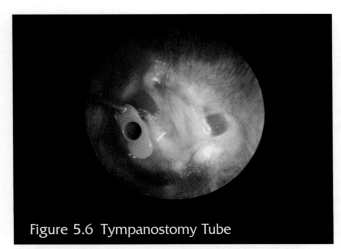

Figure 5.6 Tympanostomy Tube

Typical appearance of a tympanostomy tube in the tympanic membrane. These tubes will migrate to the periphery and eventually drop out. Occasionally, they will be found in the external ear canal. (Courtesy of C. Bruce MacDonald, MD.)

patient antibiotics during a single event, have chronic otitis media (OM) with or without acute exacerbations, or have failed prophylactic antibiotics warrant referral to an otolaryngologist for further evaluation, an audiogram, and possible tympanostomy tubes (Fig. 5.6).

Clinical Pearls

1. In children, recurrent OM is often due to food allergies.
2. Only 4% of children under 2 years old with OM develop temperatures greater than 104°F. Children with temperatures higher than 104°F or with signs of systemic toxicity should be closely evaluated for other causes of the illness before attributing the fever to OM.

Associated Clinical Features

Bullous myringitis is a direct inflammation and infection of the tympanic membrane (TM) secondary to a viral or bacterial agent. Vesicles filled with blood or serosanguinous fluid or bullae on an erythematous tympanic membrane are the hallmark of bullous myringitis (Fig. 5.7). Frequently a concomitant otitis media with effusion is noted. Common bacterial agents are *Mycoplasma pneumoniae, Streptococcus pneumoniae,* and *Haemophilus influenzae.*

The onset of bullous myringitis is preceded by an upper respiratory tract infection and is heralded by sudden onset of severe ear pain, scant serosanguinous drainage from the ear canal, and frequently some degree of hearing loss. Otoscopy reveals bullae on either the inner or outer surface of the TM, often filled with red bloody fluid. Patients presenting with fever, hearing loss, and purulent drainage are more likely to have other concomitant infections, such as otitis media and otitis externa.

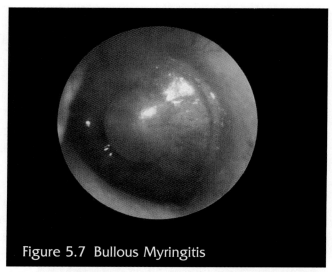

Figure 5.7 Bullous Myringitis

A large fluid-filled bulla is seen distorting the surface of the tympanic membrane. (Courtesy of Richard A. Chole, MD, PhD.)

Differential Diagnosis

Barotrauma is usually associated with swimming, diving, or airplane travel. Herpes zoster oticus produces facial nerve palsy and facial pain. Otitis externa causes edema of the external auditory canal and drainage, whereas otitis media may distort the TM but rarely causes bullae.

Emergency Department Treatment and Disposition

Differentiation between viral and bacterial etiologies for tympanic membrane bullae is difficult but, fortunately, seldom necessary. Although most episodes resolve spontaneously, many physicians prescribe antibiotics, such as trimethoprim-sulfamethoxazole or a macrolide. Warm compresses, topical or strong systemic analgesics, and oral decongestants may provide symptomatic relief. Referral is not necessary in most cases unless rupture of the bullae is required for pain relief.

Clinical Pearl

1. Facial nerve paralysis associated with clear, fluid-filled TM vesicles is characteristic of herpes zoster oticus.

Associated Clinical Features

Contrary to the origin suggested by their name, cholesteatomas are not neoplasms but rather epidermoid inclusion cysts: collections of desquamating stratified squamous epithelium found in the middle ear or mastoid air cells. Congenital cholesteatomas are most frequently found in children and young adults. Acquired cholesteatomas originate from perforations of the tympanic membrane, usually marginally or in the pars flaccida, allowing migration of stratified squamous epithelium from the external auditory canal into the middle ear.

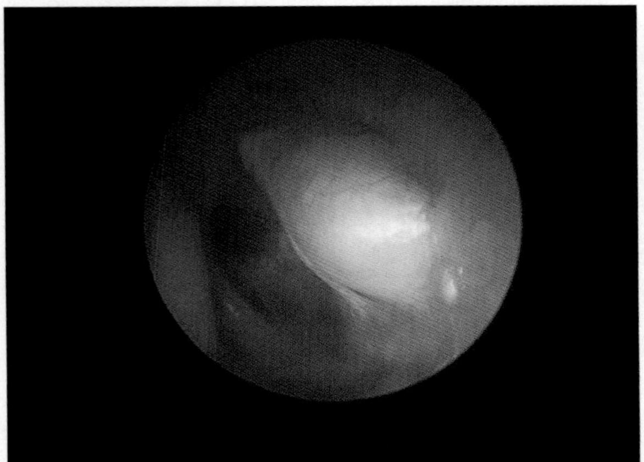

Cholesteatomas can be locally destructive of the middle ear ossicles and tympanic membrane and, through the production of collagenases, erode into the temporal bone, inner ear structures, mastoid sinus, or posterior fossa dura. Delays in treatment can lead to permanent conductive hearing loss or infectious complications.

Patients present with progressive hearing loss, foul-smelling ear drainage, and, in advanced stages, pain, headache, dizziness, facial paralysis, fever, or vertigo. Many cholesteatomas have an insidious progression without associated pain or symptoms. Cholesteatomas are seen on otoscopy as either a retraction pocket containing white debris or a yellow crust on the tympanic membrane with or without a perforation (Figs. 5.8 and 5.9). A middle ear cholesteatoma appears as a pearly white or yellow middle ear mass behind the tympanic membrane, producing a focal bulge, in contrast to the more diffuse displacement of the tympanic membrane seen in otitis media. Radiographs and computed tomography (CT) scans may reveal bony destruction.

Osteomas (sometimes called exostoses) are benign bone overgrowths of the external auditory canal (EAC) found deep in the meatus. Osteomas are often seen in patients with recurrent cold

Figure 5.8 Congenital Cholesteatoma

A congenital cholesteatoma is seen behind an intact tympanic membrane. (Courtesy of C. Bruce McDonald, MD.)

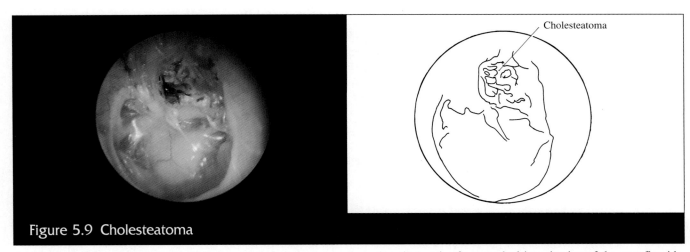

Figure 5.9 Cholesteatoma

A cholesteatoma is seen in this ear. Primary acquired cholesteatomas are thought to arise from gradual invagination of the pars flaccida, usually secondary to trauma. Note the yellow epithelial debris from the cholesteatoma in the area of the pars flaccida. Often there is an effusion and debris, which can distort the anatomy on otoscopy. (Courtesy of C. Bruce MacDonald, MD.)

122

water exposures, such as swimmers and divers. Osteomas are seen on otoscopy as single or multiple round shiny swellings of the bony external auditory canal (Fig. 5.10). A secondary cerumen impaction or an otitis externa may obscure the examination.

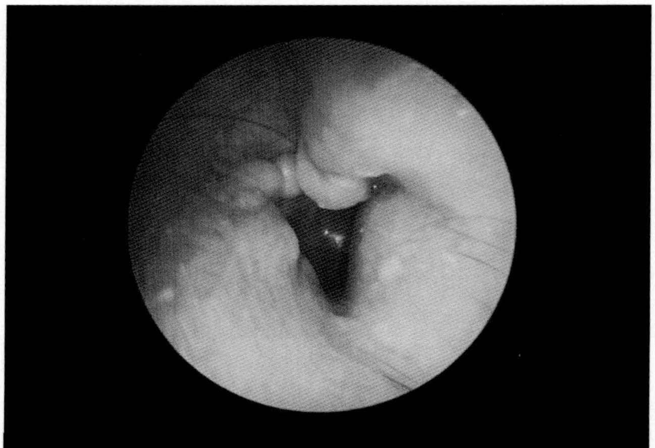

Differential Diagnosis

Wax particles and EAC foreign bodies may resemble cholesteatomas on otoscopy. Furuncles are painful to palpation, whereas otitis externa and otitis media cause EAC drainage and middle ear effusions, respectively.

Emergency Department Treatment and Disposition

Early diagnosis of cholesteatomas is essential for proper referral. Water avoidance as well as topical and sometimes systemic antibiotics are important. Small cholesteatomas found in retraction pockets can be excised and a tympanostomy tube placed to equilibrate middle ear pressures. More extensive cholesteatomas may require surgical excision, tympanoplasty, and radical mastoidectomy. Osteomas require no medical or surgical management unless they become symptomatic.

Figure 5.10 Osteomas

Multiple osteomas almost occlude the external auditory canal. The tympanic membrane can be seen in the center, past the osteomas. These lesions are often seen in patients who are cold water swimmers. (Courtesy of C. Bruce MacDonald, MD.)

Clinical Pearls

1. Persistent pain associated with headache, facial motor weakness, nystagmus, or vertigo suggests inner ear or intracranial involvement.
2. Polyps found on the tympanic membrane can indicate the presence of a cholesteatoma and require further evaluation to exclude its presence.

Associated Clinical Features

Acute tympanic membrane (TM) perforations are often the result of direct penetrating trauma, water or air pressure changes (barotrauma, blast injuries), chronic otitis media, corrosives, thermal injuries (electricity, lightning, heated objects), and iatrogenic causes (foreign-body removal, tympanostomy tubes). TM perforations are occasionally complicated by damage to the ossicular chain that produces a more complete conductive hearing loss, temporal bone injuries, and cranial nerve damage.

Patients complain of a sudden onset of ear pain, vertigo, tinnitus, and altered hearing after a specific event. Patients with posterior perforations present with a more profound deafness than those with anterior perforations. Physical examination of the TM reveals a slit-shaped tear or larger perforation with an irregular border. An acute perforation can have blood on the perforation margin and blood or clot in the canal (Fig. 5.11). The margins are smooth in subacute or chronic perforations.

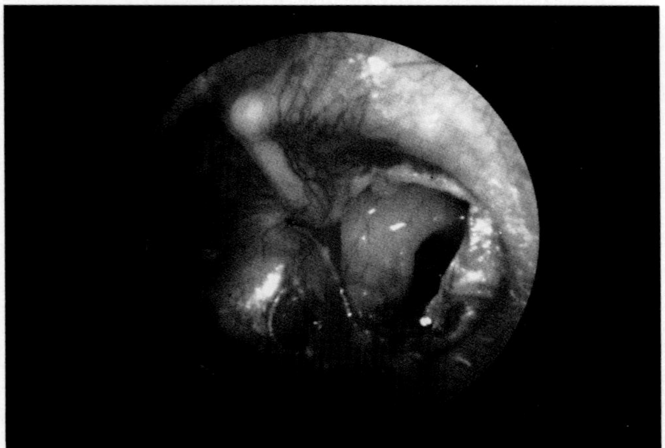

Figure 5.11 Acute Tympanic Membrane Perforation

An acute tympanic membrane perforation is seen. Note the sharp edges of the ruptured tympanic membrane. (Courtesy of Richard A. Chole, MD, PhD.)

Differential Diagnosis

Congenital malformations, chronic perforations, residual perforations from tympanostomy tubes, and retraction pockets have more regular borders and no bleeding or TM erythema.

Emergency Department Treatment and Disposition

Treatment of acute tympanic membrane perforations is tailored to the mechanism. All easily removable foreign bodies should be extracted. Corrosive exposures require face, eye, and ear decontamination. Antibiotics and irrigation do not improve the rate or completeness of healing unless the injury is associated with OM. Systemic antibiotics should be used for perforations associated with OM, penetrating injury, and possibly water-sport injuries (see "Otitis Media," above). Topical steroids impede perforation closure.

Patients are instructed to avoid allowing water to get into the ear while the perforation is healing and to return if symptoms of infection appear. All TM perforations should be referred to an otolaryngologist for follow-up for possible myringoplasty. Even though nearly 80% of all TM perforations heal spontaneously, some do not, and complications can develop.

Clinical Pearls

1. Cortisporin eardrops of any formulation have been shown to retard spontaneous healing and should be avoided.
2. Traumatic TM perforation associated with cranial nerve deficits or persistent vertigo requires immediate ear/nose/throat (ENT) consultation for possible temporal bone fractures or injury to the round or oval window.

Associated Clinical Features

Otitis externa (OE), or "swimmer's ear," is an inflammation and infection (bacterial or fungal) of the auricle and external auditory canal (EAC). Typical symptoms include otalgia, pruritus, otorrhea, and hearing loss. Physical examination reveals EAC hyperemia and edema (Fig. 5.12), otorrhea, malodorous discharge, occlusion from debris and swelling, pain with manipulation of the tragus, and periauricular lymphadenopathy.

Several factors predispose the EAC to infection: increased humidity and heat, water immersion, foreign bodies, trauma, hearing aids, and cerumen impaction. Bacterial OE is primarily an infection due to *Pseudomonas* species or *Staphylococcus aureus*. Diabetics are particularly prone to infections by *Pseudomonas, Candida albicans,* and, less commonly, *Aspergillus niger* (Fig. 5.13).

Differential Diagnosis

Cholesteatomas and foreign bodies can produce a secondary OE. Periauricular cellulitis, herpes zoster oticus (Fig. 5.14), and malignant otitis externa have auricular and facial involvement. EAC dermatitis, eczema, and furuncles rarely produce EAC drainage.

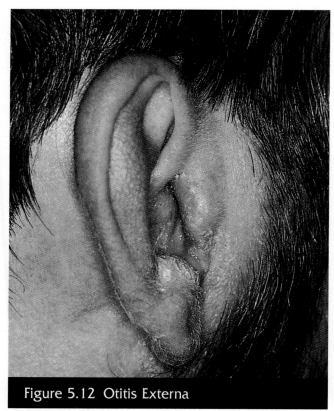

Figure 5.12 Otitis Externa

A discharge is seen coming from the external auditory canal, which is swollen and almost completely occluded. An ear wick placed in the EAC facilitates delivery of topical antibiotic suspension and drainage of debris. (Courtesy of Frank Birinyi, MD.)

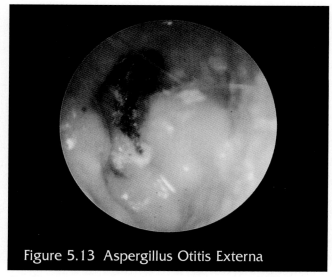

Figure 5.13 Aspergillus Otitis Externa

Chronic otitis externa with copious debris, including black spores from *Aspergillus niger,* cottony fungal elements, and wet debris. This patient had been treated with topical and systemic antibiotics. (Courtesy of C. Bruce MacDonald, MD.)

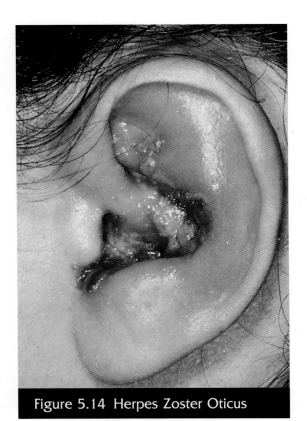

Figure 5.14 Herpes Zoster Oticus

Erythema and drainage coming from the EAC is seen in this patient with herpes zoster oticus. Otitis externa can have a similar appearance but does not have vesicles, as seen in this patient. (Courtesy of Robin T. Cotton, MD.)

Emergency Department Treatment and Disposition

Saline irrigation and suctioning is recommended to thoroughly evaluate the EAC. Topical antibiotic *suspensions* (containing polymyxin, neomycin, and hydrocortisone or ciprofloxacin) with ear wicks are effective. Topical *solutions* are not pH-balanced and thus are irritating and may cause inflammation in the middle ear if a perforation is present. Systemic antibiotics are not indicated unless extension into the periauricular tissues is noted. Patients should avoid swimming and prevent water from entering the ear while bathing. Dry heat aids in resolution, and analgesics provide symptomatic relief. Follow-up should be arranged in 10 days for routine cases.

Clinical Pearls

1. Resistant cases may have an allergic or edematous component. These typically present with a dry, scaly, itchy EAC and are recurrent and chronic in nature.
2. Drying the EAC after water exposure with a 50:50 mixture of isopropyl alcohol and water or with acetic acid (white vinegar) minimizes recurrence. If the TM is possibly perforated, isopropyl alcohol should be avoided.
3. Often the symptoms are out of proportion to the visible findings, necessitating narcotic analgesia.

Associated Clinical Features

Mastoiditis or acute coalescent mastoiditis is an infection or inflammation of the mastoid air cells that usually results from extension of purulent otitis media with progressive destruction and coalescence of air cells. Medial wall erosion can cause cavernous sinus thrombosis, facial nerve palsy, meningitis, brain abscess, and sepsis. With the use of antibiotics for acute otitis media, the incidence of mastoiditis has fallen sharply.

Patients present with fever, chills, postauricular ear pain, and frequently discharge from the external auditory canal. Patients may have tenderness, erythema, swelling, and fluctuance over the mastoid process; lateral displacement of the pinna (Fig. 5.15); erythema of the posterior-superior external auditory canal wall; and purulent otorrhea through a tympanic membrane perforation.

Differential Diagnosis

Postauricular abscesses, furuncles, suppurative adenitis, lymphadenitis, and, rarely, carcinomas of the mastoid can present with signs and symptoms of acute mastoiditis.

Emergency Department Treatment and Disposition

Initial evaluation includes a thorough head, neck, and cranial nerve examination while mastoid radiographs may demonstrate coalescence of the mastoid air cells. Computed tomography, the diagnostic procedure of choice, may reveal bony extension and intracranial involvement.

Penicillinase-resistant penicillins, amoxicillin-clavulanic acid, second-generation cephalosporins, and the newer macrolides are effective in mild cases of mastoiditis. Severe cases require parenteral semisynthetic penicillins, cephalosporins, or vancomycin. Mastoiditis requires close follow-up and prompt consultation.

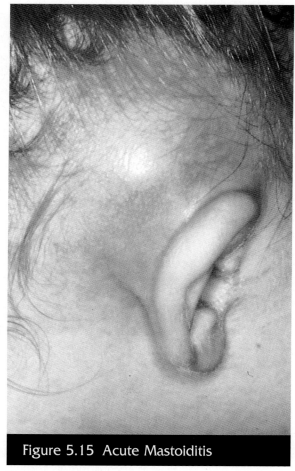

Figure 5.15 Acute Mastoiditis

Postauricular swelling and redness in a young girl with acute mastoiditis. (Courtesy of Robin T. Cotton, MD.)

Clinical Pearls

1. Most patients require admission for parenteral antibiotics to cover *Haemophilus influenzae, Moraxella catarrhalis,* streptococcal species, and *Staphylococcus aureus.*
2. Surgical irrigation and debridement and possibly mastoidectomy are reserved for refractory cases.
3. Delays in treatment can result in significant morbidity and mortality.
4. Chronic mastoiditis describes chronic otorrhea of at least 2 months duration. It is often associated with craniofacial anomalies.

Associated Clinical Features

Perichondritis is an infection of the auricular cartilage. It can result from direct trauma; traumatic hematomas; thermal injuries, typically frostbite; foreign bodies in the external auditory canal; chronic otitis media; otitis externa; skin infections; chronic mastoiditis; acupuncture and surgical procedures on the ear. Destruction and necrosis of the auricular cartilage can lead to a flaccid, flat ear.

The microbiology of perichondritis reflects the source of infection. Infections of skin structures and trauma involve streptococci and staphylococci. Ear and mastoid sources frequently involve gram-negative organisms. Untreated perichondritis in elderly diabetic and immunocompromised patients can lead to malignant external otitis.

Patients present with severe pain and diffuse swelling of the ear. Physical examination reveals an erythematous, swollen, warm and tender pinna (Fig. 5.16). Advanced cases can progress to necrosis of the ear cartilage (chondritis) and spreading cellulitis.

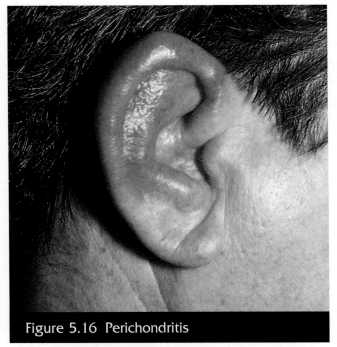

Figure 5.16 Perichondritis

The pinna is swollen and erythematous. No concomitant otitis externa, mastoiditis, or furuncle is noted. (Courtesy of Lawrence B. Stack, MD.)

Differential Diagnosis

Periauricular cellulitis can mimic perichondritis but has facial involvement. Auricular hematomas follow direct trauma. Contact dermatitis can develop from topical ear medications and jewelry. The first episode of relapsing polychondritis may be difficult to distinguish from perichondritis. The absence of fever and history of previous cartilage involvement suggests relapsing polychondritis.

Emergency Department Treatment and Disposition

Immediate treatment of perichondritis is essential to preserve the external ear cartilage. Early perichondritis is treated by irrigation and debridement of any abscess, with administration of broad-spectrum antibiotics such as penicillinase-resistant penicillins, amoxicillin-clavulanate, or ciprofloxacin. Topical antibiotics are ineffective. A compressive mastoid and auricular dressing is beneficial. Strict follow-up is essential to prevent treatment failure and progression of infection. Advanced perichondritis requires high-dose parenteral antibiotics and early specialist referral for surgical irrigation and debridement.

Clinical Pearl

1. Early diagnosis and treatment are necessary to avoid permanent deformity of the pinna.

Associated Clinical Features

Septal hematomas are an uncommon complication of direct trauma to the nose. While often associated with fracture of the nasal septum with or without concomitant nasal bone fracture, the trauma is typically minor. Septal hematomas may also result from septal surgery or rhinoplasty. Regardless of the mechanism, bleeding from submucosal blood vessels leads to an accumulation of blood between the mucoperichondrium and the septal cartilage. Pressure exerted by the hematoma on the septal cartilage and its blood supply may lead to ischemic avascular necrosis of the underlying cartilage, causing destruction of the cartilage and deformity of the distal nose (saddle deformity). The hematoma and any necrotic cartilage may then serve as a nidus for infection, resulting in a septal abscess.

In addition to the cosmetic nasal deformity, septal hematomas and deformity may lead to chronic sinus infections, recurrent epistaxis, and sleep disturbances. Rarely, septal abscesses can result in more serious complications such as cavernous sinus thrombosis and meningitis. Since the original trauma is often minor, patients may present days to weeks after the injury. Young children and infants may present with poor feeding, fever, and rhinorrhea, while older children and adults may note bleeding, headache, and more focal pain. Patients with obvious nasal fractures tend to present earlier.

On nasal examination, the hematoma appears as a large, red, round swelling originating off the septum and occluding most of the nasal cavity (Fig. 5.17). The mass is very painful to palpation and may cause the outer aspects of the nose to be tender as well. Septal abscesses tend to be more painful and larger than uncomplicated hematomas. Constitutional symptoms such as fever are frequently present. The microbiology of septal abscesses reflects the normal flora of the nasal cavity. *Staphylococcus aureus,* group A β-hemolytic streptococcus, *Haemophilus influenzae,* and *Streptococcus pneumoniae* are the organisms most commonly isolated.

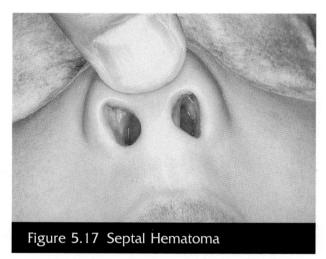

Figure 5.17 Septal Hematoma

A septal hematoma is seen in both nares in this child. (Courtesy of Robin T. Cotton, MD.)

Differential Diagnosis

Septal abscesses, foreign bodies, and nasal polyps may also appear as masses in the nasal cavity.

Emergency Department Treatment and Disposition

An index of suspicion and prompt recognition are essential in diagnosing septal hematomas. Once identified, prompt referral to an otolaryngologist is mandatory for incision of the hematoma and drainage through the mucosal surface. Purulent drainage should be sent for microbiology and culture.

Many authors recommend packing of the nasal cavity to prevent further accumulation. Other surgeons use temporary drains, such as a Penrose, while still others place dissolvable sutures in the mucoperichondrium to prevent hematoma reaccumulation.

Clinical Pearls

1. Intranasal examination in all patients with a history of nasal trauma regardless of severity is crucial.
2. Antibiotics are required in septal hematomas with a clinical suspicion for a secondary infection or abscess.
3. The physician must explore the possibility of child abuse in young children and infants with septal hematomas and abscesses.

Associated Clinical Features

Herpes zoster oticus (HZO), or Ramsay Hunt syndrome, is the second most common cause of facial paralysis, representing 3 to 12% of such patients. The syndrome consists of facial and neck pain, acoustic symptoms, and facial palsy associated with the reactivation of varicella zoster in the facial nerve and geniculate ganglion (Figs. 5.18 and 5.19; see also Fig. 5.14). Patients first note a pruritus, followed by pain out of proportion to the physical examination over the face and ear. Patients may note vertigo, hearing loss (sensorineural) from involvement of the eighth cranial nerve, tinnitus, rapid onset of facial paralysis, decrease in salivation, loss of taste sensation over the posterolateral tongue, and vesicles on the ear, external auditory canal, and face.

Differential Diagnosis

Cerebrovascular accidents develop acutely and do not produce pain in the face or external auditory canal. Facial paralysis from temporal bone fractures is associated with antecedent trauma.

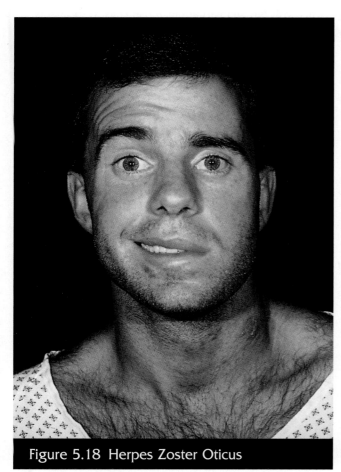

Figure 5.18 Herpes Zoster Oticus

Facial palsy in a young adult. Note the vesicular eruptions on the neck. (Courtesy of Frank Birinyi, MD.)

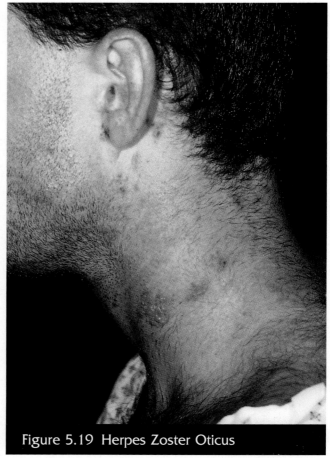

Figure 5.19 Herpes Zoster Oticus

On closer examination, the vesicles extend up the neck to the external auditory canal. (Courtesy of Frank Birinyi, MD.)

Ménière's disease can be confused with early HZO but is painless and does not cause facial paralysis.

Emergency Department Treatment and Disposition

The diagnosis of HZO is based largely on history and physical examination. Tzanck preparations may be difficult because of the vesicles' location. Magnetic resonance imaging (MRI) with contrast may show enhancement of the geniculate ganglion and facial nerve, but it is not required to make the diagnosis.

Oral acyclovir, 800 mg five times a day for 7 to 10 days, or famciclovir, 500 mg tid for 7 days in combination with oral steroids (such as prednisone 60 to 80 mg/day) are the mainstays for HZO treatment. It is important to protect the involved eye from corneal abrasions and ulcerations by using lubricating drops.

Clinical Pearl

1. The prognosis for facial paralysis due to HZO is worse than that for Bell's palsy. Approximately 10 and 66% of patients with full and partial facial paralysis, respectively, recover fully. The prognosis improves if the symptoms of HZO are preceded by the vesicular eruption.

Associated Clinical Features

The seventh cranial or facial nerve provides innervation of the facial muscles via the five branches of the motor root; it innervates the submandibular, sublingual, and lacrimal glands as well as the taste organs on the anterior two-thirds of the tongue and provides sensation to the pinna of the ear. A seventh-nerve palsy may occur as an isolated finding or as part of a constellation of symptoms. Facial palsies are classified as being either central or peripheral. Central seventh-nerve lesions occur before or proximal to the seventh-nerve nucleus in the pons. Lesions that occur distal to the nucleus are classified as peripheral lesions. The hallmark of central lesions is the sparing of the ipsilateral frontalis muscle (Fig. 5.20), since it receives innervation in the nucleus from both ipsilateral and contralateral motor cortices. Peripheral injuries involve the entire side of the face, including the forehead (Fig. 5.21).

The most common etiology of seventh-nerve dysfunction is Bell's palsy, an idiopathic facial nerve dysfunction. Bell's palsy is most likely a viral or postviral syndrome, with 60% of patients having a viral prodrome. Bell's palsy shows no age, sex, or racial predilection. The incidence is higher in pregnant women, diabetics, and those with a family history of Bell's palsy. It is bilateral in less than 1% of patients.

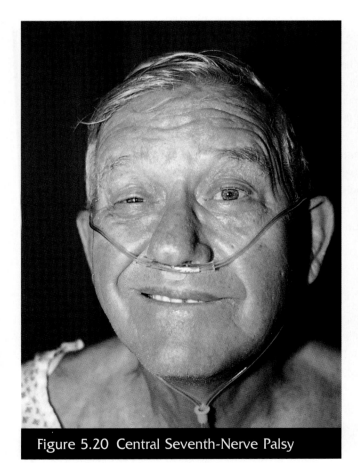

Figure 5.20 Central Seventh-Nerve Palsy

Central facial nerve paralysis with forehead sparing. (Courtesy of Frank Birinyi, MD.)

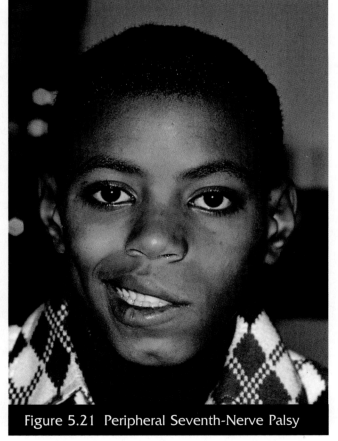

Figure 5.21 Peripheral Seventh-Nerve Palsy

A peripheral nerve paralysis involving the entire ipsilateral face, including the forehead, is seen in this patient with Bell's palsy. (Courtesy of Robin T. Cotton, MD.)

Patients with Bell's palsy have an acute onset of facial weakness and may note numbness or pain on the ipsilateral face, ear, tongue, and neck as well as a decrease or loss of ipsilateral tearing and saliva flow. Hearing in Bell's palsy is preserved.

The prognosis for facial nerve palsies is variable. Facial weakness—as compared with complete paralysis—has a better prognosis for full recovery. Facial palsies due to herpes zoster have a protracted course, and many do not fully resolve. In comparison, 80% of patients with Bell's palsy due to other causes completely recover within 3 months. The recurrence rate of Bell's palsy is 7 to 10%.

Differential Diagnosis

Acoustic neuromas and central nervous system masses have gradual progression of symptoms and cause other neurologic findings. Neurologic disorders—such as Guillain-Barré syndrome, multiple sclerosis, neurosarcoid, and cerebrovascular accidents—also cause additional neurologic sequelae. Temporal bone fractures are associated with trauma. The differential diagnosis also includes infections (otitis media, otitis externa, HIV) and parotid tumors.

Emergency Department Treatment and Disposition

Initial evaluation is directed by the history. The examination should include a thorough examination of the ear (including sensorineural or conductive hearing loss), the eye (including lacrimation), and the cranial nerves. Motor function of the seventh cranial nerve is evaluated by having the patient raise his or her eyebrows, smile, pucker, and frown. No single laboratory test is diagnostic. Screening CT or MRI of the head is of little value in the absence of additional findings on physical examination.

Most authors empirically recommend steroids and antiherpetic antivirals for Bell's palsy. A typical regimen is prednisone, 60 mg a day for 10 days, then tapered, in combination with acylovir, famcylovir, or valacyclovir. If treated within the first 3 weeks, steroids may decrease the sequelae of Bell's palsy. In all facial nerve palsies, eye lubricants and taping or patching of the eye at night help prevent keratitis and ulceration. Referral to a specialist should be made for follow-up care.

Clinical Pearls

1. Facial nerve paralysis is a symptom, not a diagnosis. The etiology of the paralysis must be known before a diagnosis can be made.
2. If a provisional diagnosis of Bell's palsy is made and no resolution of symptoms occurs, the diagnosis must be reconsidered. In patients misdiagnosed with Bell's palsy, tumors are the most common missed etiology.
3. Lacrimation is tested by the Schirmer's or litmus test. Asymmetry may indicate a lesion proximal to the geniculate ganglion.

Associated Clinical Features

Angioedema is clinically characterized by acute onset of well-demarcated cutaneous swelling of the face, lips, and tongue; edema of the mucous membranes of the mouth, throat, or abdominal viscera; or nonpitting edema of the hands and feet. Angioedema is classified as either hereditary, allergic, or idiopathic. Hereditary angioedema is an autosomal dominant trait associated with a deficiency of serum inhibitor of the activated first component of complement (C1). Allergic angioedema can result from medications [nonsteroidal anti-inflammatory drugs (NSAIDs), contrast agents], environmental antigens (Hymenoptera), or local trauma. Whatever the cause, angioedema can be a life-threatening illness. Complications of angioedema range from dysphagia and dysphonia to respiratory distress, airway obstruction (Fig. 5.22), and death. Of special interest is angiotensin converting enzyme (ACE) inhibitor–induced angioedema. Angioedema due to ACE inhibitors has a predilection for involvement of the lips (Fig. 5.23), face, tongue, and glottis. Standard treatment practices for allergic urticaria often fail to improve ACE inhibitor–induced angioedema; in those who do improve, rebound is frequently seen.

Differential Diagnosis

Anaphylaxis and asthma occur in patients with histories of similar events and involve the lower airways. Patients with epiglottitis, Ludwig's angina, and peritonsillar or retropharyngeal abscesses often have a preceding pharyngeal or odontogenic infection and present with systemic symptoms of infection, such as fever and chills.

Emergency Department Treatment and Disposition

Initial treatment of angioedema is airway management. Most patients do not require intervention, but frequent reassessment of the patient's airway is mandatory. Airway interventions include nasopharyngeal intubation, endotracheal intubation (often difficult due to lingual and oral obstruction), or nasotracheal intubation (either blindly or with fiberoptics), or a cricothyrotomy.

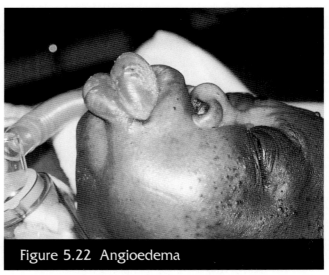

Figure 5.22 Angioedema

Severe angioedema of the face and tongue requiring emergent cricothyrotomy. (Courtesy of W. Brian Gibler, MD.)

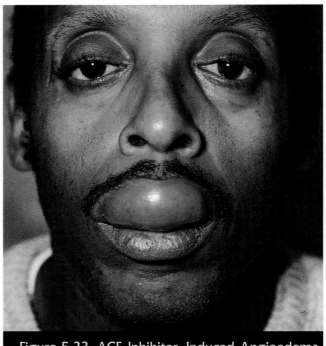

Figure 5.23 ACE Inhibitor–Induced Angioedema

Angioedema of the upper lip in a man who had been taking an ACE inhibitor for 2 years. The patient had no previous episodes. (Courtesy of Kevin J. Knoop, MD, MS.)

Acute angioedema is treated similarly to an allergic reaction. Depending on the severity of symptoms, it can be treated with steroids, antihistamines—both H_1 and H_2 blockers—and subcutaneous epinephrine. Chronic angioedema responds better to corticosteroids and H_2 blockers, but airway protection remains the primary focus of emergency treatment. Hereditary angioedema is more refractory to medical interventions; epinephrine, corticosteroids, and antihistamines provide little relief.

Disposition depends on the severity and resolution of symptoms. Patients whose symptoms significantly improve or show no progression after 4 h of observation may be discharged home on a short course of oral steroids and antihistamines. Any medication which may have caused the angioedema should be discontinued. Angioedema with airway involvement requires admission to a monitored environment, with surgical airway instruments always at the bedside.

Clinical Pearls

1. Do not underestimate the degree of airway involvement; act early to preserve airway patency.
2. Angioedema can also cause gastrointestinal and neurologic involvement.
3. Early response to medical intervention does not preclude rebound of symptoms to a greater extent than at presentation.
4. Patients who have been using ACE inhibitors for months or years can still develop angioedema.

Associated Clinical Features

Pharyngitis is an inflammation and frequently an infection of the pharynx and its lymphoid tissues, which make up Waldeyer's ring. Most causes of pharyngitis are infectious and self-limited, with viral infections accounting for 90% of all cases. Common bacterial agents include group A beta-hemolytic streptococci (GABHS, responsible for up to 50% of bacterial cases), other streptococci, *Mycoplasma pneumoniae, Neisseria gonorrhea,* and *Corynebacterium diphtheriae.* In immunocompromised patients and patients on antibiotics, *Candida* species can cause thrush. Sore throats that last longer than 2 weeks should increase suspicion for either a deep-space neck infection or a neoplastic cause.

Patients with bacterial and especially GABHS pharyngitis present with an acute onset of sore throat and fever and frequently nausea, vomiting, headache, and abdominal cramping. On examination, they may have a mild to moderate fever, an erythematous posterior pharynx and palatine tonsils, tender cervical lymphadenopathy, and palatal petechiae (Fig. 5.24). Classically, the tonsils have a white or yellow exudate with debris in the crypts; however, many patients may not have exudate on examination. Viral pharyngitis is typically more benign, with a gradual onset, lower temperature, and less impressive erythema and swelling of the pharynx. Except for infectious mononucleosis, which can take weeks to resolve, most cases of viral pharyngitis are self-limited, with spontaneous resolution in a matter of days. Lingual and adenoid tonsillitis may also be present (Fig. 5.25).

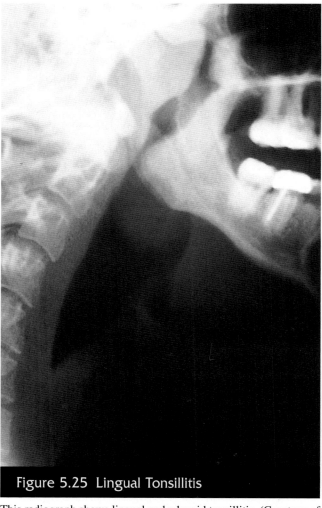

Figure 5.25 Lingual Tonsillitis

This radiograph shows lingual and adenoid tonsillitis. (Courtesy of Edward C. Jauch, MD, MS.)

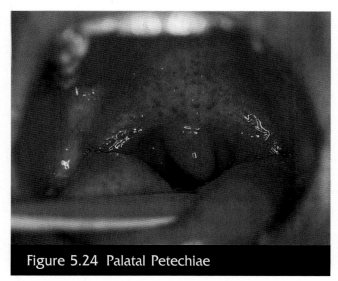

Figure 5.24 Palatal Petechiae

Palatal petechiae and erythema of the tonsillar pillars in a patient with streptococcal pharyngitis. (Courtesy of Kevin J. Knoop, MD, MS.)

Differential Diagnosis

Deep-space neck infections, diphtheria, epiglottitis, infectious mononucleosis, and Ludwig's angina are other infectious causes of sore throats that should be considered. Allergic rhinitis, angioedema, and pharyngeal neoplasms are noninfectious causes of similar pharyngeal symptoms. Foreign bodies and local pharyngeal trauma produce similar symptoms but usually have an antecedent event.

Emergency Department Treatment and Disposition

Treatment is largely symptomatic except for antibiotics and rehydration. Patients with known or suspected GABHS require antibiotics primarily to prevent the severe sequelae of the infection, including rheumatic fever and glomerulonephritis, and suppurative complications. Current first-line antibiotic therapies remain a single dose of intramuscular benzathine penicillin or oral penicillin for 10 days. Patients allergic to penicillin should receive erythromycin for primary prophylaxis against rheumatic fever. Other suitable antibiotics include azithromycin or clarithromycin and second-generation cephalosporins. Analgesics, antipyretics, and throat sprays or gargles can provide symptomatic relief.

Clinical Pearls

1. The physical examination should not end at the neck. Auscultation of the chest, palpation of the abdomen, and examination of the skin are also important.
2. Sore throats or chronic pharyngitis that lasts more than 2 weeks must be referred for further evaluation to rule out possible neoplastic or neurologic causes, especially in patients over 50 years old who have a smoking or chewing tobacco history.
3. Recurrent tonsillitis in children merits referral for possible adenoid-tonsillectomy.
4. Amoxicillin should be avoided if infectious mononucleosis is a possibility, as a diffuse maculopapular rash will occur in up to 80%.
5. Pharyngitis itself may be a prodrome for other pathologic conditions, such as measles, scarlet fever, and influenza.

Associated Clinical Features

Diphtheria is a highly contagious disease caused by the exotoxin-producing bacterium *Corynebacterium diphtheriae*. It is transmitted either by direct contact or through respiratory aerosolization in coughing or sneezing. Many adults are now susceptible to diphtheria because their vaccine-induced immunity decreases over time or owing to decreased opportunity for naturally acquired immunity. Because of this, recent outbreaks have involved adolescents and adults rather than children.

Prior to the widespread implementation of childhood vaccines in the 1940s, diphtheria was associated with significant childhood mortality. While the United States has only episodic cases of diphtheria, the incidence worldwide is increasing dramatically because of decreased immunization rates in developing countries. In the new republics of the former Soviet Union, over 160,000 new cases and 5000 deaths were reported in the recent epidemic.

Diphtheria most commonly affects the mucosa of the upper respiratory tract and less commonly the mucosa of the nasopharynx, nares, or tracheobronchial tract. Diphtheria typically produces an ulcerated pharyngeal mucosa with a white to gray inflammatory pseudomembrane (Fig. 5.26), classically with a "wet mouse" odor. Patients present with symptoms, in order of frequency, of fever, sore throat, weakness, pain with swallowing, change in voice, loss of appetite, neck swelling, difficulty breathing, and nasal discharge.

While the organism remains localized to the mucosa, hematogenous spread of the exotoxin typically produces myocarditis or peripheral neuropathies. Deaths from diphtheria occur either from tracheobronchial obstruction by the pseudomembrane acutely or cardiac complications during the several weeks after the primary infection.

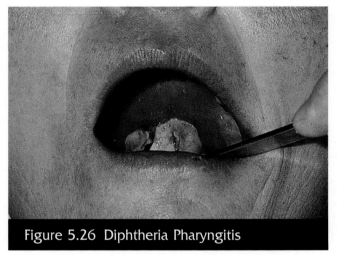

Figure 5.26 Diphtheria Pharyngitis

An exudative pharyngitis with a gray pseudomembrane is seen in this patient with diphtheria. (Courtesy of Peter Strebel, MBChB, MPH, and the *Journal of Infectious Diseases.*)

Differential Diagnosis

The differential diagnosis for exudative pharyngitis is broad (see "Pharyngitis," above). Other pathogens that can cause a membranous pharyngitis include *Streptococcus* species, Epstein-Barr virus and cytomegalovirus, and *Candida*.

Emergency Department Treatment and Disposition

The diagnosis of diphtheria is initially made clinically. The definitive diagnosis is made by successful isolation and toxigenicity testing of *C. diphtheriae*. Cultures should be taken from beneath the membrane and rapidly placed on a special culture medium containing tellurite. Histopathologic analysis may also confirm the disease. The Centers for Disease Control and Prevention (CDC) is investigating a new polymerase chain reaction (PCR) test for the presence of the diphtheria toxin gene.

Treatment is dependent on making the appropriate diagnosis. Antitoxin, only available from the CDC (telephone: 404-639-2889), is the mainstay of therapy and must be given before laboratory confirmation. Similarly, erythromycin or penicillin, the drugs of choice in treating diphtheria, should be given promptly when diphtheria is suspected. The recommended treatment course for either agent is 14 days. Antibiotics have been shown to decrease both exotoxin production and spread of the bacterium.

Many patients require hospital admission for airway precautions, pulmonary support, and intravenous hydration and antibiotics. Strict isolation is essential for patients with diphtheria, along with proper disposal of all articles soiled by a patient. All cases should reported to local public health officials to assist in identifying contacts.

Clinical Pearls

1. Outcome is improved with early treatment; thus the diagnosis of diphtheria must be made clinically and treatment begun empirically before bacteriologic confirmation.
2. Patients with a membranous pharyngitis need to be questioned regarding immunization, exposures, and travel history.
3. All contacts should have a booster dose of vaccine (TD or Td, depending on age) while nonimmune contacts should also be given prophylactic antibiotics after a throat swab.
4. Travelers to endemic areas must be current with their diphtheria vaccinations.

Associated Clinical Features

Peritonsillar abscess, or quinsy, is the most common deep neck infection. Although most occur in young adults, immunocompromised and diabetic patients are at increased risk. Most abscesses develop as a complication of tonsillitis or pharyngitis, but they can also result from odontogenic spread, recent dental procedures, and local mucosal trauma. They recur in 10 to 15% of patients.

The pathogens involved are similar to those causing tonsillitis, especially streptococcal species, but many infections are polymicrobial and involve anaerobic bacteria. Patients present with a fever, severe sore throat that is often out of proportion to physical findings, localization of symptoms to one side of the throat, trismus, drooling, dysphagia, dysphonia, fetid breath, and ipsilateral ear pain.

During the early stages, the tonsil and anterior pillar are erythematous, appear full, and may be shifted medially. Later, the uvula and soft palate are shifted to the contralateral side (Fig. 5.27). The tonsillar pillar may feel fluctuant and tender on palpation.

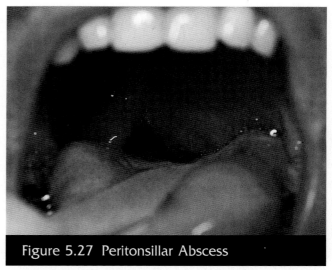

Figure 5.27 Peritonsillar Abscess

Acute peritonsillar abscess showing medial displacement of the uvula, palatine tonsil, and anterior pillar. Some trismus is present, as demonstrated by patient's inability to open the mouth maximally. (Courtesy of Kevin J. Knoop, MD, MS.)

Differential Diagnosis

Ludwig's angina, odontogenic neck infections, peritonsillar cellulitis, and retropharyngeal abscesses can be confused with peritonsillar abscesses. Angioedema has a rapid onset of symptoms, whereas oral neoplasms develop slowly.

Emergency Department Treatment and Disposition

Most patients with signs of an abscess can have a needle aspiration performed as the sole surgical drainage procedure and can expect a satisfactory outcome. Alternative surgical drainage procedures—including incision and drainage and abscess tonsillectomy—can be performed by an otolaryngologist or oral surgeon. Most can be managed as outpatients on oral antibiotics following drainage. Patients who are immunocompromised, have airway involvement, appear toxic, or cannot tolerate oral intake require admission for rehydration, parenteral antibiotics, and specialty consultation.

Studies to date are divided on the incidence of penicillin-resistant organisms in peritonsillar abscesses. Although penicillin alone is arguably a good first choice, penicillin and metronidazole, amoxicillin with clavulanate, clindamycin, or third-generation cephalosporins are also suitable antibiotic choices.

Clinical Pearl

1. The value of culturing aspirates is questionable, with a review of several studies showing no clinical benefit from the cultures unless the patient is immunocompromised.

Associated Clinical Features

The uvula is the fleshy midline extension of the soft palate that hangs from the roof of the mouth. Except for idiopathic, the two most common causes of uvular enlargement are infections and angioedema. Most patients complain of a sore throat, a gagging sensation, or a foreign-body sensation in the back of the mouth.

The infectious etiologies of uvulitis are bacterial, including *Haemophilus influenzae* and streptococci; fungal, such as *Candida albicans;* and viral. Infections of the uvula are typically extensions from adjacent infections, such as epiglottitis, tonsillitis, peritonsillar abscesses, and pharyngitis.

With infectious uvulitis, patients note fever, odynophagia, trismus, facial pain, hoarseness, neck pain, and headache. On examination the uvula is red, firm, swollen, and very tender to palpation.

Angioedema of the uvula, known as Quincke's disease, can be hereditary, acquired, or idiopathic. Medications, allergens, thermal stimuli, pressure, and iatrogenic or accidental trauma can initiate angioedema. In addition to the swollen uvula, patients may note pruritus, urticaria, and wheezing. With uvular edema, the angioedema may involve the face, tongue, and oropharynx. Airway compromise is more common in angioedema of the uvula. The uvula with angioedema appears pale, boggy, and edematous, resembling a large white grape (uvular hydrops) (Fig. 5.28).

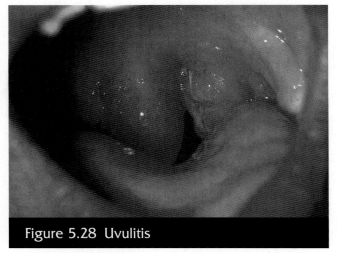

Figure 5.28 Uvulitis

Angioedema of the uvula, known as Quincke's disease. (Courtesy of Robin T. Cotton, MD.)

Differential Diagnosis

Benign polyps and neoplasms cause asymmetry of the palate or uvula. Cellulitis and peritonsillar abscesses may also cause uvular distortion.

Emergency Department Treatment and Disposition

Most cases of uvulitis are benign and self-limited. Angioedematous uvulitis is treated like any angioedema. Administration of steroids, antihistamines—both H_1 and H_2 blockers, and epinephrine, either subcutaneously or nebulized, may provide symptomatic relief. For infectious uvulitis, antibiotic coverage is dictated by the primary source of infection. For odontogenic infections, pharyngitis, or tonsillitis with uvulitis, penicillin, clindamycin, or amoxicillin with clavulanate are effective. Epiglottitis associated with uvulitis requires potent *H. influenzae* coverage, such as third-generation cephalosporins. Admission is based on severity of airway compromise and accompanying infections.

Clinical Pearls

1. Although the incidence of concomitant epiglottitis has decreased dramatically, any airway symptom dictates an evaluation of the hypopharynx, either by soft tissue lateral neck radiograph, fiber-optic nasopharyngoscope, or direct laryngoscopy.
2. If the uvula itself is causing enough airway compromise, uvular decompression by longitudinal incisions or a partial uvulectomy can be performed.

Associated Clinical Features

Epiglottitis or supraglottitis is an infection of the supraglottic structures including the epiglottis, aryepiglottic folds, arytenoids, and periepiglottic soft tissues. Bacterial epiglottitis, a rare but potentially fatal infection, is caused primarily by *Haemophilus influenzae,* but *Streptococcus pneumoniae, Staphylococcus aureus,* and β-hemolytic streptococcus have been isolated. The advent of the *H. influenzae* B vaccination for infants has changed what used to be a disease primarily of children, with a peak age range from 2 to 6 years, to one found increasingly in adults. Bacterial epiglottitis occurs most commonly in the winter and spring but may appear at any time.

Patients, especially children, with acute epiglottitis appear quite ill. They present with sore throat, fever, drooling, severe dysphagia, dyspnea, muffled or hoarse voice, and occasionally inspiratory stridor. Patients with severe respiratory distress assume the "tripod" position: sitting upright with the neck extended, arms supporting the trunk, and the jaw thrust forward. This position maximizes airway patency and caliber. Adults typically have an indolent course with a prodromal viral illness, but many children have a sudden onset and rapid progression to respiratory distress.

Differential Diagnosis

Croup, bacterial tracheitis, lingual tonsillitis, and retropharyngeal abscesses are other infectious causes of respiratory distress. Angioedema and foreign bodies cause a sudden onset of acute respiratory distress without antecedent illnesses.

Acquired and congenital subglottic stenosis and intrinsic and extrinsic masses may produce similar airway symptoms.

Emergency Department Treatment and Disposition

Airway management is paramount. Even prior to diagnosis, children should be calmed, comforted by a parent, and allowed to assume whatever position they feel is most comfortable. Anesthesiology and ENT should be consulted immediately. Indications for intubation are clinical, but severe stridor and respiratory distress are clear reasons to intervene. Nasotracheal intubation in children is preferred but not when performed blindly. Needle cricothyrotomy can provide temporary oxygenation until a surgical airway is provided.

Radiographs of the neck may reveal the classic "thumb" sign, a thickened epiglottis on the lateral soft-tissue neck radiograph (Fig. 5.29). Visualization of the epiglottis is possible in the stable adult patient via direct and indirect laryngoscopy and fiberoptic nasopharyngoscopy (Fig. 5.30). The airway orifice may be difficult to see because of the extreme distortion of tissues. In children, the top of the swollen

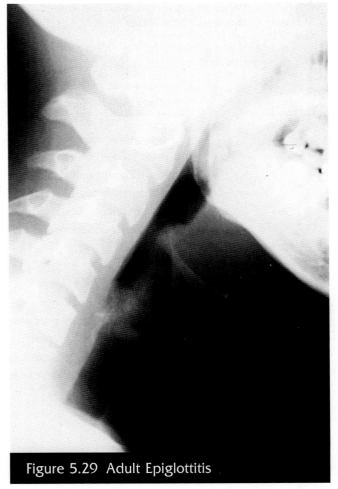

Figure 5.29 Adult Epiglottitis

Soft-tissue lateral neck radiograph of an adult with epiglottitis demonstrating the classic "thumb" sign of a swollen epiglottis. (Courtesy of Kevin J. Knoop, MD, MS.)

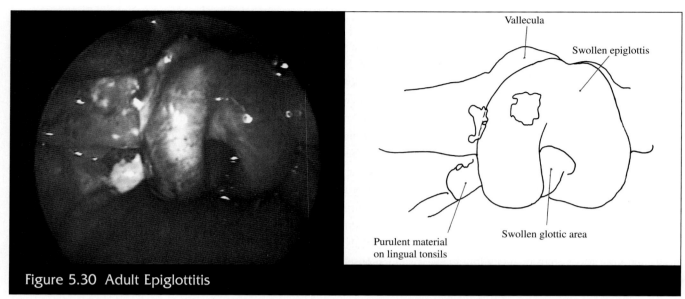

Figure 5.30 Adult Epiglottitis

Fiberoptic laryngoscopy showing a red, edematous epiglottis and glottic area with marked airway compromise in an adult with epiglottitis. (Courtesy of Timothy L. Smith, MD.)

epiglottis may be visualized on careful oral examination, whereas pharyngoscopy is typically reserved for an experienced anesthesiologist or otolaryngologist in a controlled setting.

The mainstay of epiglottitis treatment is antibiotics. Second- and third-generation parenteral cephalosporins and ampicillin with sulbactam have proven efficacy in treating epiglottitis.

Steroids or epinephrine, either nebulized or subcutaneous, may provide some improvement in edema. Recently, helium and oxygen gas mixtures—which, owing to their lower density compared with air, improve the work of breathing and flow rates—have shown promise in delaying or even preventing intubation in some patients.

In addition to airway compromise, complications of epiglottitis include epiglottic abscesses, meningitis, pulmonary edema, pneumonia, and empyema (associated with *H. influenzae*).

Clinical Pearls

1. Transport of patients with suspected epiglottitis must be done by an experienced transport team. The airway must be secured before transport of all but the most stable patients.
2. During intubation, pushing on the patient's chest may cause a bubble to form at the airway orifice, guiding placement of the tube.
3. Failure to intervene prior to loss of the airway carries a sixfold increase in mortality.

Associated Clinical Features

Ranulas are mucoceles (mucous retention cysts) that develop in the floor of the mouth, arising from obstructed sublingual or submandibular ducts or smaller minor salivary glands. At first the cysts are small and barely noticeable, but over time they can expand outward or deeper into the neck (plunging ranula). Large cysts can displace the tongue forward and upward, making the patient uncomfortable. Unlike those with sialolithiasis, patients with ranulas may not always notice an increase in swelling associated with eating. Physical examination reveals a soft, minimally tender, translucent cyst with dilated veins running over its surface (Fig. 5.31). Unlike carcinomas, no ulceration is noted with ranulas, and they are generally softer.

Differential Diagnosis

Torus mandibularis is a hard bony growth off the lingual surface of the mandible. Obstruction of major salivary glands is often painful and intermittent. Carcinomas of the mouth are slower-growing and firm. Abscesses and local cellulitis also produce sublingual swelling.

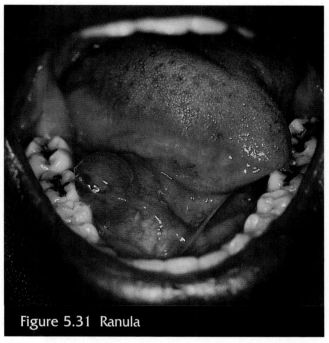

Figure 5.31 Ranula

Sublingual ranula, or mucocele, lateral to Wharton's duct. The patient was asymptomatic except for being aware of the lesion. (Courtesy of Kevin J. Knoop, MD, MS.)

Emergency Department Treatment and Disposition

Recognition by the physician is essential for proper referral. Definitive treatment is excision or marsupialization, although needle aspiration of the cyst can provide temporary relief. Unless there is a secondary infection, no antibiotic coverage is required.

Clinical Pearls

1. Most ranulas are painless and are incidental findings on routine examinations.
2. Ranulas often recur, requiring total excision of the offending salivary gland.

Associated Clinical Features

Sialoadenitis is a general term describing inflammation of any salivary gland. The three major salivary gland pairs are the parotid, submandibular, and sublingual. There are also numerous smaller salivary glands that empty into the oral cavity and all are capable of becoming inflamed. Salivary gland disorders have a broad spectrum of causes, including acute and chronic infections; metabolic, systemic, and endocrine disorders; infiltrative processes; obstructions; allergic inflammation; and neoplastic diseases. Key features in the history are the duration and course of the symptoms, complaints of pain, and unilateral or bilateral location.

Both viral and bacterial infections of the salivary gland can lead to enlarged, swollen, painful masses. Suppurative sialoadenitis is most commonly caused by *Staphylococcus aureus* and is found in patients who are elderly, diabetic, or have poor oral hygiene. It may also follow episodes of dehydration, such as those due to surgery or debilitation. Viral sialoadenitis, such as mumps parotitis, is the most common cause. It occurs with a concomitant viral illness and is usually bilateral, whereas bacterial infections are primarily unilateral.

Obstructive sialoadenitis occurs from a stone or calculus in the salivary gland or duct, most commonly in the submandibular gland. The flow of saliva is obstructed, causing swelling, pain, and firmness. Patients with sialolithiasis note general xerostomia and recurrent worsening of swelling and pain during mealtime.

A thorough head and neck examination is essential, especially a bimanual examination of the major salivary glands. In suppurative sialoadenitis, purulent drainage may be expressed from the submandibular duct (Wharton's) or parotid duct (Stensen's), and the glands are very tender and painful to examination (Figs. 5.32, 5.33). Sialolithiasis can manifest as enlargement of the ducts with minimal saliva expressed on stripping and, rarely, a palpable or visible stone (Fig. 5.34) or duct thickening. Facial radiographs are of limited utility. Ultrasound or CT may be useful to detect abscesses.

Differential Diagnosis

Tumors of the face and oropharynx, particularly primary salivary neoplasms and secondary lymphatic metastases, develop slowly and produce firm, minimally tender nodules and clear saliva. Cutaneous and odontogenic infections, angioedema variants, and lymphadenitis may mimic sialoadenitis.

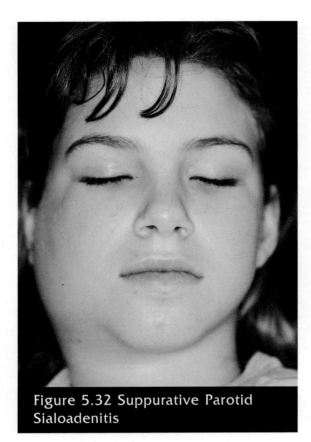

Figure 5.32 Suppurative Parotid Sialoadenitis

Painful swelling over the right parotid initially had clear saliva from Stensen's duct. (Courtesy of Kevin J. Knoop, MD, MS.)

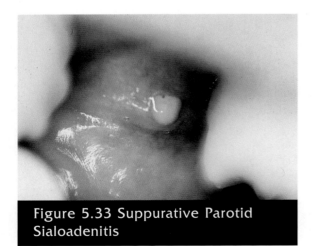

Figure 5.33 Suppurative Parotid Sialoadenitis

After applying firm pressure on the cheek, purulent discharge is seen coming from Stensen's duct. (Courtesy of Kevin J. Knoop, MD, MS.)

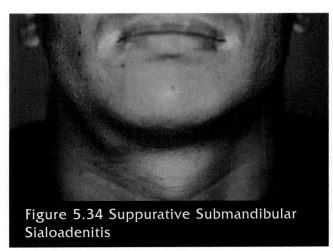

Figure 5.34 Suppurative Submandibular Sialoadenitis

Unilateral submandibular swelling. (Courtesy of Jeffery D. Bondesson, MD.)

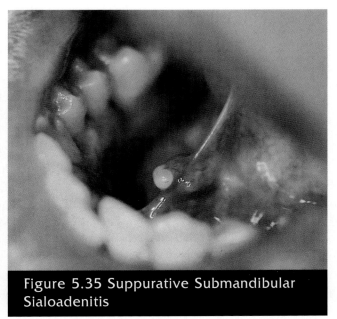

Figure 5.35 Suppurative Submandibular Sialoadenitis

After applying firm pressure, purulent discharge is seen coming from Wharton's duct. (Courtesy of Jeffery D. Bondesson, MD.)

Emergency Department Treatment and Disposition

Treatment of suppurative sialoadenitis (Figs. 5.34, 5.35) requires antibiotics with coverage of *Staphylococcus* and oral flora, rehydration, proper oral hygiene, sialogogues, local heat, and occasionally surgical irrigation and drainage of abscesses. Obstructive sialoadenitis is rarely an emergency. Most salivary stones (Fig. 5.36) pass spontaneously without complication, and patients can be discharged home on lozenges to stimulate salivary secretions and expel the stone. Prompt follow-up of sialoadenitis is essential to prevent possible morbidity and mortality associated with infections or neoplasms.

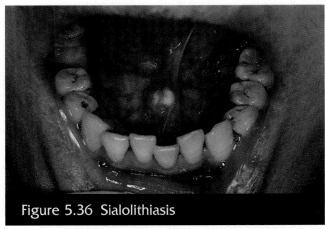

Figure 5.36 Sialolithiasis

A stone is seen at the orifice of Wharton's duct. (Courtesy of David P. Kretzschmar, DDS, MS.)

Clinical Pearls

1. Examine secretions of both mouth and eyes and elicit any history of dry eyes, keratoconjunctivitis, cutaneous lesions, or rheumatoid arthritis to establish the diagnosis of a systemic disorder.
2. Medications such as antihistamines, psychotropic drugs, and those possessing atropine-like side effects can cause xerostomia.
3. Lack of improvement on antibiotics suggests an abscess or multiple loculated abscesses that require drainage.

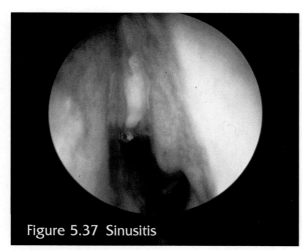

Figure 5.37 Sinusitis

Purulent drainage from the maxillary sinus ostium in a patient with maxillary sinusitis. Drainage may not always be apparent, since the ostium may be occluded from swelling and inflammation. (Courtesy of Robin T. Cotton, MD.)

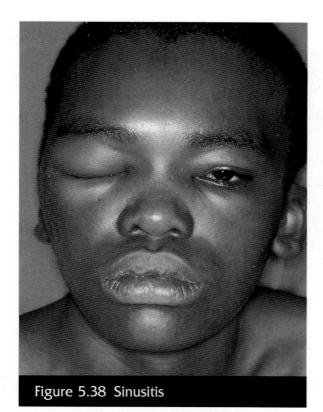

Figure 5.38 Sinusitis

Adolescent with pansinusitis complicated by periorbital cellulitis. The patient was also found to have osteomyelitis of the frontal cortex (Pott's puffy tumor). (Courtesy of Robin T. Cotton, MD.)

Associated Clinical Features

Sinusitis is an inflammation of the paranasal sinuses. Sinusitis can be classified as acute, subacute, or chronic; purulent or sterile; and allergic or nonallergic. All share an impairment of mucus clearance. Most cases of bacterial sinusitis are associated with antecedent viral upper respiratory tract infection.

Maxillary sinusitis is the most common form of sinusitis and is associated with paranasal facial pain, maxillary dental pain, purulent rhinorrhea (Fig. 5.37), retroocular pain, and conjunctivitis. Ethmoid sinusitis is more common in children and produces a low-grade fever and periorbital pain. Frontal sinusitis can cause a severe headache above the eyes, which is exacerbated by leaning forward; a low-grade fever; upper lid edema; and rhinorrhea. Sphenoid sinusitis is fortunately rare. Patients classically complain of a vertex headache and retroocular pain. Owing to its intracranial location, sphenoid sinusitis can involve several cranial nerves, the pituitary gland, and the cavernous sinus. Involvement of all sinus cavities is referred to as pansinusitis. Important complications of sinusitis include periorbital and orbital cellulitis, cavernous sinus thrombosis, and intracranial abscess (Figs. 5.38 and 5.39).

Patients with Pott's puffy tumor (a rare osteomyelitis of the cranium from direct extension of a frontal sinusitis) present with a boggy, tender swelling above the eye.

A careful history is important in patients presumed to have sinusitis. Recent steroid use, prodromal viral illness, dental work, and facial trauma are important temporal events. A history of septal deviation or defects, cystic fibrosis, smoking, and cocaine use also increases the risk of sinusitis.

Imaging modalities include transillumination of the maxillary sinuses, plain radiographs, CT, and MRI. CT is the most sensitive and specific technique and allows for better delineation of the sphenoid and ethmoid sinuses.

Common bacterial isolates are *Haemophilus influenzae*, *Streptococcus pneumoniae* (together representing 60 to 70% of all bacterial causes), *Streptococcus pyogenes*, *Staphylococcus aureus*, and *Moraxella catarrhalis*. Immunocompromised patients are susceptible to fungal infections, including *Aspergillus* and *mucor* species.

Differential Diagnosis

Other infections—including facial cellulitis, early herpes zoster, odontogenic infections, and otitis media—may produce similar signs and symptoms. Neoplasms and trigeminal neuralgia should also be considered.

Emergency Department Treatment and Disposition

For acute bacterial sinusitis, amoxicillin, macrolides, and trimethoprim-sulfamethoxazole are appropriate agents. Refractory cases or immunocompromised patients require broader-spectrum antibiotics such as amoxicillin with clavulanate, clarithromycin, second- or third-generation cephalosporins, or the newer fluoroquinolones. Treatment for up to 3 weeks may be necessary.

Decongestants reduce local edema, increase air movement within the sinuses, and decrease local secretions. A short course of topical oxymetazoline or phenylephrine as well as oral pseudoephedrine for 10 days helps minimize secretions and assists in maintaining ostia patency. Humidified air, steam, or saline nasal sprays also facilitate drainage. Patients should be strongly encouraged to stop smoking.

Parenteral steroids are not used in acute or recurrent sinusitis. Inhaled steroids, such as triamcinolone, have a role in allergic and chronic sinusitis.

Referral or follow-up by an otolaryngologist or primary care provider should be made for all patients within 3 weeks for routine cases. Patients with comorbid illnesses or more complicated sinusitis should be admitted for parenteral antibiotic therapy and supportive care.

Clinical Pearls

1. Chronic sinusitis may be due to mucoid retention cysts, deviated septum, or polyps, which are often visible on plain radiographs. Refer these patients for possible surgery.
2. Physicians must consider fungal etiologies in patients with comorbid illnesses.

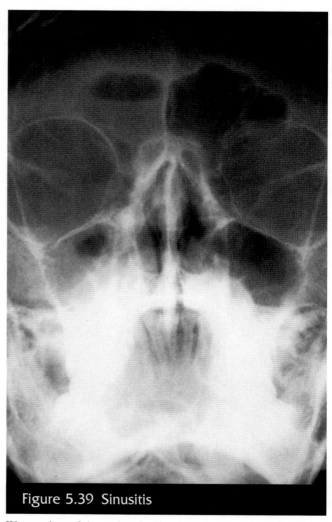

Figure 5.39 Sinusitis

Waters view of the patient in Fig. 5.37 showing an air-fluid level in the right frontal and bilateral maxillary sinuses. (Courtesy of Robin T. Cotton, MD.)

ORAL TRAUMA

CHAPTER 6

MOUTH

Edwin D. Turner*
Edward C. Jauch

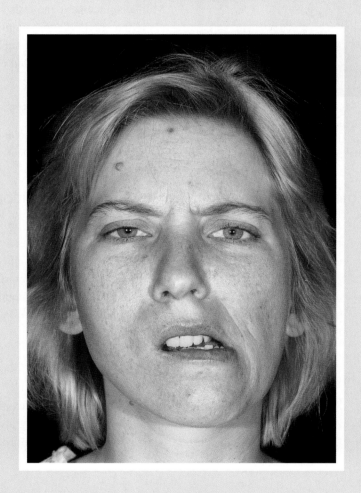

*The authors acknowledge Sara-Jo Gahm, MD, for portions of this chapter written for the first edition of this book.

Oral Trauma

TOOTH SUBLUXATION

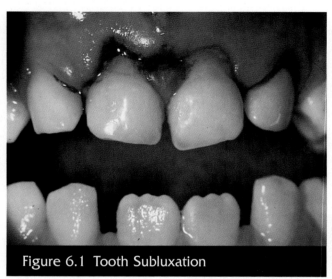

Figure 6.1 Tooth Subluxation

Note the presence of blood along the crevice of the gingival margin of both central incisors—an indication of subluxation following trauma. Mild displacement of the subluxated teeth is noted. (Courtesy of James F. Steiner, DDS.)

Associated Clinical Features

Tooth subluxation refers to the loosening of a tooth in its alveolar socket. Traumatic oral injury is a common mechanism by which dental subluxation occurs; however, infection and chronic periodontal disease may also produce loosening of teeth. Gingival lacerations and alveolar fractures are commonly associated with dental subluxations. Subluxated, or loosened, teeth are diagnosed by applying gentle pressure to the teeth with a tongue blade or fingertip. Mild displacement may also be noted (Fig. 6.1). Blood along the crevice of the gingiva, where the tooth meets the gingiva, is also a sign of subluxation. Various degrees of tooth mobility may be noted on examination.

Differential Diagnosis

Dental impaction and alveolar ridge fracture should be considered and ruled out clinically and with radiographs.

Emergency Department Treatment and Disposition

1. *Primary teeth*: If the subluxated tooth is forced into close proximity to the underlying permanent tooth, extraction by a dentist or oral surgeon is indicated. Otherwise, the patient should be instructed to follow a soft diet for 1 to 2 weeks, allowing the tooth to reimplant.
2. *Permanent teeth*: If the tooth is unstable, it should be temporarily immobilized. This may be accomplished with gauze packing, a figure-eight suture around the tooth and an adjacent tooth, aluminum foil, or a special periodontal dressing (Coe-Pak). The patient should be referred for dental follow-up.

Clinical Pearls

1. Any evidence of tooth mobility following trauma is a subluxation by definition.
2. Always consider the possibility of an associated underlying alveolar fracture.
3. Clinically subluxated teeth may actually represent an occult root fracture.

Associated Clinical Features

Impacted or intruded teeth result when a tooth is forced deeper into the alveolar socket or surrounding tissues as a result of trauma (Fig. 6.2). The force causing the impaction may be directly on the incisal or occlusal surface of the tooth. The tooth appears shorter than its contralateral partner. The primary dentition is more prone to impaction than permanent teeth. An impacted tooth may be partially visible or completely hidden by the gingiva and buried in the alveolar process. Completely impacted teeth may erroneously be considered avulsed until a radiograph demonstrates the intruded position. The apex of a completely impacted permanent central incisor may be driven through the alveolar bone into the floor of the nostril, causing a nosebleed. The apex of the incisor may be noted on examination of the nostril floor. Primary dentition apices tend to be driven into the thin vestibular bone. Other associated injuries include possible alveolar fractures, dental crown or root fractures, as well as oral mucosal and gingival lacerations. Dental pulp necrosis occurs in 15 to 50% of cases.

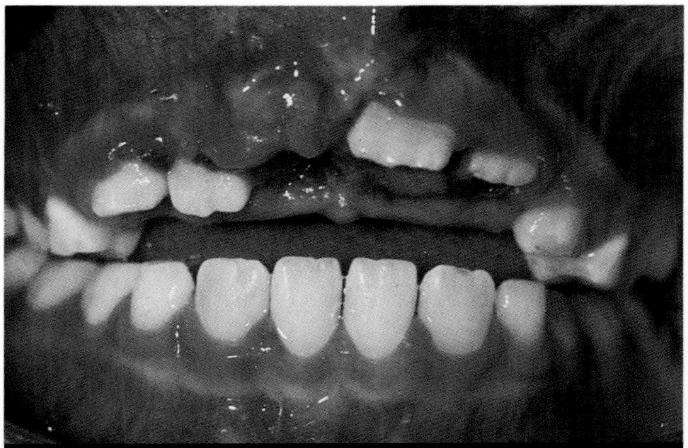

Figure 6.2 Tooth Intrusion

This impaction injury with multiple anterior maxillary tooth involvement shows various degrees of tooth impaction. Also note the complete absence of a central incisor. This may indicate a complete intrusion into the alveolar socket or an avulsion of the tooth. Radiographic studies are required when a tooth's location is in question. (Courtesy of James F. Steiner, DDS.)

Differential Diagnosis

Tooth avulsions and fractures should be considered in the differential diagnosis because of a similar mechanism of injury. Completely impacted teeth may simulate an avulsed tooth in appearance. Lateral luxation may result in teeth that appear shortened and angulated or may simulate a partial impaction. Traumatic injury to gingiva around a normal erupting tooth may be mistaken for an impaction. Impacted teeth tend to emit a high metallic sound on percussion testing with a metallic instrument, similar to ankylosed teeth. Normal teeth do not produce a metallic sound, whereas subluxated teeth produce a dull sound on percussion. Radiographs also aid in differentiating these dental injuries.

Emergency Department Treatment and Disposition

Primary teeth that are impacted usually reerupt and reposition spontaneously within 1 to 3 months. Surgical intervention is indicated if spontaneous reduction does not occur within this time frame. Any intruded primary tooth whose apex is displaced toward or impacts on the follicle of its permanent successor should be extracted. These patients should have dental follow-up and be monitored clinically and radiographically for 1 year. Permanent teeth do not reerupt. Surgical reduction is indicated to prevent complications such as external root resorption and loss of supporting bone. Orthodontic repositioning and splinting is generally carried out over 3 to 4 weeks. Follow-up for a minimum of 1 year is recommended.

Clinical Pearls

1. An undiagnosed impacted tooth is predisposed to infection and can have a poor cosmetic result.
2. The maxillary incisors are the most commonly affected teeth.
3. Only the immature primary teeth will reerupt; the permanent teeth will not.

Associated Clinical Features

Avulsion is the total displacement of a tooth from its socket (Fig. 6.3). There is usually a history of trauma; however, infectious etiologies can also cause an avulsion. Complete disruption of the periodontal ligament fibers from the affected tooth occurs as a result. Various degrees of bleeding from the socket and surrounding gingiva may be noted. Depending on the mechanism of injury, there may be an associated underlying alveolar fracture. Prompt inquiry into the location of any unaccountable tooth is indicated. Radiographic evaluation to rule out aspiration or soft tissue entrapment is indicated when the tooth's location is in question.

Differential Diagnosis

Complete tooth impactions may appear to be an avulsion. Dental fractures with retained tooth fragments in the alveolar socket may also simulate an avulsion. Radiographs should be taken to rule out an intrusion or dentoalveolar fracture.

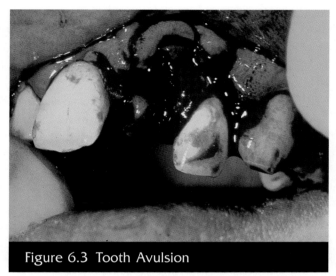

Figure 6.3 Tooth Avulsion

Avulsion injury with angulation and displacement of teeth from the alveolar socket. (Courtesy of James F. Steiner, DDS.)

Emergency Department Treatment and Disposition

Permanent teeth should be replaced in their sockets as soon as possible. The tooth should first be rinsed with saline but not scrubbed, and the root should not be handled. Successful reimplantation depends on the survival of periodontal ligament fibers, which are attached to the root of the avulsed tooth. The tooth should be placed in the socket and emergent dental consultation obtained. Antibiotics against mouth flora (penicillin, clindamycin) should be administered, as well as tetanus prophylaxis. If not replaced, the avulsed tooth should be stored in the mouth of the patient or parent or in a container of milk. Normal saline can be used, but water should not be used. Hank's solution is the ideal storage medium for the avulsed tooth until reimplantation. Primary teeth are not reimplanted, but follow-up should be obtained, as a procedure may be needed to maintain tooth spacing until the permanent tooth erupts.

Clinical Pearls

1. Reimplantation of primary avulsed teeth in patients younger than 6 years may interfere with eruptions of permanent teeth because of ankylosing and fusion to the bone.
2. Successful reimplantation of an avulsed tooth is best achieved within the first 30 min after an avulsion.
3. Storage and transport media in decreasing order for preserving tooth viability include Hank's balanced salt solution or a tissue culture medium (Save-A-Tooth), cool low-fat or skim milk, saline, and saliva.

Associated Clinical Features

Anatomically, each tooth has crown and root portions. Externally, the crown is covered with white enamel and the root portion with cementum. The cementoenamel junction (cervical line) is where the crown and root meet. The yellow-to-tan dentin is the second innermost layer and composes the bulk of the tooth. The red-to-pink pulp tissue is located in the center of the tooth and furnishes the neurovascular supply to the tooth. The Ellis classification system, while considered by some as inadequate, is still commonly used to describe tooth fractures above the cervical line in anterior teeth (Fig. 6.4):

Ellis class I: Involves the enamel only (Fig. 6.5).
Ellis class II: Involves the enamel plus exposure of the dentin (Fig. 6.6). The patient may complain of temperature sensitivity.
Ellis class III: Fracture extends into the pulp. A pink or bloody discoloration on the fracture surface is diagnostic of this type of fracture (Fig. 6.7). The patient may have severe pain but may also have no pain due to loss of nerve function.

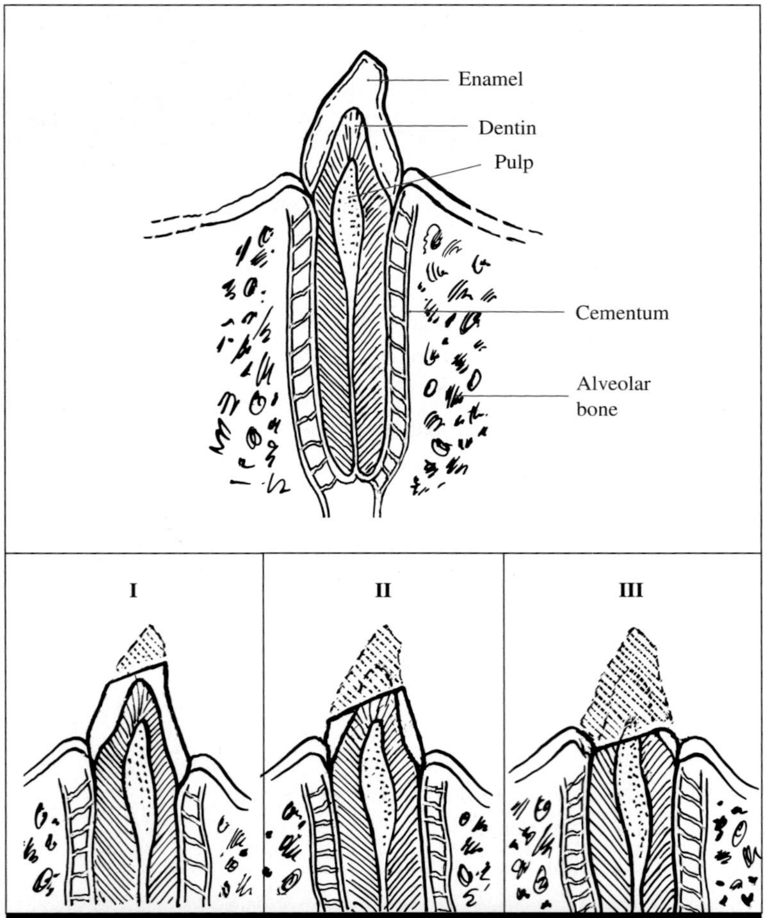

Tooth fractures may also occur below the cementoenamel junction. These dental root fractures are commonly missed on initial evaluation. Bleeding may be observed at the gingival crevice with associated tooth tenderness on percussion.

Differential Diagnosis

Subluxation, alveolar fracture, avulsion, or a traumatic impaction are in the differential. Dental fractures may also be occult and occur below the gum line or at the level of root. Radiographic evaluation will aid in differentiating these conditions.

Emergency Department Treatment and Disposition

Ellis class I: Pain control should be initiated. Rough tooth edges may be smoothed with an emery board. Immediate dental referral within 24 h is indicated when soft tissue injury is caused by sharp pieces of the tooth.
Ellis class II: Patients under 12 years of age have less dentin than older patients and are at risk for infection of the pulp. They should

Figure 6.4 Tooth Fractures

Enamel, dentin, and pulp are the anatomic landmarks used in the Ellis classification of tooth fractures.

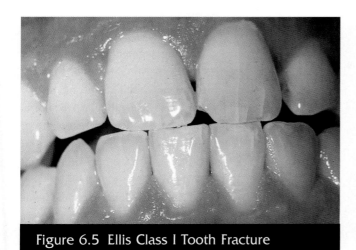

Figure 6.5 Ellis Class I Tooth Fracture

Note the fracture of the left upper central incisor. The sole involvement of the enamel is consistent with an Ellis type I injury. (Courtesy of James F. Steiner, DDS.)

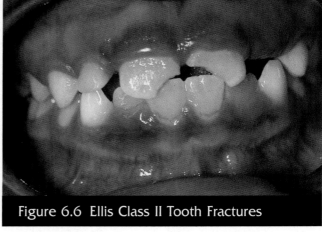

Figure 6.6 Ellis Class II Tooth Fractures

Bilateral maxillary central incisor injuries with exposed enamel and dentin consistent with an Ellis class II fracture. (Courtesy of James F. Steiner, DDS.)

have a calcium hydroxide dressing placed, coverage with gauze or aluminum foil, and see a dentist within 24 h. Older patients should be advised to see a dentist within 24 to 48 h.

Ellis class III: This is considered a dental emergency, and immediate dental consultation is indicated. Delay in treatment may result in severe pain and abscess formation.

Root Fractures: Early reduction, immobilization, and splinting are indicated once diagnosed. A commercial stabilizing compound (Coe-Pak) is available for this purpose. Dental referral is advised within 24 to 48 h. Most teeth sustaining root fractures maintain pulpal vitality and tend to heal.

Clinical Pearls

1. Check for tooth mobility on initial examination to aid in differentiating mobility involving the entire tooth from involvement of only the incisal segment.
2. Consider nonaccidental trauma when dental injuries occur in young children.

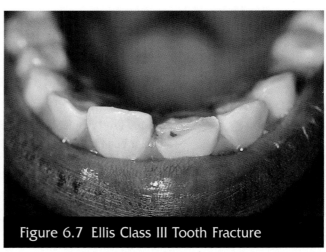

Figure 6.7 Ellis Class III Tooth Fracture

A fracture demonstrating blood at the exposed dental pulp. This sign is pathognomonic for an Ellis class III fracture. (Courtesy of Kevin J. Knoop, MD, MS.)

ALVEOLAR RIDGE FRACTURE

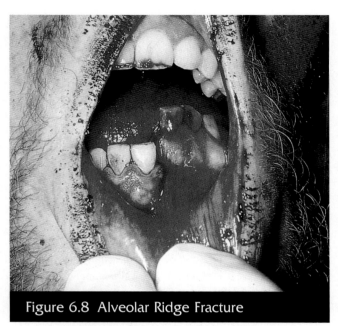

Figure 6.8 Alveolar Ridge Fracture

Note the exposed alveolar bone segment and associated multiple tooth involvement. Attempts should be made to maximally preserve all viable tissue. (Courtesy of Alan B. Storrow, MD.)

Associated Clinical Features

The alveolus is the tooth-bearing segment of the mandible and maxilla. Fracture of the alveolar process tends to occur more often in the thinner maxilla than in the mandible. However, the most common type of mandibular fracture is an alveolar fracture. The anterior alveolar processes are at greatest risk for fracture due to more direct exposure to trauma (Fig. 6.8). Exposed pieces of bone may be noted in alveolar fractures. Various degrees of tooth mobility and gingival bleeding may be noted. Both subluxation and avulsion of teeth may be associated with underlying alveolar fractures of the mandible or maxilla.

Differential Diagnosis

Fractures of the mandible and maxilla may both present with pain, deformity, malocclusion, and bleeding, which may resemble an alveolar fracture. Gingival lacerations with significant tissue damage may be associated with an underlying fracture and should be considered.

Emergency Department Treatment and Disposition

Preservation of as much viable tissue as possible is important. Do not remove any segment of alveolus firmly attached to the mucoperiosteum. Significant cosmetic deformity may result from alveolar bone loss. The involved alveolar segment should have a saline-soaked gauze applied with gentle direct pressure. Any avulsed teeth should also be preserved. The patient's tetanus status should be addressed. Antibiotic therapy with penicillin, clindamycin, or a cephalosporin should also be considered, particularly if bony fragments are exposed. Oral surgery consultation should be obtained for possible wire stabilization, arch bar fixation, and follow-up.

Clinical Pearls

1. Always consider the possibility of an associated cervical spine injury when evaluating patients with facial trauma.
2. If an avulsed tooth is associated with an alveolar fracture, the clinician should inquire about its location. If unaccounted for, consider the possibility of aspiration or soft tissue entrapment.

Associated Clinical Features

Dislocation generally results from direct trauma to the chin while the mouth is open or, more commonly, in predisposed individuals after a vigorous yawn. Opening the mouth excessively wide while eating or laughing may also result in dislocation. Acute dislocation occurs when the mandibular condyles displace forward and become locked anterior to the articular eminence. Muscle spasm contributes to prevention of spontaneous relocation. Weakness of the temporomandibular ligament, an overstretched joint capsule, and a shallow articular eminence are predisposing factors. Patients usually present with an inability to close an open mouth (Fig. 6.9). Other associated symptoms include pain, discomfort, and facial swelling near the temporomandibular joint (TMJ). Difficulty speaking and swallowing is common. Anterior dislocations are most common; however, posterior dislocation may occur with significant force in association with a basilar skull fracture. Unilateral dislocation results in deviation of the mandible to the unaffected side (Fig. 6.10).

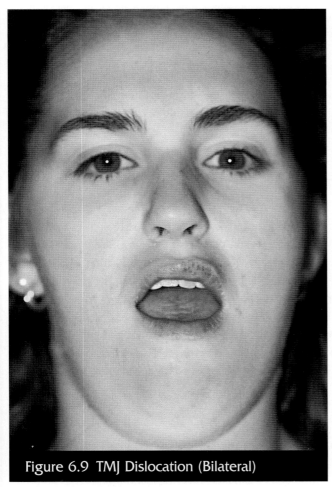

Figure 6.9 TMJ Dislocation (Bilateral)

This patient awoke from sleep with the inability to close her mouth. Note the dry lips and tongue secondary to prolonged exposure. Symmetric dislocations are more common than unilateral injury (Courtesy of Warren K. Russell, MD.)

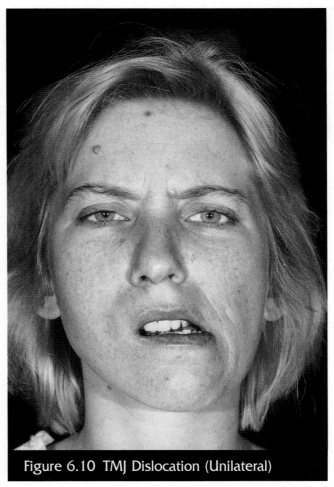

Figure 6.10 TMJ Dislocation (Unilateral)

Note the asymmetric jaw deviation toward the unaffected side. Always consider the possibility of an associated underlying fracture or cervical spine injury. (Courtesy of Frank Birinyi, MD.)

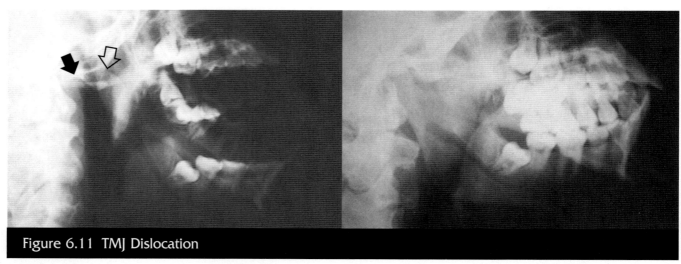

Figure 6.11 TMJ Dislocation

A. Radiographic demonstration of an anterior TMJ dislocation. The location of the condyle is indicated by the open arrow. The position of the mandibular notch is indicated by the closed arrow. B. Postreduction radiograph showing normal positioning of the condyle in the mandibular notch. (Courtesy of Edwin D. Turner, MD.)

Differential Diagnosis

TMJ hemarthrosis, dystonic reactions, and hysterical dislocation can mimic the true process of TMJ dislocation. Unilateral or bilateral mandibular fractures should also be strongly considered, particularly if there is a history of facial trauma.

Emergency Department Treatment and Disposition

Acute reduction of pain, muscle spasm, and anxiety is achieved using reassurance, analgesics, and muscle relaxants. Panorex or TMJ x-ray films (pre- and postreduction) are obtained to exclude a fracture (Fig. 6.11). The patient is typically treated in the sitting position. While facing the patient, the physician grasps the angles of the mandible with both hands. The thumbs are wrapped in gauze for protection and rest on the occlusive surfaces of the molars while downward and backward pressure is applied until the condyle slides back into the articular eminence. Instruct the patient to avoid excessively wide mouth opening while eating and yawning for 3 to 4 weeks. Apply warm compresses to the TMJ areas. A soft diet for 1 week is advised, as is the use of nonsteroidal anti-inflammatory drugs as needed. Dental follow-up should be arranged.

Clinical Pearls

1. Approximately 70% of the general population can subluxate the mandible partially and then spontaneously reduce it.
2. TMJ dysfunction secondary to a neuroleptic or antipsychotic medication–related dystonic reaction is treated with diphenhydramine or benztropine.
3. When trauma is the cause of TMJ dislocation, maintain a high index of suspicion for cervical spine injury.

Associated Clinical Features

Tongue lacerations are usually the result of oral trauma and tongue biting (Fig. 6.12). Injuries to the tongue or mouth floor can cause serious hemorrhage and potential airway compromise. Careful examination of the oral cavity for associated injuries is necessary. Specifically, the injury or absence of teeth should be ascertained. Dorsal tongue lacerations may be associated with a concurrent ventral laceration sustained from the mandibular teeth. Closely inspect the wound for possibly entrapped dental elements.

Differential Diagnosis

Superficial tongue abrasions, oral mucosal, and gingival lacerations may all bleed profusely and cause difficulty localizing the exact source. Any of the aforementioned lacerations may also accompany a tongue laceration. A detailed examination of the entire oral cavity is indicated.

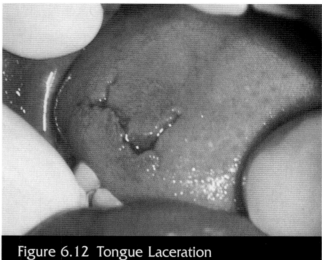

Figure 6.12 Tongue Laceration

A stellate tongue laceration that does not require suturing is shown. The ventral aspect of the tongue should be examined for additional lacerations sustained from the mandibular teeth. (Courtesy of James F. Steiner, DDS.)

Emergency Department Treatment and Disposition

Most lacerations to the tongue do not mandate surgical repair. A generous blood supply results in spontaneous repair of most tongue defects. An exception to this rule is lacerations involving the tip, where rapid healing may produce a "forked tongue." Lacerations greater than 1 cm in length that gape widely, actively bleed, or those involving a lateral margin are best stabilized by a few well-placed sutures; 4-0 black silk or preferably absorbable suture (such as chromic gut) should be used. Place sutures using large bites to include both mucosa and muscle. Laceration repair, if opted for in children, is best carried out in a controlled environment under appropriate anesthesia. Anesthesia of the anterior two-thirds of the tongue is obtained using a regional inferior alveolar nerve block (blocks the lingual nerve on the ipsilateral side). Local anesthesia may also be used. Tongue lacerations involving the floor of the mouth or having persistent bleeding may result in tongue swelling and airway compromise. Consultation for admission with airway surveillance may be indicated.

Clinical Pearls

1. If repair is elected, use an absorbable or braided suture material. Multiple well-secured knots should be placed, as tongue motion tends to untie suture material.
2. Extensive complex tongue lacerations are at risk for infection and should be prophylactically treated with antibiotics for oropharyngeal flora.

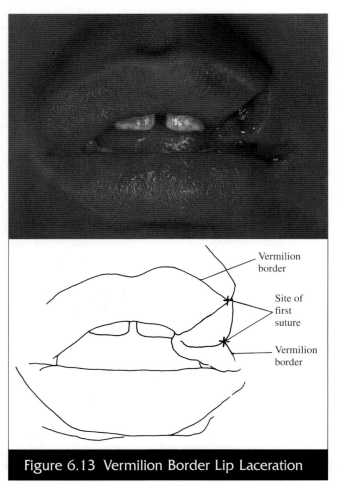

Figure 6.13 Vermilion Border Lip Laceration

A lip laceration with disruption of the vermilion border. Wound repair begins at the vermilion-skin junction for a good cosmetic result. (Courtesy of Kevin J. Knoop, MD, MS.)

Associated Clinical Features

Anatomically, the vermilion border of the lips represents a transition area from mucosal tissue to skin. Lip lacerations involving the vermilion border (Fig. 6.13) present a unique clinical situation, since inadequate repair may cause an unacceptable cosmetic result. Marked tissue edema is frequently noted with most lip trauma, which may distort the anatomy. Vermilion border lacerations may be partial or full thickness through the lip to the mucosal surface. An associated underlying gingival or dental injury is a common finding.

Differential Diagnosis

Vermilion border lip hematomas, abrasions, and soft tissue swelling may mimic a true laceration involving the vermilion border. Careful examination of the facial and mucosal surfaces of the lip help differentiate these entities.

Emergency Department Treatment and Disposition

Accurate vermilion margin reapproximation is the goal of lip repairs. An unapproximated vermilion margin of 2 mm or greater results in a cosmetic deformity and occasionally a puckering defect. A regional block of the mental or infraorbital nerve is recommended for anesthesia to avoid additional tissue edema and anatomic distortion produced by local infiltration. After closure of the deeper tissue, the first skin suture is always placed at the vermilion border to reestablish the anatomic margin. Using 5-0 or 6-0 nylon, suturing should continue along the vermilion surface until the moist mucous membrane is noted. Deep or through-and-through lacerations involving the vermilion border should be closed in layers. The deep muscular and dermal layer may be closed with 3-0 or 4-0 chromic or Vicryl sutures, and the skin with 6-0 nylon sutures. Mucosal layers are loosely reapproximated with 4-0 absorbable suture or silk. The patient should be given wound care instructions. Follow-up for wound evaluation and possible suture removal in 5 to 7 days should be arranged.

Clinical Pearls

1. A vermilion border with as little as 2 mm of malalignment may produce a cosmetically noticed defect.
2. Always place the first skin suture in the vermilion border in any lip laceration involving this area.

Odontogenic Infections

Associated Clinical Features

Gingival abscesses tend to involve the marginal gingiva and result from entrapment of food and plaque debris in a gingival pocket with subsequent staphylococcal, streptococcal, anaerobic, or mixed bacterial overgrowth, leading to abscess formation. Localized swelling, erythema, tenderness, and possible fluctuance in the space between the tooth and the gingiva (the so-called pocket) is the usual location. There may be spontaneous purulent drainage from the gingival margin, or an area of pointing may be seen. In cases of acute gingival abscess formation, pus may be expressed from the gingival margin by gentle digital pressure. When the gingival abscess involves the deeper supporting periodontal structures, it is referred to as a periodontal abscess (Fig. 6.14). This may present as a fluctuant vestibular abscess or with a draining sinus that opens onto the gingival surface.

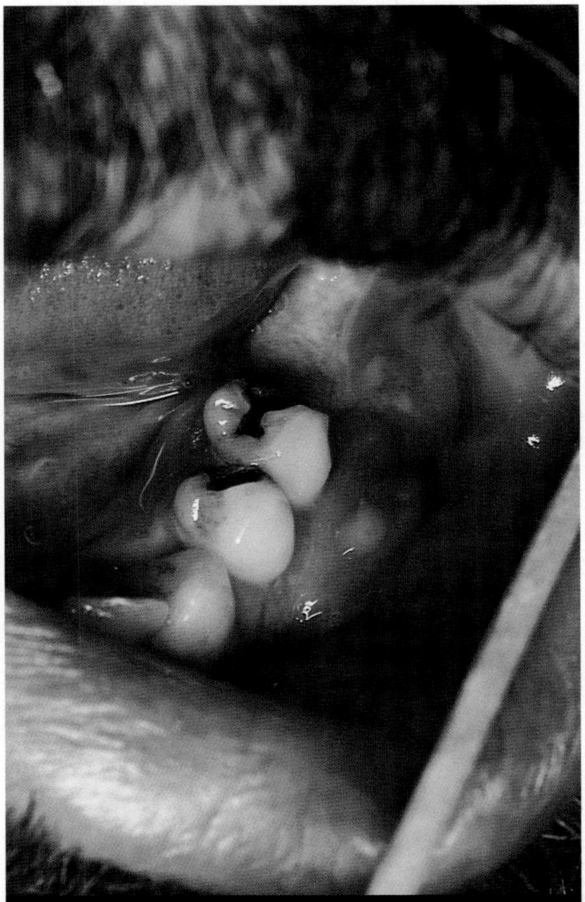

Differential Diagnosis

Periapical abscesses are deep and not obvious on inspection. They usually present as tenderness to percussion or pain with chewing over the involved tooth. A parulis may also simulate a gingival abscess; however, a parulis represents the cutaneous manifestation of a deeper periapical abscess. Unlike a parulis or periapical abscesses, gingival abscesses are not usually associated with dental caries or fillings. Pericoronal abscesses tend to involve the gingiva overlying a partially erupted third molar.

Figure 6.14 Periodontal Abscess

Localized gingival swelling, erythema, and fluctuance are seen in this periodontal abscess with spontaneous purulent drainage. (Courtesy of Kevin J. Knoop, MD, MS.)

Emergency Department Treatment and Disposition

The initial management is a small incision with drainage and warm saline irrigation. Removal of entrapped food and debris is performed. Oral antibiotic therapy with penicillin, clindamycin, tetracyclines, or macrolides is recommended. Analgesics should be provided along with dental follow-up. The patient's tetanus status should be addressed.

Clinical Pearls

1. Patients with gingival abscesses are usually afebrile.
2. Consider more extensive abscess formation and oral disease processes in the febrile toxic-appearing patient.
3. Patients with chronic, deep periodontal abscesses complain of dull, gnawing pain as well as a desire to bite down on and grind the tooth.

Associated Clinical Features

Acute pain, swelling, and mild tooth elevation is characteristic of a periapical abscess. Exquisite sensitivity to percussion or chewing on the involved tooth is a common sign. The involved tooth may have had a root canal treatment, a filling, or a dental carie. Periapical abscesses may enlarge over time and "point," internally on the lingual or buccal mucosal surfaces or extraorally with swelling and redness of the overlying skin (Fig. 6.15). Occasionally these lesions may tract up to the alveolar periosteum and gingival surface to form a parulis ("gumboil") (Fig. 6.16). Radiographically, these abscesses appear as well-circumscribed areas of radiolucency at the dental apex or along the lateral aspect of the root (Fig. 6.17). Early acute periapical abscesses may not demonstrate any radiographic changes. Both deep periodontal and periapical abscesses may have sinuses draining purulent material onto the gingival surface. If the infection is allowed to progress, it can erode through the nearest cortical bone, manifesting itself in a variety of locations (Fig. 6.18).

Differential Diagnosis

Gingival or deep periodontal abscess, buccal space abscess, and unilateral sublingual, parapharyngeal, and submandibular space abscesses should all be considered in the differential diagnosis. All the aforementioned may present with oral pain, tenderness, facial swelling, and possible fever. Panorex films, dental radiographs, or a computed tomography (CT) scan may aid in making the diagnosis.

Emergency Department Treatment and Disposition

Nonsteroidal anti-inflammatory drugs (NSAIDs) or oral narcotics for pain should be administered as well as oropharyngeal antibiotic therapy. A regional nerve block may be performed with a local anesthetic agent for more immediate temporary relief. Administer tetanus toxoid if indicated. Dental consultation or follow-up in 1 to 2 days is recommended for endodontic evaluation or possible extraction of the involved tooth. Incision and drainage along with saline irrigation and prompt referral constitutes the initial treatment of a parulis.

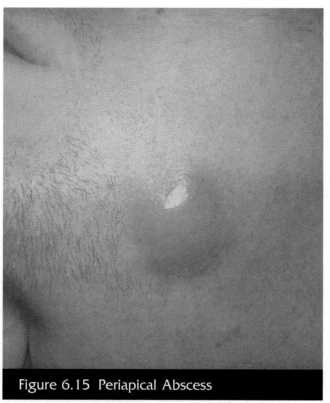

Figure 6.15 Periapical Abscess

This periapical abscess points externally, to the overlying skin. (Courtesy of Robin Cotton, MD.)

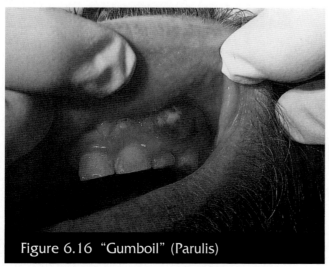

Figure 6.16 "Gumboil" (Parulis)

This lesion is an extension of a periapical abscess. It is differentiated from a periodontal abscess by tenderness to percussion. (Courtesy of Alan B. Storrow, MD.)

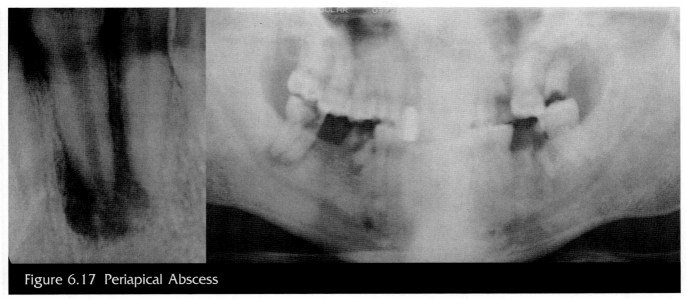

Figure 6.17 Periapical Abscess

A. Note the well-defined radiolucent area at the apex and lateral root of the tooth in this radiograph. (Courtesy of James L. Kretzschmar, DDS, MS.) B. This panorex film shows several areas consistent with periapical abscesses. (Courtesy of David P. Kretzschmar, DDS, MS.)

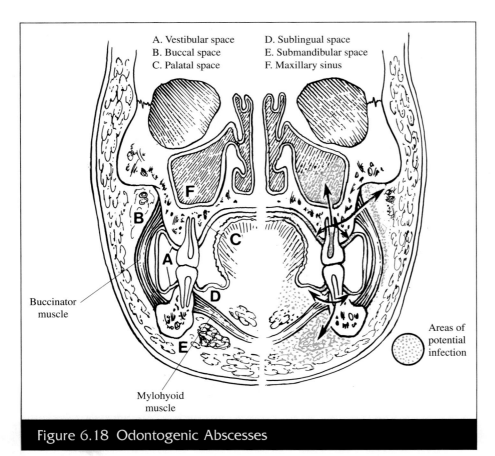

A. Vestibular space   D. Sublingual space
B. Buccal space   E. Submandibular space
C. Palatal space   F. Maxillary sinus

Buccinator muscle

Mylohyoid muscle

Areas of potential infection

Figure 6.18 Odontogenic Abscesses

As infection progresses from the pulp at the tooth apex, it erodes through the bone and can express itself in a variety of places. This illustration notes several possible locations or spaces. (Adapted with permission from Cummings C, Schuller D (eds): *Otolaryngology Head and Neck Surgery*. Chicago: Mosby-Year Book; 1986.)

Clinical Pearls

1. More than one tooth may be involved simultaneously.
2. Exquisite tenderness and pain on tooth percussion is a key feature on physical examination and identifies the involved tooth.
3. Periapical abscesses are almost always associated with carious or nonviable teeth.

Associated Clinical Features

A partially erupted or impacted third molar (wisdom tooth) is the most common site of pericoronitis and pericoronal abscesses. The accumulation of food and debris between the overlying gingival flap and crown of the tooth sets up the foci for pericoronitis and subsequent abscess formation. The gingival flap becomes irritated and inflamed. The area is also repeatedly traumatized by the opposing molar tooth and may interfere with complete jaw closure as swelling and tenderness increase. The inflamed gingival process may eventually become infected and form a fluctuant abscess (Fig. 6.19). Foul taste, inability to close the jaw, and fever may occur. Swelling of the cheek and angle of the jaw as well as localized lymphadenopathy are also characteristic. More advanced disease may spread posteriorly to the base of the tongue and oropharyngeal area. Potential spread into the deep cervical spaces is also an important concern with extensive processes.

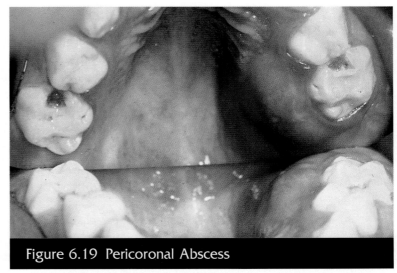

Figure 6.19 Pericoronal Abscess

Note the inflammed fluctuant gingival tissue approximating the incompletely erupted third molar. (Courtesy of James F. Steiner, DDS.)

Differential Diagnosis

Ludwig's angina, peritonsillar abscess, gingival abscess, buccal space abscess, and a severe periapical abscess may all present similarly to a pericoronal abscess. Ludwig's angina and peritonsillar abscesses are, in fact, potential sequelae of acute pericoronitis and pericoronal abscesses.

Emergency Department Treatment and Disposition

Superficial incision and drainage with warm saline irrigation may be performed initially in the ED. Adequate analgesia and antibiotic coverage should be provided. Consultation or referral to an oral maxillofacial surgeon for follow-up is indicated for possible extraction of the involved teeth.

Clinical Pearls

1. Pericoronitis and abscess formation rarely occur in the pediatric population and tend to be late adolescent and adult processes.
2. The mandibular third molar is the most commonly involved tooth.
3. Airway compromise is a potential complication with posterior extension of a pericoronal abscess.

Associated Clinical Features

The buccal space lies anatomically between the buccinator muscle and the overlying superficial fascia and skin. The maxillary second and third molars are the usual source of infection contributing to buccal space abscesses. Infection from the involved teeth erodes through the maxillary alveolar bone superiorly into the buccal space (Fig. 6.20). Rarely, the third mandibular molar may be the source. In this instance, the infection erodes through the mandibular alveolar bone inferiorly into the buccal space. These patients present with unilateral facial swelling, redness, and tenderness to the cheek (Fig. 6.21). Trismus is generally not present.

Differential Diagnosis

Canine space abscess, parapharyngeal abscess, facial cellulitis, Ludwig's angina, and masticator space abscess formation are all conditions that may resemble buccal space abscesses. Parotid gland enlargement due to mumps and suppurative bacterial parotitis should also be considered. The former lacks erythema and warmth of the overlying skin, while the latter is accompanied by trismus and the ability to express pus from Stensen's duct. Inspection of all the maxillary and third mandibular molar teeth is essential to help make the diagnosis. CT scan can aid in localizing the space involved.

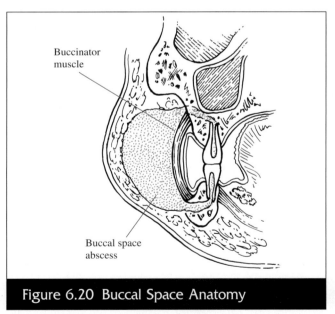

Figure 6.20 Buccal Space Anatomy

The buccal space lies between the buccinator muscle and the overlying skin and superficial fascia. This potential space may become involved by maxillary or mandibular molars. (Adapted with permission from Cummings C, Schuller D (eds): *Otolaryngology Head and Neck Surgery*, 2d ed. Chicago: Mosby-Year Book; 1993.)

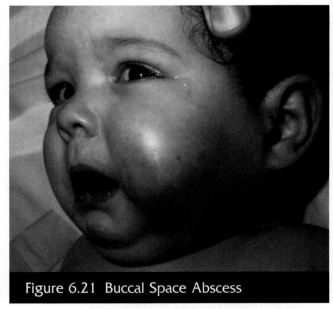

Figure 6.21 Buccal Space Abscess

Note the ovoid cheek swelling with sparing of the nasolabial fold. This finding, along with accompanying redness and tenderness, helps to identify buccal space abscess formation. (Courtesy of Michael J. Nowicki, MD.)

Emergency Department Treatment and Disposition

Parenteral antibiotic therapy with penicillin, clindamycin, or a third-generation cephalosporin is recommended. Antibiotic coverage for anaerobic organisms may also be added to the treatment regimen. NSAIDs or mild oral narcotic analgesics should be provided as indicated. Dental or oral surgical consultation is necessary for intramural abscess drainage and endodontic therapy versus extraction of the involved molar teeth.

Clinical Pearls

1. Ovoid cheek swelling with sparing of the nasolabial fold helps to identify buccal space abscesses and differentiates it from canine space abscesses.
2. Odontogenic infections of the second or third maxillary molars is the most common source for buccal space abscesses.

Associated Clinical Features

The canine space lies between the anterior surface of the maxilla and levator labii superioris muscle of the face. The origin of these abscesses can be from upper anterior teeth and bicuspids, although it is almost exclusively from the maxillary canine tooth. Erosion of maxillary tooth infection through the alveolar bone into the canine space leads to abscess formation, although cutaneous infections from the upper lip and nose are a rare source. Unilateral facial redness, pain, and swelling lateral to the nose with obliteration of the nasolabial fold is characteristic (Fig. 6.22). Severe upper lip and lower eyelid swelling may cause eye closure and drooling at the corner of the mouth.

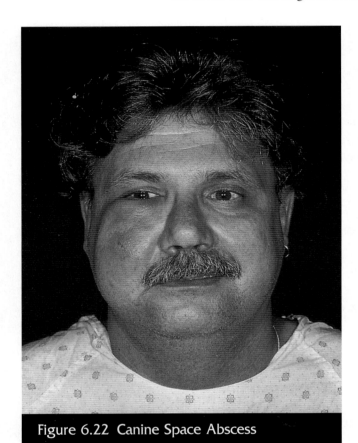

Figure 6.22 Canine Space Abscess

Unilateral facial swelling lateral to the nose with associated redness and the typical loss of the nasolabial fold is shown. The maxillary canine tooth is usually the source of this process. (Courtesy of Frank Birinyi, MD.)

Differential Diagnosis

Buccal space infection, facial cellulitis, and maxillary sinusitis may present with various clinical features similar to canine space abscesses. Examination of the anterior maxillary teeth may provide very helpful clues to the origin and diagnosis of canine space abscesses. CT scan and sinus x-rays may aid in defining these lesions.

Emergency Department Treatment and Disposition

Parenteral antibiotic therapy to include anaerobic coverage is indicated for treatment. Dental or oral surgical consultation for intramural incision and drainage represents the most definitive treatment for canine space abscesses. Extraction or endodontic treatment of the involved anterior maxillary teeth is usually necessary.

Clinical Pearls

1. The maxillary canine (cuspid) teeth are the most common source for canine space abscesses.
2. Although these patients may drool when significant upper lip swelling is present, they typically do not have trismus, dysphagia, or odynophagia.
3. Loss of the nasolabial fold is characteristic of canine space abscesses.

Associated Clinical Features

Ludwig's angina is defined as bilateral cellulitis of the submandibular and sublingual spaces (see Fig. 6.18) with associated tongue elevation (Figs. 6.23 and 6.24). A characteristic painful, brawny induration is present rather than fluctuance in the involved tissue. The posterior mandibular molars represent the usual odontogenic origin for the infection. *Streptococcus, Staphylococcus,* and *Bacteroides* species are the most common offending pathogens. Affected individuals are usually 20 to 60 years old, with a male predominance. These patients are usually febrile and may demonstrate impressive trismus, dysphonia, and odynophagia. Dysphagia and drooling are secondary to tongue displacement and oropharyngeal swelling. Potential airway compromise or spread of the infection to the deep cervical layers and the mediastinum is possible. The presence of dyspnea or cyanosis is a later, more ominous sign, which indicates impending airway closure.

Differential Diagnosis

Peritonsillar abscesses, epiglottitis, and parapharyngeal and retropharyngeal abscesses all have clinical features similar in presentation to Ludwig's angina. Oropharyngeal examination is often uncomfortable and difficult in all the aforementioned conditions. Caution should be used if epiglottitis is suspected.

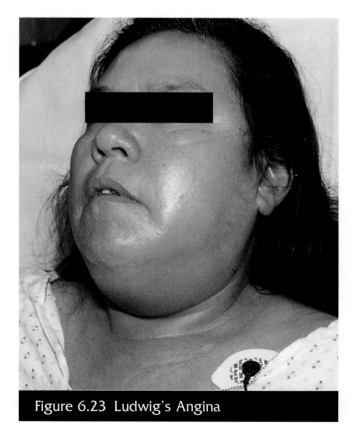

Figure 6.23 Ludwig's Angina

Note the diffuse submandibular swelling and fullness. Direct palpation of this area would reveal a characteristic brawny induration. Potential airway compromise is a key concern in all patients with Ludwig's angina. (Courtesy of Jeffrey Finkelstein, MD.)

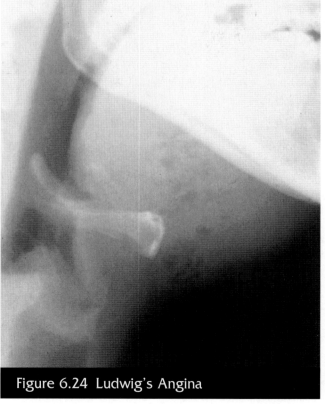

Figure 6.24 Ludwig's Angina

Note the presence of subcutaneous gas in the abscessed submandibular area on this radiograph of a patient with Ludwig's angina. (Courtesy of Edward C. Jauch, MD, MS.)

Emergency Department Treatment and Disposition

Acute laryngospasm with airway compromise is a potentially life-threatening complication and concern with Ludwig's angina; therefore, plans for definitive airway management should be prepared. Up to one-third require intubation or surgical airway placement. Parenteral antibiotic therapy can be initiated with penicillin or a third-generation cephalosporin. Coverage for anaerobic organisms should also be provided with clindamycin or metronidazole. The role of steroids is controversial and ill defined for potential airway edema in this setting. Parenteral analgesic should be given as needed. The definitive treatment is intraoperative surgical drainage of the abscess. Computed tomography (CT) or magnetic resonance imaging (MRI) can be used to identify abscess location. Admission to the intensive care unit is indicated for airway surveillance and management. Oral and maxillofacial surgical or otolaryngologic consultation is prudent.

Clinical Pearls

1. The second mandibular molar is the most common site of origin for Ludwig's angina.
2. Admission of these patients to the intensive care unit is almost always indicated because of the potential for airway compromise.
3. Intraoperative surgical incision and drainage is the definitive treatment.
4. Brawny submandibular induration and tongue elevation are common and characteristic clinical findings.
5. Acute laryngospasm with sudden total airway obstruction may be precipitated by attempts at oral or blind nasal intubation.

Associated Clinical Features

The parapharyngeal space is also known as the lateral pharyngeal or pharyngomaxillary space. Anatomically it is a pyramid-shaped space with its apex at the hyoid bone and base at the base of the skull. Laterally it is bound by the internal pterygoid muscle and parotid gland with the superior pharyngeal constrictor muscle medially. The posterior aspect of this space is in close proximity with the carotid sheath and cranial nerves IX through XII. Presenting symptoms include fever, dysphagia, odynophagia, drooling, and ipsilateral otalgia. Unilateral neck and jaw angle facial swelling, in association with rigidity and limited neck motion, is common (Fig. 6.25). Potentially disastrous complications that have been associated with infections of this space include cranial neuropathies, jugular vein septic thrombophlebitis, and erosion into the carotid artery. The origin of parapharyngeal abscesses may be from infected tonsils, sinuses and teeth, or lymphatic spread.

Differential Diagnosis

Buccal space abscess, Ludwig's angina, peritonsillar and retropharyngeal abscesses, and parotitis represent clinical conditions to consider. A CT scan provides more specific information and aids in making the diagnosis.

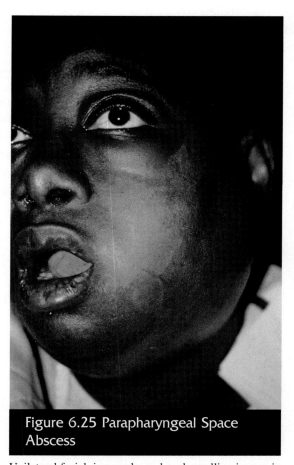

Figure 6.25 Parapharyngeal Space Abscess

Unilateral facial, jaw angle, and neck swelling is seen in this patient. Nuchal rigidity may also be present. (Courtesy of Sara-Jo Gahm, MD.)

Emergency Department Treatment and Disposition

Preparations for definitive airway management via endotracheal intubation or surgery is vital. Early recognition and anticipation of other potentially disastrous complications should be considered and managed appropriately. Broad-spectrum antibiotic coverage for mixed aerobic and anaerobic infections should be initiated. Radiologic modalities used to assess parapharyngeal and other deep space neck infections include contrast-enhanced CT, ultrasound, plain radiography, and MRI. Otolaryngologic or oral surgical consultation is warranted for definitive intraoperative incision and drainage of the abscess.

Clinical Pearls

1. Suspected oropharyngeal abscesses in association with neuropathy in cranial nerves IX through XII is pathognomonic of parapharyngeal abscesses.
2. Bacterial pharyngitis represents the most common source of parapharyngeal abscesses.

Oral Conditions

TRENCH MOUTH
(ACUTE NECROTIZING ULCERATIVE GINGIVITIS)

Associated Clinical Features

Painful, severely edematous interdental papillae is characteristic of acute necrotizing ulcerative gingivitis (ANUG). Other associated features include the presence of ulcers with an overlying grayish pseudomembrane and "punched out" appearance (Fig. 6.26). The inflamed gingival tissue is very friable, necrotic, and represents an acute destructive disease process of the periodontium. Fever, malaise, and regional lymphadenopathy are commonly associated signs. Patients may also complain of foul breath and a strong metallic taste. Poor oral hygiene, emotional stress, smoking, and immunocompromised states (e.g., HIV, steroid use, diabetes) all may contribute to predisposition for ANUG. Anaerobic *Fusobacterium* and spirochetes are the predominate bacterial organisms involved. The anterior incisor and posterior molar gingival regions are the most commonly affected oral tissue.

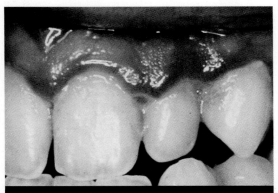

Figure 6.26 Acute Necrotizing Ulcerative Gingivitis

Note the inflamed, friable, and necrotic gingival tissue. An overlying grayish pseudomembrane or punched out ulcerations of the interdental papillae are pathognomonic. (Courtesy of David P. Kretzschmar, DDS, MS.)

Differential Diagnosis

Acute herpetic gingivostomatitis, aphthous stomatitis, desquamative gingivitis, gonococcal and streptococcal gingivostomatitis, and chronic periodontal disease all represent oral diseases that may mimic ANUG. Differentiating these oral conditions from one another is based primarily on history and a thorough oropharyngeal examination.

Emergency Department Treatment and Disposition

Initial management includes warm saline irrigation. Systemic analgesics and topical anesthetics such as viscous lidocaine may facilitate oral hygiene measures. Antibiotic treatment is initiated immediately with oropharyngeal coverage. Dilute 1.5 to 2% hydrogen peroxide or chlorhexidine oral rinses are also helpful. Follow-up with a dentist or periodontist in 1 to 2 days is recommended. Patients with more advanced disease may require admission and oral surgical consultation.

Clinical Pearls

1. Dramatic relief of symptoms within 24 h of initiating antibiotics and supportive treatment is characteristic.
2. Periodontal abscesses and underlying alveolar bone destruction are common complications of ANUG and require dental follow-up.
3. There is no evidence that ANUG is a communicable disease.
4. Gingivitis is a nontender inflammatory disorder.
5. Consider HIV testing in patients with ANUG refractory to antibiotic therapy.

Associated Clinical Features

Bulimia nervosa is an eating disorder—thought to be psychological in origin—with significant associated physical complications. It is characterized by binge eating with self-induced vomiting, laxative use, dieting, and exercise to prevent weight gain. Patients with bulimia are at significant risk for damage to the dental enamel and dentin as a result of repeated episodes of vomiting. Chronic exposure to regurgitated acidic gastric contents represents the main mechanism of injury, which is aggravated by tongue movement. The lingual dental surfaces are most commonly affected (Fig. 6.27). In severe cases, all surfaces of the teeth may be affected. Buccal dental surface erosions may be noted as a result of excessive consumption of fruit (i.e., lemons) and juices by some bulimic patients. Trauma to the oral and esophageal mucosa may also result from induced vomiting. The quantity, buffering capacity, and pH of both the resting and stimulated saliva are found to be reduced. Salivary gland enlargement, most commonly the parotid, may occur in bulimic persons as well. Unexplained elevation of serum amylase, hypokalemia, esophagitis, menstrual irregularities, and fluctuating weight are other complications noted with bulimia.

Differential Diagnosis

Included in the differential diagnosis of acid tooth erosion are conditions that involve vomiting, such as pregnancy, stricture or spasm of the esophagus, and disturbances of gastrointestinal tract peristalsis. Xerostomia is a condition of excessive mouth dryness (associated with Sjögren's syndrome) and can also accelerate the process of enamel loss. Conditions resulting in short-term episodes of vomiting do not have severe destructive effects on the dentition. Dental abrasions and erosions, singly or in combination, may result in a considerable loss of tooth structure. Tooth erosions may be brought about by the use of chewing tobacco (Fig. 6.28), eating betel nuts, dentifrice, bruxism, abnormal swallowing, and clenching.

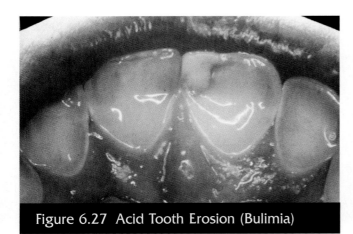

Figure 6.27 Acid Tooth Erosion (Bulimia)

Erosive dentin exposure of the maxillary teeth secondary to chronic vomiting. The involvement of the lingual dental surfaces is characteristic of bulimia. (Courtesy of David P. Kretzschmar, DDS, MS.)

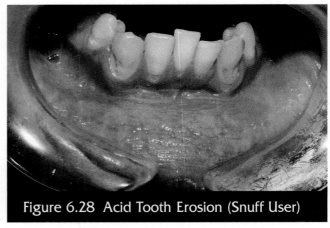

Figure 6.28 Acid Tooth Erosion (Snuff User)

Note the typical dentin exposure on the buccal dental surfaces resulting from prolonged snuff use and its accompanying acid erosion. (Courtesy of David P. Kretzschmar, DDS, MS.)

Emergency Department Treatment and Disposition

Dental treatment should begin with vigorous oral hygiene to prevent further destruction of tooth structures. Regular professional fluoride treatments to cover exposed dentin should be instituted, as well as pain treatment. With the exception of temporary cosmetic procedures, definitive dental treatment should be deferred until the patient is adequately stabilized psychologically. The initial ED management of patients with bulimia should address any medical complication of the disorder like hypokalemia, metabolic acidosis, and its associated cardiac, renal, and central nervous system effects. Hospitalization to stabilize medical complications and provide nutritional support may be indicated. A multidisciplinary team approach is necessary and should involve psychiatry, internal medicine, and dental consultation as needed.

Clinical Pearls

1. The lingual surfaces of the teeth are the most commonly involved tooth surfaces.
2. Attrition or bruxism tends to cause enamel loss from occlusal and incisal dental surfaces.
3. The labial and buccal surfaces of the teeth tend to show enamel loss from repeat or prolonged chemical contact (e.g., lemon sucking or tobacco products).

Associated Clinical Features

White, flaky, curd-like plaques covering the tongue and buccal mucosa with an erythematous base is typical of thrush (Fig. 6.29). These lesions tend to be painless; however, painful inflammatory erosions or ulcers may be noted, particularly in adults. Decreased oral intake secondary to pain is common. Colonization of surface epithelium by *Candida* may be opportunistic as a result of an altered oral milieu. Predisposing factors include antibiotic use, corticosteroids, radiation to the head and neck, extremes of ages, patients with immunologic deficiencies, and chronic irritation (e.g., denture use and xerostomia).

Differential Diagnosis

Hairy leukoplakia, lingual lichen planus, flecks of milk or food debris, and liquid antacid adhering to the tongue may be confused with candidiasis. Hairy leukoplakia cannot be brushed off with a tongue depressor. This helps differentiate this process from thrush or residue from ingested materials. Microscopic examination of the removed specimen for the presence of hyphae in potassium hydroxide mount will aid in the identification of *Candida*.

Emergency Department Treatment and Disposition

Nystatin oral tablets, nystatin suspension, or clotrimazole oral troches are usually adequate therapy. Topical analgesic cocktails may also provide comfort for patients (e.g., Maalox, diphenhydramine, viscous lidocaine oral rinse).

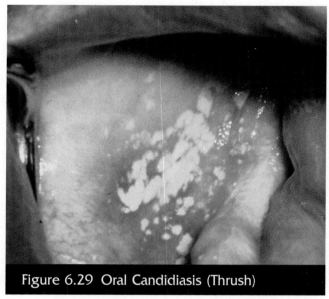

Figure 6.29 Oral Candidiasis (Thrush)

Whitish plaques are seen here on the buccal mucosa. These plaques are easily removed with a tongue blade, differentiating them from lichen planus or leukoplakia. (Courtesy of James F. Steiner, DDS.)

Clinical Pearls

1. Thrush is most common in premature infants and immunosuppressed patients.
2. In young adults, thrush may be the first sign of AIDS; a history of HIV risk factors should be elicited.
3. Failure of oral candidiasis to respond to topical antifungal agents may suggest an immune deficiency.

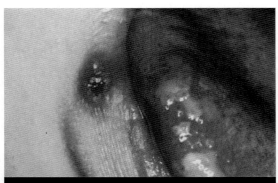

Figure 6.30 Herpes Simplex Virus (HSV) Stomatitis

Note the vermilion border and lingual lesions that are common in this condition. A prodromal period of fever, malaise, and cervical adenopathy may herald the onset of these painful ulcerations. (Courtesy of James F. Steiner, DDS.)

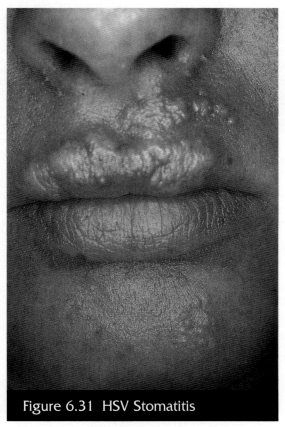

Figure 6.31 HSV Stomatitis

Extensive vesicular lesions along the vermilion border and surrounding tissues are consistent with HSV infection. (Courtesy of Frank Birinyi, MD.)

Associated Clinical Features

Oral herpes simplex may present acutely as a primary gingivostomatitis or as a recurrence. Painful vesicular eruptions on the oral mucosa, tongue, palate, vermilion borders, and gingiva are highly characteristic (Figs. 6.30, 6.31). A 2- to 3-day prodromal period of malaise, fever, and cervical adenopathy is common. The vesicular lesions rupture to form a tender ulcer with yellow crusting and an erythematous margin. Pain may be severe enough to cause drooling and odynophagia, which can discourage eating and drinking, particularly in children. The disease tends to run its course in a 7- to 10-day period with resolution of the lesions without scarring. Recurrent herpes labialis may present with an aura of burning, itching, or tingling prior to vesicle formation. Oral trauma, sunburn, stress, and any variety of febrile illnesses can precipitate this condition.

Differential Diagnosis

Oral erythema multiforme or Stevens-Johnson syndrome, aphthous lesions, oral pemphigus, and hand-foot-mouth (HFM) syndrome are in the differential diagnosis. It should be noted that aphthous ulcers tend to occur on movable oral mucosa and rarely on immovable mucosa (i.e., hard palate and gingiva). The vermilion border is a characteristic location for herpes labialis as opposed to aphthous lesions. Posterior oropharyngeal ulcerations with associated hand and foot lesions help to define HFM syndrome. Painful hemorrhagic oral ulcers in association with anorectal and conjunctival lesions aid in identifying erythema multiforme or Stevens-Johnson syndrome. Oral pemphigus is commonly found in elderly patients. Cutaneous skin bullae and several weeks of vague constitutional symptoms are also characteristic of pemphigus. A thorough history is invaluable in differentiating the aforementioned disorders.

Emergency Department Treatment and Disposition

Supportive care with rehydration and pain control are the mainstays of therapy. Temporary pain relief may be achieved with topical analgesics. Viscous lidocaine, 2%, may be used as an oral rinse, 5 mL every 3 to 4 h. Oral antiviral agents may be useful in adults with primary infections. Topical acyclovir ointment may also be of use by preventing viral spreading and acting as a lubricant to prevent lip cracking and bleeding. Secondary infection of herpetic lesions should be treated with oral penicillin or erythromycin.

Clinical Pearls

1. Oral herpetic lesions tend to occur on the vermilion border, gingiva, and hard palate.
2. Fatal viremia and systemic involvement may occur in infants and children with herpetic gingivostomatitis.
3. Primary acute oral herpetic infection occurs most commonly in children and young adults.
4. Corticosteroid use is contraindicated in herpetic gingivostomatitis because of potential worsening of the condition.

Associated Clinical Features

Aphthous ulcers are painful mucosal lesions varying in size from 1 to 15 mm. A prodromal burning sensation in the affected area may be noted 2 to 48 h before an ulcer is noted. The initial lesion is a small white papule that ulcerates and enlarges over the subsequent 48 to 72 h (Fig. 6.32). The lesions are typically round or ovoid with a raised yellow border and surrounding erythema. Multiple aphthous ulcers may occur on the lips, tongue, buccal mucosa, floor of the mouth, or soft palate (Fig. 6.33). Spontaneous healing of lesions occurs in 7 to 10 days without scarring. The exact etiology of aphthous lesions is unknown. Deficiencies of vitamin B_{12}, folic acid, and iron as well as viruses have been implicated. Stress, local trauma, and immunocompromised states have all been cited as possible precipitating factors.

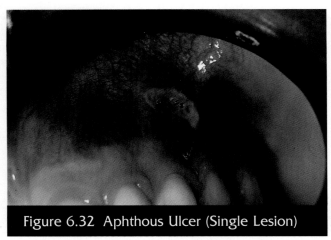

Figure 6.32 Aphthous Ulcer (Single Lesion)

Raised yellow borders with surrounding erythema are typical of aphthous ulcers. (Courtesy of James F. Steiner, DDS.)

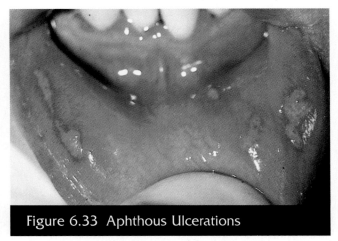

Figure 6.33 Aphthous Ulcerations

Note the multiple ulcers of various sizes located on the lip and gingival mucosa. These lesions rarely occur on the immobile oral mucosa of the gingiva or hard palate. (Courtesy of James F. Steiner, DDS.)

Differential Diagnosis

Primary or recurrent herpetic oral lesions may present with an almost identical prodrome and similar appearance to aphthous ulcerations. Herpetic lesions, unlike aphthous ones, tend to occur on the gingiva, hard palate, and vermilion border. Oral erythema multiforme may also present similarly to aphthous stomatitis; however, like oral herpes, it may tend to present with multiple vesicles in the early stages. Stevens-Johnson syndrome represents a severe form of erythema multiforme characterized by hemorrhagic anogenital and conjunctival lesions as well as oral lesions. Herpangina results from coxsackie and echoviruses with oral ulcerations typically involving the posterior pharynx. Oral pemphigus should also be considered in the differential. Behçet's syndrome can present with recurrent oral lesions, genital ulcers and uveitis.

Emergency Department Treatment and Disposition

Supportive care, rehydration, and pain control constitutes the focus of therapy. A topical anesthetic agent such as 2% viscous lidocaine as an oral rinse every 3 to 4 h is palliative. Oral rinses containing antihistamines and liquid antacid mixtures provide comfort. Use of oral antimicrobial rinses containing 0.12% chlorhexidine (Peridex) or tetracycline is effective in promoting healing. Protective dental paste (Orabase) may be applied every 6 h to prevent irritation of lesions. Triamcinolone acetonide in an emollient dental paste applied three to four times daily may also reduce pain and promote healing of the lesions.

Clinical Pearls

1. Aphthous ulcers may be associated with Crohn's disease.
2. Women are more commonly affected by aphthous lesions than men.
3. The first aphthous episode occurs most commonly in the second decade of life.
4. Aphthous lesions almost never occur on the gums or hard palate.

Associated Clinical Features

Reddened, hypertrophied lingual papillae, called strawberry tongue, is associated primarily with scarlet fever, which is caused by group A streptococcus. The tongue initially appears white with the erythematous papillae sticking through the white exudate. After several days, the white coating is lost and the tongue appears bright red (Fig. 6.34). Other signs of group A streptococcal infection include fever, an exudative pharyngitis, a scarlatiniform rash, and the presence of Pastia's lines (petechial linear rash in the skin folds (see Fig. 14.30)).

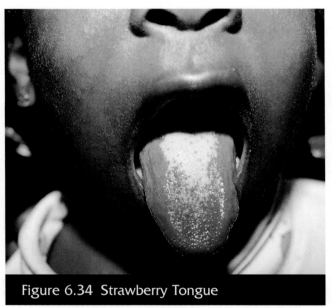

Figure 6.34 Strawberry Tongue

Note the white exudate with bulging red papillae. The white coating is eventually lost after several days, and the tongue then appears bright red. (Courtesy of Michael J. Nowicki, MD.)

Differential Diagnosis

Kawasaki syndrome may also present with an injected pharynx and an erythematous strawberry-like tongue. It is essential to make the distinction between streptococcal infection and Kawasaki syndrome, since the latter is associated with a high incidence of coronary artery aneurysm if left untreated. Also consider toxic shock syndrome (TSS), in which one-half to three-fourths of patients tend to have pharyngitis with a strawberry-red tongue. Patients with TSS also have skin rashes, as with scarlet fever; however, the rash in TSS is macular and "sunburn-like." Erythema multiforme can also be associated with fever, pharyngeal erythema, and lingual lesions; however, it has a more distinct pathognomonic cutaneous rash (called target or iris lesions).

Emergency Department Treatment and Disposition

Penicillin or a macrolide is the drug of choice for group A streptococci. Pharyngeal cultures are useful for confirming the diagnosis. Antistreptolysin O (ASO) titers can be used for confirmation in the convalescent stage if the diagnosis is in question. Rapid streptococcal immunoassay testing may help expedite the diagnosis.

Clinical Pearls

1. A coarse, palpable, sandpaper-like rash of the skin is highly characteristic of scarlet fever.
2. Strawberry tongue initially appears white in color, with prominent red papillae bulging through the white exudate. After several days, the tongue becomes completely beefy red.
3. Erythrogenic toxin elaborated by the streptococcal organism is responsible for producing the exanthem and enanthem of scarlet fever.

Associated Clinical Features

Tori are benign nodular overgrowths of the cortical bone. Although their physical appearance can be somewhat alarming to those unfamiliar with this entity, there is generally no need for concern. These bony protuberances occur in the midline of the palate where the maxilla fuses (Fig. 6.35). Tori may also be located on the mandible, typically on the lingual aspect of the molar teeth. Tori are covered by a thin epithelium, which is easily traumatized and ulcerated. These ulcerations tend to heal very slowly because of the poor vascularization of the tori. Torus palatinus, in particular, is slow-growing and may occur at any age; however, it is most commonly noted prior to age 30 in adults. Torus palatinus affects women twice as frequently as men.

Differential Diagnosis

There are a variety of oral conditions that may be confused with mandibular or palatal tori. Gingival fibromatosis, fibroma formation secondary to irritation, granulomas, abscesses, and oral neurofibromatosis located on the palate may all be similar in appearance to torus palatinus. Nodular bony enlargement in the oral cavity may also result from fibrous dysplasia, osteomas, and Paget's disease. Oral malignancies may also manifest themselves on the palate as primary lesions. Biopsies, oral radiographs, and CT scans may aid in differentiating these conditions.

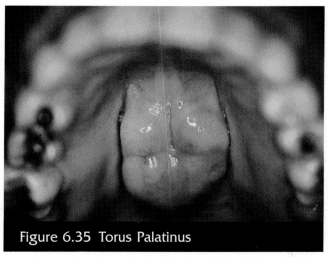

Figure 6.35 Torus Palatinus

Note the nodular appearance and characteristic central palatal location. Abrasions and ulcerations can occur on the thin overlying epithelium secondary to trauma by food and oral objects. (Courtesy of Kevin J. Knoop, MD, MS.)

Emergency Department Treatment and Disposition

Tori are normal structural variants and do not represent any inflammatory or neoplastic process. Therefore, they are of no clinical significance and require no treatment unless associated with a complication. Tori may enlarge enough to interfere with eating or speaking and impair proper fitting of dental prosthesis. For some patients the mere presence of torus palatinus may be bothersome and undesirable. Oral and maxillofacial consultation is indicated for suspected malignancies or lesions of questionable origin.

Clinical Pearls

1. Torus palatinus almost always occurs in the midline of the hard palate.
2. Both torus palatinus and torus mandibularis are nontender and otherwise asymptomatic.

Associated Clinical Features

Black hairy tongue represents a benign reactive process characterized by hyperplasia and dark pigmentation of the tongue's filiform papillae (Fig. 6.36). The elongated filiform papillae may reach up to 2 cm in length and vary in actual degree of pigmentation from light tan to black. Predisposing factors may include excessive smoking, poor oral hygiene, and the use of broad-spectrum oral antibiotics. Pigment from consumed food, beverages, and tobacco products stains the entrapped food debris and desquamated papillary keratin. Some antibiotics may alter normal oral microflora and promote the growth of chromogenic organisms, also contributing to the tongue's discoloration. The darkly pigmented filament-like papillae give the tongue a black, hairy appearance. Males are more often affected than females; this condition very rarely occurs in children. Alteration of taste perception and halitosis may be a consequence of this disorder.

Differential Diagnosis

Geographic tongue and orolingual candidiasis may resemble more lightly pigmented forms of black hairy tongue (BHT). Similarly, dark discoloration of normal tongue papillae may also mimic BHT clinically. This exogenous pigmentation of normal papillae may come from ingested food dyes and certain medications, such as bismuth-containing compounds (Fig. 6.37), keto-

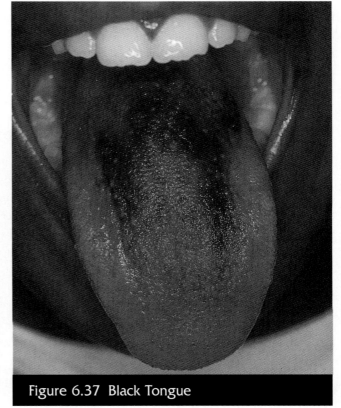

Figure 6.37 Black Tongue

Deposition of black pigment secondary to bismuth ingestion. This patient ingested Pepto-Bismol. (Courtesy of Kevin J. Knoop, MD, MS.)

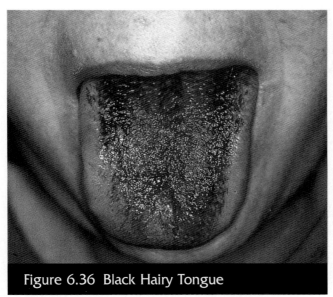

Figure 6.36 Black Hairy Tongue

Hyperplasia of the filiform papillae on the dorsum of the tongue accompanied by deposition of dark pigment is characteristic of black hairy tongue. (Courtesy of the Department of Dermatology, National Naval Medical Center, Bethesda, MD.)

conazole, and azidothymidine. The lack of hyperplastic filiform papillae with additional pigmentation of other oral mucosal surfaces may aid in distinguishing these conditions.

Emergency Department Treatment and Disposition

Improved oral hygiene with gentle tongue brushing and a reduction in the ingestion of exogenous pigment-containing substance represent the cornerstone of treatment. Removal of other predisposing factors (e.g., antibiotic withdrawal and smoking cessation) will also promote resolution of this condition. The use of topically applied retinoid preparations and antifungal agents has been advocated for more refractory instances.

Clinical Pearls

1. BHT always involves the dorsal aspect of the tongue anterior to the circumvallate papillae.
2. This is a benign condition and is rarely symptomatic.
3. The tongue is not always black and can be as light as a tan or yellow color.

CHAPTER 7

CHEST
AND ABDOMEN

Stephen Corbett
Lawrence B. Stack
Kevin J. Knoop

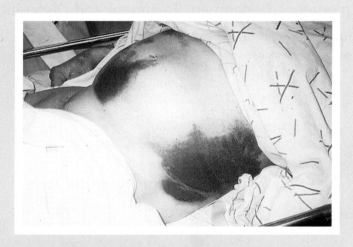

Chest and Abdominal Trauma

TRAUMATIC ASPHYXIA

Associated Clinical Features

Traumatic asphyxia is due to a sudden increase in intrathoracic pressure against a closed glottis. The elevated pressure is transmitted to the veins, venules, and capillaries of the head, neck, extremities, and upper torso, resulting in capillary rupture. Survivors demonstrate plethora, ecchymoses, petechiae (Figs. 7.1 and 7.2), and subconjunctival hemorrhages. Severe cases may produce CNS injury with seizures, posturing, and paraplegia.

Differential Diagnosis

Sudden traumatic compression of the superior vena cava produces obstruction similar to that seen in the superior vena cava syndrome. Both demonstrate a violaceous discoloration of the face and neck. History will confirm the diagnosis.

Emergency Department Treatment and Disposition

Treatment is supportive, with attention to other concurrent injuries. Long-term morbidity is related to the associated injuries.

Clinical Pearls

1. Facial petechiae are known as Tardieu's spots.
2. Be alert for associated rib and vertebral fractures.

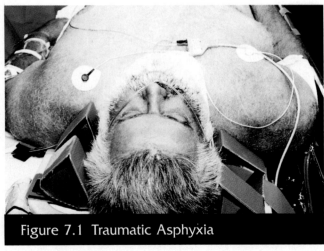

Figure 7.1 Traumatic Asphyxia

This 45-year-old male was pinned when the truck he was working under fell on his chest. He was unable to breathe for 3 to 4 min until his coworkers rescued him. The violaceous coloration of the shoulders, face, and upper chest is apparent. (Courtesy of Stephen Corbett, MD.)

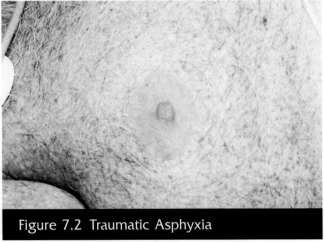

Figure 7.2 Traumatic Asphyxia

A closer view showing the petechial nature of this rash. The patient was observed in the hospital overnight and recovered completely. (Courtesy of Stephen Corbett, MD.)

TENSION PNEUMOTHORAX WITH NEEDLE THORACENTESIS

Associated Clinical Features

A tension pneumothorax results when air is able to enter but not exit the pleural space. Air in the pleural space accumulates and compresses the ipsilateral lung and vena cava, with a rapid decrease in cardiac output. The contralateral lung may suffer ventilation/perfusion($\dot{V}/\dot{Q}$) mismatch. Subcutaneous air, tracheal deviation, jugulovenous distention (JVD), and diminished or hyperresonant ipsilateral breath sounds can be clues. Subcutaneous emphysema may be visible on the neck and chest and is easily diagnosed by palpation. The released air from a tension pneumothorax can be heard escaping from a needle thoracostomy.

Differential Diagnosis

Cardiac tamponade, congestive heart failure with pulmonary edema, esophageal intubation, and anaphylaxis should be considered.

Emergency Department Treatment and Disposition

Treatment requires rapid recognition of the tension pneumothorax, frequently without benefit of chest radiographs. A large-bore needle (at least 14 gauge) should be placed over the superior rib surface of the second interspace in the midclavicular line (Fig. 7.3). A rush of air with improvement of vital signs confirms the diagnosis. A syringe loaded with sterile saline allows visualization of air return but is not mandatory. If there is no immediate improvement, do not hesitate to place a second needle in the next interspace. A chest tube should be placed as soon as possible. Ventilation with appropriate inspiratory/expiratory ratio would prevent further occurrences.

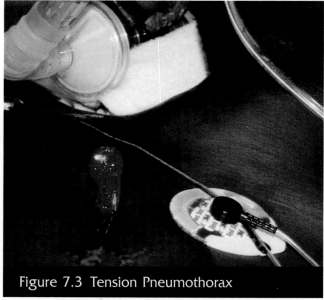

Figure 7.3 Tension Pneumothorax

A 35-year-old male with severe asthma suffered respiratory arrest during transport by ambulance. He was intubated on arrival but soon became hard to ventilate and developed subcutaneous emphysema followed by hypotension. Needle thoracostomy produced a rush of air and bubbling from the needle with stabilization of vital signs. (Courtesy of Stephen Corbett, MD.)

Clinical Pearls

1. Do not overventilate patients with obstructive pulmonary disease. "Stacking" breaths trap air in the lungs and predispose to bleb rupture and pneumothorax. The pathophysiology of this disease requires a prolonged expiratory phase.
2. The diagnosis of a tension pneumothorax is made clinically and should be treated immediately with a needle thoracostomy and ultimately a tube thoracostomy.

CARDIAC TAMPONADE WITH PERICARDIOCENTESIS

Associated Clinical Features

Beck's triad of acute cardiac tamponade includes jugulovenous distention (JVD) from an elevated central venous pressure (CVP), hypotension, and muffled heart sounds. In trauma, only one-third of patients with cardiac tamponade demonstrate this classic triad, although 90% have at least one of the signs. The simultaneous appearance of all three physical signs is a late manifestation of tamponade and usually seen just prior to cardiac arrest. Other symptoms include shortness of breath, orthopnea, dyspnea on exertion, syncope, and symptoms of inadequate perfusion.

Differential Diagnosis

Patients with a chronic pericardial effusion have an elevated CVP and a small, quiet heart but are relatively asymptomatic and without hypotension.

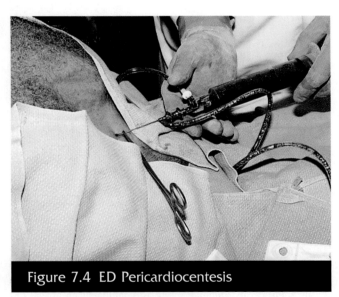

Figure 7.4 ED Pericardiocentesis

A positive pericardiocentesis in a patient with a sudden onset of shortness of breath and electrical alternans. (Courtesy of Lawrence B. Stack, MD.)

Emergency Department Treatment and Disposition

The clinical diagnosis of tamponade requires suspicion and a careful evaluation of the signs and, when available, imaging techniques. Two-dimensional echocardiography represents the ultimate standard for diagnosis. ED pericardiocentesis (Fig. 7.4) is a diagnostic and resuscitative procedure in patients with suspected cardiac tamponade. Goals of ED pericardiocentesis include identification of pericardial effusion and removal of blood from the pericardial space to relieve the tamponade.

Clinical Pearls

1. An electrical alternans seen on a 12-lead ECG suggests pericardial effusion.
2. Beck's triad for acute cardiac tamponade is a late manifestation and is seen in only 30% of trauma patients.

Associated Clinical Features

ED thoracotomy is a resuscitative procedure performed in patients with penetrating chest trauma who have lost signs of life in the presence of prehospital or ED personnel. Resuscitative thoracotomy (Fig. 7.5) in the ED has specific goals once the chest is opened: relief of cardiac tamponade, support of cardiac function (internal cardiac compressions, cross-clamping the aorta to improve coronary perfusion, and internal defibrillation), and control of hemorrhage from the heart, pulmonary vessels, thoracic wall, and great vessels.

Differential Diagnosis

Few conditions present that require immediate ED thoracotomy. A trauma patient who has lost vital signs prior to arrival of prehospital personnel is deceased and not a candidate for this procedure.

Emergency Department Treatment and Disposition

Patients with penetrating thoracic trauma who lose their vital signs en route to the ED should receive an immediate thoracotomy on arrival by the most experienced provider. Patients with penetrating thoracic trauma whose blood pressure cannot be maintained above 70 mmHg with aggressive fluid and blood management should be considered for ED thoracotomy. Patients with blunt trauma who lose their vital signs en route to the ED should not undergo an ED thoracotomy, since they rarely survive. Surgical support should be notified as soon as possible.

Clinical Pearls

1. Injuries potentially responsive to resuscitative ED thoracotomy include cardiac tamponade, pulmonary parenchymal and tracheobronchial injuries, large-vessel injuries, air embolism, and penetrating heart injuries.
2. Resuscitative ED thoracotomy should be performed immediately once the indications have been met, since the likelihood of survival is greater when this is performed earlier in the resuscitation.

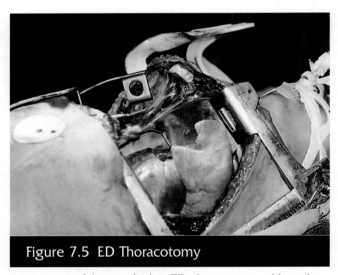

Figure 7.5 ED Thoracotomy

An unsuccessful resuscitative ED thoracotomy with pericardiotomy in a patient with penetrating chest trauma who lost signs of life in the field after the paramedics arrived at the scene. (Courtesy of Alan B. Storrow, MD.)

191

Associated Clinical Features

Diagnostic peritoneal lavage (DPL) was introduced in 1965 as a simple, fast, and reliable technique to identify hemoperitoneum in patients with blunt and penetrating abdominal trauma. It is performed by placing a catheter into the peritoneum, aspirating for gross blood, and introducing 1 L of crystalloid if the initial aspiration is negative (Fig. 7.6). The lavage fluid is then withdrawn and white and red cell blood counts are obtained. Interpretation of the results is based on the type of trauma. A "grossly positive" DPL is evident when 10 mL of blood is obtained on the initial aspiration. The procedure is considered positive in blunt abdominal trauma when >100,000 RBC/mm^3 or >500 WBC/mm^3 are present in the lavage fluid. In penetrating abdominal trauma, the procedure is considered positive when >10,000 RBC/mm^3 are present (up to 100,000 RBC/mm^3 is used by some). Lavage fluid containing intestinal contents is evidence of perforating bowel injury.

Indications for DPL in blunt trauma include equivocal examination with significant abdominal trauma, unreliable examination (intoxication, spinal trauma, head injury), unexplained hypotension with suspected abdominal injury, and when serial examinations are not possible (in patients going to the operating room for other injuries).

Indications for DPL in penetrating trauma include patients in whom the need for celiotomy is unclear, tangential wounds in which peritoneal penetration is uncertain, stab wounds in which

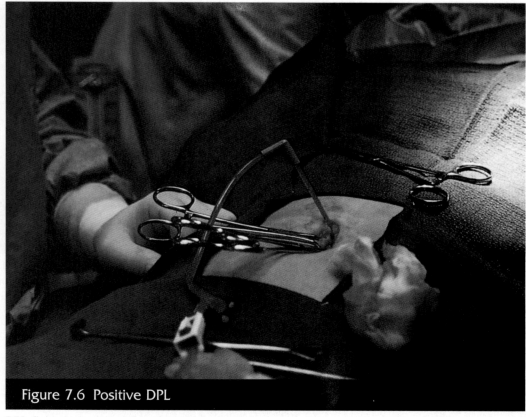

Figure 7.6 Positive DPL

DPL fluid obtained from this patient with blunt trauma was microscopically positive. Initial aspiration was negative. (Courtesy of Kevin J. Knoop, MD, MS.)

there are no peritoneal signs or signs of peritoneal penetration, and low chest wounds to identify diaphragmatic injury.

Contraindications to DPL include any condition in which a celiotomy is clearly indicated, since this would delay definitive treatment.

Differential Diagnosis

Injuries that may not be diagnosed with DPL include subcapsular liver or spleen hematomas, injury to a hollow viscus, ruptured diaphragm, and ruptured bladder. Retroperitoneal injuries (pancreatic, duodenal) are not diagnosed with DPL.

Emergency Department Treatment and Disposition

A positive DPL is an indication for celiotomy. Patients with negative DPLs are observed or discharged based on a variety of factors including injury mechanism, comorbid disease states, and concurrent traumatic injuries.

Clinical Pearls

1. Intraperitoneal blood (30 mL) will typically give a DPL result of $\geq 100,000$ RBC/mm^3.
2. Controversy exists over the positive cell count in penetrating abdominal trauma, since the range for a positive result can vary between centers from 1000 to 100,000 RBC/mm^3.
3. If transfer is indicated, a sample of DPL fluid should accompany the patient.

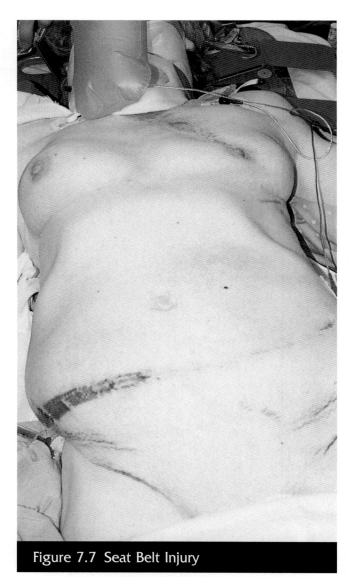

Figure 7.7 Seat Belt Injury

Ecchymosis from the three-point seat belt is clearly seen. The injuries identified are multiple rib fractures and multiple hematomas of the small bowel wall. (Courtesy of Stephen Corbett, MD.)

Associated Clinical Features

Seat belts have reduced mortality and the severity of trauma due to motor vehicle accidents; however, they occasionally produce injury. Injuries caused by the standard three-point restraint harness (Fig. 7.7) are most commonly rib fractures. Injuries caused by the older lap belts include abdominal injuries such as bowel contusion or perforation and lumbar fractures.

Differential Diagnosis

A careful primary and secondary survey identifies most injuries caused by seat belt use. Difficult diagnosis occurs in the case of bowel perforation or diaphragmatic rupture, in which signs and symptoms may not occur until hours or days after the initial injury.

Emergency Department Treatment and Disposition

Patients with a mechanism for significant trauma or with other injuries requiring admission should be admitted for observation or definitive treatment. Patients discharged home from the ED should be given appropriate precautions to monitor for a delayed injury presentation.

Clinical Pearls

1. Maintain a high suspicion for intraabdominal injury when ecchymosis from a seat belt is seen in a trauma victim.
2. When lap belt bruises are present, there is a higher incidence of bowel injury.

Associated Clinical Features

Bluish to purplish periumbilical discoloration (Cullen's sign) and left flank discoloration (Grey-Turner's sign) represent retroperitoneal hemorrhage that has dissected through fascial planes to the skin (Fig. 7.8). Retroperitoneal blood may also extravasate into the perineum, causing a scrotal hematoma or inguinal mass. This hemorrhage may represent a hemodynamically significant bleed.

Differential Diagnosis

Cullen's sign and Grey-Turner's sign are most frequently associated with hemorrhagic pancreatitis (seen in 1 to 2% of cases), and typically are seen 2 to 3 days after onset of acute pancreatitis. These signs may also be seen in ruptured ectopic pregnancy, severe trauma, leaking or ruptured abdominal aortic aneurysm, coagulopathy, or any other condition associated with bleeding into the retroperitoneum.

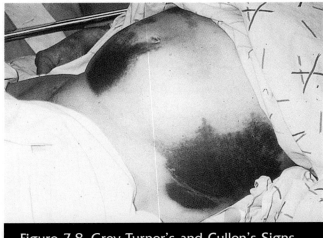

Figure 7.8 Grey-Turner's and Cullen's Signs

This patient displays both flank and periumbilical ecchymoses characteristic of Grey-Turner's and Cullen's signs. (Courtesy of Michael Ritter, MD.)

Emergency Department Treatment and Disposition

Treatment of patients with Grey-Turner's sign or Cullen's sign depends on the etiology of the hemorrhage. Because the hemorrhage may represent a hemodynamically significant bleed, cardiovascular stabilization after airway stabilization is of the utmost importance. Once the patient has been stabilized, the source of bleeding can be elicited by selected laboratory [complete blood cell count (CBC), amylase, lipase, human chorionic gonadotropin (HCG)] and diagnostic studies [ultrasound, computed tomography (CT)]. Because of the severity of diseases associated with Grey-Turner's and Cullen's signs, these patients are usually admitted to the hospital.

Clinical Pearls

1. Grey-Turner's sign (flank discoloration) and Cullen's sign (periumbilical discoloration) are due to retroperitoneal bleeding that has dissected through fascial planes.
2. These signs are typically seen 2 to 3 days after the acute event.
3. These signs are seen in only 1 to 2% of patients with hemorrhagic pancreatitis.

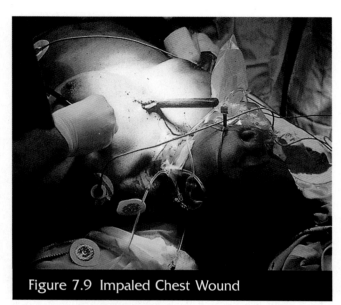

Figure 7.9 Impaled Chest Wound

This patient was stabbed in the chest with a butcher knife in a family dispute. The knife was stabilized by EMS providers at the scene and removed in the operating room. Injury was isolated to the right atrium. (Courtesy of Kevin J. Knoop, MD, MS.)

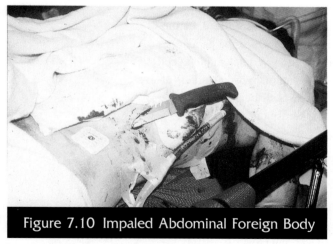

Figure 7.10 Impaled Abdominal Foreign Body

Impaled knife to the left abdomen. (Courtesy of Ian Jones, MD.)

Associated Clinical Features

Stab wounds cause injury to tissue in their path. Stab wounds to the chest, in addition to causing pneumo- or hemothorax, may also cause life-threatening injuries to the heart and major blood vessels (Fig. 7.9). One-third of stab wounds to the abdomen (Fig. 7.10) penetrate the peritoneal cavity. Half of those injuries that penetrate the peritoneum require surgical intervention. The path of the stab wound is difficult to determine if the inflicting object has been removed. The size of the external wound frequently underestimates the internal injury. Impaled foreign bodies to the chest or abdomen pose a complex problem. The object inflicting the injury may also be preventing significant blood loss and therefore should be removed by the trauma surgeon in the operating room.

Differential Diagnosis

Determining whether the impaled object has violated the peritoneum or if injury to a significant structure has occurred can be determined by local wound exploration or diagnostic peritoneal lavage (DPL), depending on the stability of the patient and location of the wound (see Fig. 7.13).

Emergency Department Treatment and Disposition

Initial stabilization of the patient (intravenous fluid resuscitation, oxygen, monitoring), obtaining appropriate laboratory studies including blood type and cross-matching, and resource mobilization (trauma team) are important steps in the initial management of penetrating chest or abdominal trauma. Prior to surgical evaluation, stabilization of the impaled foreign object should be performed to prevent further injury.

Clinical Pearl

1. Impaled chest or abdominal foreign bodies should be removed only by the trauma surgeon in a controlled setting.

Associated Clinical Features

Evisceration of abdominal contents (Fig. 7.11) usually occurs after a stab or slash wound to the abdomen (Fig. 7.12). It is an indication for celiotomy (laparotomy). Other indications for celiotomy in penetrating abdominal trauma include peritoneal injury; unexplained shock; evidence of blood in the stomach, bladder, or rectum; and loss of bowel sounds.

Differential Diagnosis

Superficial laceration without peritoneal penetration, laceration with peritoneal penetration but no visceral injury, and laceration with peritoneal penetration and visceral injury may present with a similar mechanism and need to be differentiated. Consideration of the anatomic boundaries of the abdomen (Fig. 7.13) is important in differentiating abdominal injuries from penetrating chest or retroperitoneal injuries.

Emergency Department Treatment and Disposition

Initial stabilization (intravenous fluid resuscitation, oxygen, and monitoring), obtaining appropriate laboratory studies including a blood type and cross-matching, and resource mobilization (notifying surgical team, operating room, and anesthesiology) are important steps in the initial management of penetrating abdominal trauma. In most cases, definitive treatment is celiotomy.

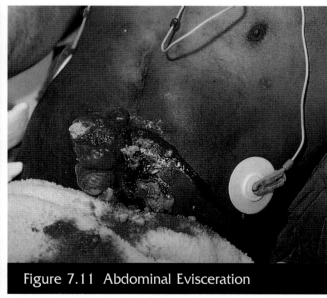

Figure 7.11 Abdominal Evisceration

Self-induced evisceration with bowel perforation and spillage of food particles is clearly seen in this photograph. This patient went directly to the operating room. (Courtesy of Lawrence B. Stack, MD.)

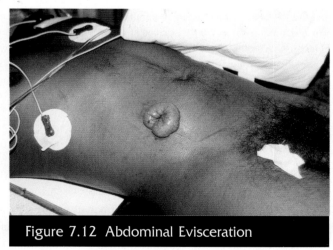

Figure 7.12 Abdominal Evisceration

Evisceration of small bowel after assault and stab wound to the right lower abdomen. (Courtesy of Frank Birinyi, MD.)

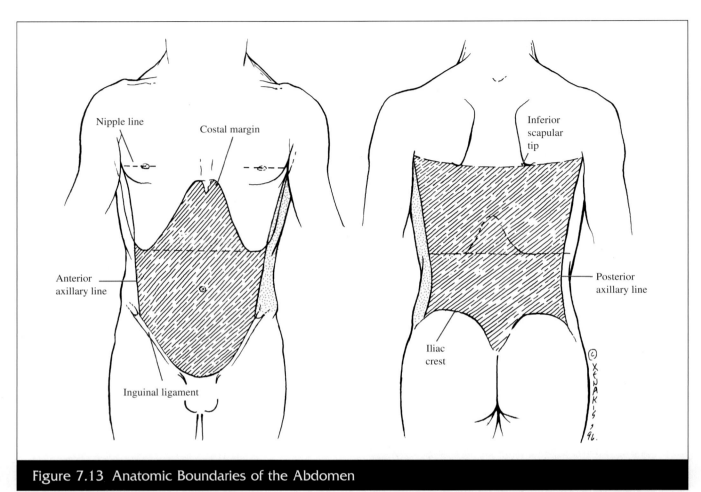

Figure 7.13 Anatomic Boundaries of the Abdomen

Anterior abdomen: Anterior costal margins superiorly, laterally by the anterior axillary lines, and inferiorly by the inguinal ligaments.
Low chest: Nipple line (fourth intercostal space) anteriorly and inferior scapular tip (seventh intercostal space) to inferior costal margins.
Flank: (Shaded blue) Anterior axillary line anteriorly, posteriorly by the posterior axillary line, inferiorly by the iliac crest, and superiorly by the inferior scapular tip. The back is bounded laterally by the posterior axillary lines.
Back: Inferior scapular tip to iliac crest and posterior axillary lines.

Clinical Pearls

1. Indications for celiotomy after penetrating wounds to the abdomen include evisceration; peritoneal signs; unexplained hypotension; blood in the stomach, bladder, or rectum; and loss of bowel sounds.
2. Selected patients with stab wounds to the abdomen and peritoneal penetration may be conservatively observed for delayed complications.
3. As many as 20% of patients with stab wounds to the abdomen can be discharged from the ED based on a negative wound exploration.

Associated Clinical Features

Blunt traumatic abdominal hernia is defined as herniation through disrupted musculature and fascia associated with adequate trauma, without skin penetration, and no evidence of a prior hernial defect at the site of injury (Fig. 7.14). This occurs when a considerable blunt force is distributed over a surface area large enough to prevent skin penetration but small enough to cause a focal defect in the underlying fascia or muscle wall. Most of these injuries are due to seat belt injures in motor vehicle crashes; handlebar injuries are the second most common cause.

Differential Diagnosis

Existing hernia, abdominal wall hematoma, and abdominal wall contusion should be considered in evaluating a patient with focal blunt trauma to the abdomen and possible hernia. Abdominal computed tomography (CT) with contrast is the diagnostic procedure of choice in the evaluation of abdominal trauma (Fig. 7.15). Ultrasound may play a limited role in the diagnosis of abdominal wall hernia.

Emergency Department Treatment and Disposition

Identification and treatment of life-threatening associated injuries takes priority over the hernia. The hernial defect should be repaired after the patient has been stabilized.

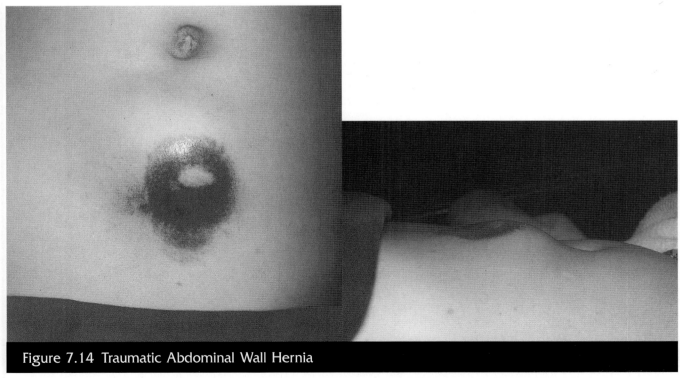

Figure 7.14 Traumatic Abdominal Wall Hernia

This 5-year-old boy suffered a traumatic hernia from a handlebar injury. (Courtesy of Lawrence B. Stack, MD.)

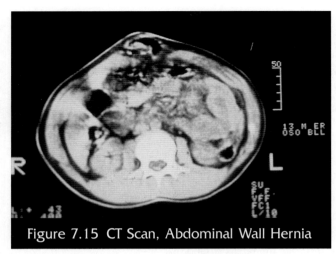

Figure 7.15 CT Scan, Abdominal Wall Hernia

Abdominal contents are seen extruding through a fascial defect. (Courtesy of Lawrence B. Stack, MD.)

Clinical Pearls

1. Abdominal hernia due to blunt trauma is a rare injury, most frequently due to seat belt injuries in motor vehicle crashes.

2. CT scan is the diagnostic procedure of choice for abdominal wall hernia.

Chest and Abdominal Conditions

Associated Clinical Features

Increased respiratory effort may be manifest by increased respiratory rate, increased chest wall excursion, and retractions of the less rigid structures of the thorax. Retractions of the sternum (Fig. 7.16), suprasternal notch (Fig. 7.17), and intercostal retractions reflect increased respiratory effort. This may be due to obstructive disease such as asthma or tracheal obstruction, pneumonia, or restrictive disease. The presence of stridor, wheezing, or rhonchi will help distinguish the cause.

Differential Diagnosis

Asthma, chronic obstructive pulmonary disease, emphysema, epiglottitis, croup, foreign-body aspiration, esophageal foreign body, bacterial tracheitis, posterior pharyngeal abscess, and anaphylaxis are all conditions that must be considered in a patient with retractions.

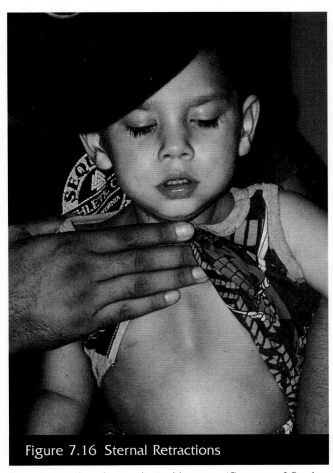

Figure 7.16 Sternal Retractions

Sternal retractions in a patient with croup. (Courtesy of Stephen Corbett, MD.)

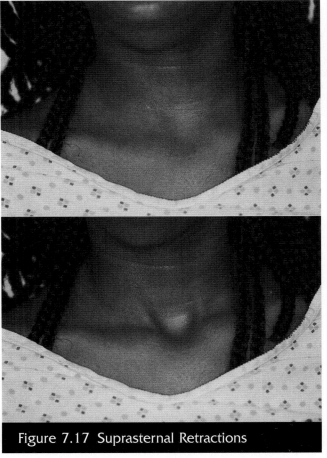

Figure 7.17 Suprasternal Retractions

Suprasternal retractions in an adolescent with severe asthma. (Courtesy of Kevin J. Knoop, MD, MS.)

Emergency Department Treatment and Disposition

An aggressive search for the cause of the retractions is required to direct therapy. Rapid evaluation of the airway for patency and breathing for oxygenation should be done immediately on presentation. High-flow oxygen by face mask is appropriate for patients in respiratory distress. Preparations for securing an airway should be underway for those patients in severe distress or respiratory failure. Routine measures for the mildly symptomatic patient depend on the cause of the retractions. For asthma or exacerbations of chronic obstructive pulmonary disease (COPD), nebulized β_2 agonists and steroid therapy may be appropriate. Patients with croup may require nebulized normal saline and possibly epinephrine or dexamethasone as initial therapy. Foreign-body aspiration requires consultation for confirmation of the suspected diagnosis and removal.

Clinical Pearls

1. Retractions are best observed with the patient at rest with the chest exposed.
2. Retractions from obstructive airway disease can be intercostal and supraclavicular and are usually accompanied by nasal flaring, increased expiratory phase, and increased respiratory rate.

Associated Clinical Features

This symptom complex develops from obstruction of venous drainage from the upper body, resulting in increased venous pressure, which leads to dilation of the collateral circulation. Superior vena cava (SVC) syndrome is most commonly caused by malignant mediastinal tumors. Dyspnea; swelling of the face, upper extremities, and trunk; chest pain, cough, or headache may be present. Physical findings include dilation of collateral veins of the trunk and upper extremities, facial edema and erythema (plethora), cyanosis, and tachypnea (Fig. 7.18).

Differential Diagnosis

Malignancy, pericarditis, pericardial tamponade, tuberculosis, and congestive heart failure should be considered.

Emergency Department Treatment and Disposition

Radiation therapy is the treatment of choice for most malignant mediastinal tumors causing SVC syndrome. Administration of corticosteroids and diuretics initiated in the ED may provide temporary relief pending definitive therapy.

Clinical Pearls

1. SVC syndrome is most commonly caused by malignant mediastinal tumors.
2. Treatment of most mediastinal tumors causing SVC syndrome is radiation therapy.
3. CT scan of the chest is the diagnostic modality of choice for patients with SVC syndrome.

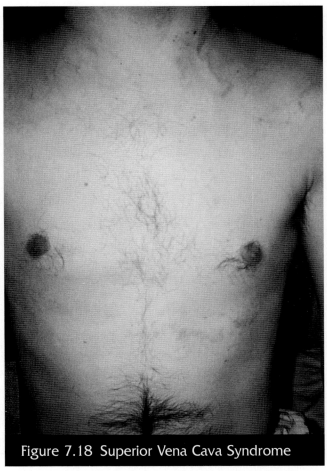

Figure 7.18 Superior Vena Cava Syndrome

A 27-year-old man with SVC syndrome. Note the prominent collateral veins of the chest and neck. (Courtesy of William K. Mallon, MD.)

Associated Clinical Features

Pancoast's tumor involves the apical lung and may affect contiguous structures such as the brachial plexus, sympathetic ganglion, vertebrae, ribs, superior vena cava, and recurrent laryngeal nerve (more common for left-sided tumors). Horner's syndrome, extremity edema, nerve deficits, hoarseness, and superior vena cava syndrome may result. Erosion of tumor through the chest wall can cause compression of venous outflow, with resultant jugulovenous distention (JVD) (Fig. 7.19).

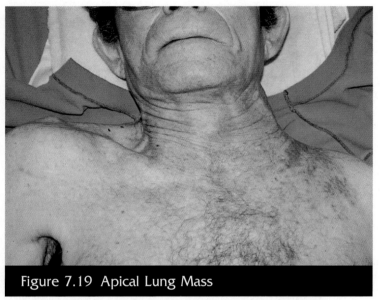

Figure 7.19 Apical Lung Mass

This 68-year-old male cigarette smoker complained of cough and weight loss. A chest radiograph shows a left apical tumor. There is erosion of the tumor into the chest wall, with an indurated supraclavicular and infraclavicular mass. Moderate JVD is apparent, suggesting venous outflow obstruction. (Courtesy of Stephen Corbett, MD.)

Differential Diagnosis

Virchow's node of abdominal carcinoma, lymphoma, vascular abnormalities, and tuberculosis should be considered.

Emergency Department Treatment and Disposition

Treatment depends on the staging and type of tumor. The superior vena cava syndrome can be treated acutely with radiation and diuretics. Thrombolytic therapy has been used successfully in some cases of acute vena caval thrombosis.

Clinical Pearls

1. Thrombosis may cause acute decompensation with edema, plethora, and airway collapse.
2. Prompt radiation therapy can be lifesaving in cases of vena caval obstruction.

Associated Clinical Features

Central venous (right atrial) pressure is reflected by distention of the internal or external jugular veins. Normal pressure is less than 3 cm of distention above the sternal angle of Louis. Distention greater than 4 cm should be considered abnormal. Evaluation begins by raising the head of the supine patient 30 to 60 degrees. The highest point of venous pulsation at the end of normal expiration is measured from the sternal angle of Louis. The presence of jugulovenous distention (JVD) (Fig. 7.20) should prompt an immediate search for possible pulmonary or cardiac pathology. The presence of crackles, murmurs, rubs, percussed hyperresonance, or crepitus may help disclose the etiology.

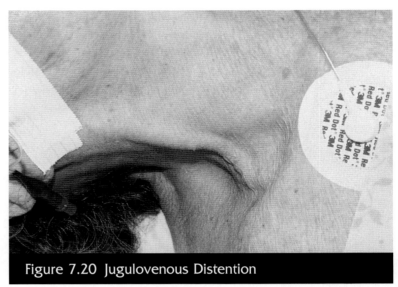

Figure 7.20 Jugulovenous Distention

An engorged external jugular vein is noted as it crosses the sternocleidomastoid muscle into the posterior triangle of the neck and disappears beneath the clavicle to join the brachiocephalic vein and the superior vena cava. This patient has severe congestive heart failure requiring intubation. (Courtesy of Stephen Corbett, MD.)

Differential Diagnosis

Causes of JVD include right ventricular failure, left ventricular failure, biventricular failure, parenchymal lung disease, pulmonary hypertension, pulmonic stenosis, restrictive pericarditis, superior vena cava syndrome, pulmonary embolus, tricuspid valve outflow obstruction, tension pneumothorax, increased circulating blood volume, and atrial myxoma. Temporary venous engorgement may result from Valsalva maneuver, positive pressure ventilation, and Trendelenburg position.

Emergency Department Treatment and Disposition

Treatment varies depending on the cause. Preload reduction may help in cases of congestive heart disease. Reversal of a traumatic etiology with needle thoracostomy or pericardiocentesis may be required.

Clinical Pearls

1. Right-sided myocardial infarction may produce JVD with clear lung fields.
2. JVD may be absent in the presence of the above-listed causes if hypovolemia is present.

Associated Clinical Features

Veins of the abdomen normally are scarcely visible within the abdominal wall. Engorged veins, however, are often visible through the normal abdominal wall. Engorged veins forming a knot in the area of the umbilicus are described as a caput medusae (Fig. 7.21). The extent of associated findings depends on the underlying etiology. It is usually secondary to liver cirrhosis, with subsequent portal hypertension and development of circulation circumventing the liver.

Differential Diagnosis

Emaciation, inferior vena caval obstruction, superior vena caval obstruction, portal vein obstruction, and superficial abdominal vein thrombosis can cause engorged abdominal veins.

Emergency Department Treatment and Disposition

Treatment is directed at the underlying cause. This finding by itself does not require acute treatment.

Clinical Pearl

1. Caput medusae has the same clinical significance as the more common pattern of venous engorgement.

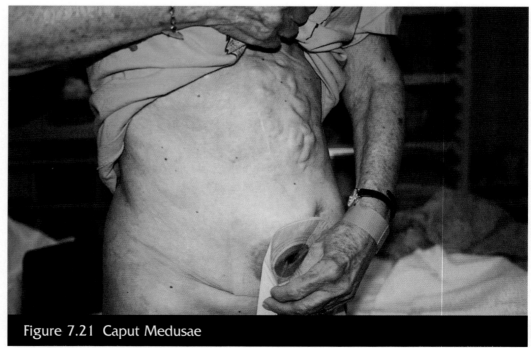

Figure 7.21 Caput Medusae

This elderly female with alcoholic cirrhosis has engorged abdominal veins in the knotted appearance consistent with caput medusae. (Courtesy of Gary Schwartz, MD.)

Associated Clinical Features

A hernia is a tissue protrusion through an abnormal body cavity opening. Most abdominal wall hernias occur at the groin and umbilicus. Incarceration is defined as the inability to reduce the protruding tissue to its normal position. Strangulation occurs when the blood supply of the hernia's contents is obstructed and tissue necrosis ensues. An *incisional* hernia (Fig. 7.22) may manifest clinically as a mass or palpable defect adjacent to a surgical incision and can be reproduced by having the patient perform Valsalva's maneuver. Obesity and wound infection, which interfere with wound healing, predispose to the formation of incisional hernias. The defect of an *indirect* inguinal hernia (Figs. 7.23, 7.24) is the internal (abdominal) inguinal ring and may be manifest in either sex by a bulge over the midpoint of the inguinal ligament that increases in size with Valsalva's maneuver. A fingertip placed into the external ring through the inguinal canal may palpate the defect. A *direct* hernia (Fig. 7.25) may be manifest by a bulge midway adjacent to the pubic tubercle and may be felt by the pad of the finger placed in the inguinal canal. The defect is in the posterior wall of the inguinal canal. Direct inguinal hernias are usually painless and occur in males.

Nausea and vomiting may be present if incarceration with bowel obstruction occurs. Strangulation can lead to fever, peritonitis, and sepsis.

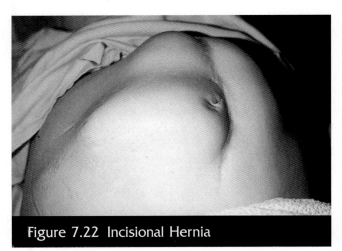

Figure 7.22 Incisional Hernia

An incisional hernia in an obese female. (Courtesy of Stephen Corbett, MD.)

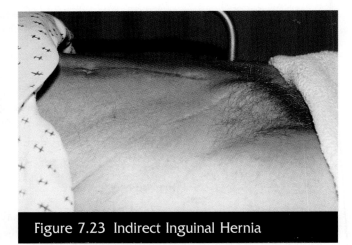

Figure 7.23 Indirect Inguinal Hernia

A recurrent indirect inguinal hernia in a female patient. (Courtesy of Frank Birinyi, MD.)

Differential Diagnosis

Tumor, aneurysm, lymphadenopathy, bowel obstruction, ascites, lipoma, femoral hernia, hydrocele, testicular torsion, and epididymitis may have similar presentations.

Emergency Department Treatment and Disposition

When patients present without clinical evidence of strangulation (fever, leukocytosis, systemic signs of toxicity), reduction should be attempted. In the presence of these signs, prompt surgical consultation is warranted for surgical reduction. Reduction in the ED is facilitated with systemic

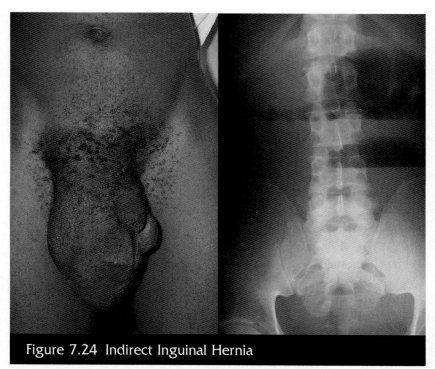

Figure 7.24 Indirect Inguinal Hernia

This 35-year-old man has an incarcerated indirect inguinal hernia (A) with small bowel obstruction (B). (Courtesy of Lawrence B. Stack, MD.)

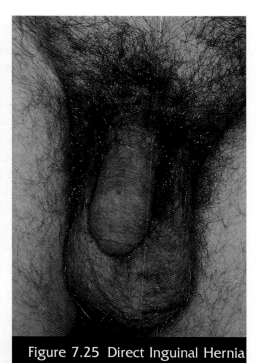

Figure 7.25 Direct Inguinal Hernia

A direct inguinal hernia. Note the bulge adjacent to the left pubic tubercle. (Courtesy of Daniel L. Savitt, MD.)

analgesia (as most patients present with significant pain), placing the patient in the supine position, and applying a cold pack to the hernia. Routine consultation for operative repair is indicated in asymptomatic patients with reducible hernias.

Clinical Pearls

1. Acutely strangulated or incarcerated hernias require immediate surgical evaluation.
2. Direct inguinal hernias are usually painless.
3. Evaluation and treatment of concomitant exacerbating conditions (cough, constipation, vomiting) prevent recurrences.

Associated Clinical Features

The umbilicus is a common site of abdominal hernias. Predisposing conditions in adults most commonly include ascites and prior abdominal surgery. The size of the defect determines the symptomatology and incidence of incarceration, with smaller defects resulting in more pronounced symptoms and an increased incidence of incarceration. Pain is located in the area of the fascial defect. Contents of the hernia may be palpable and tender. Symptoms of obstruction (nausea, vomiting, and abdominal distention) may be present. If the hernia becomes strangulated (Fig. 7.26), erythema of the overlying skin with fever and hypotension may occur.

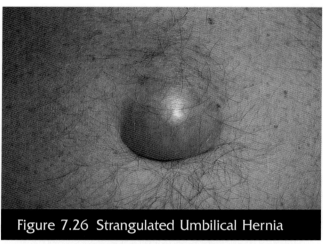

Figure 7.26 Strangulated Umbilical Hernia

The skin overlying a strangulated umbilical hernia is erythematous and tender. (Courtesy of Lawrence B. Stack, MD.)

Differential Diagnosis

An omphalocele, gastroschisis, or urachal duct cyst may present as an umbilical mass.

Emergency Department Treatment and Disposition

Reduction is attempted in the stable patient without clinical evidence of strangulation. Treatment of any predisposing conditions (i.e., abdominal paracentesis in the patient with tense ascites) may cause spontaneous reduction and avoid progression of the hernia to strangulation. Routine consultation for elective repair is indicated in asymptomatic patients with reducible hernias.

Clinical Pearls

1. Umbilical hernias in children usually resolve without treatment.
2. Umbilical hernias in adults usually become worse and require elective repair.

Associated Clinical Features

When the vestigial urachal duct is not obliterated during development, drainage can occur from the bladder to the umbilicus (Fig. 7.27). Cysts can often be palpated between the umbilicus and pubis. Besides drainage and pain, infection of the duct or cyst may occur. Rarely, adenocarcinoma may form in these remnants.

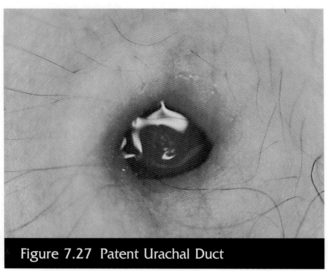

Figure 7.27 Patent Urachal Duct

This 19-year-old man presented to the ED with clear fluid (urine) draining from the umbilicus, suggestive of a patent urachal duct. (Courtesy of Kevin J. Knoop, MD, MS.)

Differential Diagnosis

Omphalocele, prune belly syndrome, exstrophy of the bladder, gastroschisis, and umbilical hernias are other abdominal wall abnormalities in children.

Emergency Department Treatment and Disposition

Acute treatment is usually not required unless an infection is evident. Routine urologic consultation for surgical revision is indicated. A retrograde study with radiopaque dye will outline the patent duct.

Clinical Pearl

1. This finding should prompt a careful search for other urogenital anomalies.

SISTER MARY JOSEPH'S NODE
(NODULAR UMBILICUS)

Associated Clinical Features

A Sister Mary Joseph's node is a metastasis manifesting as periumbilical lymphadenopathy secondary to abdominal carcinoma (Fig. 7.28). Cancers of the colon may cause pain, change in bowel habits, anemia, and obstruction. In general, left-sided cancers cause obstruction, whereas right-sided tumors may have significant metastases before they create signs and symptoms. These metastases typically involve peritoneal and omental spread with distant metastases to the liver. Spread to the umbilicus is colloquially known as the Sister Mary Joseph's node.

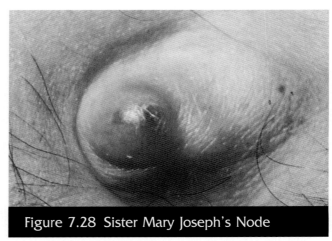

Figure 7.28 Sister Mary Joseph's Node

Sister Mary Joseph's nodule of patient with gastric carcinoma. (Courtesy of Department of Dermatology, Naval Medical Center, Portsmouth, VA.)

Differential Diagnosis

Other umbilical masses to consider include hernias, ascites, and urachal cysts.

Emergency Department Treatment and Disposition

Prompt referral for staging and treatment of the tumor is indicated. Other signs and symptoms (from obstruction, blood loss, malnutrition, and pain) should be addressed and treated.

Clinical Pearls

1. Virchow's node, presenting as a supraclavicular mass, also heralds bowel carcinoma.
2. A Sister Mary Joseph's node is commonly due to gastric carcinoma.

Associated Clinical Features

Abdominal distention may be a symptom—often described by the patient as the feeling of being bloated—or a sign, an obvious protuberance of the patient's abdomen that may or may not be out of proportion to the rest of the body. Other findings vary widely, depending on the cause. In obesity, the abdomen is uniformly rounded while an increase in girth and fat concurrently accumulates in other parts of the body. In patients with ascites, there may be shifting dullness, a fluid wave, bulging flanks, or hepatomegaly. In patients with neoplasms, there may be a palpable mass. In gravid patients, fetal heart tones may be present and fetal motion may be felt. In patients with excess gas from bowel obstruction, there may be absent or high-pitched bowel sounds and absence of bowel movements or flatus.

Differential Diagnosis

Numerous conditions present with abdominal distention. Obesity, ascites, pregnancy, neoplasms, aneurysm, tympanites (excess gas), organomegaly, and feces are important etiologies to consider in the differential.

The profile of the fluid-filled abdomen of ascites (Fig. 7.29) is a single curve from the xiphoid process to the pubic symphysis. The umbilicus may be everted, and there may be prominent superficial abdominal veins. Other physical findings suggestive of ascites include shifting dullness and a fluid wave.

The pregnant abdomen profile (Fig. 7.30) shows the outward curve to be more prominent in the lower half of the abdomen. The umbilicus may be everted in the last trimester of

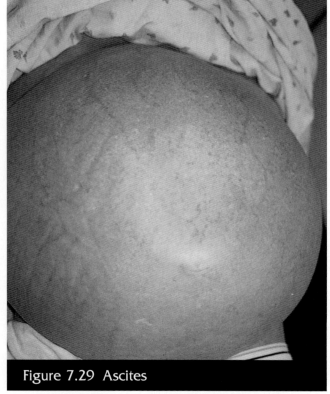

Figure 7.29 Ascites

Ascites in an alcoholic man. Note the everted umbilicus and prominent superficial abdominal veins. (Courtesy of Alan B. Storrow, MD.)

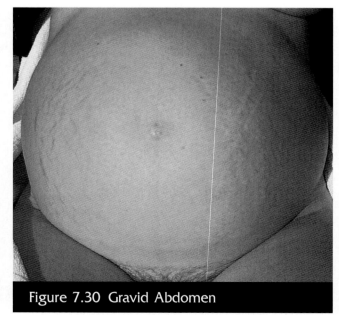

Figure 7.30 Gravid Abdomen

The abdomen of a woman at 39 weeks' gestation. Note the abdominal wall striae, everted umbilicus, and prominent superficial abdominal wall veins. (Courtesy of Stephen Corbett, MD.)

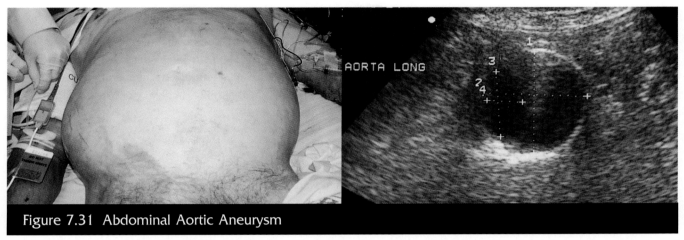

Figure 7.31 Abdominal Aortic Aneurysm

A. The abdomen of a patient with a leaking abdominal aortic aneurysm. Note the mottled abdominal wall and the prominent curvature of the right side of the abdomen. (Courtesy of Stephen Corbett, MD.) B. Abdominal aortic aneurysm seen on ultrasound in another patient. (Courtesy of Sally Santen, MD.)

pregnancy. Prominent abdominal wall veins may also be seen. The presence of fetal heart tones confirms the diagnosis.

The abdominal profile of a patient with a leaking abdominal aortic aneurysm (Fig. 7.31) shows a mottled abdominal wall reflective of hypoperfusion of this structure. There may be a curve of the midabdomen to either side of the aorta, more often on the left. Palpation of a pulsatile mass supports the diagnosis. Ultrasound or computed tomography (CT) of the abdomen will confirm the diagnosis.

Excess abdominal air (Fig. 7.32) can be located in the lumen of the stomach or intestines or free in the peritoneum. This abdominal profile is a single curve from the xiphoid process to the pubic symphysis. Nausea, vomiting, decreased bowel sounds, and colicky pain are present in a small bowel obstruction. Large bowel obstruction may be accompanied by feculent vomiting and absent production of flatus.

Emergency Department Treatment and Disposition

Treatment varies widely depending on the cause; thus emergent management is directed at determining the etiology. Life-threatening causes (aneurysm, obstruction, neoplasms) require stabilization and referral for definitive treatment.

Clinical Pearl

1. The "six f's" can categorize conditions causing abdominal distention: fat, flatus, fetus, fluid, feces, fatal growth.

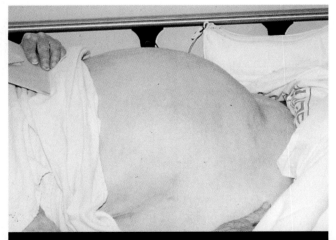

Figure 7.32 Pseudoobstruction

An 85-year-old woman was brought from a nursing home with a complaint of abdominal distention and pain for 1 to 2 days. An eventual diagnosis of Ogilvie's syndrome, or pseudoobstruction of the large bowel, was made. This is usually seen in debilitated patients and can be treated with decompression. (Courtesy of Stephen Corbett, MD.)

Associated Clinical Features

Intertrigo is a dermatitis occurring on apposed surfaces of skin, such as the creases of the neck, folds of the groin and armpit, or a panniculus (Fig. 7.33). It is characterized by a tender, red plaque with a moist, macerated surface. A candidal infection may result and often becomes secondarily infected with skin flora. Erythema, fissures, burning, itching, exudates, and fever may also accompany intertrigo.

Differential Diagnosis

Necrotizing fasciitis of the abdominal wall, cellulitis, and *Candida albicans* infection should be considered.

Emergency Department Treatment and Disposition

Local care, empiric topical antifungal treatment, and good personal hygiene are recommended. Intravenous antibiotics initiated in the ED directed against skin flora are recommended if there is secondary infection.

Clinical Pearl

1. Consider necrotizing fasciitis of the abdominal wall if the patient appears septic.

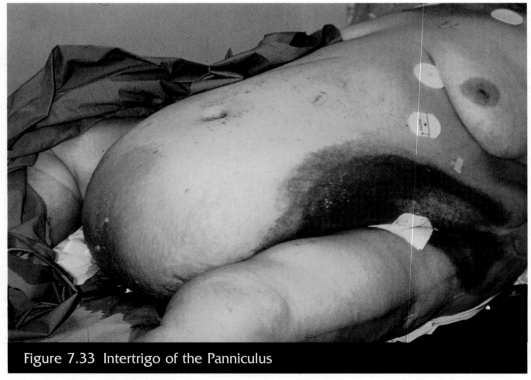

Figure 7.33 Intertrigo of the Panniculus

Note the exudate, erythema, and fissures of the abdominal wall. This patient also had fever, suggesting secondary infection. (Courtesy of Lawrence B. Stack, MD.)

Associated Clinical Features

Mild trauma may produce hematomas of the rectus sheath (Fig. 7.34). This injury results in intense abdominal pain, which can mimic an acute abdomen. The diagnosis is made by physical examination, since the ecchymosis is not always visible. Palpation of the abdominal wall reveals a tender mass that is accentuated by contraction of the rectus. Ultrasound and computed tomography (CT) may confirm the diagnosis.

Differential Diagnosis

Multiple causes of abdominal pain must be considered in the differential diagnosis. Careful examination with supplemental imaging studies, if needed, helps with the diagnosis. Two classic signs of retroperitoneal bleeding are Grey-Turner's sign (flank ecchymosis) and Cullen's sign (periumbilical ecchymosis). Hemorrhagic pancreatitis and ruptured ectopic pregnancy, respectively, should be considered.

Emergency Department Treatment and Disposition

Assuming that there is no underlying blood dyscrasia or coagulopathy, hematomas of the rectus sheath usually resolve in 1 to 2 weeks.

Clinical Pearl

1. Fothergill's sign is enhancement of a rectus sheath hematoma when the abdominal wall is tensed. The mass should not cross the midline and should be easier to palpate with abdominal muscle contractions. Intraabdominal masses are more difficult to palpate with such contractions.

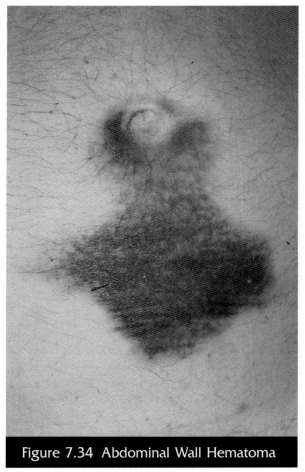

Figure 7.34 Abdominal Wall Hematoma

This 50-year-old man with chronic obstructive pulmonary disease developed right-lower-quadrant pain after an episode of coughing. A repeat examination on the second visit showed clearly visible ecchymosis. There was no coagulopathy and amylase was normal. A CT scan revealed a 10- by 8-cm hematoma in the right rectus abdominis sheath. (Courtesy of Stephen Corbett, MD.)

Associated Clinical Features

Abdominal striae are linear, depressed, pink or bluish scar-like lesions (Fig. 7.35) that may later become silver or white. They are caused by weakening of the elastic cutaneous tissues from chronic stretching. They most commonly occur on the abdomen but are also seen on the buttocks, breasts, and thighs. Striae are commonly seen in obesity, pregnancy, Cushing's syndrome, and chronic topical corticosteroid treatment. In Cushing's syndrome, a state of adrenal hypercorticism, the skin becomes fragile and easily breaks from normal stretching.

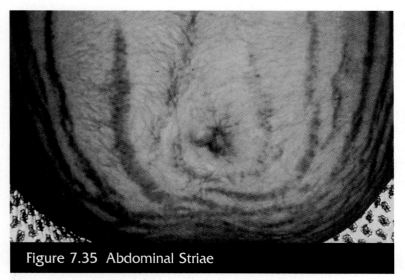

Figure 7.35 Abdominal Striae

These striae are seen in a patient with recent weight gain, moon facies, and altered mental status. The patient was diagnosed with Cushing's syndrome. (Courtesy of Geisinger Medical Center, Department of Emergency Medicine, Danville, PA.)

Differential Diagnosis

Obesity, pregnancy, Cushing's syndrome, and chronic topical corticosteroid treatment should be considered.

Emergency Department Treatment and Disposition

This finding seldom presents as a condition requiring acute treatment; thus, attention is directed to determining and treating the underlying cause.

Clinical Pearls

1. Recent striae (pink or blue) with moon facies, hypertension, renal calculi, osteoporosis, and psychiatric disorders are suggestive of Cushing's syndrome.
2. The striae caused by pregnancy typically fade with time, unlike those associated with Cushing's syndrome.

CHAPTER 8

UROLOGIC CONDITIONS

Jeffrey D. Bondesson

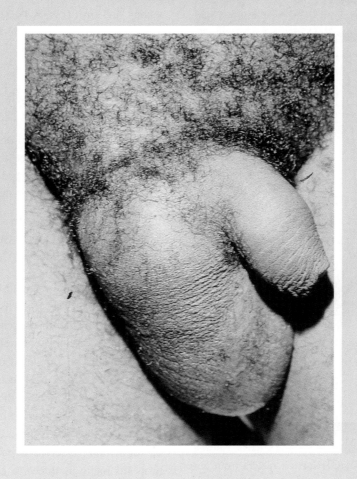

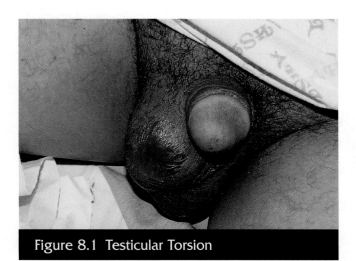

Figure 8.1 Testicular Torsion

Swollen, tender hemiscrotum, with erythema of scrotal skin and retracted testicle. (Courtesy of Stephen Corbett, MD.)

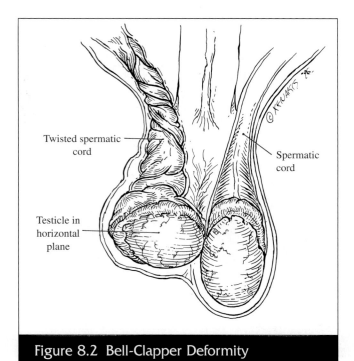

Figure 8.2 Bell-Clapper Deformity

A bell-clapper deformity in testicular torsion results from the twisting of the spermatic cord and causes the testis to be elevated, with a horizontal lie. The lack of fixation of the tunica vaginalis to the posterior scrotum predisposes the freely movable testis to rotation and subsequent torsion. An elevated testis with a horizontal lie may be seen in asymptomatic patients at risk for torsion.

Associated Clinical Features

These patients are most often young men (average age 16 to 17.5 years) who present complaining of the sudden onset of pain in one testicle. The pain is then followed by swelling of the affected testicle, reddening of the overlying scrotal skin, lower abdominal pain, nausea, and vomiting. An examination reveals a swollen, tender, retracted testicle (Fig. 8.1) that often lies in the horizontal plane (bell-clapper deformity) (Figs. 8.2 and 8.3). The spermatic cord is frequently swollen on the affected side. In delayed presentations, the entire hemiscrotum may be swollen, tender, and firm (Fig. 8.4). The urine is usually clear with a normal urinalysis. In one-third of cases there is a peripheral leukocytosis.

Differential Diagnosis

Alternative diagnoses that should be considered include acute epididymitis, torsion of the testicular appendix (Fig. 8.5), trauma, acute orchitis (mumps), hydrocele, spermatocele, varicocele, hernia, and tumor. A good history and physical examination helps narrow the diagnosis.

Emergency Department Treatment and Disposition

Urologic consultation should be obtained immediately and preparations made to go to the operating room without delay. Doppler ultrasound or technetium scanning may be helpful if these procedures will not delay surgery. In the interim, detorsion may be attempted if the patient is seen within a few hours of onset: the affected testicle should initially be opened like a book, that is, the right testicle turned counterclockwise when viewed from below and the left testicle turned clockwise when viewed from below. Pain relief should be immediate. Decreased pain should prompt additional turns (as many as three) to complete detorsion; increased pain should prompt detorsion in the opposite direction. Ancillary studies should not delay operative intervention, since testicular infarction will occur within 6 to 12 h after torsion.

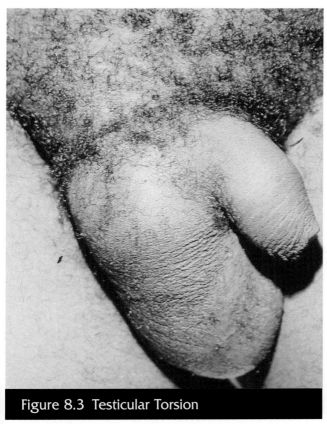

Figure 8.3 Testicular Torsion

A retracted testicle consistent with early testicular torsion is seen. (Courtesy of David W. Munter, MD, MBA.)

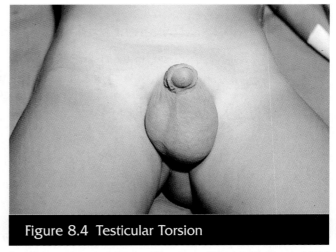

Figure 8.4 Testicular Torsion

Swollen, tender scrotal mass. (Courtesy of Patrick McKenna, MD.)

Clinical Pearls

1. The cremasteric reflex is almost always absent in testicular torsion.
2. Patients may report similar, less severe episodes that spontaneously resolved in the recent past.
3. Half of all torsions occur during sleep.
4. Abdominal or inguinal pain is sometimes present without pain to the scrotum.
5. The age of presentation has a bimodal pattern, since torsion is also more prevalent during infancy and adolescence.

TORSION OF A TESTICULAR OR EPIDIDYMAL APPENDIX

Associated Clinical Features

Small vestigial remnants in the embryology of the scrotum are often found on the superior portions of the testicle or the epididymis. These appendages, which have no known function, are occasionally on a stalk that is subject to torsion. This most commonly occurs in boys up to 16 years of age but has been reported in adults. The patient will complain of sudden pain around the superior pole of the testicle or epididymis as the appendix undergoes necrosis and inflammation. Early in the course, palpation of a firm, tender nodule in this area will confirm the diagnosis.

Differential Diagnosis

Later in the course of appendiceal torsion, swelling and pain generalize to the rest of the scrotum. At this point the condition may be difficult to differentiate from testicular torsion, acute epididymitis, or acute orchitis. Hydrocele, spermatocele, varicocele, hernia, and tumor must also be considered.

Emergency Department Treatment and Disposition

Urologic consultation should be obtained immediately. Differentiating from the more emergent testicular torsion is the key responsibility. Ancillary studies are generally not helpful in making this diagnosis unless it presents very early in its course. A urinalysis is generally normal. The characteristic physical signs of a small, tender, upper-pole nodule along with a color Doppler ultrasound showing good flow to the testicle may mitigate the need for emergent surgery. With later presentations or an equivocal ultrasound, the diagnosis may not be made with confidence before surgery. Necrotic appendices are excised if found during an exploration to rule out testicular torsion. If surgery is not deemed necessary by the urologic consultant, analgesics and rest are all that is required. The appendix will involute and calcify in 1 to 2 weeks.

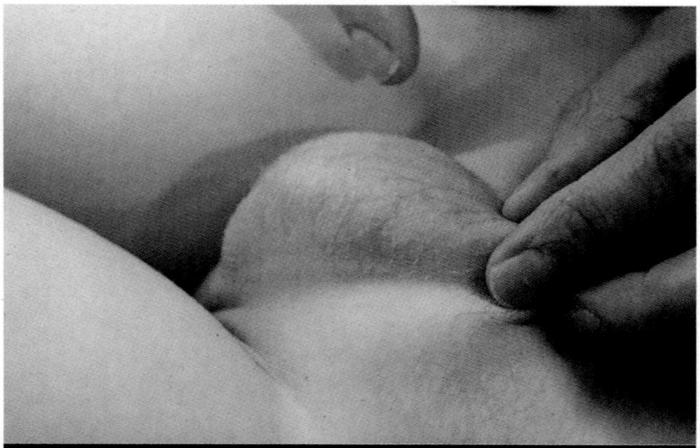

Figure 8.5 Blue-Dot Sign

A blue-dot sign is caused by torsion of the testicular appendix. It is best seen with the skin held taut over the testicular appendix. (Courtesy of Javier A. Gonzalez del Rey, MD.)

Clinical Pearls

1. Stretching of the scrotal skin across the necrotic nodule will occasionally reveal a bluish discoloration of the nodule, called the "blue-dot sign" (Fig. 8.5). This is pathognomonic for torsion of the appendix.
2. A reactive hydrocele may accompany appendiceal torsion. When the hydrocele is transilluminated, the blue-dot sign may be revealed.

Associated Clinical Features

Most hydroceles occur in older patients and develop gradually without any significant symptoms. A hydrocele generally presents as a soft, pear-shaped, fluid-filled cystic mass anterior to the testicle and epididymis that will transilluminate (Fig. 8.6). However, it can be tense and firm and will transilluminate poorly if the tunica vaginalis is thickened. Almost all hydroceles in children are communicating, resulting from the same mechanism that causes inguinal hernia. A persistent narrow processus vaginalis acts like a one-way valve, thus permitting the accumulation of dependent peritoneal fluid in the scrotum. Acute symptomatic hydroceles are more rare and can occur in association with epididymitis, trauma, or tumor.

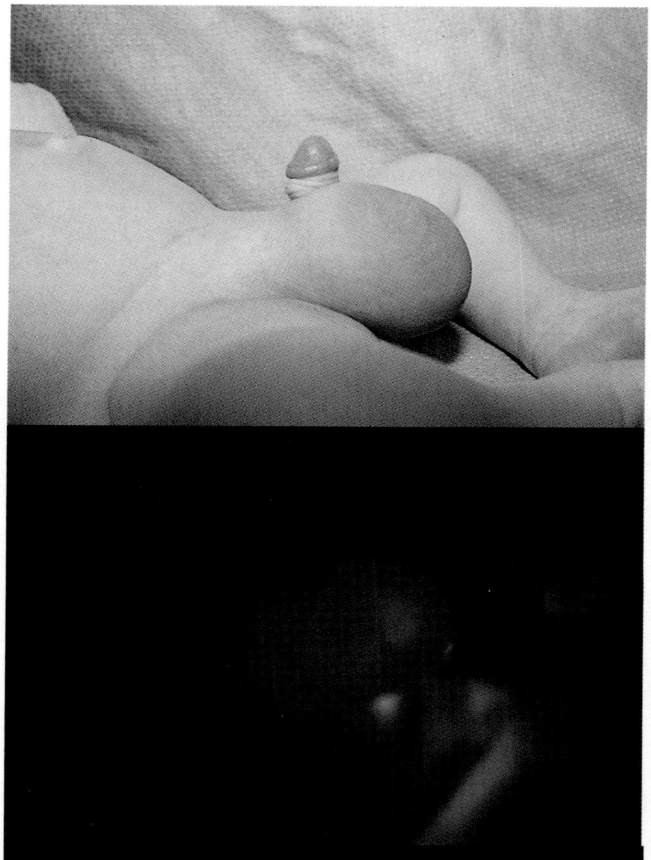

Differential Diagnosis

Painless masses that must be differentiated from hydrocele include spermatocele, varicocele, inguinal hernia, and tumor. Painful masses to be differentiated include traumatic hematocele, epididymitis, orchitis, and torsion.

Emergency Department Treatment and Disposition

In an acute hydrocele, treatment must be directed at discovering a possible underlying cause. A positive urinalysis may point toward an infectious etiology. Transillumination helps demonstrate whether the mass is cystic or solid. Ultrasound can be very helpful in imaging the scrotal contents and delineating the composition of the mass. Acute hydroceles should not be considered benign and require referral to a urologist to rule out tumor or infection. Chronic accumulations are referred to a urologist on a more routine basis for elective drainage.

Figure 8.6 Hydrocele

Painless swelling in the scrotum of a young boy (*top*). Transillumination of the swelling (*bottom*) identifies the hydrocele. (Courtesy of Michael J. Nowicki, MD.)

Clinical Pearls

1. Ten percent of testicular tumors have a reactive hydrocele as the presenting complaint.
2. An inguinal hernia with a loop of bowel in it may emit bowel sounds.
3. Hydroceles are almost never symptomatic.
4. Acute reactive hydroceles may be caused by infection, trauma, or torsion.

Associated Clinical Features

In testicular tumor, a painless, firm testicular mass (Fig. 8.7) is palpated, with the patient often complaining of a "heaviness" of his testicle. If the patient presents early, the mass will be distinct from the testis, whereas later presentations will have generalized testicular or scrotal swelling. These lesions occasionally present with pain due to infarction of the tumor.

Differential Diagnosis

Epididymitis is the most frequent misdiagnosis, which unfortunately may delay surgical intervention. When the tumor presents with infarction pain, differentiation from epididymitis or torsion can be difficult. In some cases, ultrasound can help differentiate these entities.

Emergency Department Treatment and Disposition

Patients should be promptly referred to a urologist for surgical exploration.

Clinical Pearls

1. Acute hydroceles and hematoceles should prompt the physician to consider a tumor as the cause.
2. Pain from tumor infarction is usually not as severe as pain due to torsion or epididymitis.
3. Findings of an unexplained supraclavicular lymph node, abdominal mass, or chronic nonproductive cough resistant to conventional therapy should prompt a testicular examination for tumor.

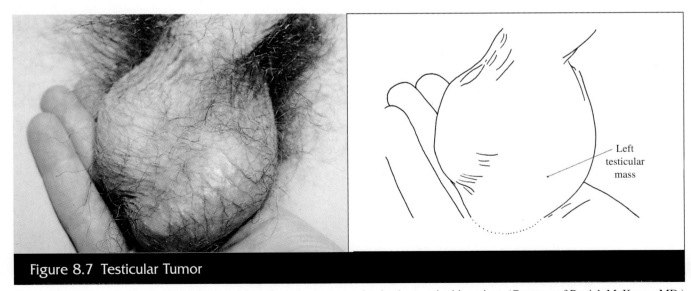

Figure 8.7 Testicular Tumor

This painless left testicular mass is highly suspicious for tumor, as proved to be the case in this patient. (Courtesy of Patrick McKenna, MD.)

Associated Clinical Features

A scrotal abscess is a suppurative mass with surrounding erythema involving the superficial layers of the scrotal wall (Fig. 8.8). The usual history is of progressive swelling of a small pustule or papule followed by increasing pain and induration or fluctuance. Constitutional symptoms and fever are generally absent.

Differential Diagnosis

An apparently superficial scrotal abscess must be distinguished from a deep scrotal abscess or early Fournier's gangrene. In the latter two cases, patients tend to appear quite ill. The erythema of the skin overlying an abscess should not be mistaken for an urticarial reaction, erythema multiforme, or drug eruption.

Emergency Department Treatment and Disposition

Using local anesthesia, simply make a stab incision and drain the abscess. The patient is then instructed to use a sitz bath and to change the dressing frequently. An alternative method of treatment is to unroof the abscess by circumferential excision. This ensures that there is adequate wound drainage. Immunocompromised patients may require intravenous antibiotics and admission.

Clinical Pearl

1. If the patient appears ill out of proportion to the superficial appearance, suspect that this mass is the point of a deep scrotal abscess.

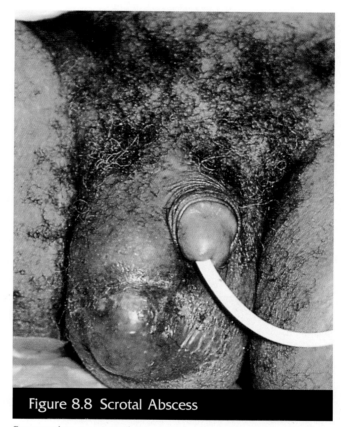

Figure 8.8 Scrotal Abscess

Suppurative mass on the scrotum. (Courtesy of David Effron, MD.)

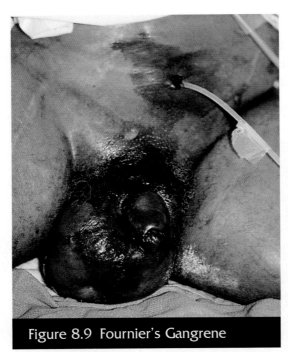

Figure 8.9 Fournier's Gangrene

Markedly swollen, necrotic, tender scrotum, perineum, and adjacent thighs are seen. (Courtesy of David Effron, MD.)

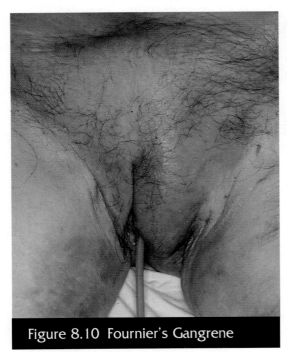

Figure 8.10 Fournier's Gangrene

Swollen, tender, erythematous labia, perineum, and inner thighs in a female patient with Fournier's gangrene. (Courtesy of Daniel L. Savitt, MD.)

Associated Clinical Features

Fournier's gangrene most frequently occurs in a middle-aged diabetic male who presents with swelling, erythema, and severe pain of the entire scrotum (Fig. 8.9), but it is also known to occur in females (Fig. 8.10). In males, the scrotal contents often cannot be palpated because of the marked inflammation. The patient has constitutional symptoms with fever and frequently is in shock. There is often a history of recent urethral instrumentation, an indwelling Foley catheter, or perirectal disease. A localized area of fluctuance cannot be appreciated.

Differential Diagnosis

The differential diagnosis includes cellulitis, superficial scrotal abscess, edema due to heart failure or lymphatic obstruction, allergic reaction, and epididymoorchitis with skin fixation.

Emergency Department Treatment and Disposition

These patients require aggressive fluid resuscitation and early surgical consultation for immediate debridement and surgical drainage. Broad-spectrum antibiotics effective against gram-positive, gram-negative, and anaerobic organisms should be given as soon as possible in the ED. There is anecdotal experience that treatment is enhanced by hyperbaric oxygen.

Clinical Pearls

1. Pain out of proportion to the clinical findings may represent an early presentation of Fournier's gangrene.
2. A plain pelvic radiograph may reveal subcutaneous air.
3. Fournier's gangrene is usually quite painful but has been known to present with only a mildly uncomfortable necrosis of the scrotal wall and exposed testis.

Associated Clinical Features

Paraphimosis is the entrapment of a retracted foreskin that cannot be reduced behind the coronal sulcus (Fig. 8.11). Pain, swelling, and erythema are common. If severe, the constriction causes edema and venous engorgement of the glans, which can lead to arterial compromise with subsequent tissue necrosis.

Differential Diagnosis

In contrast to paraphimosis, phimosis is the inability to retract the foreskin (Fig. 8.12), usually a chronic condition. Other diagnoses to consider include superficial balanitis, hair tourniquet, contact dermatitis, and urticaria.

Emergency Department Treatment and Disposition

Squeezing the glans firmly for 5 min to reduce the swelling can lead to successful reduction of the foreskin. Local infiltration of anesthesia with vertical incision of the constricting band should be performed by a urologist if manual reduction fails.

Clinical Pearls

1. In the presence of arterial compromise, if a urologist is not immediately available, the emergency physician should incise the constricting band.
2. The patient should be referred to a urologist for circumcision if successfully reduced.
3. Phimosis is "physiologic" in young males (generally less than 5 to 6 years old).
4. Phimosis, if "reduced" (retracted proximally over the glans), can cause a paraphimosis—a true emergency.

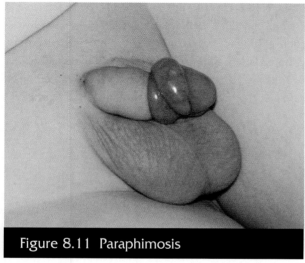

Figure 8.11 Paraphimosis

Moderate edema of retracted foreskin, which is entrapped behind the coronal sulcus. (Courtesy of Alan C. Heffner, MD.)

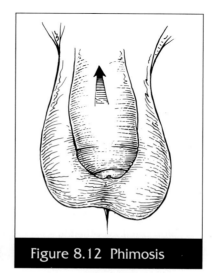

Figure 8.12 Phimosis

In phimosis, the foreskin cannot be retracted, often due to meatal stenosis and scarring.

Associated Clinical Features

These patients present with persistent, usually painful erection due to pathologic engorgement of the corpora cavernosa (Fig. 8.13). Patients may present within several hours or several days of their first symptoms. The glans penis and corpus spongiosum are generally not engorged and remain flaccid. The physiology is either arterial, which is generally traumatic, or venoocclusive. Reversible causes of venoocclusive disease include sickle cell disease, direct injection of erectile agents, and leukemic infiltration. Nonreversible causes include idiopathic ones—the most common, spinal cord lesions, and a variety of medications.

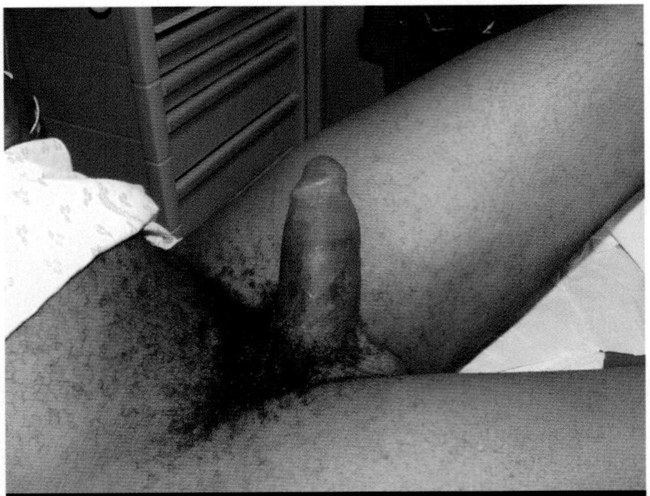

Figure 8.13 Priapism

A painful persistent erection due to pathologic engorgement of the corpora cavernosa is seen in this patient with sickle cell disease. The glans penis and corpus spongiosum are not engorged (Courtesy of Kevin J. Knoop, MD, MS.)

Differential Diagnosis

Priapism is confirmed when there is a prolonged erection with a flaccid glans and corpus spongiosum. The history and physical examination should be directed toward signs of trauma, infection, medications, drug use, and the diseases that predispose to priapism. Traumatic priapism is more flaccid and generally less painful than the venoocclusive form.

Emergency Department Treatment and Disposition

The diseases that are associated with reversible priapism should be treated. Ice packs to the perineum have traditionally been recommended but are frequently unsuccessful. Terbutaline given orally or subcutaneously occasionally reverses priapism. Aspiration of blood from the corpus cavernosum can lead to detumescence and should be followed by a compressive dressing. Injectable erectile agents can be reversed by aspiration followed by intracavernous injection of alpha-adrenergic agents such as phenylephrine. Urologic consultation should be obtained immediately for traumatic or persistent priapism despite initial treatment, with close urologic follow-up for those that are successfully reversed in the ED. Patients with persistent priapism despite treatment must frequently undergo surgery.

Clinical Pearls

1. Patients should be advised that impotence is a frequent complication of priapism, regardless of the length of the symptoms or the success of any treatment.
2. Although the glans penis and corpus spongiosum are generally not affected, urinary retention often accompanies priapism.

Associated Clinical Features

Urethral injury is rarely an isolated event; it is often associated with multiple trauma. Anterior urethral injuries are most often the result of a straddle injury and may present late (many patients are still able to void), with a local infection or sepsis from extravasated urine. Posterior urethral injuries occur in motor vehicle and motorcycle accidents and are usually the result of pelvic fractures. Patients have blood at the urethral meatus (Fig. 8.14), cannot void, and have perineal bruising. In males, the prostate is often boggy or free-floating or may not be palpable at all if there is a retroperitoneal hematoma between the prostate and the rectum.

Differential Diagnosis

Bladder rupture, higher urinary tract injuries, urethritis, and penile fracture may all present with blood at the meatus.

Emergency Department Treatment and Disposition

Urethral instrumentation such as Foley catheterization should not occur prior to a retrograde urethrogram with highly concentrated water-soluble contrast. If there is only a partial anterior tear, a gentle attempt at catheterization can be made if it is abandoned at the first sign of resistance. If catheterization is unsuccessful and whenever there is a posterior tear, a suprapubic catheter should be placed in the ED with a trocar if relief of bladder distention is required prior to operative repair.

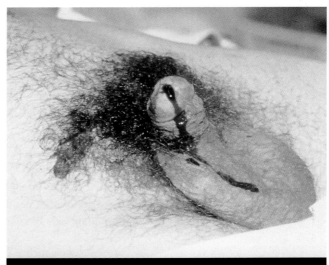

Figure 8.14 Urethral Rupture

Blood at the urethral meatus in a patient with urethral rupture secondary to trauma. (Courtesy of David Effron, MD.)

Clinical Pearls

1. Foley catheter insertion is contraindicated in patients with a suspected urethral injury prior to a retrograde urethrogram.
2. Urethral injury should be suspected in the multiple trauma patient who is unable to void or has blood at the meatus, a high-riding prostate, or perineal trauma.
3. Vaginal lacerations due to trauma in females should prompt consideration of a urethral tear.
4. Occasionally urine from an anterior urethral tear will extravasate into the scrotum, causing marked swelling.
5. Posterior injuries are frequently associated with other intraabdominal injury.

Associated Clinical Features

Patients usually present complaining of trauma during sexual arousal and often relate experiencing a sudden "snapping" sound or sensation, pain, and deformity, which is caused by a tearing of the tunica albuginea. The shaft of the penis is swollen and often angulated at the fracture site (Fig. 8.15).

Differential Diagnosis

Penile fracture can be confused with penile trauma without tear of the tunica albuginea, urethral injury, Peyronie's disease (dorsal contracture), priapism, or foreign bodies.

Emergency Department Treatment and Disposition

If the patient cannot urinate, a retrograde urethrogram may be required to rule out urethral injury (Fig. 8.16). These patients require admission and referral to a urologist, who frequently takes them immediately to the operating room for repair.

Clinical Pearls

1. Patients sometimes concoct elaborate, non-sexually-related stories surrounding the circumstances of injury, but penile fracture most commonly occurs during sexual arousal.
2. Penile implants are also subject to injury in a similar fashion.

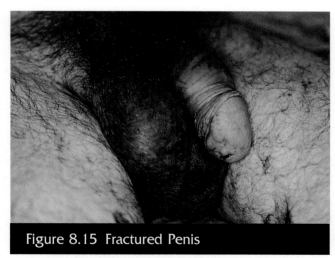

Figure 8.15 Fractured Penis

A swollen, ecchymotic penis is shown. Note the angulation at the midshaft of the penis, indicating the "fracture" site. Blood at the meatus, as shown here, is further evidence of a urethral injury. (Courtesy of Kevin J. Knoop, MD, MS.)

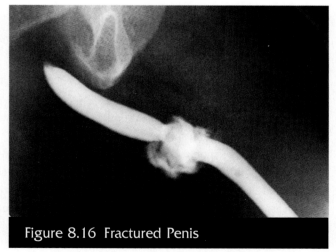

Figure 8.16 Fractured Penis

Retrograde urethrogram showing urethral injury from the fractured penis in Fig. 8.15. (Courtesy of David W. Munter, MD.)

Associated Clinical Features

In straddle injury, the patient has pain, swelling, contusion, and hematoma of the perineum or scrotum following direct blunt trauma (Figs. 8.17 and 8.18). This injury is commonly caused by a fall onto a bicycle frame cross-tube, playground equipment, or a toilet seat. Swelling can be severe enough to interfere with urination. Scrotal contents can also be contused or crushed with this injury.

Differential Diagnosis

Fournier's gangrene, cellulitis, and urticaria are similar in appearance but without the history of trauma. Sexual or physical abuse should be considered.

Emergency Department Treatment and Disposition

Treatment is supportive and includes cold packs, elevation, rest, and analgesics. If unable to void, the patient may require catheterization.

Clinical Pearls

1. Laceration of the perineum can be obscured by swelling if a careful examination is not performed.
2. Pelvic radiographs should be obtained in all perineal injuries.
3. Males and females are at high risk for urethral injuries with this type of injury.
4. Straddle injury is differentiated from abuse with a good history from a reliable caregiver that matches the injury.

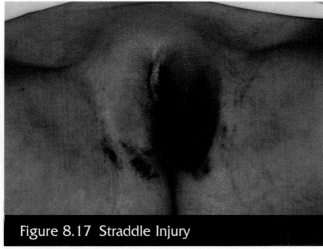

Figure 8.17 Straddle Injury

Ecchymosis, swelling, and contusion of the perineum in a 3-year-old female who tripped and fell on a large plastic toy. (Courtesy of James Mensching, MD.)

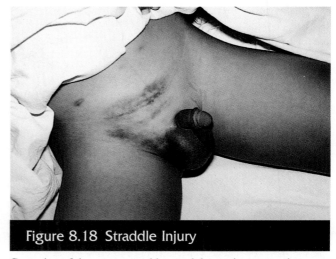

Figure 8.18 Straddle Injury

Contusion of the scrotum and lower abdomen in a young boy consistent with a straddle injury. (Courtesy of David W. Munter, MD.)

Associated Clinical Features

Balanoposthitis is an infection and inflammation of the glans penis that also involves the overlying foreskin (prepuce) (Fig. 8.19). *Balanitis* is isolated to the glans, whereas *posthitis* involves only the prepuce. Pain, erythema, and edema of the affected parts of the penis are typically present. Patients may refrain from urination secondary to dysuria, or the edema may induce meatal occlusion, leading to urinary retention or obstruction. Common etiologies include overgrowth of normal bacterial flora secondary to poor hygiene (pediatric patients), sexually transmitted diseases (adolescents and adults), and candidal infections (the elderly or immunocompromised) (Fig. 8.20).

Differential Diagnosis

The diagnosis is usually straightforward; however, the underlying etiology often must also be addressed. Examples are sexually transmitted diseases in healthy adults and diseases associated with immunocompromise (e.g. diabetes mellitus, AIDS, alcoholism). Phimosis occurs when

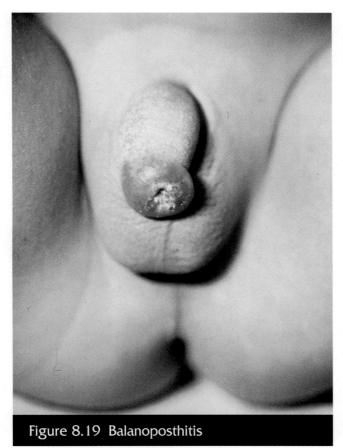

Figure 8.19 Balanoposthitis

Note the erythema, localized edema, and significantly constricted preputial orifice of the distal penis. (Courtesy of Lawrence B. Stack, MD.)

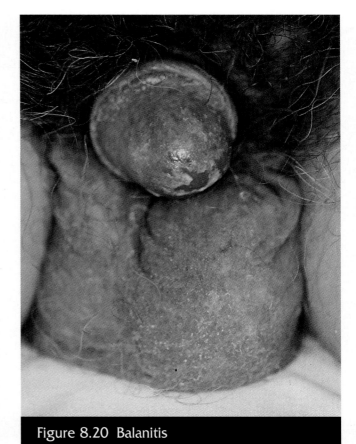

Figure 8.20 Balanitis

Candidal balanitis in an elderly patient with no other complaints. New-onset diabetes was diagnosed. (Courtesy of Kevin J. Knoop, MD, MS.)

chronic infection due to poor hygiene causes fibrosis and contracture of the preputial opening. Other diagnoses to consider include contact dermatitis, fixed drug eruptions, lichen sclerosus et atrophicus, and squamous cell carcinoma.

Emergency Department Treatment and Disposition

Treatment is directed at the suspected etiology. Warm soaks and topical antibiotics (bacitracin) are the mainstay of therapy for infectious etiologies owing to poor hygiene. Parents should be counseled about proper cleansing and handling of the prepuce. Oral or intravenous antibiotics may be indicated if there is an accompanying cellulitis. If urinary obstruction is present, catheterization may be attempted using a small catheter. If catheterization is unsuccessful, urologic consultation for emergent surgical correction of the prepuce is required. Candidal infections are treated with meticulous hygiene and topical antifungal agents. Routine urologic referral is indicated for suspected lichen sclerosus et atrophicus and squamous cell carcinoma.

Clinical Pearls

1. The inability to retract the foreskin completely is normal in young males up to age 4 or 5. Attempting to do so could cause a paraphimosis, a true emergency.
2. Placing the child in a bathtub with warm water will help alleviate difficulty with micturition assuming that no obstruction is present.
3. Candidal balanitis or balanoposthitis may be associated with an undiagnosed immunocompromised state.
4. Suspected sexually transmitted diseases require treatment for the partners as well.

CHAPTER 9

SEXUALLY TRANSMITTED DISEASES AND ANORECTAL CONDITIONS

Diane M. Birnbaumer
Lynn K. Flowers

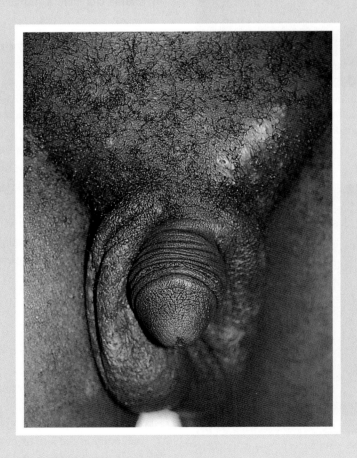

Associated Clinical Features

Lesions of primary syphilis generally appear after an incubation period of 2 to 6 weeks, but they may appear up to 3 months after exposure. The patient usually presents with a solitary round to oval painless genital ulcer (Figs. 9.1 and 9.2). However, the ulcer may be slightly painful, and several lesions are sometimes seen. The base of the genital ulcer is dry in males, moist in females; purulent fluid in the base is uncommon. The borders of the ulcer are often indurated. Patients may develop ulcers at any site of inoculation on the body. Bilateral, nontender, nonfluctuant adenopathy is common. Lesions resolve spontaneously in 3 to 12 weeks without treatment as the infection progresses to the secondary stage. Patients with primary syphilis are at risk for concurrent infection with other sexually transmitted diseases.

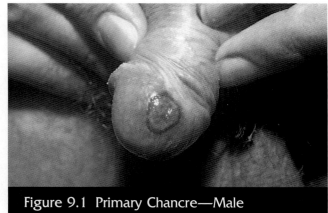

Figure 9.1 Primary Chancre—Male

This dry-based, painless ulcer with indurated borders is typical for a primary chancre in a male patient. (Courtesy of A. Wisdom: *Sexually Transmitted Diseases.* London: Mosby-Wolfe; 1992.)

Differential Diagnosis

Behçet's disease, fixed drug eruption, recurrent genital herpes, chancroid, squamous cell carcinoma, and lesions caused by trauma can have a similar appearance.

Emergency Department Treatment and Disposition

Treat with benzathine penicillin G, 2.4 million units IM once. Penicillin-allergic patients should be given doxycycline, 100 mg PO bid for 2 weeks. Other alternatives include tetracycline, 500 mg PO qid for 2 weeks; erythromycin base, 500 mg PO qid for 2 weeks; or ceftriaxone, 250 mg IM once daily for 10 days. An RPR or VDRL should be checked. Partners within the last 90 days should be treated presumptively; partners over the last 90 days should be treated on the basis of their serologic testing results. This is a reportable disease, and appropriate paperwork should be filed.

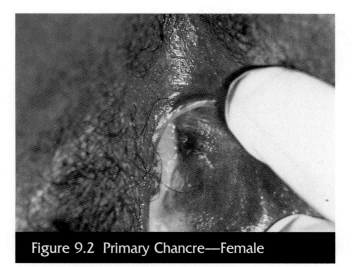

Figure 9.2 Primary Chancre—Female

A solitary, painless genital chancre with a clean base in a patient with primary syphilis. (Courtesy of the Department of Dermatology, Naval Medical Center, Portsmouth, VA.)

Clinical Pearls

1. Lesions are usually painless and solitary, but they may be slightly painful; two or three lesions may also be seen.
2. Consider dark-field examination of the lesion to rapidly confirm the diagnosis.
3. Chancres of primary syphilis can occur anywhere on the body at the site of inoculation.
4. Evaluate patients with primary syphilis for concurrent sexually transmitted diseases and treat accordingly.

Associated Clinical Features

The rash of secondary syphilis often occurs 2 to 10 weeks after resolution of the primary lesions. It begins as a nonpruritic macular rash that evolves into a papulosquamous rash involving primarily the trunk, palms, and soles (Figs. 9.3, 9.4, 9.5). The rash is often annular in shape. Diffuse, painless lymphadenopathy is also seen at this stage. Mucous patches represent mucous membrane involvement of the tongue and buccal mucosa (Fig. 9.6). Condyloma lata (Fig. 9.7) can be seen during this stage, as can patchy alopecia. The manifestations of this stage resolve without treatment in several months.

Differential Diagnosis

The differential diagnosis depends on the site involved:

Rash: Pityriasis rosea, psoriasis, lichen planus, Reiter's syndrome, viral syndrome, allergic rash
Mucous patches: Apthous ulcerations, thrush
Condyloma lata: Condyloma accuminata, squamous cell carcinoma, granuloma inguinale

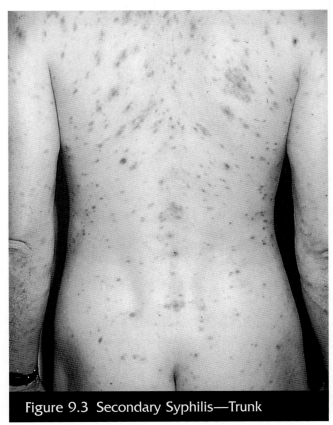

Figure 9.3 Secondary Syphilis—Trunk

Rash on trunk in secondary syphilis. (Courtesy of A. Wisdom: *Sexually Transmitted Diseases*. London: Mosby-Wolfe; 1992.)

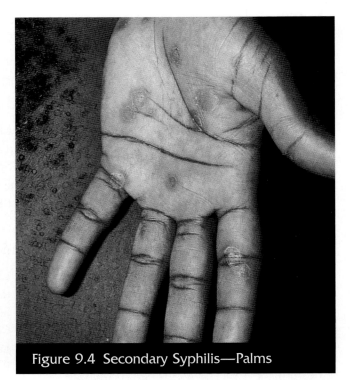

Figure 9.4 Secondary Syphilis—Palms

Papulosquamous rash of secondary syphilis. Note the annular appearance of the palmar rash. (Courtesy of H. Hunter Handsfield: *Atlas of Sexually Transmitted Diseases*. New York: McGraw-Hill; 1992.)

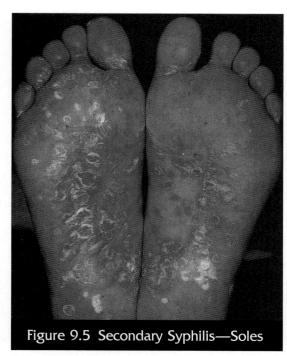

Figure 9.5 Secondary Syphilis—Soles

Hyperkeratotic plantar rash in a patient with secondary syphilis. (Courtesy of H. Hunter Handsfield: *Atlas of Sexually Transmitted Diseases.* New York: McGraw-Hill; 1992.)

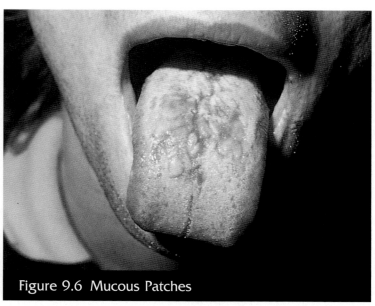

Figure 9.6 Mucous Patches

Oral involvement in secondary syphilis manifest by mucous patches. These lesions are very infectious, and dark-field examination is often positive for spirochetes. (Courtesy of Morse, Moreland, Thompson: *Atlas of Sexually Transmitted Diseases.* London: Mosby-Wolfe; 1990.)

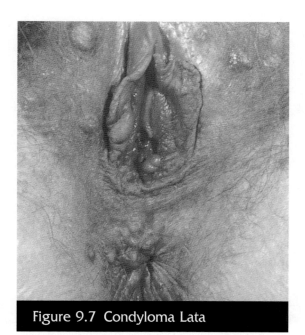

Figure 9.7 Condyloma Lata

Typical appearance of the verrucous, heaped up lesions of condyloma lata, a manifestation of secondary syphilis. (Courtesy of H. Hunter Handsfield: *Atlas of Sexually Transmitted Diseases.* New York: McGraw-Hill; 1992.)

Emergency Department Treatment and Disposition

Benzathine penicillin G, 2.4 million units IM once; penicillin allergic patients should receive doxycycline, 100 mg PO bid for 2 weeks. RPR or VDRL should be sent and titers followed to determine adequate response to therapy. Suspected and confirmed cases of syphilis must be reported to public health officials.

Clinical Pearls

1. Lesions of secondary syphilis are very infectious. It is prudent to always wear gloves when examining a patient with a rash that may be due to secondary syphilis.
2. Consider using dark-field examination of scrapings of the rash, mucous patches, and condyloma lata to make a rapid diagnosis.
3. Patients should be warned about the potential development of the Jarish-Herxheimer reaction after they are treated. This syndrome, characterized by fever, headache, malaise, and myalgias, occurs within 24 h of treatment and is caused by massive release of pyrogens by the dying spirochetes.

Associated Clinical Features

Gonorrhea often becomes manifest after a short incubation period of 2 to 5 days. In men, urethritis is characterized by purulent, usually copious urethral discharge (Fig. 9.8) with dysuria; however, up to 10% of men are asymptomatic. Women may also develop urethritis (Fig. 9.9) and complain of dysuria. Cervicitis is often asymptomatic. If symptomatic, women may complain of increased vaginal discharge or vaginal spotting, particularly after intercourse. On speculum examination, the cervix is friable, with a mucopurulent endocervical exudate (Fig. 9.10). Patients with gonococcal conjunctivitis have chemosis and copious purulent exudate (Fig. 9.11); untreated, these patients can develop endophthalmitis and perforation of the globe. Untreated gonorrhea may disseminate and more commonly does so in women. Disseminated gonococcal infection (DGI) typically presents with a monoarticular septic arthritis usually involving the knees, ankles, elbows, or wrists. Skin lesions are necrotic pustules on an erythematous base; they may ulcerate and are more commonly found on the distal extremities (Figs. 9.12, 9.13).

Differential Diagnosis

The differential diagnosis depends on the site involved:

Urethritis and cervicitis: Chlamydia, Mycoplasma, Ureaplasma
Conjunctivitis: Bacterial conjunctivitis, chemical conjunctivitis
Arthritis: Septic arthritis, rheumatic fever, hepatitis B prodrome, immune complex disease, Reiter's syndrome, systemic lupus erythematosus
Skin lesions: Folliculitis, subacute bacterial endocarditis (septic emboli)

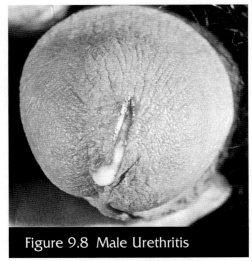

Figure 9.8 Male Urethritis

Purulent, copious urethral discharge in a patient with gonococcal urethritis. (Courtesy of H. Hunter Handsfield: *Atlas of Sexually Transmitted Diseases.* New York: McGraw-Hill; 1992.)

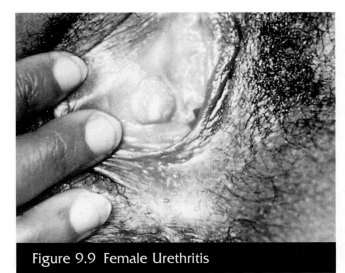

Figure 9.9 Female Urethritis

Gonococcal urethritis in a female patient. Note the purulent urethral discharge. (Courtesy of Morse, Moreland, Thompson: *Atlas of Sexually Transmitted Diseases.* London: Mosby-Wolfe; 1990.)

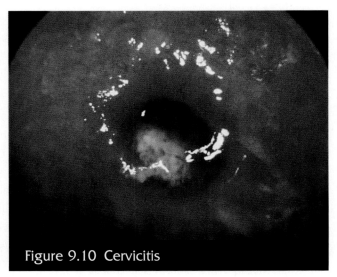

Figure 9.10 Cervicitis

Endocervical purulent exudate in an asymptomatic patient with gonococcal cervicitis. The cervix is very friable. (Courtesy of King K. Holmes, MD, from H. Hunter Handsfield: *Atlas of Sexually Transmitted Diseases.* New York: McGraw-Hill; 1992.)

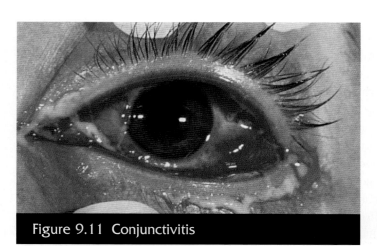

Figure 9.11 Conjunctivitis

Chemotic conjunctiva and copious purulent exudate in a patient with gonococcal conjunctivitis. (Courtesy of H. Hunter Handsfield: *Atlas of Sexually Transmitted Diseases.* New York: McGraw-Hill; 1992.)

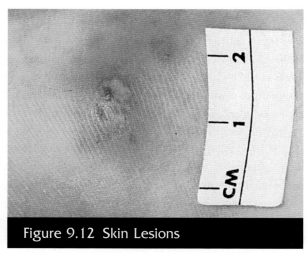

Figure 9.12 Skin Lesions

Small pustules with hemorrhage suggestive of the skin lesions of disseminated gonococcal infection. (Courtesy of H. Hunter Handsfield: *Atlas of Sexually Transmitted Diseases.* New York: McGraw-Hill; 1992.)

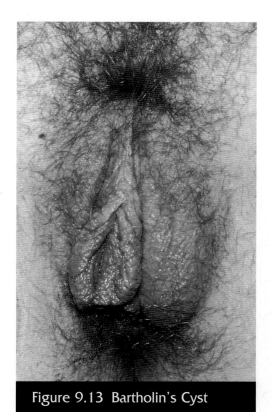

Figure 9.13 Bartholin's Cyst

Enlarged, fluctuant, tender Bartholin's abscess of the labia, usually but not always a result of gonorrhea. (Courtesy of A. Wisdom: *Sexually Transmitted Diseases.* London: Mosby-Wolfe; 1992.)

Emergency Department Treatment and Disposition

Treatment is dependent on the site of infection:

Urethritis and cervicitis: Ceftriaxone, 125 mg IM once; cefixime, 400 mg PO once; ciprofloxacin, 500 mg PO once; ofloxacin, 400 mg PO once.

Conjunctivitis: Ceftriaxone 1 g IM once; eye irrigation.

Disseminated gonococcal infection: Ceftriaxone, 1 g IV or IM daily for 7 to 10 days; may treat with 1 to 2 days of IM ceftriaxone and then change to cefixime, 400 mg PO bid, or ciprofloxacin, 500 mg PO bid, to complete a 7- to 10-day course. Sexual partners should be notified and treated. Gonorrhea is a reportable disease.

Clinical Pearls

1. Patients with gonorrhea need to be treated for concurrent infection with *Chlamydia*. Coinfection with these organisms is seen in 30% of men with urethritis and 50% of women with cervicitis.

2. Gonococcal arthritis is the most common cause of monoarticular arthritis in young, sexually active patients.

3. Suspect gonococcal conjunctivitis in patients with copious eye discharge and chemosis.

4. Cultures are the gold standard for confirming the diagnosis of gonorrhea. Selective media should be used when specimens are obtained from the cervix, pharynx, urethra, or rectum. Nonselective medium (blood agar) should be used in culturing joint fluid, blood, or cerebrospinal fluid.

Associated Clinical Features

After an incubation period of 1 to 3 weeks, males with urethritis may present with a thin, often clear urethral discharge and dysuria (Fig. 9.14). Up to 10% of these men may be asymptomatic. Women may also develop urethritis, which may only cause dysuria and be misdiagnosed as a urinary tract infection. Cervicitis in women (Fig. 9.15) is almost always asymptomatic. Women may develop pelvic inflammatory disease with upper genital tract infection. Men may develop epididymitis.

Differential Diagnosis

For urethritis and cervicitis, *Neisseria gonorrhoeae, Mycoplasma,* and *Ureaplasma* should be considered.

Emergency Department Treatment and Disposition

The preferred treatment consists of azithromycin, 1 g PO once, or doxycycline 100 mg PO bid for 7 days. Alternatives include ofloxacin, 500 mg PO bid for 7 days. Pregnant women should receive erythromycin base, 500 mg, or erythromycin ethylsuccinate 800 mg PO qid for 7 days. Partners should be examined and treated appropriately.

Clinical Pearls

1. Chlamydial infection often accompanies gonococcal infection, and patients being treated for gonorrhea should also be treated for chlamydial infection.
2. Women with chlamydial infections may be completely asymptomatic for long periods of time.
3. Consider syphilis serologic testing and HIV testing in patients presenting with sexually transmitted diseases.

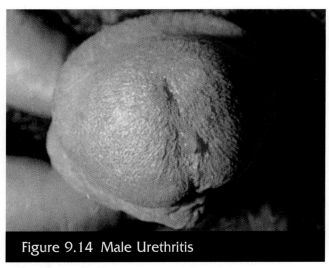

Figure 9.14 Male Urethritis

Thin urethral discharge of chlamydial urethritis. (Courtesy of Walter Stamm, MD, from H. Hunter Handsfield: *Atlas of Sexually Transmitted Diseases.* New York: McGraw-Hill; 1992.)

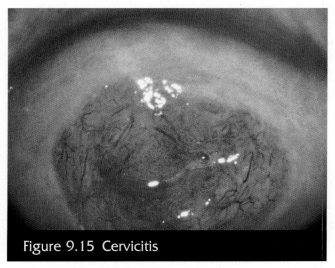

Figure 9.15 Cervicitis

Mucopurulent cervicitis from chlamydial infection. (Courtesy of H. Hunter Handsfield: *Atlas of Sexually Transmitted Diseases.* New York: McGraw-Hill; 1992.)

LYMPHOGRANULOMA VENEREUM

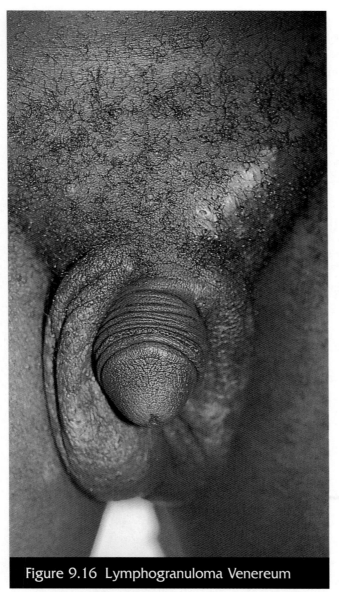

Figure 9.16 Lymphogranuloma Venereum

Unilateral left lymphadenopathy in a patient with lymphogranuloma venereum. (Courtesy of Lawrence B. Stack, MD.)

Associated Clinical Features

Lymphogranuloma venereum (LGV) is caused by a serotype of *Chlamydia trachomatis* and is primarily a disease of lymphatic tissue. Initially, LGV is often a painless genital ulceration that is not noticed by the patient more than 90% of the time. Patients often present with painful, nonfluctuant inguinal adenopathy, which is often but not always unilateral (Fig. 9.16). Lymph-adenopathy may lie above and below the inguinal ligament, causing the "groove sign" suggestive of this diagnosis. The lesion of lymphadenopathy may spontaneously open into draining sinus tracts to the skin.

Differential Diagnosis

Chancroid, granuloma inguinale, lymphoma, pyogenic or mycobacterial infection, syphilis, and cat-scratch disease may have a similar appearance.

Emergency Department Treatment and Disposition

Doxycycline, 100 mg PO bid for 3 weeks. Rarely, patients may need needle aspiration of the lymph nodes if they become fluctuant. Serologic testing is needed to confirm the diagnosis.

Clinical Pearls

1. Patients rarely note the evanescent ulcer associated with LGV.
2. The lymphadenopathy of LGV progresses over several weeks.
3. Treatment for LGV requires 3 weeks of therapy for a cure.

Associated Clinical Features

Herpes genitalis presents in several ways: symptomatic primary infection, first-episode nonprimary infection, and recurrent infection. Symptomatic primary infection occurs when the patient develops symptoms upon first acquiring the virus. Some patients may be asymptomatic when primarily infected with the virus, however, and present at a later time with their first symptomatic episode of nonprimary genital herpes. Patients with either symptomatic primary infection or first-episode nonprimary infection may develop recurrences.

Symptomatic primary genital herpes is characterized by multiple vesicles that quickly ulcerate into shallow, painful ulcers (Figs. 9.17, 9.18). The ulcers may coalesce. The lesions are accompanied by a viral syndrome with low-grade fever and myalgias. Up to 10% of patients may develop aseptic meningitis. Women may develop sacral autonomic dysfunction and require urinary catheterization because of urinary retention. The lesions last up to 3 weeks and heal without scarring.

First-episode nonprimary genital herpes and recurrent genital herpes are less dramatic (Fig. 9.19). Patients with first-episode nonprimary genital herpes do not have systemic symptoms, have solitary to several painful lesions, and resolve their symptoms in 1 to 2 weeks. Recurrences of genital herpes are often heralded by a warning prodrome of tingling or numbness in the perineal area. Vesicles and their subsequent ulcers are often solitary. The duration of symptoms is often several days and usually less than a week.

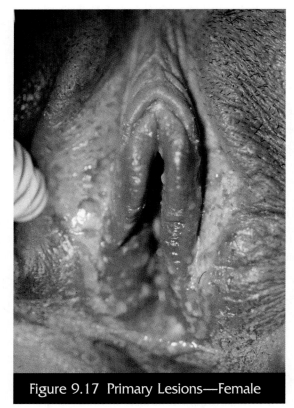

Figure 9.17 Primary Lesions—Female

Multiple coalescing superficial ulcerations of primary genital herpes. (Courtesy of Lawrence B. Stack, MD.)

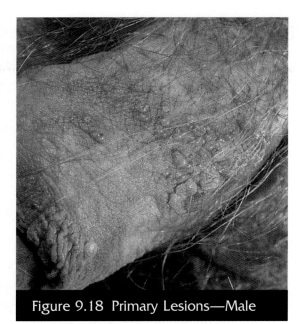

Figure 9.18 Primary Lesions—Male

Multiple genital vesicles of primary genital herpes. (Courtesy of H. Hunter Handsfield: *Atlas of Sexually Transmitted Diseases.* New York: McGraw-Hill; 1992.)

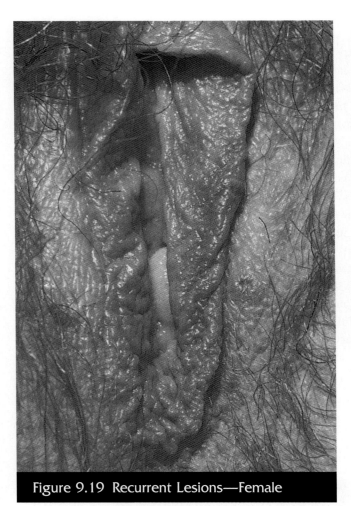

Figure 9.19 Recurrent Lesions—Female

Solitary, minimally painful lesion of recurrent genital herpes. (Courtesy of H. Hunter Handsfield: *Atlas of Sexually Transmitted Diseases.* New York: McGraw-Hill; 1992.)

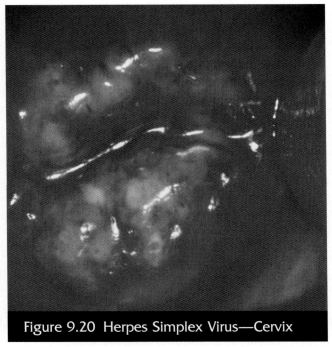

Figure 9.20 Herpes Simplex Virus—Cervix

Erosive ulcerations of the cervix in a patient with genital herpes infection. This patient may be completely asymptomatic and may transmit the disease. (Courtesy of A. Wisdom: *Sexually Transmitted Diseases.* London: Mosby-Wolfe; 1992.)

Differential Diagnosis

Pustular psoriasis, chancroid, erythema multiforme, fixed drug eruption, Behçet's disease, Stevens-Johnson syndrome, pyoderma gangrenosum, syphilis, and pyodermic infection may have a similar appearance.

Emergency Department Treatment and Disposition

Primary genital herpes: Acyclovir, 200 mg PO five times daily for 7 to 10 days or until symptoms resolve; 400 mg PO tid may be substituted for patient convenience.

Recurrent genital herpes: Acyclovir, 200 mg PO five times daily; 400 mg PO tid for 5 to 7 days; or Famciclovir, 125 mg PO bid for 5 days.

Clinical Pearls

1. Women with genital herpes must be counseled to inform their obstetrician of this history of herpes when they become pregnant.
2. Genital herpes is the most common cause of ulcerating genital lesions.
3. Patients may initially present with full-blown primary genital herpes symptoms or may have their first clinical presentation as a recurrence of an asymptomatically acquired infection (Fig. 9.20).

Associated Clinical Features

Chancroid is caused by *Haemophilus ducreyi*. After an incubation period of 2 to 10 days, this disease presents with multiple, painful, nonindurated genital ulcerations that are often deep and undermined and may have a purulent base (Fig. 9.21). Inguinal adenopathy may develop and becomes fluctuant, large, and painful (Fig. 9.22). Infected lymph nodes may rupture spontaneously. Systemic symptoms are uncommon.

Differential Diagnosis

Lymphogranuloma venereum, granuloma inguinale, herpes simplex virus, and syphilis should be considered.

Emergency Department Treatment and Disposition

Ceftriaxone, 250 mg IM once, or azithromycin, 1 g PO once. Alternatives include amoxicillin and clavulanic acid, 500 mg and 125 mg PO tid for 7 days or ciprofloxacin, 500 mg PO bid for 3 days. Large, fluctuant nodes should be aspirated to prevent rupture; incision and drainage should be avoided to prevent development of chronic draining sinus tracts. Partners should be notified of exposure to the disease.

Clinical Pearls

1. Chancroid is usually found in high-risk populations: drug-abusing, inner-city.
2. Chancroid is a diagnosis of exclusion, as culturing *H. ducreyi* requires a special medium not readily available. Genital herpes and syphilis must be ruled out.
3. The lymphadenopathy of chancroid is often very tender and fluctuant.
4. Chancroid lesions are very tender and usually multiple.

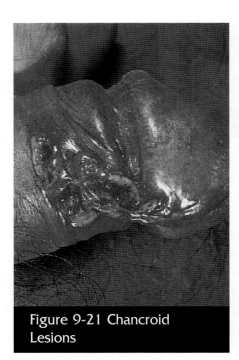

Figure 9-21 Chancroid Lesions

Multiple painful, deep ulcerations of chancroid. (Courtesy of H. Hunter Handsfield: *Atlas of Sexually Transmitted Diseases.* New York: McGraw-Hill; 1992.)

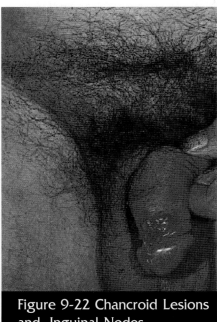

Figure 9-22 Chancroid Lesions and Inguinal Nodes

Chancroid lesions with an enlarged lymph node. On examination, this node is tender and fluctuant. (Courtesy of H. Hunter Handsfield: *Atlas of Sexually Transmitted Diseases.* New York: McGraw-Hill; 1992.)

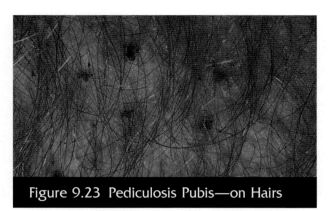

Figure 9.23 Pediculosis Pubis—on Hairs

Phthirus pubis, or the crab louse, in the pubic hair of a patient complaining of itching. Note also the nits attached to the hairs. (Courtesy of Morse, Moreland, Thompson: *Atlas of Sexually Transmitted Diseases.* London: Mosby-Wolfe; 1990.)

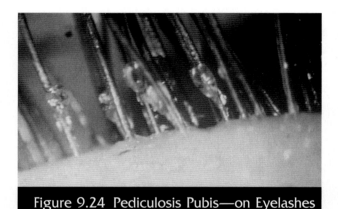

Figure 9.24 Pediculosis Pubis—on Eyelashes

Phthirus pubis lice noted in the eyelashes. (Courtesy of Spalton, Hitchings, Hunter: *Atlas of Clinical Ophthalmology,* 2d ed. London: Mosby–Year Book Europe; 1994.)

Associated Clinical Features

Pediculosis can be caused by either the body louse or the crab louse. Body lice (Fig. 17.21) are not sexually transmitted and tend to cluster around the waist, shoulders, axillae, neck, and head. They are extremely itchy; patients may present with excoriations and intense pruritus. The lice are very small and may not be easily seen. The larval form of the louse, the nit, may be mistaken for dandruff in the hair. Unlike dandruff, however, the nits are extremely adherent to the hair shaft and cannot be brushed out of the hair. The adult lice and their eggs are often found in the seams of clothing.

Pubic infestation is caused by *Phthirus pubis,* the crab louse (Figs. 9.23, 21.20). Patients may present with intense itching in the pubic area; however, as many as half of patients with this infestation may be asymptomatic. Patients may notice the lice or may note tiny rust-colored spots on their underwear, which represent bleeding from the sites of louse bites. Nits may be found at the base of pubic hairs and hatch in 5 to 10 days.

Differential Diagnosis

Tinea, contact dermatitis, scabies, and heat rash may have a similar appearance.

Emergency Department Treatment and Disposition

Lindane shampoo (Kevell) should be lathered into the pubic, perineal, and perianal hair, or lindane lotion applied in the affected areas and left on for 10 min and rinsed off. Synergized pyrethrins (RID), or synthetic pyrethrins (NIX, Elmite), may also be used. Since lindane may be toxic, pyrethrins are preferred in pregnant women and children. Treatment should be repeated in 1 week to treat any nits that may have hatched. Clothing worn or linen used in the preceding 24 h should be washed. Mechanical removal of nits attached to hairs should be attempted. Petroleum jelly or any bland ophthalmic ointment can be applied to the eyelashes twice daily for a week to treat infestation of the eyelashes (Fig. 9.24). Sexual contacts should be examined.

Clinical Pearls

1. Nits are easier to find on examination than are mature lice; the average number of lice in an infestation is only 10.
2. Patients with pediculosis pubis should be considered at risk for other sexually transmitted diseases and examined.
3. Lindane shampoo or lotion should not be used in infants under 1 year of age or in pregnant women.

Associated Clinical Features

Caused by human papillomavirus (HPV), these flesh-colored lesions may be flat, sessile, or pedunculated (Figs. 9.25, 9.26). They often have a cauliflowerlike appearance and are usually asymptomatic but may be seen or felt by patients or their sexual partners. They range in size from 1 to 4 mm to masses that may be several centimeters large (giant warts, Figs. 9.27, 9.28).

Differential Diagnosis

Condyloma lata due to secondary syphilis is the primary alternative diagnosis (Fig. 9.7). Bowen's disease, molluscum contagiosum, and carcinoma may have a similar appearance.

Emergency Department Treatment and Disposition

Local caustic agents (e.g., podophyllin) are used to treat the lesions; multiple treatment is often needed, and recurrence is common. Other therapies include cryotherapy, electrocautery, and trichloracetic acid. Laser therapy or surgery may be needed in cases of giant warts.

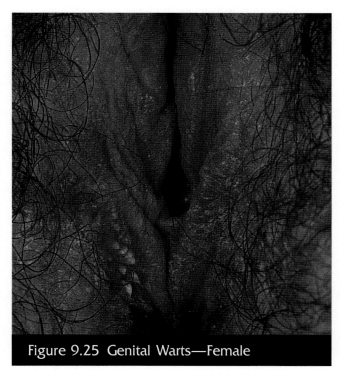

Figure 9.25 Genital Warts—Female

Verrucous lesions of the posterior fourchette in a patient with condyloma acuminata. (Used with permission from H. Hunter Handsfield: *Atlas of Sexually Transmitted Diseases.* New York: McGraw-Hill; 1992.)

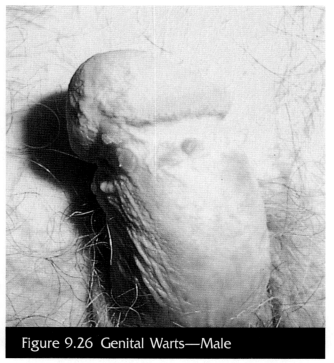

Figure 9.26 Genital Warts—Male

Typical appearance of condyloma acuminata of the glans penis. (Courtesy of Morse, Moreland, Thompson: *Atlas of Sexually Transmitted Diseases.* London: Mosby-Wolfe; 1990.)

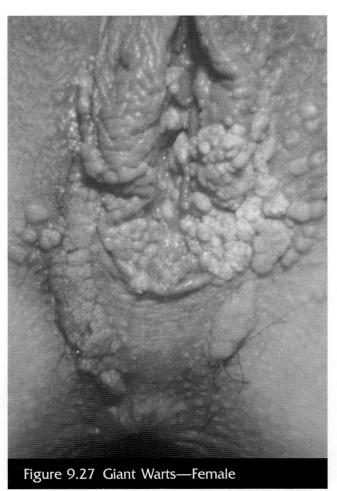

Figure 9.27 Giant Warts—Female

Giant warts of a female patient with extensive condyloma acuminata. (Courtesy of Morse, Moreland, Thompson: *Atlas of Sexually Transmitted Diseases.* London: Mosby-Wolfe; 1990.)

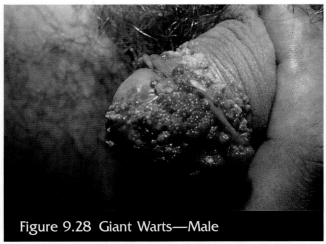

Figure 9.28 Giant Warts—Male

Giant warts in a male patient with extensive condyloma acuminata. (Courtesy of A. Wisdom: *Sexually Transmitted Diseases.* London: Mosby-Wolfe; 1992.)

Clinical Pearls

1. Evidence suggests that HPV is linked with increased risk of cervical cancer.
2. Women with genital warts need to have a Pap smear to rule out coexisting carcinoma in situ.
3. Large lesions should be biopsied to rule out cancer.
4. Patients should be advised that it may take several to many visits to completely eradicate the condyloma.
5. In cases where the diagnosis is not obvious, rule out condyloma lata (secondary syphilis) by sending serologic studies.

Anorectal Conditions

Associated Clinical Features

An anal fissure is a longitudinal tear in the skin of the anal canal and usually extends from the dentate line to the anal verge. Fissures are thought to be caused by the passage of hard or large stools with constipation, but they may also be seen with diarrhea. The fissures are typically a few millimeters wide and occur in the posterior midline (Fig. 9.29), but they can occur elsewhere. An anal fissure that is off the midline may have a secondary cause, such as inflammatory bowel disease or sexually transmitted infection. Although often seen in infants, this condition is found mostly in young and middle-aged adults. Patients present with the complaint of intense sharp, burning pain during and after bowel movements. They may also note bright red blood at the time or shortly after the passage of stool. Gentle examination with separation of the buttocks usually provides good visualization (Fig. 9.29). Anoscopy should be performed, if possible.

Differential Diagnosis

The diagnosis of inflammatory bowel disease, ulcerative colitis, or Crohn's disease should be considered, particularly if the fissure is atypical. Anal fissures may be the result of a sexually transmitted disease such as *Chlamydia,* gonorrhea, herpes, and syphilis. Tuberculosis, anal neoplasms, and sickle cell disease can also present as an anal fissure. An anal abscess and thrombosed hemorrhoids may cause similar symptoms but can usually be ruled out on physical examination.

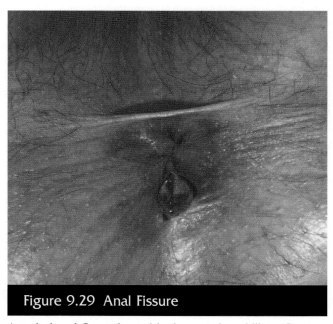

Figure 9.29 Anal Fissure

A typical anal fissure located in the posterior midline. (Courtesy of Paul J. Kovalcik, MD.)

Emergency Department Treatment and Disposition

Acute treatment of anal fissures consists of anal hygiene, bulk fiber diet supplements to soften stools, warm sitz baths, and topical anesthetics. Oral pain medication and muscle relaxants such as diazepam may be required in certain patients.

Clinical Pearls

1. Pain and involuntary sphincter spasm may preclude a routine digital or anoscopic examination and require an examination under anesthesia.
2. A proctoscopic examination should be done at some point to rule out secondary causes.
3. Most anal fissures heal spontaneously, but refractory cases may require surgical repair.

Associated Clinical Features

The perianal abscess is the most common anorectal abscess. It is associated with pain in the anal area that is exacerbated by bowel movements, straining, coughing, or palpation. On examination, a fluctuant and possibly erythematous mass is found at the perianal region (Fig. 9.30). Perianal abscesses are usually fairly superficial and easy to drain with local anesthesia. The patient may notice swelling or a pressure sensation. Perirectal abscesses tend to be more complex and are named according to the involved space: ischiorectal, intersphincteric, or supralevator (Fig. 9.31). These are fluctuant masses that are usually palpable along the rectal wall. Patients may complain of pain, fever, and mucous or bloody discharge with bowel movement.

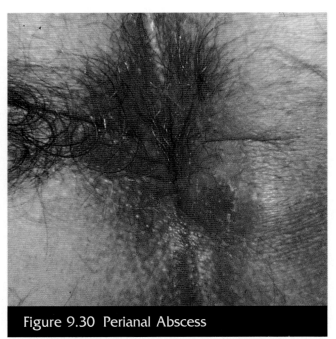

Figure 9.30 Perianal Abscess

Swelling and erythema around the anus consistent with a perianal abscess. (Courtesy of the American Society of Colon and Rectal Surgeons.)

Differential Diagnosis

Crohn's disease should be considered, because 36% of Crohn's patients have a perianal abscess at the presentation of their disease. An underlying process may exist, such as diabetes mellitus, leukemia, or other malignancy.

Emergency Department Treatment and Disposition

Incision and drainage of perianal abscesses should be performed with a small radial or cruciate incision lateral to the external sphincter. For an uncomplicated abscess, this can be accomplished under local anesthesia. The cavity should be cleared of loculations and then loosely packed with iodoform gauze, which should be removed in 24 to 48 h. All patients require outpatient follow-up. Antibiotic therapy is not indicated unless there is underlying disease affecting the patient's immunologic function or the patient appears septic. Surgical consultation should be obtained for treatment of perirectal abscesses under anesthesia.

Clinical Pearls

1. Surgical consultation and treatment may be required in the patient with a large or complicated perianal abscess or where adequate analgesia cannot be obtained.
2. Consider admission for debilitated, elderly, febrile, obese, or otherwise ill-appearing patients.
3. All patients warrant follow-up referral due to the high incidence of fistulae with anorectal abscesses.

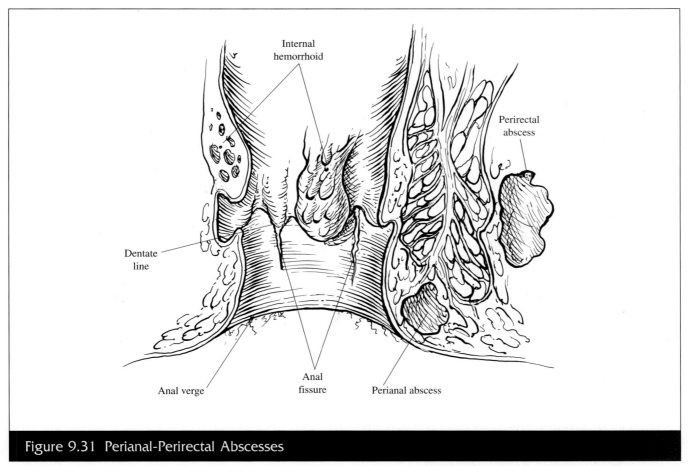

Internal
hemorrhoid

Perirectal
abscess

Dentate
line

Anal verge

Anal
fissure

Perianal abscess

Figure 9.31 Perianal-Perirectal Abscesses

The anatomy of perianal and perirectal abscesses is illustrated. Also shown are anal fissure and internal and external hemorrhoids.

Associated Clinical Features

External hemorrhoids result from the dilatation of the venules of the inferior hemorrhoidal plexus below the dentate line. They have a covering of skin, or anoderm, versus internal hemorrhoids, which have a mucosal covering. Hemorrhoids commonly present with an episode of rectal bleeding of bright red blood after defecation. This results from the passage of the fecal mass over the thin-walled venules, causing abrasions and bleeding. Symptoms from external hemorrhoids include complaints of swelling and burning rectal pain. Numerous associated factors exist, such as constipation, family history, pregnancy, portal hypertension, or increased intraabdominal pressure. Hemorrhoids are commonly found at three anatomic locations: right anterior, right posterior, and left lateral positions (Fig. 9.32). A thrombosed external hemorrhoid contains intravascular clots and causes exquisite pain the first 48 h.

Internal hemorrhoids (Figs. 9.31, 9.33) present with painless rectal bleeding or possibly the sensation of prolapse. They are graded according to the degree of prolapse, where the first degree is identifiable at the dentate line and the fourth degree shows irreducible prolapse through the anus. Internal hemorrhoids are not typically painful, whereas external hemorrhoids do cause pain.

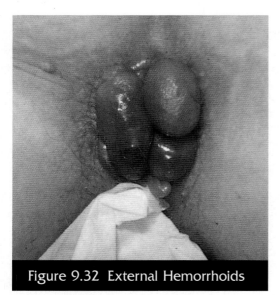

Figure 9.32 External Hemorrhoids

Multiple engorged external hemorrhoids are seen in all quadrants. (Courtesy of the American Society of Colon and Rectal Surgeons.)

Differential Diagnosis

Other diagnoses to consider include infection, perianal or perirectal abscess, inflammatory bowel disease, malignancy, local trauma, herpes or other sexually transmitted infection, rectal polyp, or rectal prolapse.

In the case of severe bleeding, fluid resuscitation would need to be instituted and the bleeding vessel located, clamped, and ligated. The treatment for less severe cases warrants more conservative therapy, including increased dietary fiber, increased fluid intake, hot sitz baths, bed rest, and nonnarcotic pain medication. Advanced cases may require surgical consultation and treatment. ED treatment of thrombosed external hemorrhoids includes an elliptical excision and extrusion of the clot under local anesthesia.

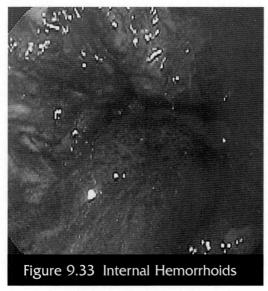

Figure 9.33 Internal Hemorrhoids

Internal hemorrhoids are seen in this endoscopic view of the rectum. (Courtesy of Virender K. Sharman, MD.)

Clinical Pearls

1. Many patients with any anorectal problem complain of hemorrhoids. Therefore, careful examination and consideration of the differential diagnosis should be undertaken with each patient.
2. Having the patient strain during the examination may reveal bleeding or prolapse that might otherwise go unnoticed.
3. Hemorrhoids are a rare cause of anorectal pruritus.

Associated Clinical Features

Rectal prolapse occurs when anorectal tissue slides through the anal orifice; it can include mucosa or a full-thickness layer. This is due to several anatomic features, including laxity of the pelvic floor, weak anal sphincters, and lack of mesorectal fixation. Patients complain of bleeding, mucous discharge, rectal pressure, or a mass (Fig. 9.34). Problems with fecal incontinence, constipation, and rectal ulceration are common as well. Prolapse may be associated with an increased familial incidence, chronic cough, dysentery, or parasitic infection.

Differential Diagnosis

Other diagnoses to consider include foreign body, tumor, perianal or perirectal abscess, rectal polyp, or engorged external hemorrhoids.

Emergency Department Treatment and Disposition

Usually reduction is possible with gentle manual pressure. However, if this cannot be accomplished, surgical consultation and admission are needed. Surgical treatment is also indicated with a complete prolapse. All patients should undergo an anoscopic and sigmoidoscopic examination at some point; if rectal bleeding is a problem, full colonic evaluation should be completed.

Clinical Pearls

1. This is commonly seen in children with cystic fibrosis (22%); therefore, all children with rectal prolapse should have a sweat chloride test.
2. Examination of rectal prolapse reveals concentric mucosal rings and a sulcus between the anal canal and the rectum, whereas prolapsed hemorrhoids are separated by radial grooves and the sulcus is absent.
3. To confirm the diagnosis, prolapse may be reproduced by having the patient bear down.

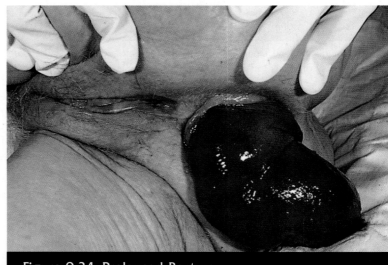

Figure 9.34 Prolapsed Rectum

The rectum is completely prolapsed in this elderly patient. (Courtesy of Alan B. Storrow, MD.)

Associated Clinical Features

Pilonidal abscesses are typically seen at or just superior to the gluteal fold (Fig. 9.35) and are more common in teenage and young adult males. Patients complain of localized pain, swelling, and drainage but usually do not have systemic symptoms. The abscess begins with the formation of a small opening in the skin that develops into a cystic structure involving surrounding hairs. This opening is occluded by hair or keratin, creating a closed space that does not allow drainage. The acute abscess contains mixed organisms including *Staphylococcus aureus* and *Streptococcus,* but anaerobes and gram-negative organisms may also be present.

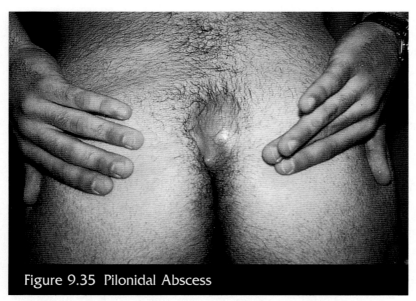

Figure 9.35 Pilonidal Abscess

Redness, fluctuance, and tenderness in the gluteal cleft seen with a pilonidal abscess. (Courtesy of Louis La Vopa, MD.)

Differential Diagnosis

Evidence of cellulitis in the sacrococcygeal area may result from a simple abscess or furuncle. However, other causes should be considered, such as anal fistulae, hidradenitis, inflammatory bowel disease, or tuberculosis.

Emergency Department Treatment and Disposition

An acutely fluctuant abscess requires incision and drainage under local anesthesia with removal of pus and debris. The patient should be instructed on meticulous wound care and sitz baths. Antibiotic therapy is not indicated unless the patient is immunocompromised. Surgical referral is given, particularly with a chronic or recurrent cyst, which may require surgical excision and closure.

Clinical Pearls

1. Pilonidal abscesses almost always occur in the midline but can have sinus tracts extending off the midline.
2. Pilonidal disease is three times more common in men than in women.

Associated Clinical Features

The diagnosis of rectal foreign body is usually made by history and confirmed by digital examination. Most often the foreign body is inserted (Fig. 9.36), but it is possible to have an ingested foreign body trapped in the rectum. The most serious complication of a rectal foreign body is perforation of the rectum or distal colon. The patient must be carefully evaluated for evidence of perforation with x-rays demonstrating free air and clinically for the presentation of an acute abdomen. Perforation above the peritoneal reflection is associated with free air in the abdominal cavity and peritoneal signs. Perforation below the peritoneal reflection presents with more insidious signs of pain and infection in the perianal or perineal region. It is important to determine the size, shape, and number of objects to assess the risk of perforation. In children, rectal foreign bodies usually present as rectal bleeding.

Differential Diagnosis

Depending on the clinical scenario, the diagnoses of sexual assault or child abuse should be considered.

Emergency Department Treatment and Disposition

Removal can often take place in the ED with sedation of the patient and local anesthesia of the anal sphincter. If the risk of perforation appears high or adequate relaxation and anesthesia cannot be obtained, then the patient is prepared for emergency surgery. After removal, proctoscopic or sigmoidoscopic examination is recommended to rule out perforation or laceration.

Clinical Pearls

1. A Foley catheter or an endotracheal tube may be used to release the vacuum effect of some foreign bodies, and the balloon can be inflated and aid in the removal.
2. A rectal foreign body in a child should raise the suspicion of abuse.

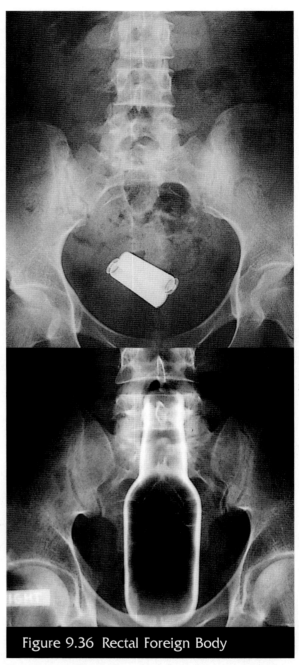

Figure 9.36 Rectal Foreign Body

Top: The metallic outline of two batteries is seen in this x-ray. *Bottom*: This foreign body (a 7-oz beer bottle) required removal in the operating room. [Courtesy of David W. Munter, MD (*top*), and Kevin J. Knoop, MD, MS (*bottom*).]

Associated Clinical Features

Gastrointestinal bleeding commonly presents with the alteration of stool color. By definition, melena is the passage of dark, pitchlike stools stained with blood pigments (Fig. 9.37). Generally, but not always, melena results from bleeding into the upper gastrointestinal tract proximal to the ligament of Treitz. Black stools have been seen with as little as 60 mL of blood in the upper gastrointestinal tract, but melena typically does not develop until 100 to 200 mL is present. Melena can be found in lower bleeds with decreased transit time, as with an obstruction distal to the site of bleeding.

Differential Diagnosis

Melenic stools may occur from swallowed blood, as from epistaxis or other oropharyngeal bleeding. Dark or black stools can also be seen with the ingestion of bismuth salicylate, food coloring, and iron supplements.

Emergency Department Treatment and Disposition

Patients with melenic stools should be evaluated in a monitored setting and undergo assessment for signs and symptoms of hypovolemia and treated accordingly. At least one large-bore intravenous line should be placed and saline infused. Depending on the patient's stability, type-specific packed red blood cells or other blood products may be required. Abdominal radiographs are done to look for free air in the peritoneum, and gastric aspiration should be done to assess for active gastric bleeding. Stable patients who present with melena may be admitted to the ward. Evidence of unstable vital signs, continued bleeding, severe anemia, or comorbid disease warrants admission to the intensive care unit. Consultation with a gastroenterologist should be sought unless patients require more than two units of blood for resuscitation, which would call for surgical intervention.

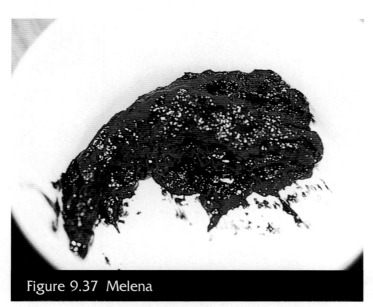

Figure 9.37 Melena

The black, tarry appearance of melena in a patient with a duodenal ulcer. (Courtesy of Alan B. Storrow, MD.)

Clinical Pearls

1. Melena is the most common presenting symptom of bleeding from peptic ulcer disease.
2. Melena represents approximately 200 mL of blood loss in the gastrointestinal tract.

CHAPTER 10

GYNECOLOGIC AND OBSTETRIC CONDITIONS

Robert G. Buckley
Kevin J. Knoop

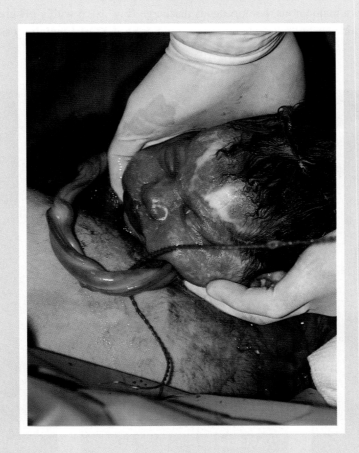

Gynecologic Conditions

Associated Clinical Features

Candidal vaginitis is characterized by a thick, curdy, white discharge (Fig. 10.1) and vulvar discomfort. Intense vulvar erythema, pruritus, or burning are often present. A microscopic slide prepared with 10% potassium hydroxide yielding characteristic branch chain hyphae and spores establishes the diagnosis (Fig. 20.13). The pH of the discharge is less than 4.5. Predisposing factors that should be considered include oral contraceptive, antibiotic, or corticosteroid use; pregnancy; and diabetes. Sexually transmitted diseases are not usually associated with isolated candidal vaginitis.

Trichomonas vaginitis presents as a persistent, thin, copious discharge that is often frothy (Fig. 10.2), green, or foul-smelling. The pH of these secretions is greater than 4.5. The amount of vaginal and cervical erythema and inflammation varies considerably; thus the diagnosis depends on the presence of motile flagellates on normal saline wet-mount microscopy. Occasionally, multiple petechiae on the vaginal wall (strawberry spots) or cervix (strawberry cervix) are seen.

Bacterial vaginosis (previously termed *Haemophilus* or *Gardnerella* vaginitis) is characterized by a malodorous, homogeneous discharge (Fig. 10.3) with a pH greater than 4.5 and a transient amine (fishy) odor when mixed with a drop of KOH solution (positive sniff test). The presence

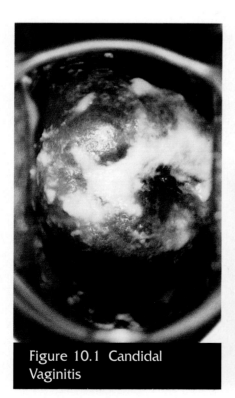

Figure 10.1 Candidal Vaginitis

Thick, curdy white discharge secondary to candidal vaginitis. (Courtesy of Kevin J. Knoop, MS, MD.)

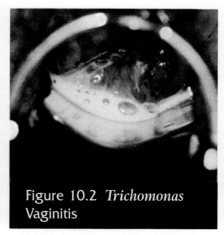

Figure 10.2 *Trichomonas* **Vaginitis**

Thin vaginal discharge suggestive of *Trichomonas* vaginitis. (Courtesy of H. Hunter Handsfield: *Atlas of Sexually Transmitted Diseases.* New York: McGraw-Hill; 1992.)

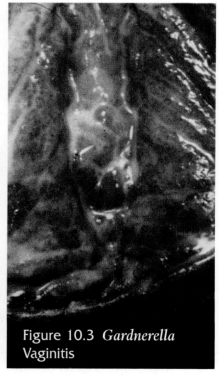

Figure 10.3 *Gardnerella* **Vaginitis**

Thin, milky white discharge suggestive of *Gardnerella* vaginitis. (Courtesy of Curatek Pharmaceuticals.)

of clue cells on normal saline wet mount establishes the diagnosis (Fig. 20.14). Other associated vaginal or abdominal complaints are minimal and, if significant, may represent another disease process.

Differential Diagnosis

Vaginal foreign bodies, especially in prepubescent girls, may present with a heavy white discharge but would be unaccompanied by vulvar erythema or the microscopic appearance of hyphae. Atrophic vaginitis is commonly found in postmenopausal women and is distinguished from candidal vaginitis by mucosal dryness, atrophy, dyspareunia, minimal discharge, and itching. Other considerations include contact dermatitis, local irritation secondary to tight-fitting underwear, and contact dermatitis from toiletry items.

Emergency Department Treatment and Disposition

For *candidal vaginitis,* various regimens of topical antifungal agents are the mainstay of treatment (clotrimazole 1% cream, one applicatorful inserted high into the vaginal vault for 7 nights, clotrimazole, two 100-mg vaginal tablets for 3 nights or one 500-mg vaginal tablet for single-dose treatment). Oral fluconazole (Diflucan, 150 mg as a single dose) is also effective. Nystatin vaginal tablets (100,000 U daily for 2 weeks) are generally considered safe for use in the first trimester of pregnancy.

For *Trichomonas vaginitis,* a single, one-time dose of metronidazole (2 g) is generally curative. Alternatively, 500 mg given twice daily can be used for recurrent or refractory cases. Metronidazole is contraindicted in pregnancy and is associated with an Antabuse-like reaction when taken with alcohol. For the pregnant patient, clotrimazole (100-mg vaginal suppositories daily for 7 to 14 days) may provide symptomatic relief.

For *bacterial vaginosis,* metronidazole (500 mg twice daily for 7 days) is recommended in the nonpregnant patient. Amoxicillin (500 mg tid for 7 days) or clindamycin (300 mg bid) for 7 days is a safe but less effective alternative during pregnancy. Treatment for asymptomatic infection or for male sexual partners is not generally recommended.

Clinical Pearls

1. Diabetes mellitus or immunosuppression should be considered in refractory or recurrent cases of candidal vaginitis.
2. A history of balanitis in the sexual partner should be sought and treated if present.
3. *Trichomonas* should be considered a sexually transmitted disease. It is generally recommended, therefore, that concomitant culturing for gonorrhea and *Chlamydia* be performed. Serologic testing for syphilis, HIV, and hepatitis B should be considered.
4. Patients treated with metronidazole should abstain from alcohol for the duration of treatment and for at least 24 h after their last dose.

Associated Clinical Features

The patient's chief complaint is often a purulent vaginal discharge. Speculum examination reveals a purulent, viscous discharge emanating from the cervical os (Fig. 10.4). Otherwise, a purulent discharge may be seen on a cervical swab. A Gram's stain may reveal either gram-negative intracellular diplococci consistent with *Neisseria gonorrhoeae* (Fig. 20.11) or be nonspecific, consistent with *Chlamydia trachomatis,* a coinfectant with the gonococcus about 50% of the time. The diagnosis of pelvic inflammatory disease should be considered, when accompanied by symptoms of lower abdominal pain and signs of pelvic peritonitis such as cervical motion and adnexal tenderness.

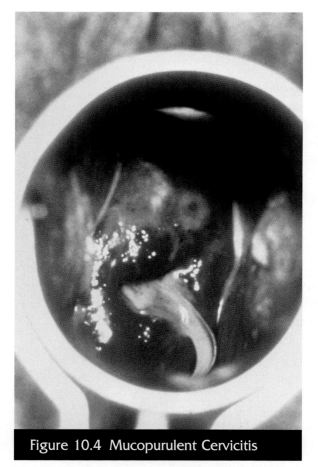

Figure 10.4 Mucopurulent Cervicitis

Viscous, opaque discharge emanating from the cervical os, consistent with mucopurulent cervicitis. The string from an intrauterine device is seen descending through the os in this patient. (Courtesy of Sue Rist, FNP.)

Differential Diagnosis

Physiologic cervical mucous discharge at the time of ovulation may occur but is generally clear, with few white blood cells on Gram's stain.

Emergency Department Treatment and Disposition

Cultures for *Chlamydia trachomatis* and *N. gonorrhoeae* should be obtained prior to initiation of therapy. Ceftriaxone (125 mg as a single intramuscular dose) provides coverage for *N. gonorrhoeae*. Single-dose oral quinolones (ciprofloxacin, 500 mg, or ofloxacin, 400 mg) can be used in penicillin-allergic patients. Doxycycline (100 mg) or ofloxacin (300 mg) bid for 7 days or a single 1-g dose of azithromycin provides coverage for *Chlamydia*. Erythromycin (base 500 mg qid for 7 days) is the alternative for pregnant patients.

Clinical Pearls

1. The discharge of candidal, trichomonal, or *Gardnerella* vaginitis is almost never limited solely to the cervix.
2. Mucopurulent cervicitis is almost always secondary to a sexually transmitted disease; thus sexual partners should be treated as well.
3. Refer all patients for formal gynecologic follow-up after culture and treatment, since early cervical neoplasia may have a similar appearance.

Associated Clinical Features

Bartholin's glands and ducts are located over the lower third of the introitus near the labia minora. A cyst or abscess can result from an obstructed duct, which usually occurs secondary to scarring from trauma, delivery, or episiotomy. Infection of the cyst is usually with mixed vaginal or fecal flora (*Escherichia coli*) but may also contain *Neisseria gonorrhoeae* and *Chlamydia trachomatis*. Progressive enlargement and infection lead to increasing pain, swelling, and dyspareunia. A tender, fluctuant cystic mass with surrounding labial edema is easily appreciated on examination (Fig. 10.5).

Differential Diagnosis

Epidermal inclusion cysts and sebaceous cysts of the labia majora may look similar but are generally smaller. When they are inflamed or infected, maximal fluctuance generally points toward the external aspect of the labium, as opposed to Bartholin's gland cysts, which point medially. Occlusion and infection of apocrine sweat glands can lead to subcutaneous abscess formation—known as hidradenitis suppurativa. Vulvar hematoma, leiomyoma, lipoma, and fibromas may occasionally be confused with a noninfected Bartholin's cyst. Vulvar cancer usually arises in postmenopausal women and is generally either ulcerated, excoriated, or exophytic.

Emergency Department Treatment and Disposition

Simple incision and drainage (Fig. 10.6) followed by sitz baths provide the most effective and expeditious relief on an emergency basis. Unfortunately, reocclusion and reaccumulation of cystic swelling are common. Definitive therapy of recurrent Bartholin's gland cysts involves marsupialization by suturing the introital mucosa to the inner cyst wall.

Clinical Pearls

1. Antibiotics, although commonly used, are usually not required.
2. Placement of a Word catheter into the cyst cavity (Fig. 10.7) decreases the incidence of reocclusion, but it must be allowed to remain in place for up to 6 weeks to ensure epithelialization of the drainage tract.

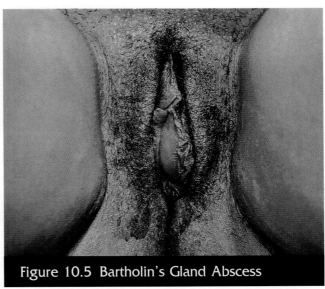

Figure 10.5 Bartholin's Gland Abscess

Typical appearance of a Bartholin's gland abscess with the labial fluctuance pointing medially. (Courtesy of the Medical Photography Department, Naval Medical Center, San Diego, CA.)

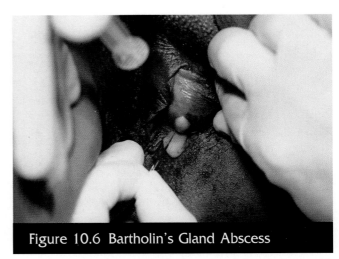

Figure 10.6 Bartholin's Gland Abscess

Medial incision of the cyst yielding purulent fluid, consistent with a Bartholin's gland abscess. (Courtesy of the Medical Photography Department, Naval Medical Center, San Diego, CA.)

259

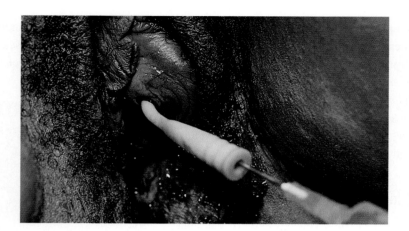

Figure 10.7 Bartholin's Gland Abscess

Insertion and inflation of a Word catheter into the cyst cavity. The free end of the catheter can be tucked into the vagina for long-term placement, allowing for epithelialization of the incision site. (Courtesy of the Medical Photography Department, Naval Medical Center, San Diego, CA.)

Associated Clinical Features

Spontaneous abortion is associated with vaginal bleeding and abdominal discomfort. Severe pain, heavy bleeding with the passage of clots or tissue (Fig. 10.8), and hypotension may also be present. *Threatened abortion* is diagnosed when mild cramping and vaginal bleeding are not accompanied by the complete or partial extrusion of tissue, cervical dilation, or ectopic pregnancy. Uterine cramping with progressive dilation of the cervix, with or without partial extrusion of the products of conception, indicates the presence of an *inevitable abortion* (Fig. 10.9). In an *incomplete abortion,* some elements of the conceptus have passed, yet retained intrauterine tissue leads to ongoing uterine cramping, cervical dilation, and persistent bleeding.

Differential Diagnosis

Ectopic pregnancy should be considered in all first-trimester females with lower abdominal pain or vaginal bleeding. The presence of frank tissue passage or cervical dilation essentially excludes this diagnosis. Large blood clots or an intrauterine decidual cast (Fig. 10.10), however, may occasionally be mistaken for products of conception.

Emergency Department Treatment and Disposition

Intravenous access, fluid resuscitation, cross-matching of blood, and urgent gynecologic consultation should be implemented in the presence of severe pain, heavy bleeding, or hypovolemia. All tissue should be sent to pathology for definitive identification. Occasionally, patients who initially

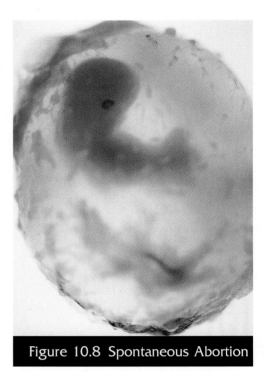

Figure 10.8 Spontaneous Abortion

Passage of tissue in a spontaneous abortion at 4 weeks. (Courtesy of Lawrence B. Stack, MD.)

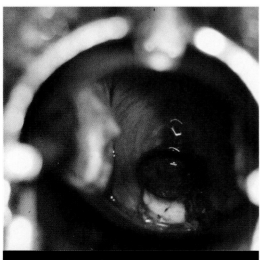

Figure 10.9 Spontaneous Abortion

◀— Dilation of the cervical os with partial extrusion of tissue in the setting of an inevitable abortion. (Courtesy of Robert Buckley, MD.)

A decidual cast or —▶ organized clot may occasionally be mistaken for products of conception. (Courtesy of the Medical Photography Department, Naval Medical Center, San Diego, CA.)

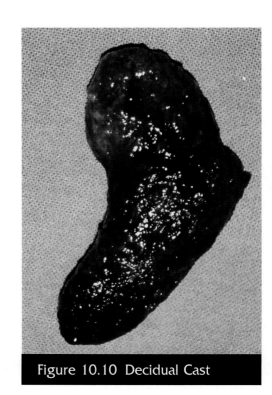

Figure 10.10 Decidual Cast

have an open cervical os will rapidly expel the remaining products of conception, with subsequent resolution of all pain and bleeding. These patients may be discharged from the ED with the diagnosis of completed abortion if otherwise clinically stable. Anti-Rh immunoglobulin (RhoGAM) should be administered in all cases of vaginal bleeding in the pregnant patient where the mother is Rh-negative and the father is Rh-positive.

Clinical Pearls

1. The passage of large clots usually indicates rapid heavy bleeding.
2. *Completed abortion* is characterized by the passage of tissue, followed by resolution of bleeding and closure of the cervical os.
3. Fever, leukocytosis, pelvic tenderness, and malodorous cervical discharge should suggest *septic abortion*.

Associated Clinical Features

Patients who present for examination and treatment following an incident of sexual assault are ideally cared for by a multidisciplinary team capable of addressing the immediate medical and psychosocial needs of the patient in concert with forensic and legal requirements. A thorough general examination may reveal associated contusions and other soft tissue injuries. A meticulous inspection of the perineum, rectum, vaginal fornices, vagina, and cervix is required to identify inflicted injuries. Toluidine staining and colposcopy are often useful in enhancing less apparent injuries such as those to the posterior fourchette following sexual assault (Fig. 10.11). These are most commonly found between the 3 and 9 o'clock distribution when the patient is examined in the dorsal lithotomy position. Perianal lacerations (Fig. 10.12) may also be seen as toluidine-enhanced linear tears (Fig. 10.13). Examination of the cervix and posterior vaginal vault may reveal injuries to those structures (Fig. 10.14).

Differential Diagnosis

Perineal injuries from accidental trauma may be indistinguishable from those of sexual assault and should be interpreted in the context of the history. The assessment of assault or rape is technically a legal one; therefore the examiner should be careful to document the medical appearance of the wounds rather than speculate as to the specific mechanism by which each injury occurred.

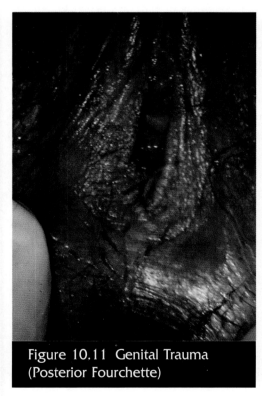

Figure 10.11 Genital Trauma (Posterior Fourchette)

Linear tears to the posterior fourchette—due to sexual assault—enhanced by toluidine staining. (Courtesy of Hillary J. Larkin, PA-C, and Lauri A. Paolinetti, PA-C.)

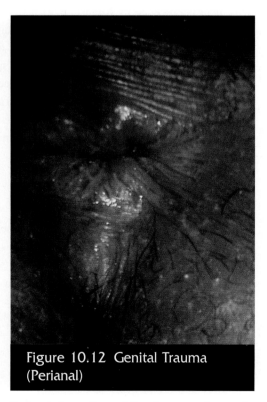

Figure 10.12 Genital Trauma (Perianal)

Perianal lacerations following sexual assault. (Courtesy of Hillary J. Larkin, PA-C, and Lauri A. Paolinetti, PA-C.)

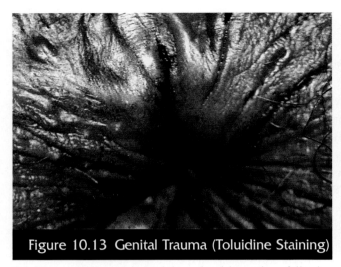

Figure 10.13 Genital Trauma (Toluidine Staining)

Toluidine staining showing subtle perianal lacerations following forceful anal penetration. (Courtesy of Aurora Mendez, RN.)

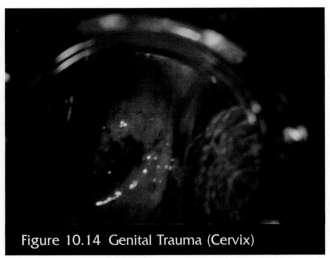

Figure 10.14 Genital Trauma (Cervix)

Cervical trauma in an elderly victim of sexual assault. Petechiae and freshly bleeding abrasions are noted from 10 to 3 o'clock. (Courtesy of Hillary J. Larkin, PA-C, and Lauri A. Paolinetti, PA-C.)

Emergency Department Treatment and Disposition

Treatment is preceded by forensic evidence gathering, consisting of a Wood's lamp examination to identify semen for collection, pubic hair sampling and combing, vaginal and cervical smears (air-dried), a cervical and vaginal wet mount to identify sperm, vaginal aspirate to test for acid phosphatase, and rectal or buccal swabs for sperm. A prepackaged kit with directions may be available to facilitate the collection of evidence.

Cervical cultures for *Chlamydia* and *Neisseria gonorrhoea* should be obtained as well as serum testing for syphilis, hepatitis, and HIV. Empiric antibiotic coverage against sexually transmitted diseases should be provided and an oral contraceptive offered (after confirming a nonpregnant state) to prevent unwanted pregnancy.

Clinical Pearls

1. The medical care of the patient who has been sexually assaulted should ideally be performed by experienced supportive staff familiar with the details of forensic evidence gathering and colposcopic photography.
2. Normal findings on physical examination and no sperm on wet preparation do *not* exclude the possibility of assault.

Associated Clinical Features

Uterine prolapse is defined as the propulsion of the uterus through the pelvic floor or vaginal introitus. In first-degree prolapse, the cervix descends into the lower third of the vagina; in second-degree prolapse, the cervix usually protrudes through the introitus; whereas in third-degree prolapse, or procidentia, the entire uterus is externalized with inversion of the vagina (Fig. 10.15). Symptoms include a sensation of inguinal traction, low back pain, urinary incontinence, and the presence of a vaginal mass.

Differential Diagnosis

Uterine prolapse can occasionally be confused with a cystocele, enterocele, or soft tissue tumor. These disorders, which may all be accompanied by introital bulging, are easily distinguished by the absence of cervicouterine descent.

Emergency Department Treatment and Disposition

Patients with first- or second-degree prolapse should be referred to a gynecologist for pessary placement or surgical correction. With procidentia, the uterus should be manually reduced into the vaginal vault and the patient placed at bed rest until evaluated by a gynecologic consultant.

Clinical Pearl

1. With procidentia, the exposed uterus is prone to abrasion and possible secondary infection.

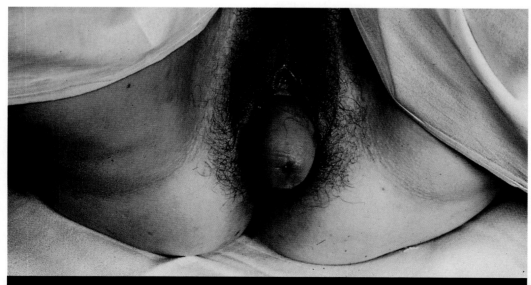

Figure 10.15 Third-Degree Uterine Prolapse

Note the protrusion of the entire uterus with cervix visible through the vaginal introitus. (Courtesy of Matthew Backer, Jr., MD.)

Associated Clinical Features

A cystocele occurs when there is relaxation and bulging of the posterior bladder wall and trigone into the vagina (Fig. 10.16) and is usually due to birth trauma. Patients complain of bulging or fullness over the introitus that is worsened with Valsalva (Fig. 10.17) and relieved with recumbency. It is often associated with urinary incontinence or symptoms of incomplete emptying. Most cystoceles, however, are asymptomatic. Examination reveals a thin-walled bulging of the anterior vaginal wall, which, in severe cases, may pass through the introitus with Valsalva.

Differential Diagnosis

An enterocele may lead to a similar bulging of the anterior vaginal wall but is much less common and is generally limited to those patients who have had a hysterectomy. Rectocele, uterine prolapse, and soft tissue tumors should also be considered.

Emergency Department Treatment and Disposition

Larger cystoceles or those associated with urinary symptomatology, pain, or bothersome bulging should be referred to a gynecologist for further evaluation.

Clinical Pearl

1. Most cystoceles are asymptomatic and are detected incidentally at the time of pelvic examination.

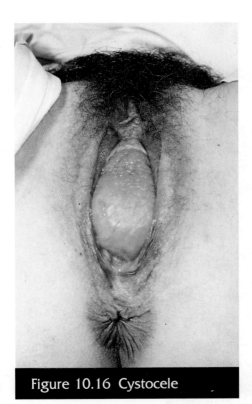

Figure 10.16 Cystocele

Cystocele with bulging of the posterior bladder wall into the vagina. (Courtesy of Matthew Backer, Jr., MD.)

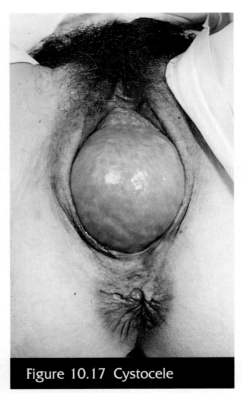

Figure 10.17 Cystocele

Cystocele worsening with Valsalva. (Courtesy of Matthew Backer, Jr., MD.)

Associated Clinical Features

Most small rectoceles are completely asymptomatic, though symptoms of introital bulging, constipation, and incomplete rectal evacuation may occur. Bulging of the introitus can be seen grossly on physical examination (Fig. 10.18) and can become worse with Valsalva (Fig. 10.19). Rectovaginal examination reveals a thin-walled protrusion of the rectovaginal septum into the lower part of the vagina.

Differential Diagnosis

Cystocele, enterocele, uterine prolapse, and soft-tissue tumors should all be easily distinguished by careful inspection.

Emergency Department Treatment and Disposition

Supportive measures with hydration, laxatives, and stool softeners are generally all that is needed to relieve the patient's symptoms. Those patients with large symptomatic rectoceles who do not desire further childbearing are candidates for posterior colpoperineorrhaphy.

Clinical Pearl

1. A rectocele is the herniation of the rectovaginal wall and is usually due to childbirth.

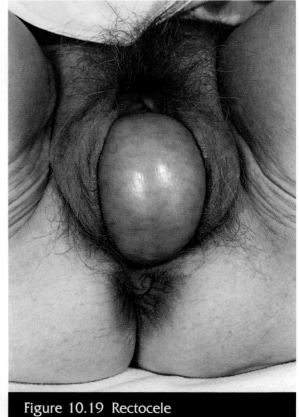

Figure 10.19 Rectocele

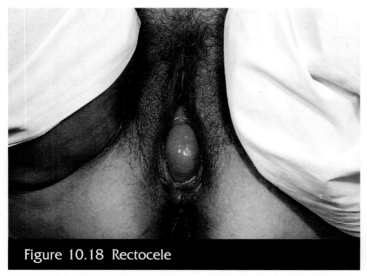

Figure 10.18 Rectocele

This is characterized by bulging of the posterior vaginal wall at the introitus. (Courtesy of Matthew Backer, Jr., MD.)

Worsening of the rectocele with Valsalva. (Courtesy of Matthew Backer, Jr., MD.)

Associated Clinical Features

The hymen is a membrane visible at the introitus that separates the vestibule externally from the vagina internally. The opening of the hymen can take on a variety of shapes—annular, semilunar, cribiform, and septate. The congenital absence of a hymenal orifice is called an imperforate hymen (IH). This condition may become evident in infants or young children as a smooth, glistening, protruding membrane due to the buildup of vaginal secretions known as a mucocolpos. More commonly, an imperforate hymen presents in adolescent girls with primary amenorrhea and recurrent abdominal pain. The buildup of menstrual blood and secretions behind the hymen is called hematocolpos and may become large enough to cause urinary retention by pressing on the bladder neck.

Physical examination reveals a smooth, dome-shaped, bluish-red bulging membrane (Fig. 10.20). A large, smooth, cystic mass can often be palpated anteriorly on digital rectal examination. Occasionally, the buildup of blood may spill over through the fallopian tubes into the peritoneal cavity, resulting in signs of pelvic or abdominal peritonitis.

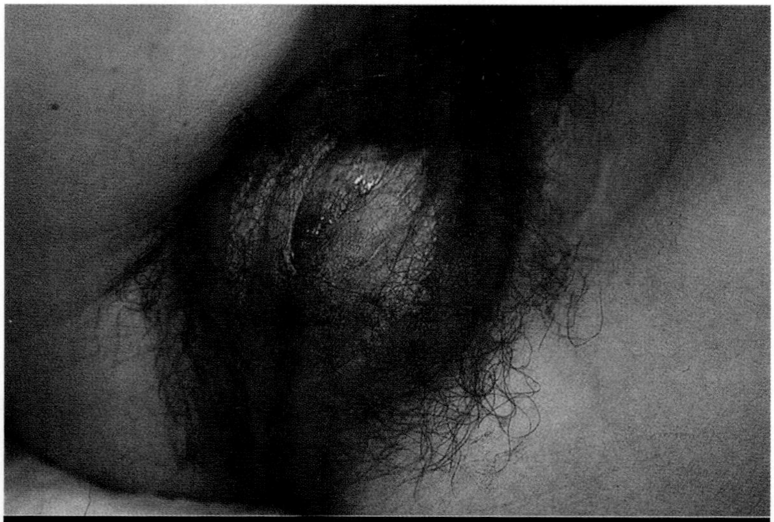

Figure 10.20 Imperforate Hymen

A bulging mass at the introitus is seen in this patient with abdominal distention and amenorrhea. The imperforate hymen was diagnosed, with subsequent incision and drainage of the hematocolpos. (Courtesy of Mark Eich, MD.)

Differential Diagnosis

A complete transverse septum, located in the midvagina, presents similarly to IH but is generally not visible to simple inspection. Partial and complete vaginal agenesis may be confused with IH in preadolescents. Both cystocele and rectocele present as bulging masses at the introitus (see Figs. 10.16, 10.18) but occur almost exclusively in multiparous women, thus excluding IH from consideration. The presentation of a bulging membrane at the introitus may be briefly confused with a bulging amniotic sac—history and abdominal examination, however, should allow this possibility to be quickly excluded.

Emergency Department Treatment and Disposition

Imperforate hymen as well as other abnormalities of the vaginal outlet should be referred to a gynecologist for definitive treatment. This includes incision of the hymen to allow drainage of the hematocolpos. Those instances detected in preadolescence should ideally be referred to a practitioner who specializes in pediatric cases.

Clinical Pearl

1. An imperforate hymen presents in adolescent girls with primary amenorrhea and recurrent abdominal pain.

Associated Clinical Features

Ectopic pregnancy is the leading cause of maternal obstetric morbidity in the first trimester of pregnancy. Presentations commonly include mild vaginal bleeding and lower abdominal pain, but patients can present in shock secondary to massive hemorrhage. The menstrual history, although often unreliable, may reveal a missed or recent abnormal menses. The presence of early signs of pregnancy (breast changes, morning sickness, fatigue) is variable. On examination, the uterus may be slightly enlarged, and adnexal tenderness is not always present. The visualization of an intrauterine pregnancy (IUP) by ultrasound (US) essentially excludes the diagnosis of ectopic pregnancy, the exception being a rare dual pregnancy (IUP and ectopic). The appearance of a gestational sac at about 5 weeks (Fig. 10.21) is the first significant finding on US *suggestive* of an IUP; however, definitive diagnosis of IUP should be deferred until a yolk sac is present (Fig. 10.22). A fetal pole develops next and can be seen on part of the yolk sac (Fig. 10.23). The double decidual sac sign is evidence of a true gestational sac and should be differentiated from the pseudogestational sac formed from a decidual cast in ectopic pregnancy (Fig. 10.24). When no gestational sac is visualized ("empty uterus") (Fig. 10.25), ectopic pregnancy cannot be distinguished from an early IUP too small to be seen on US.

Differential Diagnosis

Ectopic pregnancy should be considered in all first-trimester females presenting to the emergency department with either lower abdominal pain or tenderness or vaginal bleeding. A spontaneously completed abortion with an empty uterine cavity may lead to confusion if the beta human chorionic gonadotropin (βhCG) level is elevated above the institution's or sonographer's discriminatory zone [generally between 1000 and 2000 mIU/mL (Third International Standard)] and clinical ev-

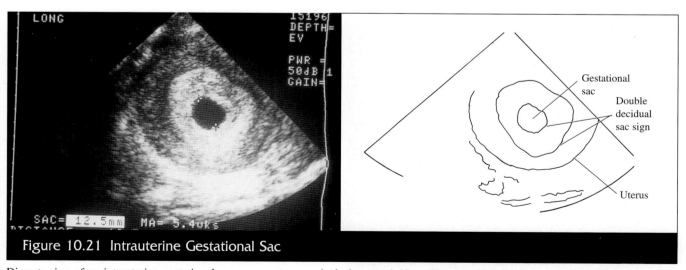

Figure 10.21 Intrauterine Gestational Sac

Discrete ring of an intrauterine gestational sac seen on transvaginal ultrasound. No yolk sac is visualized. A double decidual sac sign is seen, however, lending evidence of a true gestational sac versus a pseudogestational sac formed from a decidual cast in ectopic pregnancy. A thorough look in the adnexa is important in diagnosing ectopic pregnancy when a gestational sac is the only finding. (Courtesy of Janice Underwood.)

idence for the passage of products of conception is lacking. Alternative causes of first-trimester lower abdominal pain or vaginal bleeding include threatened or incomplete abortion, molar pregnancy, ruptured corpus luteum cyst, adnexal torsion, urinary tract infection, appendicitis, pelvic inflammatory disease, and ureteral calculi.

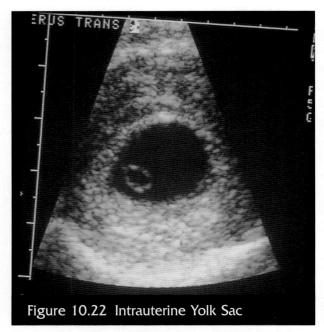

Figure 10.22 Intrauterine Yolk Sac

Discrete ring of an intrauterine yolk sac within the gestational sac seen on transvaginal ultrasound. Definitive diagnosis of IUP should be deferred until a fetal pole is present in the sac. (Courtesy of Janice Underwood.)

Emergency Department Treatment and Disposition

Unstable patients require aggressive resuscitation with fluid and blood followed by surgery. Stable patients with an ultrasound diagnosis consistent with ectopic pregnancy (Fig. 10.24) warrant immediate gynecologic consultation. Definitive therapeutic options range from observation in asymptomatic patients with declining hCG levels, traditional or laparoscopic surgery, to pharmacologic therapy with methotrexate. Despite the diminished diagnostic accuracy of ultrasound at lower levels (up to half of all ectopic pregnancies have a serum hCG level less than 2000 mIU/mL), if there is a strong clinical suspicion for ectopic pregnancy, gynecologic consultation should be considered. Those patients in whom a normal IUP is visualized can be safely discharged with early outpatient follow-up.

Clinical Pearls

1. Ectopic pregnancy should be considered in all women of reproductive age presenting with vaginal bleeding, abdominal pain or tenderness, or a missed menstrual period.

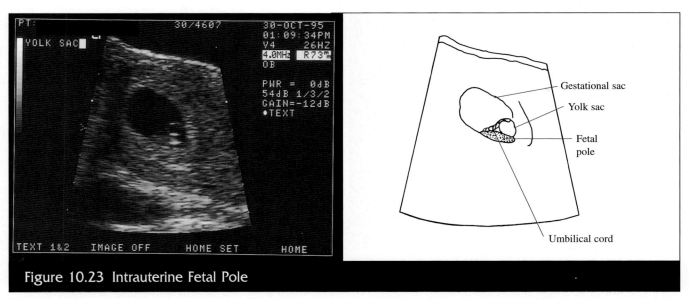

Figure 10.23 Intrauterine Fetal Pole

Ultrasound image of an intrauterine pregnancy with a fetal pole consistent with an 8-week gestation. An umbilical cord can be seen interposed between the yolk sac and the fetal pole. (Courtesy of Robert Buckley, MD.)

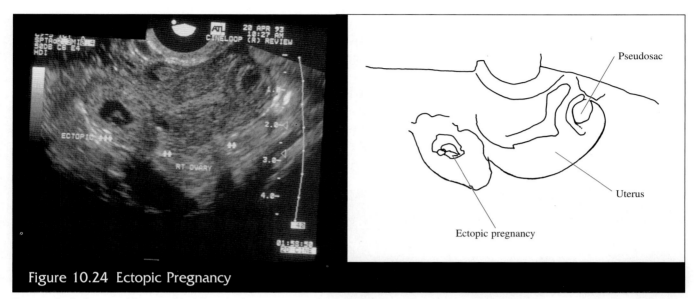

Figure 10.24 Ectopic Pregnancy

Transvaginal ultrasound image of a right ectopic pregnancy with a decidual reaction in the uterus resembling a gestational sac, or "pseudosac." Visualization of a pseudogestational, or "single," sac sign could be consistent with an early gestational sac or an ectopic pregnancy with a uterine decidual cast. (Courtesy of Janice Underwood.)

2. Failure to visualize an intrauterine pregnancy by transvaginal ultrasonography by the time the serum hCG level has reached approximately 1000 mIU/mL or by abdominal ultrasound once it has reached a level of approximately 6000 mIU/mL is highly suggestive of the diagnosis of ectopic pregnancy.

3. The ability of ultrasound and quantitative βhCG to diagnose ectopic pregnancy is highly dependent on the resolution of the machine, the skill of the examiner, and the βhCG assay used. Thus, every institution and examiner must develop a specific "discriminatory zone," the level of βhCG on which to base diagnostic decisions.

4. A decidual cast in the uterus of an ectopic pregnancy may resemble a gestational sac of an intrauterine pregnancy on ultrasound.

5. Consider ectopic pregnancy in any female of reproductive age presenting with syncope.

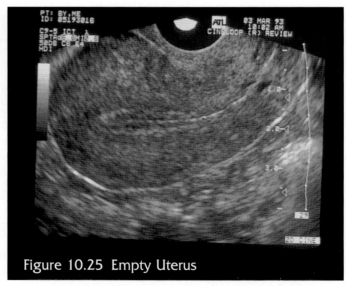

Figure 10.25 Empty Uterus

Transvaginal ultrasound image of an apparently empty uterus. Ectopic pregnancy should be strongly suspected if a transvaginal ultrasound reveals an empty uterus in the setting of a serum quantitative hCG level above the institution's discriminatory zone. (Courtesy of Janice Underwood.)

Associated Clinical Features

Molar pregnancy is part of a spectrum of gestational trophoblastic tumors that include benign hydatidiform moles, locally invasive moles, and choriocarcinoma. The classic clinical presentation is painless first- or early second-trimester vaginal bleeding with a uterine size larger than the estimated gestational age based on the last menstrual period. Additional clinical findings include nausea and vomiting, though this is often indistinguishable from that found in normal pregnancy.

Signs of preeclampsia in the first trimester or early second trimester (hypertension, headache, proteinuria, and edema), are highly suggestive of this diagnosis. Hyperthyroidism can be found in roughly 5% of cases. Acute respiratory distress may occur owing to embolization of trophoblastic tissue into the pulmonary vasculature, thyrotoxicosis, or simply fluid overload.

Moles commonly produce serum hCG levels greater than 100,000 mIU/mL. The diagnosis is made by ultrasound. Figure 10.26 demonstrates the classic finding of multiple intrauterine echoes with no fetus.

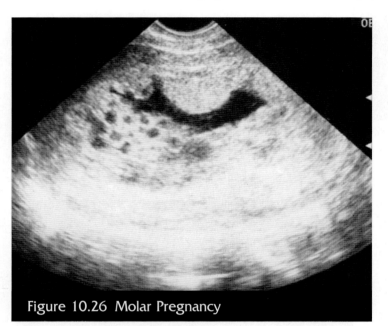

Figure 10.26 Molar Pregnancy

"Snowstorm" pattern demonstrating multiple intrauterine echoes with no fetus is seen on transvaginal ultrasonography in a patient with a molar pregnancy. Serum βHCG was > 180,000 mIU/mL. (Courtesy of Robin Marshall, MD.)

Differential Diagnosis

Spontaneous abortion and ectopic pregnancy are much more common that molar disease and can generally be differentiated based on typical ultrasound findings accompanied by markedly elevated serum hCG levels.

Emergency Department Treatment and Disposition

Gynecologic consultation for dilatation and curettage (D & C) should be obtained in all cases. For patients who are reliable for follow-up, suction curettage may be performed in an outpatient setting when the uterine size is less than 16 weeks and there is no evidence of preeclampsia, hyperthyroidism, or respiratory distress.

All cases must have close outpatient monitoring of serum hCG levels to rule out the presence of malignant gestational trophoblastic disease.

Clinical Pearls

1. All patients with pregnancies of less than 20 weeks' gestation with clinical findings of preeclampsia should have gestational trophoblastic disease ruled out.
2. A "snowstorm" pattern on ultrasonography demonstrating multiple intrauterine echoes with no fetus coupled with a high hCG level is typical of molar pregnancy.

Obstetric Conditions

THIRD-TRIMESTER BLUNT ABDOMINAL TRAUMA

Associated Clinical Features

Trauma is a major cause of maternal and fetal mortality. In addition to the common injuries to a solid organ and/or hollow viscus associated with blunt abdominal trauma, special consideration should be given to the possibility of preterm labor, fetal-maternal hemorrhage, uterine rupture, and, most importantly, abruptio placentae. Abruptio placentae is defined as the premature separation of the placenta from the site of uterine implantation. It is found in up to 50% of major blunt trauma patients and up to 5% of those with apparent minor injuries. There are generally signs of uterine hyperactivity and fetal distress when significant placental detachment occurs. Most patients have vaginal bleeding, although the margins of detachment are above the cervical os in up to 20%, who therefore have little or no vaginal bleeding. Laboratory evidence of a consumptive coagulopathy is occasionally seen with significant abruption. Electronic fetal monitoring is of paramount importance in all cases of significant trauma in patients beyond 20 weeks' gestation. As the pregnancy progresses toward term, a normal heart rate averages between 120 and 160 bpm. Rapid, frequent fluctuations in the baseline are characteristic of normal "reactivity" (Fig. 10.27). The loss of this reactivity can occur during a normal sleep cycle, following narcotic administration, or, most importantly, in the setting of fetal hypoxia or distress (Fig. 10.28). Decelerations are transient reductions in the fetal heart rate. Late decelerations begin after the contraction begins and return to baseline well after it ends, with the nadir of the deceleration occurring after the peak of the uterine contraction. Late decelerations should suggest fetal hypoxia, especially when they are accompanied by a loss of normal baseline beat-to-beat variability (Fig. 10.29). Variable decelerations are characterized by deep, broad decreases in fetal heart rate, often falling below 100 bpm (Fig. 10.30). They can occur slightly before, during, or after the onset of a uterine contraction, hence the term *variable*. Variable decelerations are caused by the transient compression of the umbilical cord during a contraction and are rarely associated with

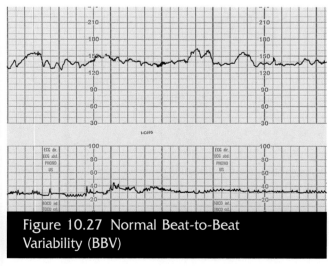

Figure 10.27 Normal Beat-to-Beat Variability (BBV)

A normal reactive fetal monitor strip showing a baseline heart rate between 120 and 160 with fluctuations in the short- and long-term heart rate. (Courtesy of Timothy Jahn, MD.)

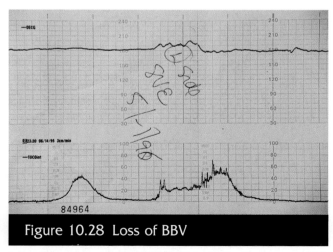

Figure 10.28 Loss of BBV

Loss of beat-to-beat variability (BBV) in the fetal heart rate, which may forewarn of fetal distress. This same pattern may also be seen during a normal sleep cycle or following maternal narcotic administration. (Courtesy of Gerard Van Houdt, MD.)

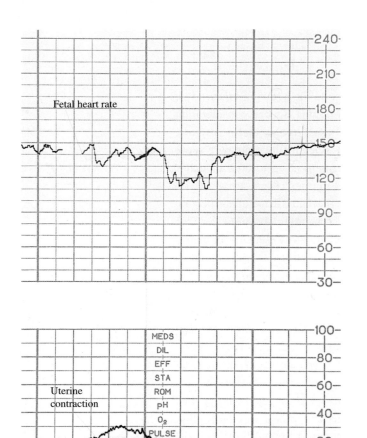

Figure 10.29 Late Deceleration

The nadir of a late deceleration always follows the peak of the uterine contraction with the heart rate approaching the baseline after the completion of the uterine contraction; this is suggestive of hypoxia. (Courtesy of James Palombaro, MD.)

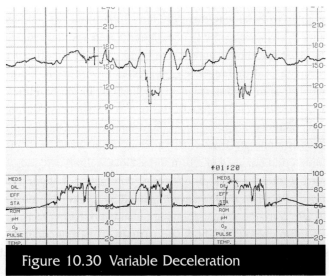

Figure 10.30 Variable Deceleration

Variable decelerations are due to cord compression. They are characterized by a rapid onset and recovery and may occur slightly before, during, or after the onset of the contraction. (Courtesy of John O. Boyle, MD.)

significant hypoxia or acidosis unless they are frequent or prolonged. They are most commonly appreciated during the second stage of labor, when forceful uterine compression transiently occludes the umbilical cord as the infant is propelled through the birth canal.

Differential Diagnosis

Another alternative cause of bright red vaginal bleeding in the third trimester of pregnancy is placenta previa. This can generally be differentiated from abruption by the visualization of a low-lying placenta on ultrasound.

Emergency Department Treatment and Disposition

An obstetrician should be consulted immediately in all trauma patients beyond 20 weeks' gestation. Blood for type- and cross-matching, complete blood count, prothrombin time (PT), partial thromboplastin time (PTT), fibrinogen, and fibrin degradation products or D-dimer should be obtained. It is generally recommended that patients undergo continuous tocofetal monitoring for a minimum of 4 h to rule out preterm labor or fetal distress. Ultrasound is essential in visualizing placental abruption. Indications for emergency cesarean section include placental abruption, signs of ongoing fetal distress, or uncontrolled maternal hemorrhage.

Clinical Pearls

1. Ecchymotic markings imparted by a significant blunt force (Fig. 10.31) are not always present on a gravid abdomen; thus, a careful history of the mechanism of trauma and associated complaints is essential.
2. Anti-Rh immunoglobulin should be administered for all cases of significant third-trimester blunt abdominal trauma if the mother is Rh-negative and the father is Rh-positive.

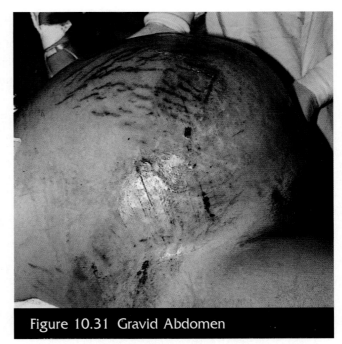

Figure 10.31 Gravid Abdomen

A third-trimester gravid abdomen with ecchymotic markings imparted by a significant blunt force. Fetal assessment should occur simultaneously with maternal resuscitation. (Courtesy of John Fildes, MD.)

Associated Clinical Features

Patients beyond the 20th week of pregnancy presenting with a history of uncontrolled leakage of fluid should undergo sterile speculum examination to determine the presence of amniotic fluid. The diagnosis of membrane rupture can be made by observing the passage of fluid from the cervix or pooling in the vaginal vault. Without gross evidence of rupture, secretions from the vaginal vault can be placed on a slide and allowed to air dry. The characteristic arborization, or ferning pattern (Fig. 10.32), is diagnostic of amniotic fluid, thus rupture of the membranes. In addition, the secretions can be applied to nitrazine paper. The pH of normal vaginal secretions generally falls between 4.5 and 5.5, whereas amniotic fluid generally ranges between 7.0 and 7.5, yielding a dark blue tint.

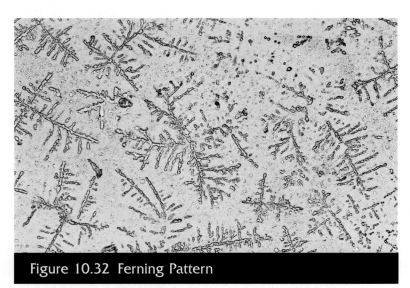

Figure 10.32 Ferning Pattern

The arborization pattern found when a drop of amniotic fluid is allowed to air dry on a microscope slide, known as ferning. (Courtesy of Robert Buckley, MD.)

Differential Diagnosis

Urinary incontinence is the most common alternative diagnosis in a third-trimester patient who presents with a history of possible membrane rupture. The passage of the cervical mucous plug, known as bloody show, may rarely be confused with the passage of amniotic fluid. Although a small, subclinical amniotic fluid leak can never be completely excluded, the presence of an acid pH, the absence of gross fluid in the vaginal vault, and ferning all point against the diagnosis of membrane rupture.

Emergency Department Treatment and Disposition

All patients with confirmed ruptured fetal membranes should be admitted to the labor and delivery area and the obstetric consultant notified, irrespective of the presence or absence of uterine contractions. The greatest risk to the fetus before 37 weeks is preterm delivery. The fetus at term is at risk for infection secondary to chorioamnionitis if the time from membrane rupture to vaginal delivery exceeds 24 h.

Clinical Pearls

1. With a strong suspicion of membrane rupture by history and no objective evidence of amniotic fluid on examination, a large sterile pad may be placed on the perineum and the patient reexamined after brief ambulation. This assumes the absence of uterine contractions and the presence of a reactive fetal monitor strip.
2. Umbilical cord prolapse should be excluded with a speculum examination in all cases of membrane rupture.

Associated Clinical Features

The second stage of labor begins when the cervix is fully dilated, allowing for the gradual descent of the head toward the vaginal outlet. As the head approaches the perineum, the labia begin to separate with each contraction and then recede once the contraction subsides. *Crowning* is the term applied when the head separates the labial margins without receding at the end of the contraction (Fig. 10.33).

Emergency Department Treatment and Disposition

The appearance of crowning heralds imminent vaginal delivery. Equipment for delivery and neonatal resuscitation should be brought to the bedside. Both the on-call obstetric consultant and pediatrician should be notified while preparations are being made for ED delivery.

Clinical Pearls

1. Primigravida patients may still require multiple sets of contractions and pushing to fully expel the head through the vaginal outlet.
2. If meconium secretions are detected well before delivery, continuous electronic tocofetal monitoring should be begun and the obstetric and pediatric consultants notified.

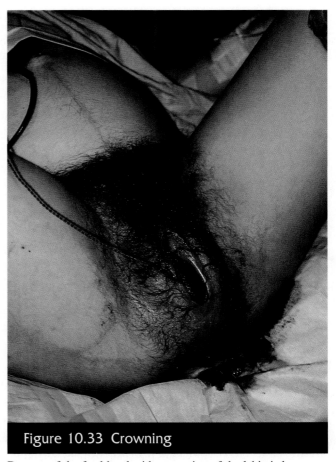

Figure 10.33 Crowning

Descent of the fetal head with separation of the labia is known as crowning and heralds imminent vertex delivery. (Courtesy of William Leninger, MD.)

Associated Clinical Features

A gravid female with regular forceful contractions and the urge to strain (push) can present without warning. Crowning may be present and heralds imminent vaginal delivery. Important historical questions include the number of previous pregnancies, a diagnosis of twin gestations, and whether there is a history of prenatal care or complications. The presence of greenish brown fetal stool, known as meconium, is associated with fetal hypoxia and is a clinical indicator of fetal distress. Fetal bradycardia or late decelerations (Fig. 10.29) may be present and are also evidence of fetal distress.

Differential Diagnosis

Complications (discussed below) should be considered when the progress of delivery is altered or when the presenting part is something other than the occiput. Twin gestations should be considered in all emergency deliveries and asked about early in the history.

Emergency Department Treatment and Disposition

Intravenous access, oxygen, and equipment for delivery and neonatal resuscitation (suction, oxygen, warming light, etc.) are immediately obtained as preparation for the impending delivery.

Delivery of the Head

As the vertex passes through the vaginal outlet, extension of the head occurs, followed by the appearance of the forehead and chin. Extension and delivery of the fetal head can be facilitated by applying gentle pressure upward on the chin through the perineum—known as the modified Ritgen maneuver (Fig. 10.34). Simultaneously, the fingers of the other hand can be used to elevate the scalp to help extend the head. Once the head has been delivered, the occiput promptly rotates toward a left or right lateral position. At this stage, the nuchal region should be swept to

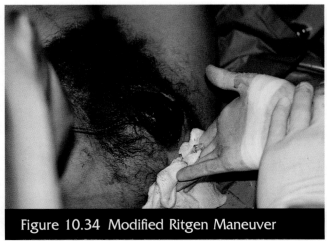

Figure 10.34 Modified Ritgen Maneuver

Modified Ritgen maneuver: upward pressure is applied on the fetal chin through the perineum. (Courtesy of William Leninger, MD.)

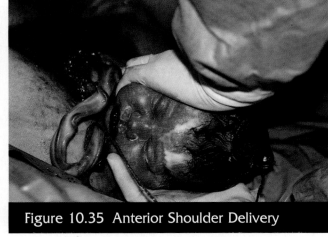

Figure 10.35 Anterior Shoulder Delivery

Delivery of the anterior shoulder is facilitated with downward traction. (Courtesy of William Leninger, MD.)

detect the presence of a nuchal umbilical cord (see Fig. 10.45). Before the delivery of the shoulders, the nasopharynx should be gently suctioned with a bulb syringe to clear away any blood or amniotic debris. If thick meconium is present, deeper and more thorough suctioning of the posterior pharynx and glottic region should be accomplished with a mechanical suction trap, since aspiration of thick meconium by the newborn can lead to pneumonitis and hypoxia.

Delivery of the Shoulders

Delivery of the shoulders generally occurs spontaneously with little manipulation. Occasionally, gentle downward traction applied by grasping the sides of the head with two hands eases the delivery of the anterior shoulder (Fig. 10.35). The head can then be directed upward to permit the delivery of the posterior shoulder (Fig. 10.36). Following delivery of both shoulders, the body and legs are easily delivered. Attention is then directed toward the immediate care of the newborn. The cord is doubly clamped and ligated (Fig. 10.37) and inspected for three vessels: two umbilical arteries and one umbilical vein (Fig. 10.38). The child's pediatrician should be notified

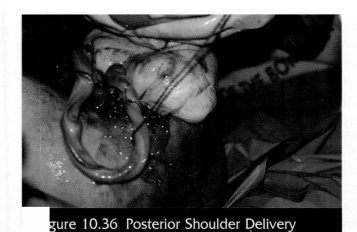

gure 10.36 Posterior Shoulder Delivery

Delivery of the posterior shoulder with upward traction. (Courtesy of William Leninger, MD.)

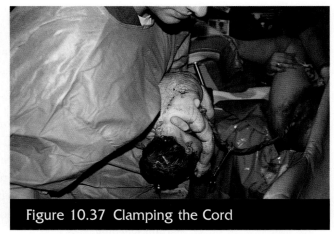

Figure 10.37 Clamping the Cord

The cord is clamped immediately after delivery. (Courtesy of William Leninger, MD.)

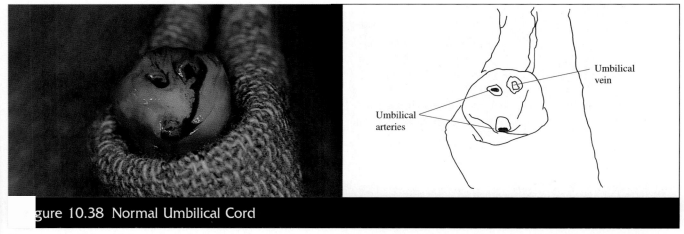

gure 10.38 Normal Umbilical Cord

Cross-sectional view of the two arteries and single vein of a normal three-vessel umbilical cord. (Courtesy of Jennifer Jagoe, MD.)

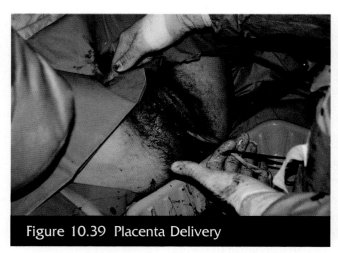

Figure 10.39 Placenta Delivery

Gentle traction is applied to the cord while the opposite hand massages the uterus. (Courtesy of William Leninger, MD.)

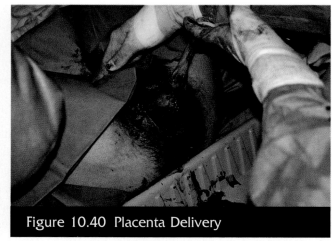

Figure 10.40 Placenta Delivery

Delivery of the placenta. (Courtesy of William Leninger, MD.)

if a two-vessel umbilical cord is found at delivery. The newborn is immediately placed under a warming lamp for drying and gentle stimulation while being observed for signs of distress (heart rate < 100, limp muscle tone, poor color, weak cry).

Delivery of the Placenta

Following delivery, gentle traction can be placed on the cord while the opposite hand is used to massage the uterine fundus (Fig. 10.39). The placenta will generally be delivered within 15 to 20 min (Fig. 10.40) and should be grossly inspected. Retention of small fragments should be suspected when inspection of the placenta reveals evidence of a missing segment or cotyledon (Fig. 10.41). The attending obstetric consultant should be notified, since retained placental fragments often warrant manual exploration of the uterus, especially in the context of persistent postpartum bleeding.

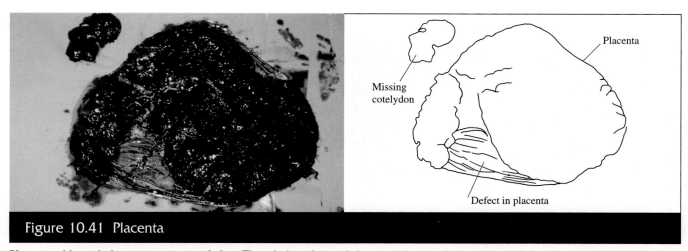

Figure 10.41 Placenta

Placenta with a missing segment or cotyledon. The missing placental tissue can be seen in the upper left-hand corner of the photograph. (Courtesy of John O. Boyle, MD.)

Clinical Pearls

1. Both obstetric and pediatric consultants should be alerted that preparations are being made for ED delivery.
2. A two-vessel cord may be found in about 1 in 500 singleton deliveries and is associated with an increased incidence of congenital defects.
3. Retained placental fragments should be considered in the setting of postpartum hemorrhage or endometritis.

Associated Clinical Features

In an overt cord prolapse, a loop of umbilical cord is visualized either at the introitus (Fig. 10.42) or on speculum examination following membrane rupture (Fig. 10.43). Alternatively, a small loop of cord may be palpated at the cervical os. In a funic cord prolapse, a loop of umbilical cord is palpated directly through intact fetal membranes. Occult prolapse occurs when the umbilical cord descends between the presenting part and the lower uterine segment but is not visible or directly palpable on examination. Intermittent compression of the umbilical cord with each uterine contraction may be detected by the presence of variable decelerations of the fetal monitor (see Fig. 10.30). The new onset of variable decelerations should always prompt immediate cervical examination to rule out an overt cord prolapse. Severe persistent bradycardia may ensue if cord compression is sustained beyond the duration of the contraction, which is often the case in an overt prolapse.

Differential Diagnosis

Rarely, an inexperienced examiner may mistake a presenting hand or foot for a prolapsed cord. This may be clarified by careful digital or speculum examination.

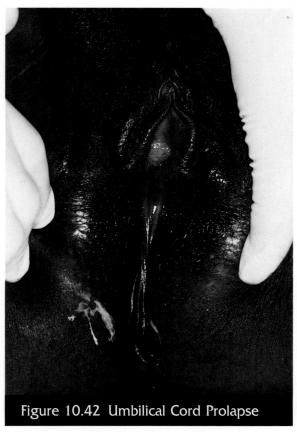

Figure 10.42 Umbilical Cord Prolapse

Prolapsed umbilical cord visible at the vaginal introitus in a patient with twin gestations. (Courtesy of Kevin J. Knoop, MD, MS.)

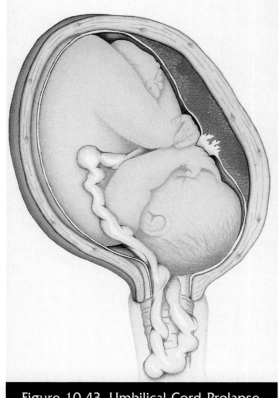

Figure 10.43 Umbilical Cord Prolapse

Schematic drawing of an overt prolapse of the umbilical cord through a partially dilated cervical os. (Courtesy of Judy Christensen.)

Emergency Department Treatment and Disposition

Prolapse of the umbilical cord presents an immediate threat to the fetal circulation and constitutes an obstetric emergency. If an overt prolapse is detected in the ED, the patient should immediately be placed in a knee-chest position and continuous upward pressure applied by the examining hand to relieve the pressure of the presenting part on the lower uterine segment. An obstetrician should be summoned immediately and the patient taken directly to the operating room for cesarean delivery. Continuous upward pressure should be applied to the presenting part of the fetus at all times during transport. Occasionally, precipitous vaginal delivery may ensue in the ED shortly after a cord prolapse is detected. Resuscitative equipment should be available in anticipation of a physiologically compromised infant. If a funic prolapse is appreciated in the ED, an obstetrician should be notified and the patient prepared for cesarean delivery. Under no circumstance should the membranes be broken. Occult prolapse is rarely appreciated in the ED.

Clinical Pearl

1. Pelvic examination to exclude umbilical cord prolapse should be performed immediately following rupture of membranes, the appearance of variable decelerations, or the detection of bradycardia.

Associated Clinical Features

The incidence of singleton breech presentation is approximately 3% but rises to higher than 20% in preterm infants weighing less than 2000 g. In a frank breech, both hips are flexed and both knees extended. In a complete breech, both hips and knees are flexed, whereas a footling breech has one or both legs extended below the buttocks. Frank breech is most common in full-term deliveries, whereas footling presentation can be found in up to half of all preterm deliveries. Breech deliveries carry a much higher mortality rate than cephalic deliveries. Complications of breech delivery include umbilical cord prolapse, nuchal arm obstruction, and difficulty in delivery of the following head (Fig. 10.44).

Emergency Department Treatment and Disposition

The specific maneuvers for breech extraction are beyond the scope of this text. If breech delivery appears imminent, support and gentle traction should be applied as the various parts spontaneously pass through the vaginal outlet, keeping in mind that the biparietal diameter is greater than either the bitrochanteric or bisacromial diameter.

Clinical Pearl

1. Immediate obstetric consultation should be obtained in all breech deliveries.

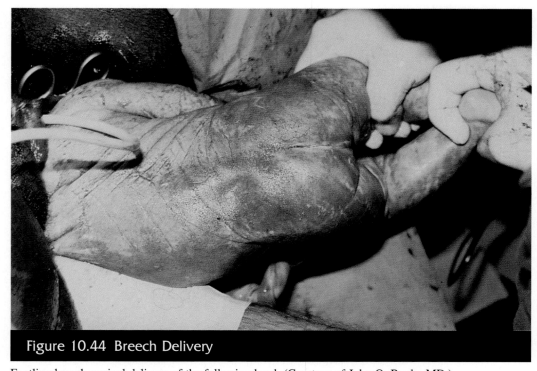

Figure 10.44 Breech Delivery

Footling breech vaginal delivery of the following head. (Courtesy of John O. Boyle, MD.)

Associated Clinical Features

The circumferential wrapping of the umbilical cord around the child's neck occurs in about 20% of all deliveries (Fig. 10.45). Tight approximation of the cord around the infant's neck can lead to transient disruption of uterine blood flow during contractions, leading to variable decelerations noted on the fetal heart rate monitor (Fig. 10.30); it may also impede delivery once the head passes through the introitus.

Emergency Department Treatment and Disposition

Once a cord is identified around the neck, it should be slipped over the head using the index and middle fingers. Occasionally two coils are identified.

Clinical Pearl

1. A loosely applied cord should be pulled over the child's head. If the cord is wrapped too tightly, it can be clamped and ligated on the perineum, followed by the immediate delivery of the shoulders and body.

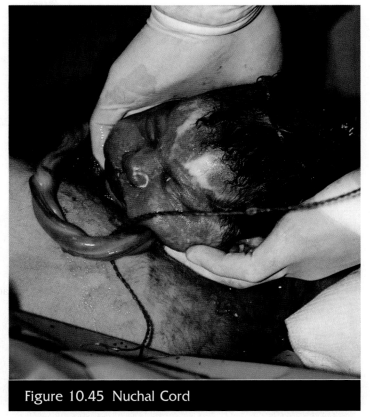

Figure 10.45 Nuchal Cord

A loose nuchal cord is seen around the neck. (Courtesy of William Leninger, MD.)

Associated Clinical Features

Shoulder dystocia is defined as failure to deliver the shoulders, following delivery of the head, because of impaction of the fetal shoulders against the pelvic outlet (Fig. 10.46). Risk factors include gestational diabetes, prior delivery of large infants, and postterm delivery.

Emergency Department Treatment and Disposition

Shoulder dystocia is an acute obstetric emergency, with the immediate life threat being asphyxia from prolonged delivery. An obstetrician should be summoned immediately. Equipment for neonatal resuscitation should be set up and, ideally, a pediatric consultant should be summoned. In the absence of an obstetric consultant, a wide episiotomy should be performed. The least invasive maneuver is to forcefully flex the mother's knees toward her chest (McRobert's maneuver). This extreme dorsal lithotomy position occasionally allows for the appropriate engagement of the fetal shoulders. If this is unsuccessful, a Wood's maneuver can be attempted by hooking two fingers behind the infant's posterior scapula and rotating the entire body in a screwlike manner. As the posterior shoulder rotates upward, it can generally be delivered past the symphysis pubis. If the Wood's maneuver fails to deliver the anterior shoulder, delivery of the posterior arm may be attempted by inserting two fingers into the sacral fossa and bringing down the entire posterior arm by flexing it at the elbow. The remaining anterior shoulder should then deliver, either spontaneously or else following rotation into the oblique position to facilitate its delivery.

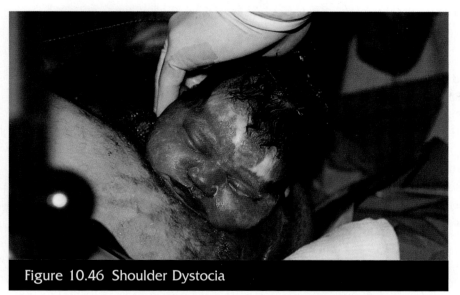

Figure 10.46 Shoulder Dystocia

Firm approximation of the fetal head against the vaginal outlet consistent with shoulder dystocia. (Courtesy of William Leninger, MD.)

Clinical Pearls

1. Shoulder dystocia is an acute obstetric emergency that requires quick action:

   Call for help.
   Cut a wide episiotomy.
   Perform McRobert's maneuver.
   Rotate the posterior shoulder.

2. After delivery, look for fracture of the clavicles or humerus and possible brachial plexus injury.

Associated Clinical Features

Lacerations to the perineum occur commonly following a rapid, uncontrolled expulsion of the fetal head. Postpartum perineal lacerations range from minor to severe.

Differential Diagnosis

Perineal lacerations due to birth trauma are categorized into four groups. First-degree lacerations are limited to the mucosa, skin, and superficial subcutaneous and submucosal tissues (Fig. 10.47). Second-degree lacerations penetrate deeper into the superficial fascia and transverse perineal musculature (Fig. 10.48). In addition to these structures, a third-degree laceration disrupts the anal sphincter, whereas a fourth-degree laceration extends into the rectal lumen (Fig. 10.49).

Emergency Department Treatment and Disposition

In precipitous ED deliveries, the repair of the episiotomy and/or perineal lacerations can often be performed by the obstetric consultant, the details of repair being beyond the scope of this book.

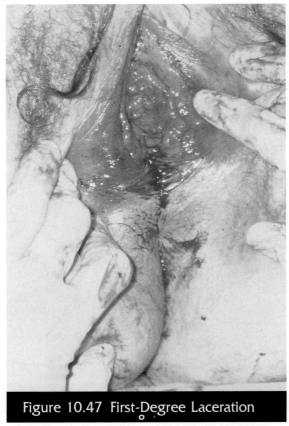

Figure 10.47 First-Degree Laceration

First-degree laceration limited to the mucosa, skin, and superficial subcutaneous and submucosal tissues. There is no involvement of the underlying fascia and muscle. (Courtesy of Jerry Van Houdt, MD.)

287

Clinical Pearl

1. Perineal laceration repair fundamentally involves the sequential anatomic reapproximation, using absorbable suture material, of the rectal mucosa, anal sphincter, transverse perineal musculature, vaginal mucosa, and skin.

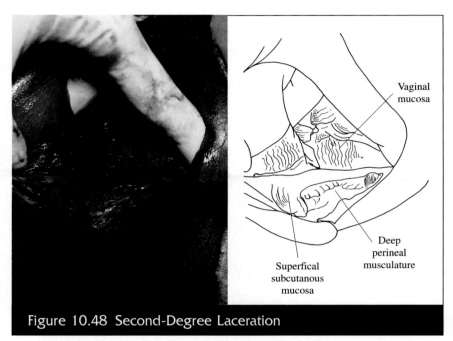

Figure 10.48 Second-Degree Laceration

There is disruption of the hymenal ring and the deep perineal musculature, extending into the vaginal mucosa and transversalis fascia, but no involvement of the anal sphincter or mucosa. (Courtesy of Pamela Ambroz, MD.)

Fourth-degree perineal laceration revealing wide separation of the perineal fascia and anal sphincter. The examiner's small finger is in the rectal lumen, showing extension of the tear proximally. (Courtesy of Timothy Jahn, MD.)

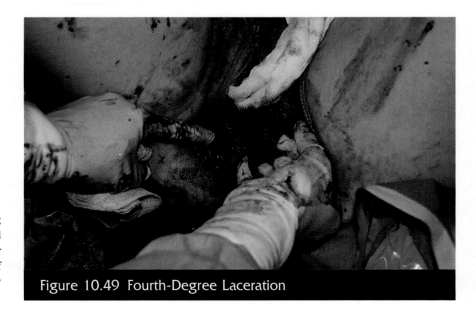

Figure 10.49 Fourth-Degree Laceration

CHAPTER 11

EXTREMITY TRAUMA

Deborah Gutman
Daniel L. Savitt
Alan B. Storrow

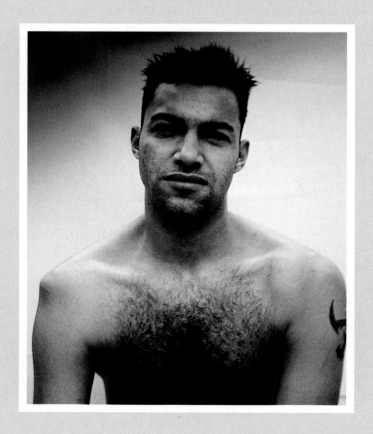

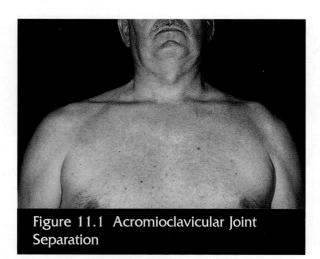

Figure 11.1 Acromioclavicular Joint Separation

Subtle prominence of the left distal clavicle. The upward displacement of the clavicle is due to stretching or disruption of the suspending ligaments. (Courtesy of Frank Birinyi, MD.)

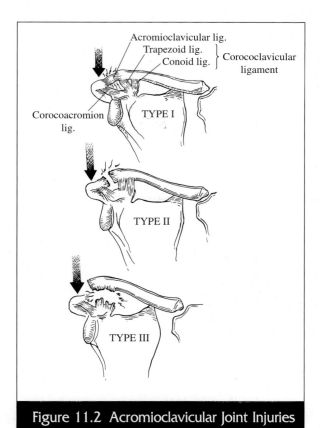

Figure 11.2 Acromioclavicular Joint Injuries

Classification of acromioclavicular joint injuries. (Adapted with permission from Rockwood CA, Green DP, Bucholz RW: *Rockwood and Green's Fractures in Adults,* 3d ed. Philadelphia: Lippincott; 1991.)

Associated Clinical Features

Injury to the acromioclavicular (AC) joint is a common finding in the ED, resulting from direct trauma with an adducted arm or indirectly from a fall on an outstretched arm with pressure directed to the joint (Fig. 11.1). There are three degrees of injury (Fig. 11.2). A first-degree injury is equivalent to a sprain. There is an incomplete tear of the ligament. Radiographs are negative. A second-degree injury consists of subluxation of the AC joint and disruption of the ligament. Subluxation of the clavicle from the acromion, of less than 50% the diameter of the clavicle, is only evident on stress radiographs. Complete disruption of the AC, coracoacromial, and coracoclavicular ligaments is a third-degree injury. Radiographs reveal more than 50% displacement of the clavicle from the acromion. All patients complain of pain at the joint site with moderate to severe amounts of swelling. Stress radiographs are obtained by suspending 5 to 10 lb of weight from each arm and taking a bilateral anteroposterior (AP) shoulder film. The joint space and any subluxation are easily visualized.

Differential Diagnosis

Clavicular fracture, scapular fracture, rotator cuff injury, shoulder dislocation, contusion, or isolated coracoclavicular ligament damage can be confused with AC joint separation.

Emergency Department Treatment and Disposition

First- and second-degree injuries are treated with rest, ice, analgesics, and a simple sling until acute pain with movement is relieved. Third-degree injury treatment is controversial. Many experts advocate immobilization with a sling for 3 weeks, whereas others advocate operative repair. Orthopedic referral is essential for all third-degree injuries.

Clinical Pearls

1. The AC joint stress test is an accurate means of testing for AC joint separation. The patient is instructed to bring the arm across the chest and try to align the opposite shoulder with the elbow. The production of pain over the AC joint confirms the diagnosis.
2. Since first- and second-degree separations are managed conservatively, stress views rarely alter management.

Associated Clinical Features

Anterior shoulder dislocations are the most common dislocation seen in the ED. They are caused by external rotation and abduction that disrupts the capsule and glenohumeral ligaments. The affected extremity is held in slight abduction and external rotation. Often, the patient supports the dislocated shoulder with the other arm. The acromion becomes prominent and there is a squared-off box-like appearance to the top of the shoulder. The rounded contour of the deltoid is lost (Fig. 11.3). These patients complain of shoulder pain and refuse to move the shoulder on the affected side. Many patients will appear diaphoretic and pale. A neurologic examination of the upper extremity should be performed to rule out associated injury, most commonly of the axillary nerve (sensation over the deltoid). Radiographic examination is necessary to evaluate for associated fracture (Fig. 11.4). Posterior shoulder dislocations are commonly missed because of subtle radiographic findings (Figs. 11.5 and 11.6). The arm is held internally rotated and adducted. There is no external rotation. On examination, a posterior prominence exists. Posterior dislocations commonly occur during seizures. The Hill-Sachs deformity (an impaction of the humeral head) can occur in a significant percentage (11 to 50%) of these patients.

Differential Diagnosis

Acromioclavicular separation, fracture of the greater tuberosity, humeral fracture, and fracture of the humeral head are commonly mistaken for a shoulder dislocation prior to radiographic examination.

Emergency Department Treatment and Disposition

Closed reduction is the treatment of choice and may require conscious sedation. There are many methods to reduce shoulder dislocations, including Stimson, traction-countertraction, and external rotation. Neurovascular and radiographic examination should occur before and after reduction. The patient should be placed in a sling and swathe after reduction. The shoulder should remain immobilized for 2 to 5 weeks (shorter periods for older patients owing to their greater propensity to develop shoulder stiffness).

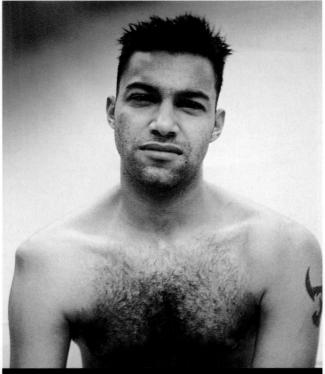

Figure 11.3 Anterior Shoulder Dislocation

This right anterior shoulder dislocation occurred when the patient fell while playing basketball. There is an obvious contour deformity as well as prominence of the acromion. (Courtesy of Kevin J. Knoop, MD, MS.)

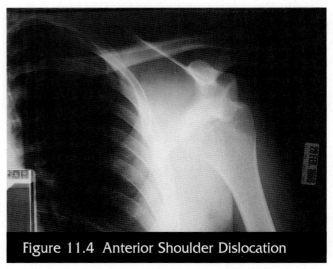

Figure 11.4 Anterior Shoulder Dislocation

Radiographic evaluation of this anterior shoulder dislocation demonstrates that the humeral head is not in the glenoid fossa but is located anterior and inferior to it. (Courtesy of Kevin J. Knoop, MD, MS.)

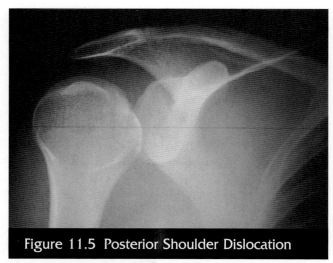

Figure 11.5 Posterior Shoulder Dislocation

AP radiograph of this rare type of shoulder dislocation. Because of internal rotation of the greater tuberosity, the humeral head appears like a dip of ice cream on a cone, thus called the "ice cream cone sign." (Courtesy of Alan B. Storrow, MD.)

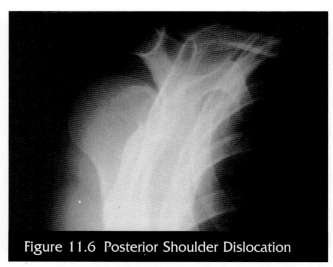

Figure 11.6 Posterior Shoulder Dislocation

A scapular Y view of the same patient in Fig. 11.5 confirms the diagnosis. (Courtesy of Alan B. Storrow, MD.)

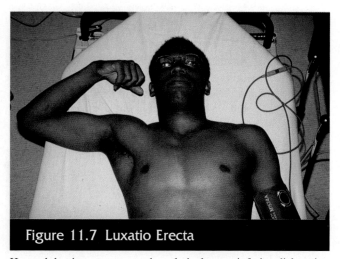

Figure 11.7 Luxatio Erecta

Hyperabduction may cause the relatively rare inferior dislocation known as luxatio erecta. The patient presents with the arm held in elevation and the humeral head may be palpated along the lateral chest wall. (Courtesy of Kevin J. Knoop, MD, MS.)

Clinical Pearls

1. Patients with a dislocated shoulder usually cannot touch the contralateral shoulder with the hand of the affected side.
2. Relaxation of the pectoral musculature is an excellent aid in shoulder reduction. This can be accomplished by manual massage of the muscle. Some patients can relax this muscle voluntarily when asked to do so (e.g., weightlifters).
3. Luxatio erecta (Fig. 11.7) is inferior glenohumeral dislocation. The humeral head is forced below the inferior aspect of the glenoid fossa. These patients present with the arm locked 180 degrees overhead.

Associated Clinical Features

Rupture of the biceps may occur anywhere along its route. It occurs most commonly in the dominant extremity of men between 40 and 60 years of age when an unexpected extension force is applied to the flexed arm. It may be associated with chronic bicipital tenosynovitis. When it occurs proximally, the patient notes a sharp pain in the bicipital groove and the muscle may be noted to contract within the arm (Fig. 11.8). It may be helpful to have the patient hold his or her arm abducted and externally rotated at 90 degrees. Flexion at the elbow will cause the biceps to move away from the shoulder. Rupture may also occur at the tendon insertion into the radial tuberosity at the elbow, often in an area of preexisting tendon degeneration. This diagnosis is made on the basis of a history of a painful, tearing sensation in the antecubital region. A snap or pop may also occur. The ability to palpate the tendon in the antecubital fossa may indicate partial tearing of the biceps tendon.

Differential Diagnosis

Muscle strain, partial tendon rupture, and deep venous thrombosis should be considered.

Emergency Department Treatment and Disposition

Nonoperative treatment consists of gentle range-of-motion exercises, anti-inflammatory medication, and physical therapy. This type of treatment results in restoring about 60% of normal strength of the biceps tendon. Operative treatment of proximal or distal ruptures is indicated for patients who wish to try to restore normal strength to the biceps tendon.

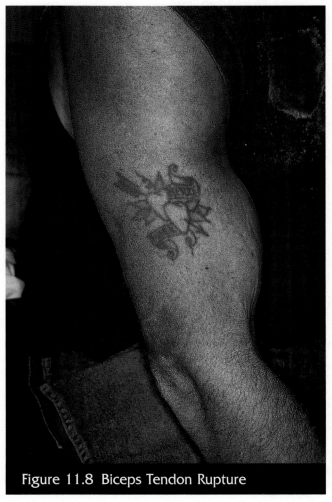

Figure 11.8 Biceps Tendon Rupture

The biceps is noted to contract within the arm after biceps tendon rupture. (Courtesy of Daniel L. Savitt, MD.)

Clinical Pearls

1. Early surgical reattachment to the coracoid, bicipital groove, or radial tuberosity is recommended for optimal results.
2. Rupture in the belly of the biceps is treated conservatively.

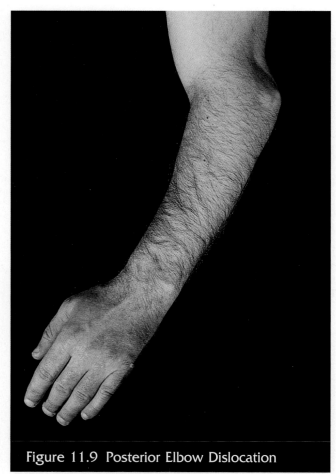

Figure 11.9 Posterior Elbow Dislocation

This patient dislocated his elbow while playing basketball. Note the flexed position of the elbow and the prominence of the olecranon. (Courtesy of Frank Birinyi, MD.)

Associated Clinical Features

Dislocations of the elbow can be anterior, posterior, medial, or lateral. All dislocations require immediate reduction to relieve pain and prevent circulatory compromise. Elbow dislocations are caused by a considerable amount of force, and approximately 40% have an associated fracture. Posterior dislocation is the most common (Fig. 11.9), occurring after a fall on an outstretched hand. The arm is extended and abducted. The elbow is held in a flexed position and is swollen, tender, and deformed. The olecranon is very prominent. Neurovascular status must be evaluated immediately because of associated injury. Anterior dislocations are rare. They occur if the elbow is in a flexed position and is hit from behind on the olecranon. The elbow is extended with the forearm supinated and elongated. The upper arm appears shortened. Injury to nerves and vessels is more common with anterior dislocation.

Differential Diagnosis

Contusion, radial or ulnar fracture, or supracondylar fracture of the humerus are commonly confused with an elbow dislocation until examined radiographically.

Emergency Department Treatment and Disposition

Most patients require analgesia and muscle relaxants prior to reduction. After reduction, the elbow should be immobilized in 90 to 120 degrees of flexion in a posterior splint and sling. Neurologic and radiographic examination should occur after any attempt at reduction. The patient should be observed in the ED for vascular compromise. Elbow dislocations with associated fractures may make closed reduction difficult and also leave the joint unstable. In these cases, consultation with an orthopedic surgeon is recommended prior to reduction attempts.

Clinical Pearls

1. Patients should not be placed in a circular cast because of the necessity for reexamination.
2. Factors that increase the index of suspicion for arterial injury include pulselessness prior to reduction, open dislocations, and concurrent serious traumatic injury.
3. The ulnar nerve is the most common nerve injured.
4. For posterior dislocations, palpate the two epicondyles and the tip of the olecranon. If they are in the same plane, a supracondylar fracture is likely. If the olecranon is displaced, a dislocation is likely.

Associated Clinical Features

Direct trauma or fall on an outstretched hand may result in elbow fractures. The patient is usually unable to extend the elbow but has pain on supination/pronation. AP, lateral and oblique views of the elbow should visualize most elbow fractures. The radial head should be aligned with the capitellum on all views (Fig. 11.10). The presence of a "fat pad" sign on x-ray can be indicative of trauma. The anterior fat pad may be seen on normal radiographs but may be displaced anteriorly and superiorly by effusion or hemarthrosis (sail sign). The posterior fat pad is not normally visualized and if seen is indicative of effusion or hemarthrosis (Fig. 11.11).

Supracondylar fractures often occur in patients 5 to 10 years old. At this age the tensile strength of the collateral ligaments and the joint capsule of the elbow are greater than the bone itself. Neurovascular insult occurs in 7% of supracondylar fractures, with the radial, median, and ulnar nerves equally injured. Ulnar nerve impingement may occur, causing distal neuropraxia or injury.

Capitellum fractures occur from direct forces, a fall on an outstretched arm, or as an indirect result of posterior elbow dislocation. With a force directed at the radial head, shearing of the capitellum causes anterior displacement of the fracture segment. Radiographically, the joint capsule depicts a swelling along the anteriorly displaced fragment. This fracture is commonly asso-

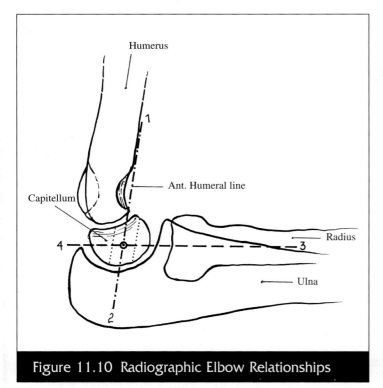

Figure 11.10 Radiographic Elbow Relationships

The anterior humeral line (1–2) should normally pass through the middle third of the capitellum. With an extension-type supracondylar fracture, this line will transect the anterior third of the capitellum or pass anterior to it. The radiocapitellar line (drawn through the center of the radius, 3–4) should also pass through the center of the capitellum. Disruption of this relationship may indicate fracture of the radial neck or dislocation.

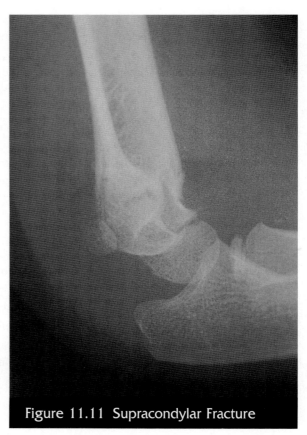

Figure 11.11 Supracondylar Fracture

This radiograph shows both a pronounced anterior fat pad (sail sign) and posterior fat pad indicative of a supracondylar fracture. (Courtesy of Alan B. Storrow, MD.)

ciated with fractures of the radial head, which are common but may be subtle and require a high index of suspicion.

Differential Diagnosis

Posterior elbow dislocation, nursemaid's elbow, and inter- or transcondylar fractures should be considered.

Emergency Department Treatment and Disposition

Treatment of supracondylar fractures is influenced by angulation and displacement as well as associated soft tissue injuries (especially neurovascular). Adult patients usually require surgical intervention. In general, an orthopedic consultant best handles decisions regarding reduction of significantly angulated and displaced fractures. If neurovascular compromise exists, the emergency physician may need to apply forearm traction to reestablish distal pulses. If the pulse is not restored with traction, emergent operative intervention for brachial artery exploration or fasciotomy is indicated. The indications for primary open reduction are (1) those fractures in which there is inability to obtain a satisfactory closed reduction; (2) vascular injury; or (3) an associated fracture of the humerus or forearm in the same limb. In children, nondisplaced, nonangulated fractures can be splinted (90 degrees of flexion); angulated fractures require reduction and splinting; and displaced fractures require reduction and percutaneous pinning on an urgent basis, within 12 to 24 h. Fractures of the capitellum and radial head are treated with immobilization in a posterior long arm splint with the elbow in 90 degrees of flexion and the forearm in supination, analgesics, and control of swelling. Complications of displaced capitellum fractures include arthritis, avascular necrosis, and decreased range of motion. More severe fractures may need radial head excision to prevent malunion and joint malfunction. Patients with uncomplicated fractures may begin range-of-motion exercises within 3 to 7 days to reduce the risk of permanent loss of elbow motion from joint contracture. Intraarticular fractures, which may require radial head excision or fixation, should be referred to an orthopedist within 1 week for definitive management.

Clinical Pearls

1. Ten percent of children with supracondylar fractures temporarily lose their radial pulse due to joint swelling after injury. This usually resolves and does not present long-term sequelae.
2. Capitellum and radial head fractures often occur together.
3. Bleeding around the elbow raises suspicion of an open fracture or open joint and requires urgent orthopedic consultation.
4. The presence of a joint effusion with a history of trauma is presumptive evidence of a fracture.

Associated Clinical Features

Fractures of the wrist and elbow usually involve a fall onto the outstretched arm, while fractures of the forearm shaft are more commonly the result of a direct blow. Injury to one of the bones of the forearm is often associated with fracture or dislocation of the other; therefore one must examine joints above and below involved bones both radiologically and clinically when injury to one forearm bone is identified. AP and lateral views of the wrist, forearm, and elbow are required when a forearm fracture is suspected. Functional deficits in the hand are important clues to identification of occult injury to forearm nerve and vascular structures that could require immediate surgical intervention. Monteggia's fracture-dislocation (Figs. 11.12, 11.13) is an ulnar fracture (usually proximal third) with associated proximal dislocation of the radial head. Dislocation is associated with about 7% of ulnar fractures. Forearm shortening can be noted, and significant forearm swelling is often present. Such a fracture is associated with significant radial nerve injury in 17% of cases.

Galeazzi's fracture-dislocation is a fracture of the distal one-third of the radius with dislocation of the distal radioulnar joint. It occurs three times more often than a Monteggia fracture. Tenderness over the distal radioulnar joint is noted, in addition to swelling, tenderness, and possibly deformity at the fracture site.

Isolated fractures of the middle ulna may result from direct trauma and are termed nightstick fractures. High-energy injuries to the forearm may result in fractures of both the radius and ulna at midshaft, resulting in a grossly deformed and unstable injury.

Differential Diagnosis

Simple contusion, compartment syndrome, and muscular injuries should be considered.

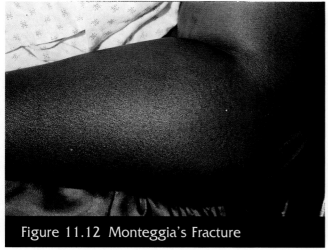

Figure 11.12 Monteggia's Fracture

Patients with a Monteggia's fracture present with swelling and pain in the forearm and often a palpable radial head in the antecubital fossa. (Courtesy of Alan B. Storrow, MD.)

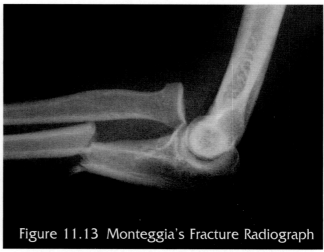

Figure 11.13 Monteggia's Fracture Radiograph

A Monteggia's fracture is defined by a fracture of the proximal one-third of the ulna combined with dislocation of the radial head. (Courtesy of Alan B. Storrow, MD.)

Emergency Department Treatment and Disposition

Both Monteggia's and Galeazzi's fracture-dislocations require orthopedic consultation and are treated with immobilization in a long-arm splint (with elbow flexed at 90 degrees). The forearm is placed in a neutral position for a Monteggia fracture and pronated for Galeazzi fracture. Treatment is usually surgical for both injuries, although children may be treated by reduction and casting.

Clinical Pearls

1. Any ulnar fracture with greater than 10 degrees of angulation or with a bony fragment displaced more than 50% of the bones' diameter is considered displaced and requires surgical correction.
2. Isolated proximal ulnar fractures are rare. Always suspect a Monteggia fracture-dislocation and closely examine the radial head for dislocation or other evidence of injury. A line drawn through the radial shaft and head must align with the capitellum in all views to exclude dislocation (see Fig. 11.10).
3. A distal ulnar styloid fracture, if found, can be a clue to a Galeazzi's fracture. It is associated with Galeazzi's injury in approximately 60% of cases.
4. Fractures of the forearm may result in compartment syndrome.

Associated Clinical Features

Falls on an outstretched arm are common and the forces involved with this mechanism of injury are often significant enough to break both the radius and the ulna. Open fractures are common, and one must look closely for overlying soft tissue injury. Distal radial fractures account for 17% of all fractures treated in the ED. In the elderly they are usually extraarticular metaphyseal fractures, whereas in younger patients they are usually intraarticular with displacement of the joint surface. There are four types of radial fractures, associated with commonly known eponyms: Colles' fracture, Smith's fracture, Barton's fracture and Hutchinson's (chauffeur's) fracture.

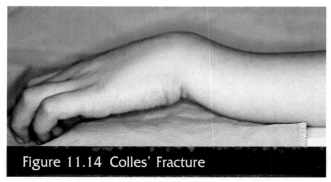

Figure 11.14 Colles' Fracture

The classic dinner-fork deformity is demonstrated in this photograph. The distal forearm is displaced dorsally. (Courtesy of Cathleen M. Vossler, MD.)

A Colles' fracture is dorsal displacement and angulation of the distal radius and is the most common wrist fracture in adults. Colles' fracture is usually an extension injury associated with significant bony displacement and obvious "dinner fork" deformity on physical examination (Fig. 11.14).

Smith's fracture is a distal metaphyseal fracture with volar displacement and angulation. This usually results from a blow to the dorsum of the wrist or hand or a hyperflexion injury. Radiography reveals distal volar displacement. Examination reveals deformity and pain in the distal radius (Figs. 11.15, 11.16, 11.17).

Barton's fracture (Fig. 11.17) is a fracture of the dorsal rim of the distal radius. The rim of the distal radius, commonly a triangular bone fragment, is displaced dorsally. It may be associated with dislocation of the radiocarpal joint.

A chauffeur's or Hutchinson's fracture (Fig. 11.17) is an avulsion fracture of the distal radial styloid that occurs from a force transmitted from the scaphoid to the styloid. It may be considered an unstable fracture secondary to an associated ligamentous injury.

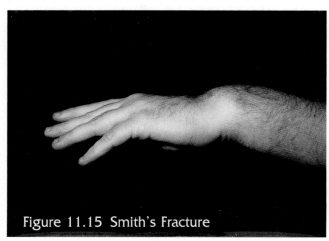

Figure 11.15 Smith's Fracture

A Smith's fracture is sometimes described as a reverse Colles'. (Courtesy of Frank Birinyi, MD.)

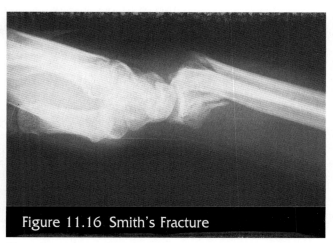

Figure 11.16 Smith's Fracture

The radiograph reveals volar displacement of the distal radial fragment together with the bones of the wrist and hand. (Courtesy of Frank Birinyi, MD.)

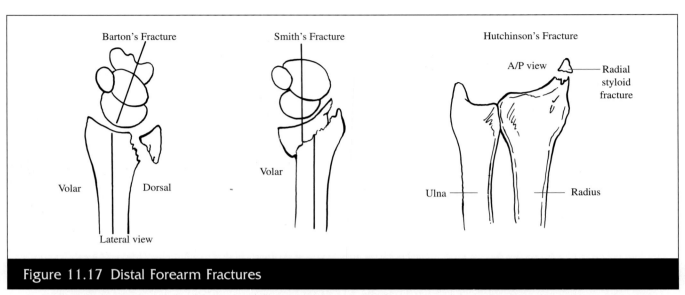

Figure 11.17 Distal Forearm Fractures

These illustrations depict three different types of distal forearm fractures: Smith's, Barton's, and Hutchinson's. (Adapted from Simon R: *Emergency Orthopedics: The Extremities.* Norwalk, CT: Appleton & Lange; 1987, pp 118–119.)

Emergency Department Treatment and Disposition

ED evaluation and management of these fractures is similar because certain fracture characteristics define instability. Comminuted, displaced, unstable, and open fractures or those with neurologic or vascular compromise require prompt orthopedic attention. In addition, fractures with greater than 20 degrees of angulation or with more than 1 cm of shortening are potentially unstable and deserve aggressive management. Initial immobilization can be accomplished with a double sugar-tong splint. Stable fractures respond well to closed reduction and casting for 6 to 8 weeks. Most closed Colles' and Smith's fractures can be managed with closed reduction in the ED with use of finger traps, local anesthesia via hematoma or Bier block, and gentle manipulation to restore anatomic alignment. Detailed discharge instructions should be given regarding symptoms of median nerve impingement, including paresthesias and hand weakness, which should prompt return to the ED.

Clinical Pearls

1. All fractures of the distal radius must be evaluated for median nerve function before and after reduction.
2. Colles' fractures warrant a high index of suspicion for intraarticular injury, especially when a radial styloid fracture is noted.
3. With a Hutchinson's fracture, associated ligamentous injuries should be sought, especially scapholunate dissociation and perilunate and lunate dislocation.

Associated Clinical Features

Carpal and carpometacarpal dislocations are serious wrist injuries usually occurring from hyperextension. Their diagnosis requires careful physical and radiographic examination. Patients complain of decreased range of motion, pain, swelling, and ecchymosis.

Lunate dislocation (Fig. 11.18) can occur in a volar or dorsal position with the lunate displaced relative to the other carpal bones (Fig. 11.19). The normal lunoradial relationship is disrupted. The median nerve is most commonly involved and should be evaluated.

If the lunoradial articulation is intact and the other carpal bones are dislocated relative to the lunate, it is termed a perilunate dislocation. (Figs. 11.20, 11.21).

Another potentially serious injury is scapholunate dislocation, often mistakenly diagnosed as a sprained wrist. Although the physical examination may be unremarkable except for wrist pain, an anteroposterior (AP) radiograph reveals a widening of the scapholunate joint space (Fig. 11.22). This space is normally less than 3 mm. A space of 4 mm or greater should prompt suspicion of

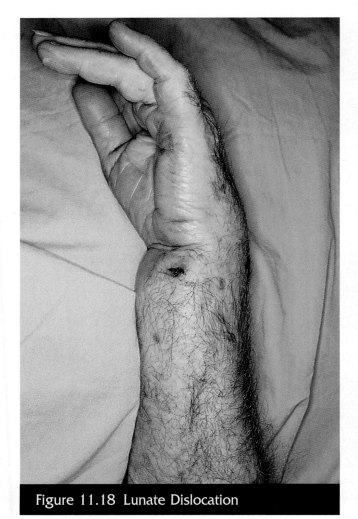

Figure 11.18 Lunate Dislocation

This photograph demonstrates swelling associated with a volar lunate dislocation. (Courtesy of Cathleen M. Vossler, MD.)

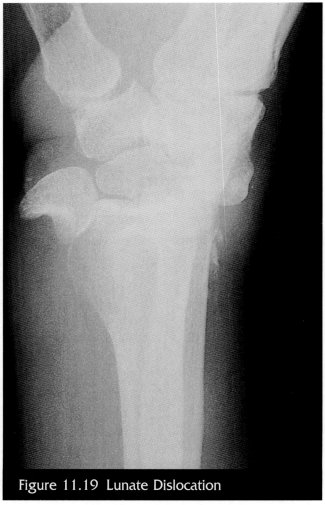

Figure 11.19 Lunate Dislocation

Radiographic examination of a dorsal lunate dislocation. (Courtesy of Cathleen M. Vossler, MD.)

this problem. In addition, the lateral radiograph may reveal an increase of the scapholunate angle to greater than 60 to 65 degrees (normal 45 to 50 degrees).

All these dislocations may present with concomitant fractures of the carpal bones or distal forearm. A scaphoid fracture is particularly troublesome, since misdiagnosis of this problem can result in later delayed healing or avascular necrosis (Fig. 11.23). This potentially serious problem is due to lack of a direct blood supply to the proximal portion of the bone. Tenderness on palpation of the anatomic snuffbox, or with axial loading, is a common finding. Unfortunately, negative radiographs do not rule out an occult scaphoid fracture.

Carpometacarpal dislocations are fortunately rare, since they are often devastating injuries requiring extensive repair (Fig. 11.24). Functional loss is marked and common.

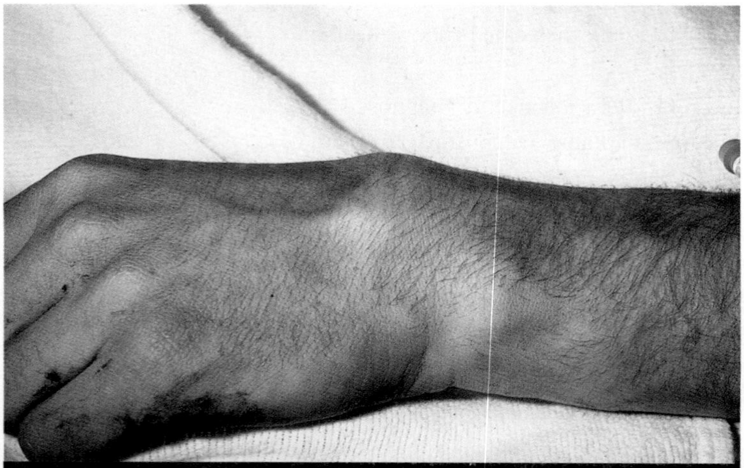

Differential Diagnosis

Arthritis, carpal tunnel syndrome, and joint infections should be considered in patients with wrist pain.

Emergency Department Treatment and Disposition

Initial management includes adequate radiographic evaluation followed by ice, elevation, and splinting. Referral to a hand specialist is essential for adequate reduction and long-term care.

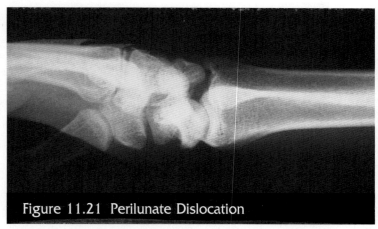

Figure 11.20 Perilunate Dislocation

This patient sustained a fall on his outstretched hand with impact on the palm. The force transmitted through the radius and lunate disrupted the lunate-capitate articulation. The capitate and other carpal bones were driven posteriorly with respect to the lunate, resulting in the prominent dorsal deformity. (Courtesy of Alan B. Storrow, MD.)

Figure 11.21 Perilunate Dislocation

This slightly oblique radiograph of the patient in Figure 11.20 reveals dorsal displacement of the carpal bones in relation to the lunate. The lunate does have slight anterior rotation, although its relationship with respect to the distal radius is intact. (Courtesy of Alan B. Storrow, MD.)

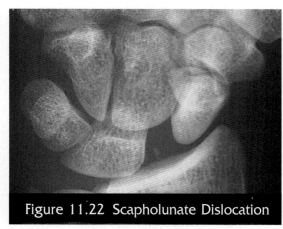

Figure 11.22 Scapholunate Dislocation

Radiographic evidence of a scapholunate dislocation. Note the widened scapholunate joint space. This injury is often misdiagnosed as simple wrist sprain. (Courtesy of Alan B. Storrow, MD.)

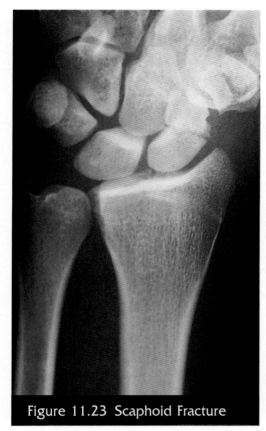

Figure 11.23 Scaphoid Fracture

Fracture of the wrist, or middle third, of the scaphoid. These injuries can be associated with delayed healing and avascular necrosis. (Courtesy of Alan B. Storrow, MD.)

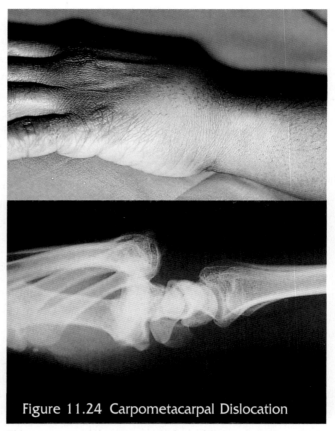

Figure 11.24 Carpometacarpal Dislocation

This uncommon injury occurred after a fall from a ladder onto an outstretched hand. Note the prominent deformity of the proximal metacarpals, II to IV, on the dorsal hand. Also note the normal prominence of the ulnar styloid, which helps the examiner in anatomic localization of the dislocation. (A). Radiographic examination of the patient depicted above (B). (Courtesy of Alan B. Storrow, MD.)

Clinical Pearls

1. A true lateral wrist radiograph best demonstrates a lunate dislocation by exhibiting the usual cup-shaped lunate bone as lying on its side and displaced either dorsally or volarly.

2. On lateral wrist radiographs, the metacarpal, capitate, lunate, and radius should all be aligned so that a line drawn through the long axis will bisect all four bones including the lunate. If this is not found, then some element of dislocation, subluxation, or ligamentous instability exists.

3. Patients in whom there is a clinical suspicion of an occult scaphoid fracture (anatomic snuff-box tenderness or axial load tenderness of the thumb without radiologic evidence of fracture) should receive a thumb spica splint and a repeat examination in 7 to 10 days.

Associated Clinical Features

The clenched fist injury classically occurs during a fight when the metacarpophalangeal (MCP) joint contacts human teeth, resulting in a laceration in the skin (Fig. 11.25). Many patients will not divulge the true circumstances surrounding the injury; therefore all wounds at the MCP joint are considered a clenched fist injury until proven otherwise. Once these wounds occur, the inoculated organisms are sealed in a warm, closed environment, allowing rapid spread and destruction. Serious complications can result, including infection, loss of function, and amputation. Most wounds are polymicrobial. Patients who present initially may have little evidence of intra-articular injury on physical examination, whereas those who present more than 18 h after injury are more likely to have evidence of infection, including pain, swelling, erythema, and purulent drainage.

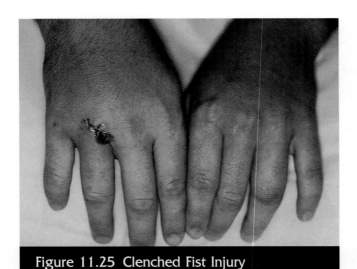

Figure 11.25 Clenched Fist Injury

The small lacerations seen in this photograph were sustained from human teeth during a fight. Note the subtle black ink bar stamp across the proximal metacarpals of the right hand; this may reveal a clue about the wound's etiology. (Courtesy of Lawrence B. Stack, MD.)

Differential Diagnosis

Abrasions or lacerations secondary to a source other than human teeth can be mistaken for a clenched fist injury.

Emergency Department Treatment and Disposition

All wounds should be irrigated, debrided, explored, elevated, and immobilized. Patients should receive antibiotics directed at both oral and skin flora. Tetanus prophylaxis is given if needed. Radiographs should be obtained to evaluate for fractures and any foreign bodies remaining in the wound. These wounds should never be closed initially. All patients require careful follow-up with a hand specialist. Reliable patients who present early, without evidence of infection or significant medical history (e.g., diabetes), and no involvement of bone, joint, or tendon may be treated on an outpatient basis. They must return in 24 h for a wound check, sooner if any signs of infection develop. Any patient who does not meet these requirements must be hospitalized for intravenous antibiotics and wound care.

Clinical Pearls

1. Complications include cellulitis, lymphangitis, septic arthritis, abscess formation, osteomyelitis, and tenosynovitis.
2. All wounds need to be examined in full flexion and extension so that tendon injuries are not missed. A tendon injury sustained with the fingers flexed will be missed if the hand is examined only in extension due to the retraction of the tendon with extension.

Associated Clinical Features

A boxer's fracture is a metacarpal neck fracture of the fifth and sometimes fourth digit, which commonly occurs after a direct blow to the metacarpophalangeal joints of the clenched fist. The proximal metacarpal bone is angulated dorsally and the metacarpal head is angulated volarly. On physical examination, the "knuckle" is missing and can be palpated on the volar surface (Figs. 11.26, 11.27). Any associated laceration should be considered secondary to impact with human teeth ("fight bite," see "Clenched Fist Injury" Fig. 11.25).

Differential Diagnosis

Fracture of the metacarpal head or metacarpal shaft, hematoma, sprain, clenched fist injury, and metacarpophalangeal dislocation are often mistaken for a boxer's fracture until radiographic evaluation is performed.

Emergency Department Treatment and Disposition

Prior to reduction, the injury must be evaluated for rotational malalignment. This is easily done by having the patient place all fingers in the palm; all fingers should point to the scaphoid bone (Fig. 11.28). Rotational deformities of greater than 15% require reduction. An ulnar nerve block provides sufficient anesthesia for the fifth metacarpal, but median and radial nerve blocks should be used for the other metacarpals. Hematoma block can be used as an alternative.

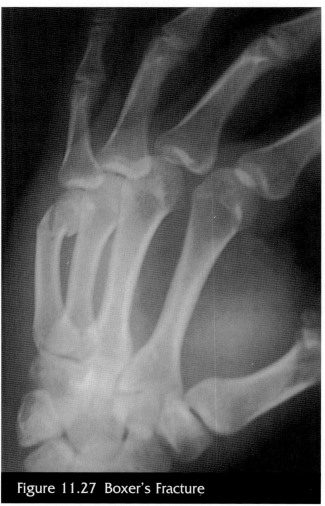

Figure 11.27 Boxer's Fracture

Radiographic examination reveals a fracture through the neck of the metacarpal and volar displacement of the fractured segment. (Courtesy of Cathleen M. Vossler, MD.)

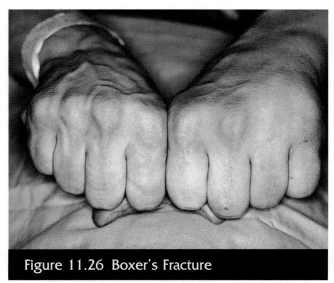

Figure 11.26 Boxer's Fracture

This boxer's fracture occurred when the patient punched a wall with his hand. There is loss of the "knuckle" when the dorsum of the hand is examined, especially noticeable when the patient makes a fist. (Courtesy of Cathleen M. Vossler, MD.)

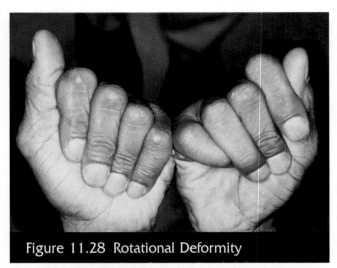

Figure 11.28 Rotational Deformity

Malpositioning of the right fifth digit due to a boxer's fracture. Normally, all the digits point toward a single spot on the scaphoid. (Courtesy of Alexander T. Trott, MD.)

Once adequate anesthesia is achieved, reduction can be attempted. A nondisplaced nonangulated fracture requires no reduction. Treatment includes ice, elevation, and immobilization in a gutter splint. For reduction, the distal interphalangeal (DIP), proximal interphalangeal (PIP), and metacarpophalangeal (MCP) joints are all held in flexion at 90 degrees. Pressure is exerted on the proximal phalanx, directed upward to push the metacarpal head dorsally back into position. At the same time, the metacarpal shaft is stabilized with pressure on the dorsum over the shaft. The patient should be splinted with the MCP at 90 degrees of flexion. Postreduction radiographs are necessary to ensure adequate reduction. Early follow-up (within 7 days) with a hand specialist is essential, since simple splinting may not adequately maintain proper reduction and fractures with higher degrees of angulation and instability may require fixation.

Clinical Pearls

1. Fractures of the second and third metacarpal neck will not tolerate any angulation and require orthopedic referral for anatomic reduction. Fractures of the fourth and fifth metacarpal neck can tolerate up to 30 and 50 degrees of angulation, respectively, before function is impaired.
2. Subtle malrotation can be recognized by looking at the alignment of the nail beds with the digits flexed. Complications include collateral ligamentous damage, extensor injury damage, and malposition or clawing of the fingers secondary to incomplete reduction.

Associated Clinical Features

Ulnar nerve injury results in the classic claw-hand deformity (Fig. 11.29) because of the wasting of small hand muscles. The deformity is formed by hyperextension of the metacarpophalangeal joint and flexion at the proximal and distal interphalangeal joints of the fourth and fifth digits. There is wasting of the interosseous and hypothenar muscles, as well as the hypothenar eminence (Fig. 11.30). The patient is unable to abduct or adduct the digits.

Median nerve damage also results in the claw-hand deformity, but to the second and third digits. Damage to the proximal portion of the nerve results in weakness of wrist flexion, forearm pronation, thumb apposition, and flexion of the first three digits. Atrophy of the thenar eminence also occurs. There is a sensory loss over the area of distribution for each nerve. These findings are not seen acutely but are chronic signs from an old injury.

Wrist drop is the most common symptom seen with *radial nerve* damage, occurring in situations of acute compression. It is frequently referred to as Saturday night palsy (as when a person who has been drinking alcohol falls asleep on an arm or with the arm over a chair and there is temporary damage to the nerve).

Differential Diagnosis

Rheumatoid arthritis, osteoarthritis, and undiagnosed proximal (cervical osteophyte) or distal (carpal tunnel syndrome) entrapment syndromes can be mistaken for peripheral nerve injury.

Emergency Department Treatment and Disposition

Treatment is aimed at recognizing the underlying cause of the nerve damage. Such causes include laceration of the nerve, compression from swelling, or hematoma formation. In the ED, splinting and appropriate referral is the treatment.

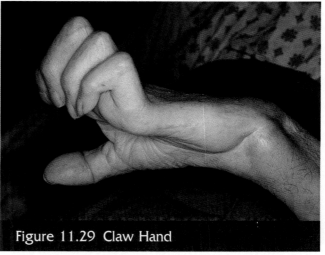

Figure 11.29 Claw Hand

This photograph demonstrates the claw-hand appearance resulting from median and ulnar nerve injury. Note metacarpophalangeal joint hyperextension. (Courtesy of Daniel L. Savitt, MD.)

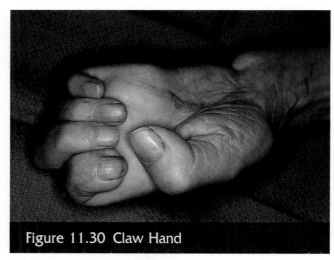

Figure 11.30 Claw Hand

Atrophy of the thenar and hypothenar eminences also occurs as a result of damage to the median and ulnar nerves, respectively. Note the concavity to the hypothenar eminence. (Courtesy of Cathleen M. Vossler, MD.)

Clinical Pearl

1. Long-term nerve injury results in muscle wasting. Prior to any nerve damage, the thenar and hypothenar eminences have a full appearance. This is lost in patients with nerve damage. Initially, there is flattening of each eminence, followed by a concave or hollow appearance.

Associated Clinical Features

These patients complain of pain, swelling, and decreased range of motion at the base of the thumb (Fig. 11.31). Bennett's fracture is an intraarticular fracture at the ulnar aspect of the base of the first metacarpal with disruption of the carpometacarpal joint (Fig. 11.32). The first metacarpal is displaced radially and proximally, with subluxation or complete dislocation (Fig. 11.33). Rolando's fracture is an intraarticular comminuted fracture at the base of the first metacarpal, with dorsal and volar fragments resulting in a Y- or T-shaped intraarticular fragment (Fig. 11.34).

Differential Diagnosis

Sprain, fracture of the first metacarpal shaft, or a gamekeeper's thumb (disruption of the ulnar collateral ligament of the metacarpophalangeal joint) are commonly mistaken for Bennett's or Rolando's fracture prior to radiographic evaluation.

Emergency Department Treatment and Disposition

The treatment of these fractures in the ED consists of ice, elevation, and immobilization in a thumb spica splint and early referral to a hand specialist. These fractures generally require operative reduction and fixation.

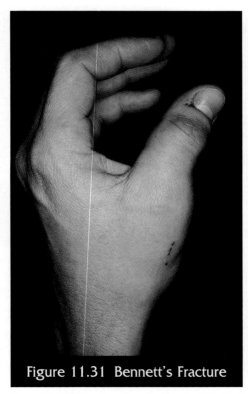

Figure 11.31 Bennett's Fracture

Bennett's fracture involves the base of the first metacarpal. The digit is swollen and ecchymotic over the affected area. (Courtesy of Daniel L. Savitt, MD.)

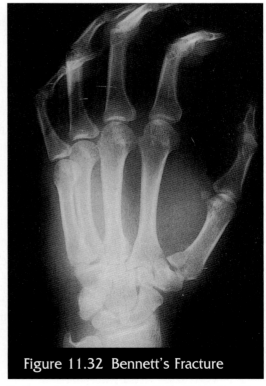

Figure 11.32 Bennett's Fracture

Radiographic examination of a Bennett's fracture illustrates an intraarticular fracture at the base of the first metacarpal with the metacarpal displaced radially and proximally. (Courtesy of Cathleen M. Vossler, MD.)

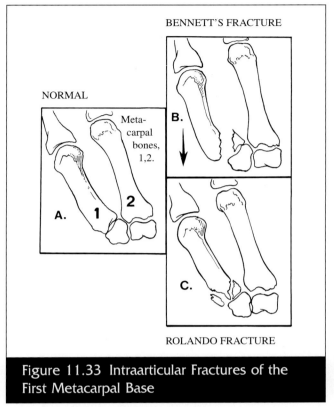

Figure 11.33 Intraarticular Fractures of the First Metacarpal Base

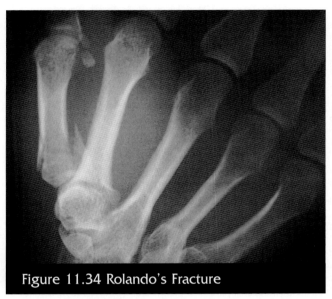

Figure 11.34 Rolando's Fracture

(A). An intraarticular fracture at the base of the first metacarpal with radial and proximal displacement is a Bennett's fracture (B). A comminuted intraarticular fracture at the base of the first metacarpal is a Rolando's fracture (C).

Note the comminuted intraarticular fracture at the base of the first metacarpal. (Courtesy of Cathleen M. Vossler, MD.)

Clinical Pearls

1. Carpometacarpal dislocations are frequently difficult to reduce and require open reduction and fixation approximately 50% of the time.
2. Osteoarthritis is a common long-term complication, even after optimal management.

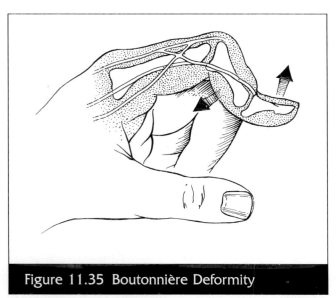

Figure 11.35 Boutonnière Deformity

This depiction of a boutonnière deformity illustrates the rupture of the central slip and the resultant subluxation of the lateral bands. The subluxation exerts a pull on the middle phalanx resulting in the deformity.

Associated Clinical Features

The boutonnière deformity is a result of injury or disruption to the insertion of the extensor tendon on the dorsal base of the middle phalanx. Common causes of this problem are proximal interphalangeal (PIP) joint contusion, forceful flexion of the PIP joint against resistance, and palmar dislocation of the PIP joint. Initially, a deformity may be absent but will develop over the course of time if the injury remains untreated. The lateral bands sublux and exert a proximal pull on the middle phalanx. The result is flexion of the PIP joint and extension of the DIP joint (Figs. 11.35, 11.36). Radiographically, a small fragment of bone may be visualized at the proximal portion of the dorsal aspect of the middle phalanx.

Swan-neck deformity occurs as a result of the shortening of interosseous muscles secondary to systemic diseases such as rheumatoid arthritis. The digit is contorted with hyperextension of the PIP and flexion of the distal interphalangeal (DIP) and metacarpophalangeal (MCP) joints (Fig. 11.37).

Differential Diagnosis

Fracture, dislocation, or tendon damage can be mistaken for a boutonnière or swan neck deformity.

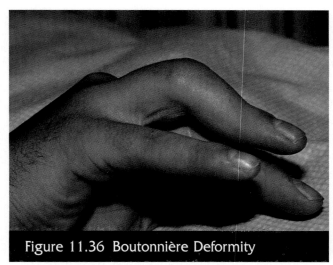

Figure 11.36 Boutonnière Deformity

A boutonnière deformity of the fourth digit. Note the flexion of the PIP joint and the extension of the DIP joint. (Courtesy of E. Lee Edstrom, MD.)

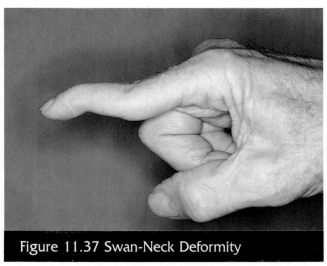

Figure 11.37 Swan-Neck Deformity

A swan-neck deformity of the index finger. Note the hyperextension of the PIP joint and the flexion of the DIP joint. (Courtesy of Cathleen M. Vossler, MD.)

Emergency Department Treatment and Disposition

In dealing with a closed injury resulting in a boutonnière deformity, immobilization of the PIP joint in extension is adequate. Splinting the MCP and DIP joints is not necessary. The splint should be used for 4 weeks, at which point active range of motion can start. Open injuries must be carefully explored and repaired. Swan-neck deformities are treated by splinting the digit to prevent further deformity. Both deformities require referral to a hand specialist.

Clinical Pearls

1. Boutonnière deformity generally develops weeks after the initial injury as the lateral bands contract; therefore, it is frequently missed in the ED. Early diagnosis can be made with the proper examination of the finger. The digit should be adequately anesthetized and then examined for range of motion and joint stability.
2. Any injury involving the dorsal PIP surface should be reexamined for development of a boutonnière deformity after 7 to 10 days.
3. Surgical repair may be required for cases where conservative therapy yields inadequate results.

Associated Clinical Features

A large number of commercial devices are able to deliver liquids and gases at high pressures. Occasionally, substances from these devices are injected into the body, especially the upper extremities. The most common devices include spray guns, diesel injectors, and hydraulic lines. The injury occurs when the device accidentally fires during cleaning or mishandling. The injury can be very misleading if seen soon after the event. On early examination, a small puncture wound or no apparent break in the skin may be found, with minimal swelling. Swelling and pain increase over time (Fig. 11.38). Vascular compromise can occur directly from compression secondary to swelling or from the inflammatory response that the body produces to the materials injected. The injected material tends to spread along fascial planes, so the extent of injury can be quite misleading and is often subtle on initial presentation.

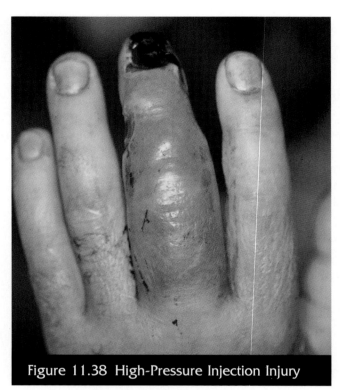

Figure 11.38 High-Pressure Injection Injury

This photograph illustrates injury incurred by a grease gun. The patient was cleaning the device and the gun accidently discharged into his hand. Note the swelling and erythema. The patient was taken to the operating room for initial debridement. (Courtesy of Richard Zienowicz, MD.)

Differential Diagnosis

Puncture wound, hematoma, or tenosynovitis can be confused with a hydraulic pressure injury.

Emergency Department Treatment and Disposition

Immediate operative debridement is the treatment of choice. Therefore, early consultation with a hand specialist is necessary. Radiographic examination evaluates for fracture and may outline spread of injected material. Tetanus and broad-spectrum antibiotics should be administered. The affected extremity should be elevated and splinted.

Clinical Pearls

1. Do not be misled by the "benign" appearance of the initial injury.
2. Delays in treatment can lead to compartment syndrome.
3. Digital blocks are contraindicated because of the potential for increased tissue pressure and compromise of tissue perfusion.

Associated Clinical Features

Phalangeal dislocations are common and can occur at all three finger joints. Distal interphalangeal (DIP) dislocations are the rarest but can occur when a force is applied to the distal phalanx. Gross deformity is noted on examination, with the distal phalanx generally displaced dorsally. Proximal interphalangeal (PIP) dislocations (Figs. 11.39, 11.40) are common and easily reducible. These are generally dislocated dorsally, caused by hyperextension, and may have associated damage to the volar plate (Fig. 11.41). PIP volar dislocations can be irreducible secondary to rupture of the extensor tendon or herniation of the proximal phalanx through the extensor mechanism, both requiring operative repair. Metacarpophalangeal (MCP) joint dorsal dislocations are often due to hyperextension.

Differential Diagnosis

Phalangeal fracture, metacarpal fracture, tendon damage, ligamentous injury, or boutonnière deformity can be confused with a phalangeal dislocation.

Emergency Department Treatment and Disposition

Digital nerve block is appropriate anesthesia for the PIP and DIP joints. Ulnar, median, or radial nerve blocks are necessary for the MCP joints. Reduction with splinting is the treatment of choice. Reduction is accomplished via hyperextension of the joint with concurrent application of horizontal traction. Flexion at the MCP joint will facilitate reduction of distal joints. Postreduction radiographs are necessary to ensure adequate reduction. The DIP joint should be splinted in slight flexion and the PIP joint in 20 degrees of flexion for 3 to 5 weeks, depending on the degree of ligamentous damage. Hand specialist follow-up is mandatory.

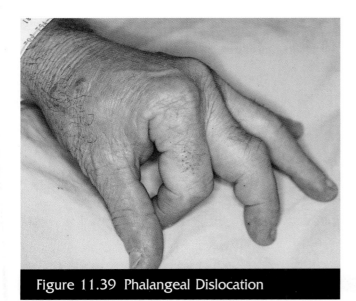

Figure 11.39 Phalangeal Dislocation

This patient dislocated the long finger PIP joint during an altercation. The PIP joint is displaced dorsally with an obvious deformity. (Courtesy of Cathleen M. Vossler, MD.)

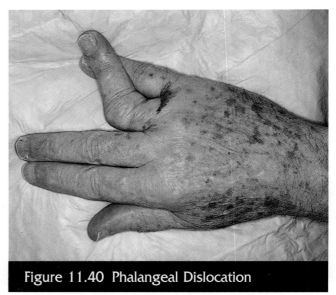

Figure 11.40 Phalangeal Dislocation

This photograph illustrates medial angulation of the ring finger, suggesting PIP dislocation. (Courtesy of Daniel L. Savitt, MD.)

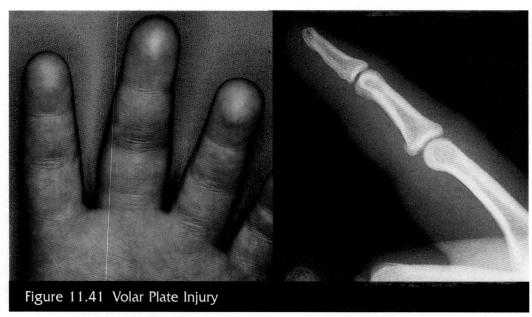

Figure 11.41 Volar Plate Injury

This photograph demonstrates the subtle PIP swelling and ecchymosis of the third (long) digit often seen with a volar plate injury (A). Hyperextension injuries cause disruption of the volar plate and result in swelling, ecchymosis, and tenderness along the volar aspect of the joint. These injuries are initially treated conservatively with splinting, but if they are unstable, operative repair is required. (Courtesy of Daniel L. Savitt, M.D.) Radiographic examination of the digit reveals a small fragment on the proximal volar surface of the PIP joint (B). (Courtesy of Cathleen M. Vossler, MD.)

Clinical Pearls

1. All joints should be tested for instability after reduction, using a digital nerve block to facilitate testing.
2. PIP joint volar dislocation can be unstable, requiring open reduction and internal fixation.
3. Joint dislocations that have volar plate entrapment may be impossible to reduce and require surgical repair for successful reduction.

Associated Clinical Features

Mallet finger commonly occurs after the distal finger, specifically the distal interphalangeal (DIP) joint, is forcibly flexed, as from a sudden blow to the tip of the extended finger. This injury represents complete avulsion or laxity of the extensor tendon from the proximal dorsum of the distal phalanx (Fig. 11.42). The patient presents with an inability to extend the distal phalanx, and it remains in a flexed position (Fig. 11.43). On radiograph, a small chip fragment on the dorsum at the DIP joint may be visualized.

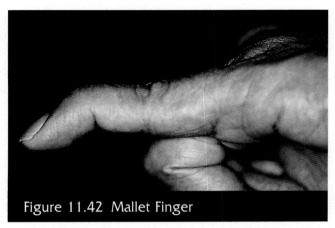

Figure 11.42 Mallet Finger

This photograph depicts a mallet finger. The distal phalanx is held in flexion and the patient is unable to extend it. (Courtesy of Kevin J. Knoop, MD, MS.)

Differential Diagnosis

Intraarticular fracture of the distal phalanx, distal tuft fracture, or extensor tendon laceration can be confused with a mallet finger.

Emergency Department Treatment and Disposition

A closed mallet finger without involvement of the joint can be treated by splinting the DIP joint in extension to mild hyperextension. True hyperextension is to be avoided. This splint should be worn for 6 to 8 weeks, at which point active range of motion begins. There is no need to splint the other joints. Motion of the PIP joint should not be blocked with the splint. Hand surgery follow-up is required.

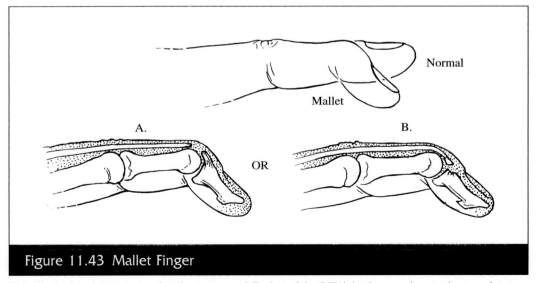

Figure 11.43 Mallet Finger

This illustration demonstrates that the unopposed flexion of the DIP joint is secondary to the complete tear of the tendon (A), or an avulsion of a small chip fragment (B).

Clinical Pearls

1. During follow-up, some patients exhibit hyperextension of the distal phalanx while out of the splint. This is due to a weakness in the volar plate. These patients should be splinted with the DIP joint in flexion and followed closely.
2. Avulsion of a significant portion of the articular surface (more than one-third) may require open reduction with internal fixation by a hand surgeon.

Associated Clinical Features

A subungual hematoma is a collection of blood found underneath the nail, usually occurring secondary to trauma to the distal fingers (Fig. 11.44). These lesions can be quite painful because of pressure beneath the nail. There can also be swelling, tenderness, and a decreased range of motion of the associated finger. Associated injuries include nail bed trauma (Fig. 11.45) and distal tuft fractures.

Differential Diagnosis

A nail bed melanoma may resemble a subungual hematoma and is differentiated from a hematoma by lack of a history of recent trauma and subsequent appearance of the "lesion."

Emergency Department Treatment and Disposition

A radiograph should be done to evaluate for possible fracture. If the subungual hematoma covers less than 25%, trephining the nail with a sterile needle or electrocautery is adequate to relieve pain by allowing drainage. Management of larger hematomas is somewhat controversial. Some authors advocate removal of the nail if the hematoma covers more than 50% of the nail or there is an associated fracture. A more recent conservative approach states that removal of the nail is best reserved for those injuries that damage the nail plate and surrounding tissues, regardless of the size of the hematoma or presence of a tuft fracture. In many cases, trephination of the nail is sufficient to relieve pain.

Clinical Pearls

1. Subungual hematomas are a sign of nail bed injury.
2. Subungual hematomas with surrounding nail bed and nail fold injuries require nail removal and evaluation of the nail bed for injury and careful repair if needed.
3. A hand-held, high-temperature, portable cautery device is a good tool for drainage of a subungual hematoma.

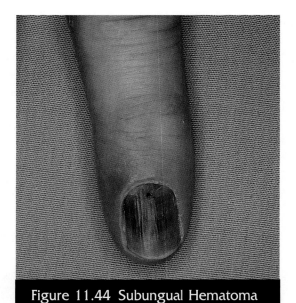

Figure 11.44 Subungual Hematoma

This subungual hematoma occurred after the patient hit his finger with a hammer. The hematoma covers approximately 50% of the subungual area. (Courtesy of Margaret P. Mueller, MD.)

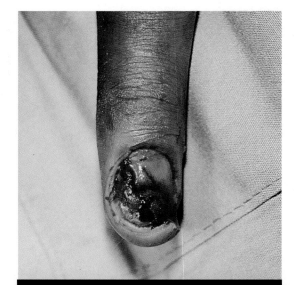

Figure 11.45 Nail Bed Laceration

Bleeding from a nail bed laceration causes a subungual hematoma. This image depicts a nail bed laceration seen after removal of the nail. (Courtesy of Alan B. Storrow, MD.)

Associated Clinical Features

Compartment syndrome develops when the pressure in a closed or inelastic fascial space increases to a point where it causes compression and dysfunction of vascular and neural structures. The five "Ps" that characterize compartment syndrome are pain, pallor, paresthesias, increased pressure, and pulselessness.

The earliest symptom is severe pain out of proportion to the physical findings. The pain is worsened with passive stretching of muscle within the compartment. Anesthesia-paresthesia is an early sign of nerve compromise. Motor weakness and pulselessness are late signs. Causes include compression, exercise, circumferential burns, frostbite, constrictive dressings, arterial bleeding, soft tissue injury, and fracture. Locations where compartment syndrome can occur include the interossei of the hand, volar and dorsal compartments of the forearm (Fig. 11.46), the gluteus medius, and anterior, peroneal, and deep posterior compartments of the leg (Fig. 11.47). A crea-

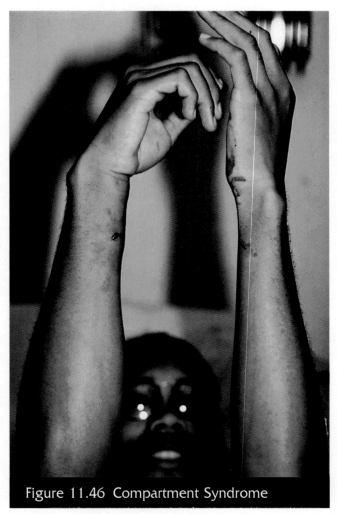

Figure 11.46 Compartment Syndrome

A swollen and tense right forearm typical for the presentation of compartment syndrome. (Courtesy of Lawrence B. Stack, MD.)

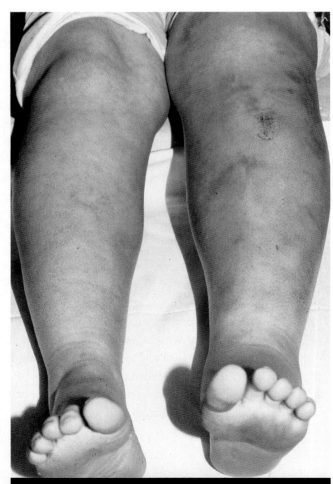

Figure 11.47 Compartment Syndrome

Anterior compartment syndrome of the left leg is manifested by anterior tibial pain, tense "woody" swelling, and erythema. Early in the course, passive plantarflexion may cause referred pain to the compartment. Later, the patient may develop foot drop. (Courtesy of Timothy Coakley, MD.)

tine phosphokinase (CPK) of 1000 to 5000 U/mL may add to suspicion of the diagnosis. Myonecrosis (Fig. 11.48) can cause myoglobinuria and renal failure.

Differential Diagnosis

Soft tissue swelling, deep venous thrombosis (DVT), neuropraxia, cellulitis, arterial intimal damage, snakebite, inflammation, or hematoma formation can be mistaken for a compartment syndrome.

Emergency Department Treatment and Disposition

The initial treatment is removal of any constrictive dressing and frequent evaluation. If there is no improvement or there are no constrictive dressings in place, decompression via a fasciotomy should be considered. Intracompartmental pressure monitoring (Fig. 11.49) should be performed to assess the need for immediate decompression. Pressures greater than 30 mmHg with signs and symptoms are suggestive of compartment syndrome, whereas pressures greater than 40 are diagnostic.

Clinical Pearls

1. The diagnosis of compartment syndrome should be made early and be based on clinical evaluation and the mechanism of injury. Crush or compression injuries should heighten suspicion.
2. The most common areas of the extremities affected by compartment syndrome are the anterior compartment of the lower leg due to proximal tibial fractures and the volar compartment of the forearm secondary to fracture of the ulna or radius and supracondylar fracture.
3. If a compartment syndrome is suspected, the compartment pressure should be measured.

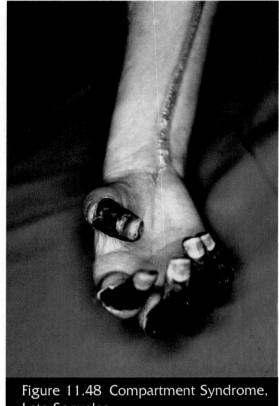

Figure 11.48 Compartment Syndrome, Late Sequelae

Muscle necrosis may result from compartment syndrome, as seen in this patient, who has undergone fasciotomy. (Courtesy of Kevin J. Knoop, MD, MS.)

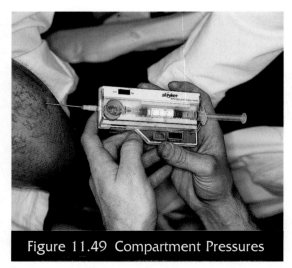

Figure 11.49 Compartment Pressures

Intracompartmental pressure monitoring can be accomplished with commercially available devices. Normal tissue pressures should be less than 10 mmHg. (Courtesy of Selim Suner, MD, MS.)

Pelvis and Hip

HIP DISLOCATIONS

Associated Clinical Features

Hip dislocations can be anterior, posterior, or central. Posterior hip dislocations are the most common, resulting from forces exerted on a flexed knee (e.g., a passenger in a motor vehicle accident whose knees hit the dashboard). The extremity is found shortened, internally rotated, and adducted (Fig. 11.50). Associated fractures occur commonly. Anterior hip dislocations occur when there is forced abduction to the femoral head, which forces the head out through a tear in the anterior capsule. Anterior dislocations can be superior (pubic) or inferior (obturator). The leg is abducted, externally rotated, and flexed with an inferior anterior hip dislocation. A superoanterior hip dislocation has the leg positioned in extension, slight abduction, and external rotation. Patients complain of severe hip pain and decreased range of motion.

Differential Diagnosis

Fractures of the femoral head, pelvis, femoral neck, acetabulum, and femoral shaft are sometimes mistaken for hip dislocations on initial examination.

Emergency Department Treatment and Disposition

Treatment for dislocations is early closed reduction using sedation, analgesia, and muscle relaxants. Anterior dislocations are reduced using strong in-line traction with the hip flexed and internally rotated, followed by abduction. Posterior dislocations are reduced using in-line traction with the hip flexed to 90 degrees, followed by gentle internal to external rotation. A neurovascular examination and radiographic evaluation should occur before and after any attempts at reduction. Orthopedic consultation should be obtained as early as possible. These patients require admission, with frequent neurovascular evaluation.

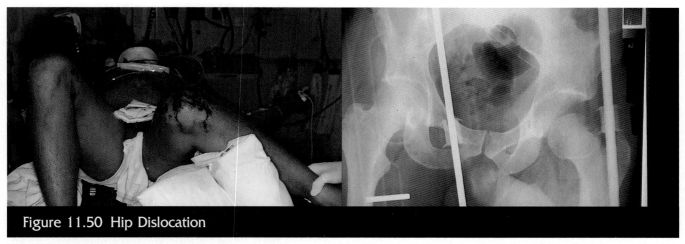

Figure 11.50 Hip Dislocation

Typical clinical appearance and patient position of a left posterior hip dislocation. Note internal rotation of the affected extremity (A). Radiograph of patient (B). (Courtesy of Cathleen M. Vossler, MD.)

Clinical Pearls

1. Complications of posterior hip dislocations include sciatic nerve injury and avascular necrosis.
2. Immediate reduction is imperative. The longer the delay in reduction, the greater the incidence of avascular necrosis.
3. Patients with prosthetic joints are at greater risk for dislocation, which can occur after only slight trauma.

Associated Clinical Features

Fractures of the femoral head and femoral neck and intertrochanteric fractures are termed *hip fractures*. For classification, hip fractures are generally divided into intracapsular (femoral head and neck fractures) and extracapsular (trochanteric, intertrochanteric, and subtrochanteric fractures) (Fig. 11.51). Accurate classification is important because of the different prognosis associated with each group. Intracapsular fractures are more likely to be associated with disruption of the vascular supply and resultant avascular necrosis. On the other hand, extracapsular fractures rarely impair the vascular supply.

All patients have complete immobility at the hip joint. Complaints include hip and groin pain, tenderness, and an inability to walk or place pressure on the affected side. There is shortening of the affected leg as well as abduction and external rotation (Fig. 11.52). Intertrochanteric fractures are associated with significant pain, a shortened extremity, marked external rotation, swelling, and ecchymosis around the hip (Fig. 11.53). Fractures of the femoral neck are suggested when the extremity is held in slight external rotation, abduction, and shortening. Dislocation of the hip is commonly associated with femoral head fractures. Patients with anterior dislocation and a femoral head fracture hold the lower extremity in abduction and external rotation. Patients with a posterior dislocation hold the extremity in adduction and internal rotation and display notable shortening.

The femoral head has a tenuous vascular supply which includes three sources: the artery of the ligamentum teres, the metaphyseal arteries, and the capsular vessels. Any injury that disturbs the anatomy of the hip can lead to compromise of this vascular supply.

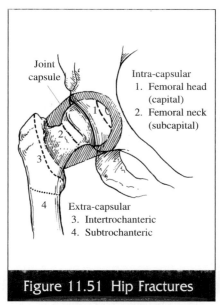

Figure 11.51 Hip Fractures

This illustration depicts the different types of proximal femoral fractures.

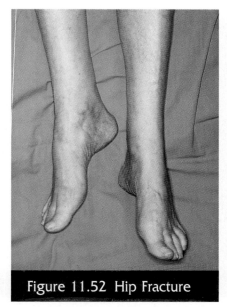

Figure 11.52 Hip Fracture

Patients with hip fractures often present with the affected extremity shortened, externally rotated, and abducted. Note the rotation and shortening in this patient with a right intertrochanteric fracture. (Courtesy of Cathleen M. Vossler, MD.)

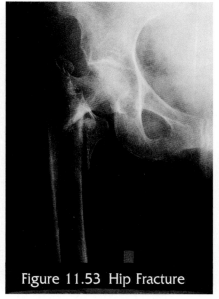

Figure 11.53 Hip Fracture

Radiographic examination reveals an intertrochanteric fracture. (Courtesy of Cathleen M. Vossler, MD.)

Shenton's line and the normal neck shaft angle of 120 to 130 degrees (obtained by measuring the angle of the intersection of lines drawn down the axis of the femoral shaft and the femoral neck) should be checked in all suspicious injuries.

Differential Diagnosis

Pelvic fracture, femoral shaft fracture, stress fracture, and hip dislocation are sometimes mistaken for a hip fracture prior to radiographic examination.

Emergency Department Treatment and Disposition

Once the patient is stabilized, the hip fracture is reduced via traction. Femoral head fracture-dislocations are an orthopedic emergency and require immediate reduction. A neurovascular examination should be carefully performed before and after any reduction attempts. Orthopedic consultation should be obtained early, since these patients will require admission and in most cases surgical reduction and fixation.

Clinical Pearls

1. Hip pain can be referred to other areas. Therefore, in any patient complaining of knee or thigh pain, consider the possibility of a hip fracture.
2. Fracture-dislocation of the femoral head requires great forces, and associated injuries such as chest, intraabdominal, and retroperitoneal injuries should be considered.
3. Intracapsular fractures usually have much less blood loss than extracapsular fractures because of hematoma containment within the capsule.
4. Fractures of the hip may be diagnosed by auscultation of differences in bone conduction between the patient's two extremities. This is performed by placing the stethoscope's diaphragm on the anterosuperior iliac spine and giving the patella several soft taps.
5. In the elderly, hip fractures are usually secondary to a fall. Be sure to address the cause of the fall to rule out a pathologic etiology (i.e., acute myocardial infarction, syncope, etc.).

Associated Clinical Features

Pelvic fractures range in severity from stable pubic rami fractures to unstable fractures with hemorrhagic shock. Pain is the most frequently encountered complaint. Blood at the urethral meatus, a high-riding prostate, gross hematuria, or a scrotal hematoma (Fig. 11.54) are all signs of associated urinary tract injury. Ecchymosis of the anterior abdominal wall, flank, sacral, or gluteal region should be regarded as a sign of serious hemorrhage. Blood found during rectal examination may indicate puncture of the wall of the rectum from a pelvic fracture. Leg shortening may also be seen. A careful neurologic examination is necessary, since there may be compromise of the sciatic, femoral, obturator, or pudendal nerves.

Differential Diagnosis

Femoral fracture, hip fracture, or intraabdominal or retroperitoneal pathology (including hemorrhage, perforated viscus) can be confused with pelvic fractures.

Emergency Department Treatment and Disposition

Management includes initial stabilization and evaluation for any life-threatening injuries. Patients may require multiple large-bore IVs and type and crossmatch with blood readily available. Hemorrhagic

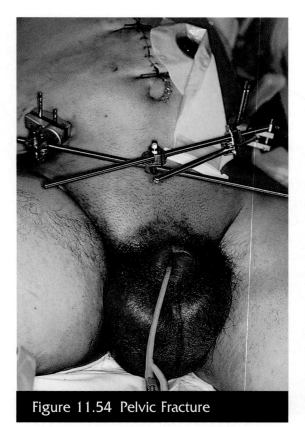

Figure 11.54 Pelvic Fracture

Pelvic fractures may require emergent external fixation to help control hemorrhage. Scrotal hematoma, or Destot's sign, suggests a pelvic fracture. (Courtesy of Cathleen M. Vossler, MD.)

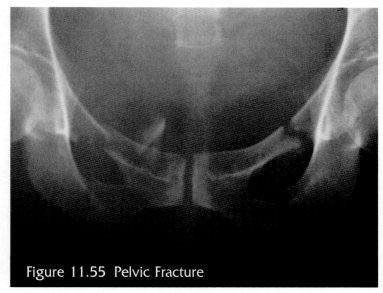

Figure 11.55 Pelvic Fracture

Radiographic examination reveals bilateral sacroiliac joint diastasis, complete transverse fracture of the sacrum, and comminuted fractures of the right superior and inferior pubic rami. (Courtesy of Cathleen M. Vossler, MD.)

shock occurs secondary to bleeding from a pelvic fracture and is the major cause of death in these patients. Retroperitoneal bleeding is unavoidable and up to 6 L of blood can easily be lost. Early orthopedic consultation is critical for emergent external fixation. Angiography should be performed to control small bleeding sites if there is continued exsanguination.

Clinical Pearls

1. MAST (medical antishock trousers) may be used to temporarily stabilize pelvic fractures.
2. Don't assume that a pelvic fracture is the sole cause of hemorrhagic shock in a patient. Look for other sources.
3. Posterior pelvic fractures are more likely to result in hemorrhage and neurovascular damage. Anterior pelvic fractures are more likely to cause urogenital damage.
4. Urinary tract injury is highly associated with pelvic fracture and must be ruled out. If there are any signs of genitourinary injury, a Foley catheter should not be placed until a retrograde urethrogram has been performed.
5. Displacement of pelvic ring fractures is usually associated with fracture or dislocation of another ring element (Fig. 11.55).

Lower Extremity

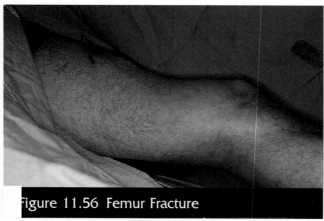

Figure 11.56 Femur Fracture

A closed midshaft femoral fracture. Note the deformity in the middle of the thigh, consistent with this injury. (Courtesy of Daniel L. Savitt, MD.)

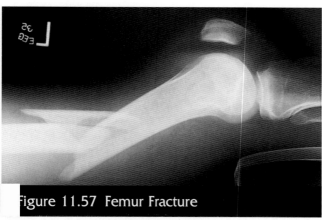

Figure 11.57 Femur Fracture

Radiographic examination reveals a comminuted displaced distal femoral fracture. (Courtesy of Cathleen M. Vossler, MD.)

Associated Clinical Features

Femoral fractures occur secondary to great forces, like those associated with motor vehicle accidents. The diagnosis is usually evident on visualization of the thigh (Fig. 11.56) and confirmed radiographically (Fig. 11.57). The position of the leg can help determine at which point the femur is fractured. Commonly associated injuries include hip fracture and dislocation as well as ligamentous injury to the knee. Hematoma formation is common.

Differential Diagnosis

Pelvic fracture, hematoma, hip fracture, hip dislocation, and contusion can be mistaken for femoral fracture prior to radiographic examination.

Emergency Department Treatment and Disposition

Initial management includes stabilization and evaluation for any life-threatening injuries. It is important to keep in mind that a large amount of blood loss can occur (average blood loss for a femoral shaft fracture is 1000 mL). These patients should have two large-bore intravenous lines and be crossmatched for blood products should they become necessary. The extremity should be immobilized and splinted with a traction device such as a Hare splint. Once this is accomplished, radiographic evaluation of the extremity should be performed. Orthopedic consultation should be obtained and admission arranged. The majority of intertrochanteric and subtrochanteric fractures require operative fixation and stabilization. An open fracture is an orthopedic emergency; these patients require tetanus prophylaxis, antibiotic coverage, and emergent irrigation and debridement in the operating room.

Clinical Pearls

1. Pain can be referred. Any injury between the lumbosacral spine and the knee can be referred to the thigh or knee.
2. Vascular compromise can occur and should be suspected with an expanding hematoma, absent or diminished pulses, or progressive neurologic signs. Neurovascular status needs to be assessed frequently.
3. Femoral shaft fractures can mask the clinical findings of a hip dislocation; thus radiographs of the pelvis and hips should be obtained routinely.

Associated Clinical Features

The quadriceps and its associated tendons predominantly extend the knee. This mechanism may be disrupted by quadriceps or patellar tendon rupture or patellar fracture. Collagen disorders, degenerative disease, tendon calcifications, and fatty tendon degeneration may predispose to these problems.

Quadriceps tendon ruptures are more common than patellar tendon ruptures and are more often seen in the elderly. Forced flexion during quadriceps contraction (as in a fall from a curb) may cause sudden buckling and pain. The patella is inferiorly displaced with proximal ecchymosis and swelling. A soft tissue defect at the distal aspect of the quadriceps may be apparent on examination (Fig. 11.58). Proximal displacement of the patella with inferior pole tenderness and swelling suggest a patellar tendon rupture (Fig. 11.59). Lateral radiographs help distinguish between the two (Fig. 11.60).

Patellar fractures may be transverse, stellate, or vertical. They may be caused by direct trauma or through avulsion secondary to the quadriceps pull against resistance. Tenderness, swelling, and sometimes a palpable defect are present.

Differential Diagnosis

Knee dislocation, patellar contusion, or proximal femoral fracture may be confused with knee extensor mechanism injuries.

Emergency Department Treatment and Disposition

An optimal outcome for quadriceps or patellar tendon rupture is realized with early consultation, immobilization, and consideration of operative repair. There are nonsurgical advocates who recommend conservative treatment.

Nondisplaced transverse patellar fractures should be treated with long-leg splinting in full extension and referral to orthopedics. Patients with displaced patellar fractures generally receive operative treatment or excision of the patella.

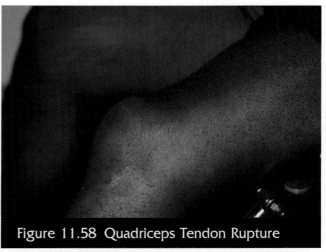

Figure 11.58 Quadriceps Tendon Rupture

Inferior displacement of the patella and a distal quadriceps defect suggest quadriceps tendon rupture. (Courtesy of Robert Trieff, MD.)

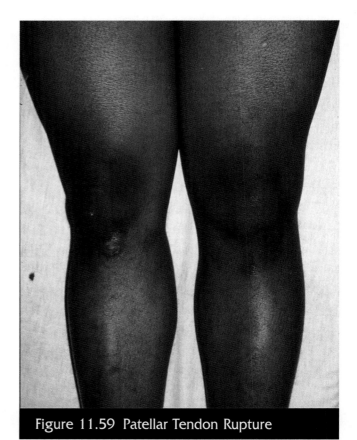

Figure 11.59 Patellar Tendon Rupture

Proximal displacement of the patella and inferior pole tenderness may be subtle, as in this patient with left patellar tendon rupture. (Courtesy of Kevin J. Knoop, MD, MS.)

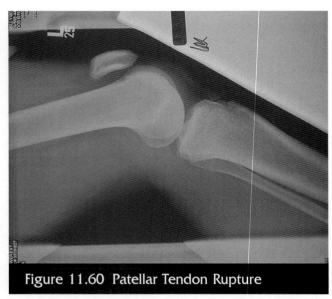

Figure 11.60 Patellar Tendon Rupture

A lateral radiograph of the patient in Fig. 11.59 reveals the proximal patellar displacement seen with complete patellar tendon rupture. (Courtesy of Kevin J. Knoop, MD, MS.)

Clinical Pearls

1. Patients with complete ruptures have loss of active extension of the knee.
2. Avulsion of the tibial tuberosity may also show a hideriding patella on physical and radiographic examination.
3. Magnetic resonance imaging may distinguish partial from complete tears.
4. Patellar fractures may be complicated by future degenerative arthritis or focal avascular necrosis.

Associated Clinical Features

Patellar dislocations result from direct trauma to the patella. A force is applied to the upper portion of the patella at the same time as a rotational force affects the knee. The most common dislocations are lateral, but horizontal, superior, and intercondylar dislocations also occur. These tend to be recurrent owing to the resultant increased laxity of the supporting structures. Patients who have had recurrent dislocations often reduce the dislocation prior to arrival at the ED. Common complaints include pain, swelling, and a deformity in the knee. Physical examination reveals fullness or deformity in the lateral aspect of the knee (Fig. 11.61). Fractures of the patella or femoral condyle occur in 5% of patients.

Differential Diagnosis

Distal femoral fracture, quadriceps rupture, patellar tendon rupture, patellar fracture, or knee dislocation can be mistaken for a patellar dislocation.

Emergency Department Treatment and Disposition

Reduction is easily accomplished and results in immediate relief of pain. Lateral dislocations are reduced by flexing the hip, extending the knee, and gently directing pressure medially on the patella. Other dislocations generally require open reduction. Radiographic examination should be obtained to document patellar position as well as evaluate for fracture. These patients require a knee immobilizer or long leg cast in full extension for 4 to 6 weeks. Orthopedic consultation should be obtained, since these patients require further evaluation.

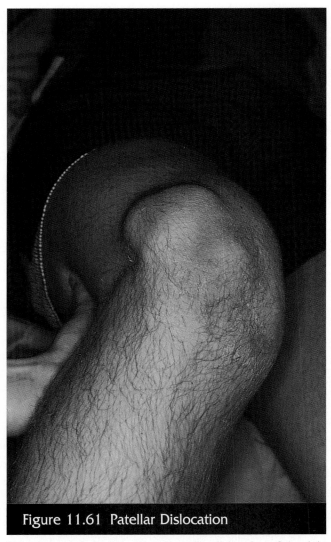

Figure 11.61 Patellar Dislocation

This photograph depicts a lateral patellar dislocation of the right knee. Note the obvious lateral deformity of the right patella. (Courtesy of Cathleen M. Vossler, MD.)

Clinical Pearls

1. A dislocated patella may reduce spontaneously prior to presentation and should be addressed as a possibility in any patient who presents with knee pain. This may be elucidated by inquiring about a knee deformity at the time of injury that is no longer present.
2. Complications of patellar dislocation include degenerative arthritis, recurrent dislocations, and fractures.
3. The patellar apprehension test should be performed on these patients: patients have the sensation that the patella will dislocate when there is lateral pressure placed on the patella, at which point they grab for their knee.

Associated Clinical Features

The peak incidence of knee dislocation is in the third decade of life. It is more common in males. Knee dislocations are classified by the direction of tibial displacement relative to the femur. They may be anterior (Fig. 11.62), posterior (Fig. 11.63), medial, lateral, or rotary. Anterior dislocations account for 50 to 60% of dislocations and usually occur after high-energy hyperextension injuries. Two-thirds of all knee dislocations are secondary to motor vehicle crashes, with the remainder from falls, from sports, and from industrial injuries. Anterior dislocations are associated with a high incidence of associated popliteal artery and peroneal nerve injuries. The affected limb will have gross deformity around the knee with swelling and immobility; peroneal nerve injury manifests itself with decreased sensation at the first web space with impaired dorsiflexion of the foot. Many of these dislocations will reduce spontaneously prior to arrival in the ED.

Differential Diagnosis

Tibia/fibular fractures, knee fractures, femoral fractures, or patellar dislocation may mimic knee dislocation.

Emergency Department Treatment and Disposition

Emergent treatment includes early reduction, immobilization, assessment of distal neurovascular function, and emergent orthopedic referral. The knee should be evaluated for valgus and varus stability at 20 degrees flexion. Reduction of anterior dislocation is accomplished by having an assistant apply longitudinal traction on the leg while keeping one hand on the tibia and simultaneously lifting the femur anteriorly back into position. A posterior splint with the knee in 15 degrees of flexion is used for immobilization and to avoid tension on the popliteal artery. The patient should be admitted for observation and arteriography. Historically, arteriography was advocated for all anterior knee dislocations even with a normal postreduction vascular examination; however, low-energy knee dislocations with normal postreduction vascular examinations

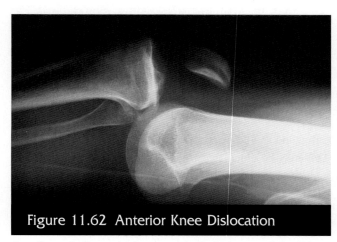

Figure 11.62 Anterior Knee Dislocation

A radiograph demonstrating anterior displacement of the tibia in relation to the femur. (Courtesy of Selim Suner, MD, MS.)

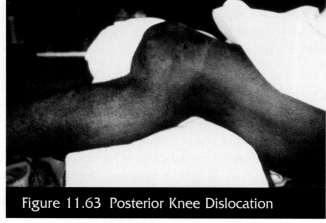

Figure 11.63 Posterior Knee Dislocation

A clinical photograph demonstrating posterior displacement of the tibia in relation to the femur. (Courtesy of Paul R. Sierzenski, MD.)

may not require arteriography and can be followed by serial examination. Duplex Doppler ultrasonography has been advocated by some authors and correlates well with arteriography but may miss intimal tears.

Clinical Pearls

1. Knee dislocations are often associated with a fracture of the proximal tibia.
2. The presence of distal pulses in the foot does not rule out an arterial injury; there is a 10% incidence of popliteal injury despite present distal pulses.
3. Vascular repair after 8 h of injury carries an amputation rate of greater than 80%.

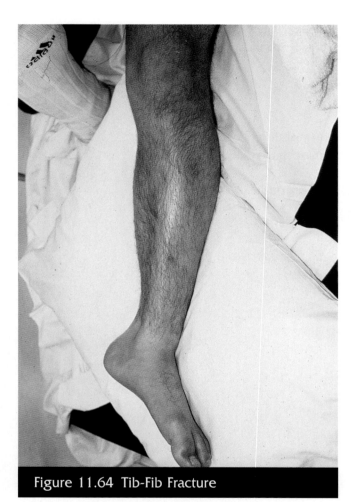

Figure 11.64 Tib-Fib Fracture

Deformity associated with a midshaft tibial and fibular fracture. (Courtesy of Kevin J. Knoop, MD, MS.)

Associated Clinical Features

The tibia sustains a high frequency of fractures secondary to direct trauma because of its subcutaneous location. Tibial fractures may be complicated by nonunion, neurovascular injury, or compartment syndrome. Suspect tibial fractures with trauma to the lower extremity, pain, and inability to bear weight. Tibial diaphyseal fractures carry a high risk for compartment syndrome, and distal neurovascular status should always be documented.

Fibular fractures may be isolated or be associated with injuries of the tibia (Fig. 11.64). Isolated fibular fractures are caused by direct trauma to the lateral aspect of the leg. Contrary to tibial fractures, complications of isolated fibular fractures are rare. The fibula is a non-weight-bearing structure, so isolated fractures are anatomically splinted by an intact tibia. Distal fibular fractures may include a disrupted ankle joint, as evidenced by a widened or nonuniform mortise on the AP radiograph.

The Maisonneuve fracture is a combination of an oblique proximal fibular fracture, disruption of the interosseous membrane and tibiofibular ligament distally, and a medial malleolar fracture or tear of the deltoid ligament. This fracture occurs when an external rotational force is applied to the foot, producing a fracture of the proximal third of the fibula. Physical examination findings include tenderness at the anteromedial ankle joint capsule or at the ankle syndesmosis in combination with proximal fibular tenderness.

Differential Diagnosis

Contusion, disseminated vascular coagulation, compartment syndrome, and sprains must be considered.

Emergency Department Treatment and Disposition

Treatment of tibial fractures depends on whether they are open or closed and on the degree of displacement. All open fractures require immediate orthopedic referral for surgical treatment and reduction. Closed fractures that cannot be reduced may also need open reduction. Patients with isolated nondisplaced tibial fractures may be splinted, started on ice therapy, and referred for outpatient treatment. Treatment of fibular fractures is dictated by the degree of pain experienced by the patient and the involvement of the ankle joint. Nondisplaced fractures can be treated with an air cast, while those with displacement should be place in a sugar-tong splint and referred for short-term orthopedic evaluation. Treatment of a Maisonneuve fracture depends on the status of the ankle mortise. An intact mortise with no joint space widening can be treated by casting. A mortise not in anatomic alignment requires open reduction.

Clinical Pearls

1. Early follow up is required for all tibial fractures owing to the risk of compartment syndrome.
2. The peroneal nerve crosses over the head of the fibula and is subject to injury with a Maisonneuve fracture.
3. Some patients with Maisonneuve fracture may complain only of ankle pain. Maisonneuve fracture represents about 1 in 20 ankle fractures, so always examine the proximal fibula in patients complaining of ankle pain.

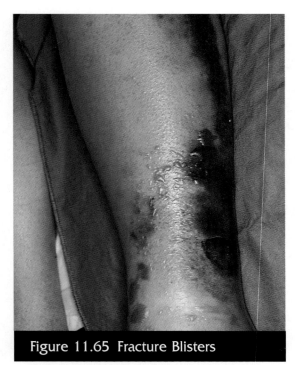

Figure 11.65 Fracture Blisters

Fracture blisters in a patient who fell down four steps on the evening prior to presentation. The patient had initially complained of ankle pain, decreased range of motion, and an inability to bear weight. Upon awakening the next morning, he noted ecchymosis, swelling, and blister formation. Radiographics revealed fracture of the fibula. (Courtesy of Daniel L. Savitt, MD.)

Associated Clinical Features

Fracture blisters are vesicles or bullae that arise secondary to swelling from soft tissue injury and fracture formation (Fig. 11.65). The most commonly affected areas include the tibia, ankle, and elbow. Patients note blister formation within 1 to 2 days after the initial trauma. Patients complain of pain, swelling, ecchymosis, and decreased range of motion. Complications include infection, deep venous thrombosis, and compartment syndrome.

Differential Diagnosis

Sprain, fracture, cellulitis, necrotizing fasciitis, compartment syndrome, or burns can be mistaken for fracture blisters.

Emergency Department Treatment and Disposition

Blisters are generally left intact, and the underlying fracture is treated.

Clinical Pearls

1. Blisters can be seen with other conditions, including barbiturate overdose; in the setting of trauma, however, they frequently indicate an underlying fracture.
2. Blisters are managed in a similar fashion to second-degree burns.

Associated Clinical Features

Rupture of the Achilles tendon occurs most frequently in middle-aged males involved in athletic activities. Three mechanisms result in this injury: a direct blow to the tendon, forceful dorsiflexion of the ankle, or increased tension on an already taut tendon. Rupture occurs 2 to 3 cm above the tendon's attachment to the calcaneus (Fig. 11.66). Patients complain of a feeling of being hit in the posterior aspect of the lower leg. They may hear or feel a pop. There is weakness when pushing off of the foot; pain, edema, and ecchymosis develop. Thompson's test can be diagnostic of an Achilles rupture (Fig. 11.67). The patient should be placed in a prone position; the gastrocnemius muscle should be grasped and squeezed. If the Achilles tendon is even partially intact, then the foot will plantarflex; if ruptured, there will be no movement of the foot.

Differential Diagnosis

Partial Achilles tendon tear, plantaris tendon rupture, ankle sprain, Achilles tendinitis, and partial gastrocnemius muscle rupture have been confused with an Achilles tendon rupture.

Emergency Department Treatment and Disposition

Treatment is either operative or conservative. In either case, the extremity is immobilized without weight bearing for 6 weeks, followed by 6 weeks of partial weight bearing. ED treatment consists of elevation, analgesia, ice, and immobilization with a posterior splint. Orthopedic consultation should be obtained so that a plan of treatment can be chosen. These patients can be discharged home with close orthopedic follow-up or can be admitted for acute repair. Partial tears are generally treated conservatively.

Clinical Pearls

1. Advantages to surgical repair are increased strength and mobility and a decreased rate of rerupture.
2. Approximately 25% of these injuries are initially misdiagnosed as ankle sprains.
3. These patients maintain the ability to plantarflex the foot in a non-weight-bearing position owing to the action of the tibialis posterior, toe flexor, and peroneal muscles.
4. Palpation of the tendon alone may not detect rupture, as the tendon sheath is often intact.

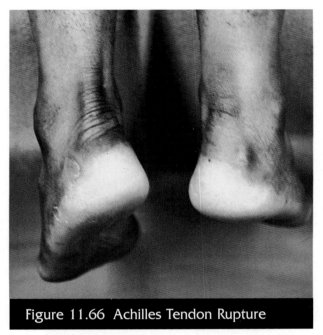

Figure 11.66 Achilles Tendon Rupture

This photograph depicts a patient with a right Achilles tendon rupture. Note the loss of the normal resting plantarflexion on the right owing to disruption of the tendon. This is seen with the patient in a nonweight-bearing position. Swelling is also apparent over the site of the tendon injury. (Courtesy of Kevin J. Knoop, MD, MS.)

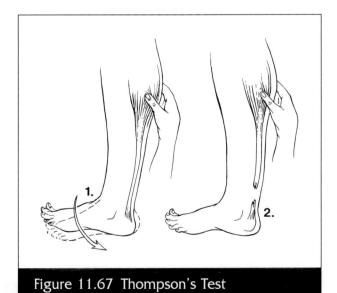

Figure 11.67 Thompson's Test

This illustration demonstrates the Thompson's test, where compression of the gastrocnemius-soleus complex normally produces plantarflexion of the foot (1). If the tendon is completely ruptured, this will not occur (2).

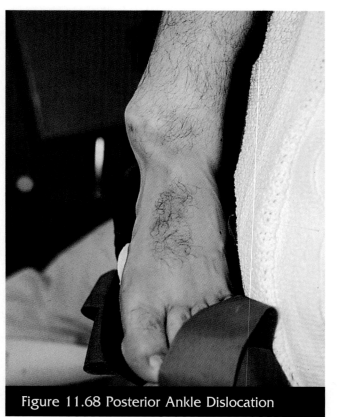

Figure 11.68 Posterior Ankle Dislocation

A posterior ankle dislocation is pictured. Radiographs showed an associated fracture. (Courtesy of Mark Madenwald, MD.)

Associated Clinical Features

Ankle dislocations require forces of great magnitude. Posterior and lateral dislocations are the most common, but the ankle can also dislocate medially, superiorly, or anteriorly (Figs. 11.68, 11.69, 11.70). A posteriorly dislocated ankle is locked in plantarflexion with the anterior tibia easily palpable. The foot has a shortened appearance, with the ankle very edematous. Anterior dislocations present with the foot dorsiflexed and elongated. Lateral dislocations present with the entire foot displaced laterally. Ankle dislocations are commonly associated with malleolar fractures.

Differential Diagnosis

Fractures of the tibia, fibula, or talus, as well as ankle sprains, are all commonly mistaken for an ankle dislocation on initial examination. A subtalar foot dislocation (Fig. 11.71) resembles ankle dislocation.

Emergency Department Treatment and Disposition

Routine radiographs should be obtained to identify any fractures. Reduction should occur before radiography if circu-

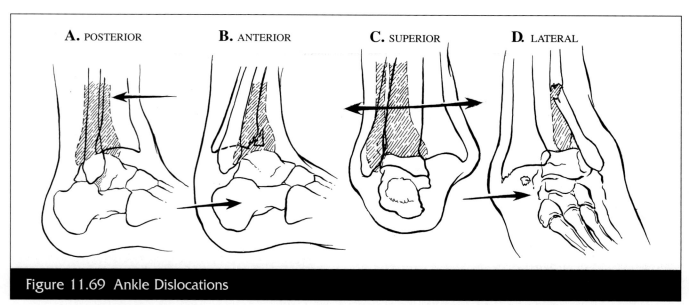

A. POSTERIOR   **B.** ANTERIOR   **C.** SUPERIOR   **D.** LATERAL

Figure 11.69 Ankle Dislocations

This illustration depicts different types of ankle dislocations. Arrows denote direction of the injury force. (Adapted with permission from Simon R: *Emergency Orthopedics: The Extremities.* New York: Appleton & Lange, 1987, p. 402.)

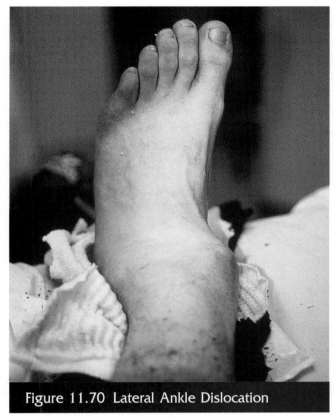

Figure 11.70 Lateral Ankle Dislocation

The foot is laterally displaced in this patient with a lateral ankle dislocation. A radiograph revealed fracture of the distal fibula. (Courtesy of Cathleen M. Vossler, MD.)

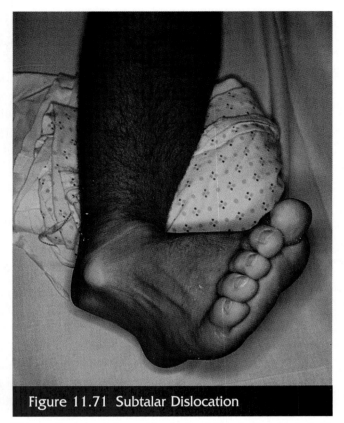

Figure 11.71 Subtalar Dislocation

This patient landed on his foot while playing basketball. Neurovascular status was intact, and the ankle was promptly reduced after x-ray showed no associated fracture. (Courtesy of Kevin J. Knoop, MD, MS.)

latory compromise exists. To reduce the ankle, gentle traction is applied to the foot, in an opposite direction of the force that caused the injury. Neurovascular status should be checked before and after any attempts at reduction or immobilization. Reduction usually requires conscious sedation, a Bier block, or general anesthesia. Patients should be placed in a posterior splint with immediate referral to an orthopedic surgeon for hospitalization.

Clinical Pearls

1. These injuries are commonly associated with malleolar fractures and often require open reduction and internal fixation.
2. Fifty percent of ankle dislocations are open and require surgical debridement.
3. There is an increased incidence of avascular necrosis following ankle dislocation.

Associated Clinical Features

The calcaneus is the most frequently fractured tarsal bone. Injuries are associated with falls from a height or twisting mechanisms. There are two types: intra- and extraarticular. Intraarticular fractures generally result from an axial load. These patients have severe heel pain in association with soft tissue swelling and ecchymosis of the pericalcaneal tissues extending to the arch. Heel contour can be distorted. Extraarticular fractures are less common and may occur secondary to twisting or avulsive muscle forces. They are divided anatomically into the following types: anterior process, tuberosity (beak or avulsion), medial process, sustentaculum tali, and body.

Differential Diagnosis

Lisfranc's fracture, midfoot or forefoot fracture, and ankle sprain must be considered.

Emergency Department Treatment and Disposition

Differentiate extraarticular (25 to 35%) fractures, which have a good prognosis, from intraarticular (70 to 75%) fractures. Oblique radiographs and computed tomography (CT) scans can be used to rule out involvement of the subtalar joint. With intraarticular fractures, a lateral foot radiograph reveals a reduction in Bohler's angle (Figs. 11.72, 11.73), the posterior angle formed by intersection of a line from posterior to middle facet and a line from anterior to middle facet. Bohler's angle is normally between 28 and 40 degrees, with an average of 30 to 35. Angles of less than 28 degrees, or more than 5 degrees less than the uninjured side, suggest a fracture.

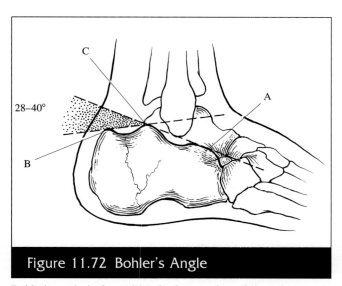

Figure 11.72 Bohler's Angle

Bohler's angle is formed by the intersection of lines drawn tangentially to the anterior (A) and posterior (B) elements of the superior surface of the calcaneus (C). A normal angle is between 28 and 40 degrees. Angles of less than 28 degrees are suggestive of a calcaneal fracture.

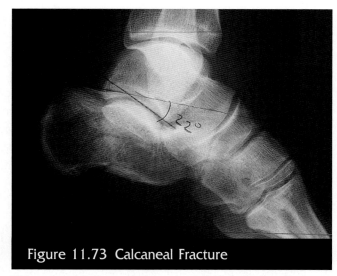

Figure 11.73 Calcaneal Fracture

This patient fell from a ladder and struck his heel. A cortical step-off is seen on the inferior aspect of the calcaneus. Bohler's angle has been calculated at approximately 22 degrees. (Courtesy of Alan B. Storrow, MD.)

Intraarticular fractures require urgent orthopedic consultation, since open reduction and internal fixation are usually necessary.

Nondisplaced extraarticular fractures not involving the subtalar joint generally heal well with bulky compressive dressings, rest, ice, elevation, and non-weight bearing for the first 6 weeks. However, some may require open reduction; therefore orthopedic referral is necessary.

Clinical Pearls

1. Calcaneal fracture warrants a diligent search for associated injuries. 20% of calcaneal fractures are associated with spinal fractures, 7% have contralateral calcaneal fractures, and 10% are associated with compartment syndromes. The subtalar joint is disrupted in 50% of cases. A high index of suspicion for thoracic aortic rupture and renal vascular pedicle disruption must be maintained when calcaneal fractures are seen.
2. Minimally displaced fractures of the anterior process are easily missed and should be suspected in a patient who does not recover appropriately from a lateral ankle sprain. If the fragment is small or diagnosis is delayed, this fragment can simply be excised.
3. CT scanning is the optimal imaging technique.

Associated Clinical Features

Ankle sprains are extremely common problems in the ED. Classification of these injuries based on physical examination and radiography helps guide management and definitive treatment.

The most common mechanism is an inversion stress that injures, in order, the joint capsule, anterior talofibular ligament, calcaneofibular ligament, and posterior talofibular ligament. Since the medial deltoid ligament is quite strong and elastic, serious eversion injuries usually result in avulsion of the medial malleolus or fracture of the lateral malleolus.

A first-degree sprain is defined by a stretch injury, or microscopic damage, to ligaments resulting in pain, tenderness, minimal swelling, and maintenance of the ability to bear weight. A second-degree sprain is defined by a partial tear of the ligamentous structures resulting in pain, swelling (Fig. 11.74), local hemorrhage (Fig. 11.75), and moderate degree of functional loss. A third-degree sprain is a complete tear of the ligament or ligaments and presents with positive stress testing, significant swelling, and an inability to bear weight.

Differential Diagnosis

Malleolar and fifth metatarsal fractures can be confused with ankle sprains prior to radiographs. Any patient with joint pain should have an infectious etiology considered.

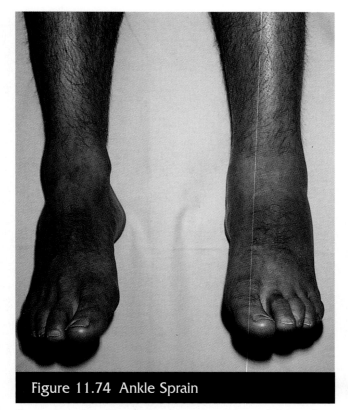

Figure 11.74 Ankle Sprain

Comparison view of a patient with a second-degree left lateral ankle sprain. Note the swelling and asymmetry of the affected area. (Courtesy of Kevin J. Knoop, MD, MS.)

Emergency Department Treatment and Disposition

First-degree injuries are treated with ice packs, elevation, woven elastic (Ace) wrap, and early mobilization. For patients with mild second-degree sprains, immobilization for 72 h followed by use of an ankle support has been advocated. More serious second-degree and all third-degree

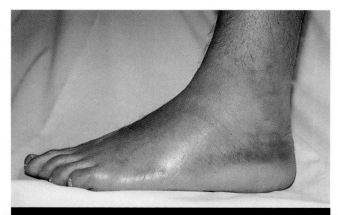

Figure 11.75 Ankle Sprain

Note the dependent ecchymosis and swelling in this patient with a second-degree left lateral ankle sprain. (Courtesy of Lawrence B. Stack, MD.)

sprains should receive immobilization, ice, and elevation and be referred to orthopedics. In younger patients, surgery is an option, although clear recommendations are lacking.

Clinical Pearls

1. Ankle injuries are the most common orthopedic problem in emergency medicine.
2. Complications of ankle sprains include instability, persistent pain, recurrent sprains, and peroneal tendon dislocation.
3. Published guidelines known as the Ottawa Ankle Rules were designed to limit unnecessary radiographs by clinical scoring.
4. The most common eversion injury is a fracture of the lateral malleolus. Since inversion injuries also produce lateral problems, the most common injuries to the ankle involve the lateral side.
5. Both malleoli, the proximal fibula, and the fifth metatarsal should be examined for injury in evaluating a patient with an ankle sprain.

Associated Clinical Features

Patients complain of pain, swelling, decreased range of motion, and tenderness over the lateral aspect of the foot (Fig. 11.76). Fractures of the fifth metatarsal base have been generically referred to as Jones fractures. However, the fractures can be divided into three types, depending on their anatomic location. Treatment is determined by this division.

The classic Jones fracture is a transverse fracture of the fifth metatarsal diaphysis (Figs. 11.77, 11.78). It occurs when a force is applied to a plantarflexed and inverted foot. It is also referred to as a stress fracture of the proximal shaft and is usually due to repetitive stress injury. Patients often have prodromal symptoms.

A fracture at the metaphyseal–diaphyseal junction has been termed a pseudo-Jones fracture. It is always an acute injury.

The last type is an avulsion fracture of the fifth metatarsal base caused by sudden inversion of the foot (Figs. 11.77, 11.79). The avulsion injury is caused by traction on the lateral cord of the plantar aponeurosis.

Differential Diagnosis

Care must be taken to avoid confusing the two sesamoid bones in this area with a fracture. The more common of the two, the os peroneum (present in approximately 15%), lies within the peroneus longus tendon. More rare is the os vesalianum, which lies in the peroneus brevis tendon. Both have smooth, rounded surfaces and usually occur bilaterally. The apophysis of the fifth metatarsal base can also be mistaken for a fracture. It usually fuses by 16 years of age, although some fail to fuse.

Other entities to consider include ankle sprain, other metatarsal fractures, and foot dislocations.

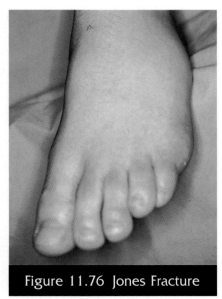

Figure 11.76 Jones Fracture

This patient sustained an injury of the fifth metatarsal and presented with pain and swelling over this site. His radiograph revealed a fracture. (Courtesy of Cathleen M. Vossler, MD.)

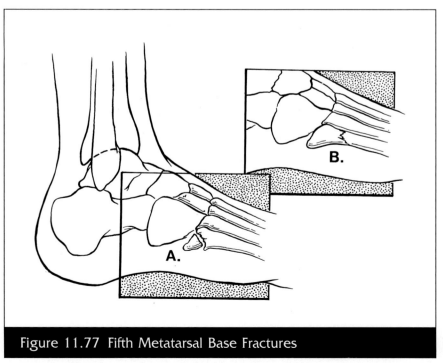

Figure 11.77 Fifth Metatarsal Base Fractures

This illustration depicts an avulsion fracture (A) and a classic Jones fracture (B).

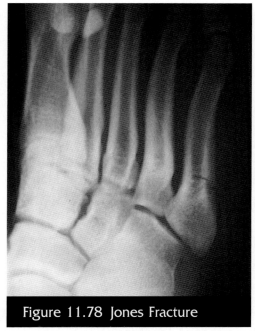

Figure 11.78 Jones Fracture

Radiograph with typical appearance for a diaphyseal fracture of the fifth metatarsal base. (Courtesy of Alan B. Storrow, MD.)

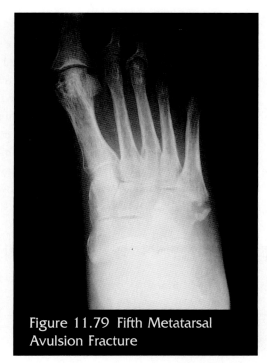

Figure 11.79 Fifth Metatarsal Avulsion Fracture

Radiograph illustrating an avulsion-type fracture of the fifth metatarsal base, sometimes referred to as a ballet dancer's fracture (see Fig. 11.77). (Courtesy of Alan B. Storrow, MD.)

Emergency Department Treatment and Disposition

A Jones fracture should be splinted and referred to orthopedics for definitive repair. It may heal slowly and cause permanent pain and disability. Surgical treatment is sometimes recommended, particularly since the stress involved with these fractures usually occurs in the sporting activities of young patients.

A pseudo-Jones fracture usually heals without complication, although more slowly than the avulsion fracture. Referral to orthopedics for a walking or non-weight-bearing cast, according to local preference, is indicated.

The avulsion fracture usually heals rapidly and seldom leads to permanent disability. Most orthopedic physicians treat these patients symptomatically with a short leg walking cast or hard-sole shoe for 2 to 3 weeks. Surgery is rarely indicated.

Clinical Pearls

1. It is important to differentiate between the different types of fractures of the fifth metatarsal base; treatment and disposition are dictated by these categories.
2. The original description of these fractures was by Sir Robert Jones, who personally sustained an injury while dancing. The avulsion fracture is sometimes referred to as the ballet dancer's fracture.
3. The classic Jones fracture has a high incidence of delayed healing and nonunion.

Associated Clinical Features

This is the most commonly misdiagnosed foot injury. The Lisfranc joint (tarsometatarsal joint) connects the midfoot and forefoot. It is defined by the articulation of the bases of the first three metatarsals with the cuneiforms and the fourth and fifth metatarsals with the cuboid. Lisfranc's ligament anchors the second metatarsal base to the medial cuneiform. Although disruption of the Lisfranc joint is typically associated with high-energy mechanisms—such as falls, vehicle crashes, and direct crush injuries—they also occur with lower-intensity mechanisms. Although the clinical presentation is variable, severe midfoot pain and the inability to bear weight are usually present (Fig. 11.80). Radiographs may reveal displacement of the metatarsals in one direction (homolateral) or a split, usually between the first and second metatarsals (divergent) (Figs. 11.81, 11.82).

Differential Diagnosis

Metatarsal fracture, navicular fracture, and contusion should be considered.

Emergency Department Treatment and Disposition

Meticulous evaluation of foot radiographs is key to diagnosis. The medial aspect of the first three metatarsals should align with the medial borders of the first three cuneiforms. The metatarsals

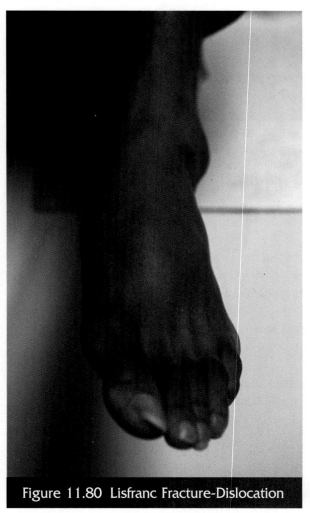

Figure 11.80 Lisfranc Fracture-Dislocation

This patient presented with extreme midfoot pain and swelling. (Courtesy of Kevin J. Knoop, MD, MS.)

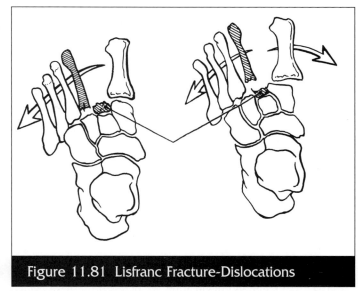

Figure 11.81 Lisfranc Fracture-Dislocations

Homolateral (*left*) and divergent (*right*) Lisfranc fracture-dislocations.

should be aligned dorsally with their respective tarsal bones on the lateral view. The medial aspect of the fourth metatarsal should align with the medial cuboid. A disruption of these anatomic relationships is suggestive of a Lisfranc injury. Also suggestive are fractures or dislocations of the cuneiform or navicular and widening of the spaces between the first and second and second and third metatarsals. Lisfranc injuries warrant orthopedic evaluation in the ED. Closed reduction can be attempted using finger traps on the toes and placing traction on the hindfoot. Postreduction displacement of more than 2 mm or a tarsometatarsal angle of greater than 15 degrees requires surgical fixation. Tenderness over the Lisfranc complex with normal radiographs can reflect a strain of the complex. Stress (weight-bearing) radiographs may unmask joint instability. Lisfranc sprains should be placed in a short-leg walking cast. Potential complications include compartment syndrome, chronic pain, loss of the metatarsal arch, reflex sympathetic dystrophy, and biomechanical difficulties.

Clinical Pearls

1. Early recognition of Lisfranc fracture-dislocations is facilitated by assessing for the normal bony alignment on x-ray and by searching for frequently associated fractures.
2. Fractures of the second metatarsal base are considered pathognomonic of a Lisfranc injury.

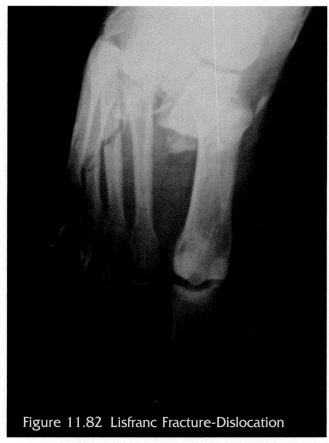

Figure 11.82 Lisfranc Fracture-Dislocation

A divergent Lisfranc fracture-dislocation. Note the disruption of the alignment of the second metatarsal and the middle cuneiform. Sometimes these injuries are not as apparent and comparison radiographs are necessary. (Courtesy of Alan B. Storrow, MD.)

Associated Clinical Features

Electricity may cause harm by heat generated through tissue resistance or directly by the current on cells. Skin, nerves, vessels, and muscles usually sustain the greatest damage. Many factors affect the severity of injury: type of current (DC or AC), current intensity, contact duration, tissue resistance, and current pathway through the body. Those at high risk for electrical injury are toddlers, those who perform risk-taking behavior, and people who work with electricity.

When electricity is deposited in the tissues, it may cause a host of injuries: contact burns (entry and exit—Fig. 11.83), thermal heating, arc burns, prolonged muscular tetany, or blunt trauma. Sudden death (asystole, respiratory arrest, ventricular fibrillation), myocardial damage, cerebral edema, neuropathies, disseminated intravascular coagulation, myoglobinuria, compartment syndrome, and various metabolic disorders have been described.

High-voltage DC or AC current typically causes a single violent muscular contraction that throws the victim from the source. As a result, blunt trauma and blast injuries may occur. Low-voltage AC currents (as from a household outlet) typically cause muscular tetany, forcing the victim to continue contact with the source.

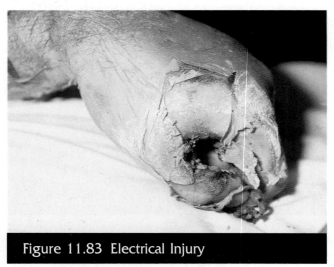

Figure 11.83 Electrical Injury

This electrical worker grabbed a high-voltage power line with his hand and sustained an electrical injury. Exit wounds may occur where the patient is grounded, often through the feet when standing. Since this is a transthoracic injury, particular attention should be paid to cardiac monitoring. (Courtesy of Alan B. Storrow, MD.)

Differential Diagnosis

Stroke, toxic ingestion, envenomation, myocardial infarction, assault, and seizures may mimic electrical injury.

Emergency Department Treatment and Disposition

After initial stabilization, consider cervical spine immobilization, oxygen administration, cardiac monitoring, and intravenous crystalloid infusion. A Foley catheter will help monitor urine output and is especially important if rhabdomyolysis is suspected.

Diagnostic testing to consider includes: ECG, CBC, urinalysis, CPK, CPK-MB, electrolytes, BUN, creatinine, and coagulation profile. Radiographic assessment is important for those with a suspicion of trauma.

Severe or high-risk injuries should be admitted to a burn or trauma center with surgical consultation. Patients with minor, brief, low-intensity exposures, with a normal ECG, normal urinalysis, and no significant burns or trauma may be considered for discharge after 6 to 8 h of observation.

Clinical Pearls

1. The low resistance of water makes its association with electricity particularly dangerous.
2. High-risk features include high-voltage exposure (>600 V), deep burns, neurologic injury, dysrhythmias, an abnormal electrocardiogram, evidence of rhabdomyolysis, suicidal intent, or significant associated trauma.

CHAPTER 12

EXTREMITY CONDITIONS

Selim Suner
Daniel L. Savitt

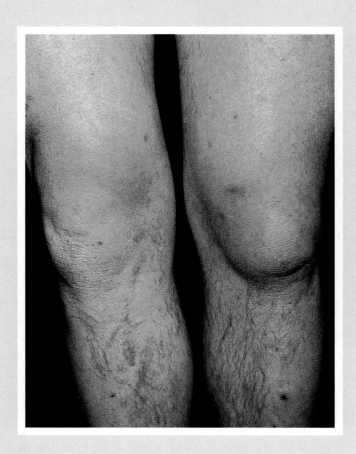

Associated Clinical Features

Cellulitis is infection of the skin or subcutaneous tissues from local invasion, traumatic wounds, or hematogenous dissemination. The local inflammatory response is characterized by erythema with poorly defined borders, edema, warmth, pain, and limitation of movement (Fig. 12.1). Fever and constitutional symptoms may be present and are commonly associated with bacteremia. Trauma, lymphatic or venous stasis, immunodeficiency, and foreign bodies are predisposing factors. There may be enlarged regional lymph nodes. Organisms commonly causing cellulitis are group A beta hemolytic *Streptococcus* and *Staphylococcus aureus* in non-intertriginous skin not associated with an ulcer, gram-negative organisms in intertriginous skin and ulcerations, and *Haemophilus influenzae* in children younger than 3 years. In immunocompromised hosts, *Escherichia coli*, *Klebsiella* species, *Enterobacter* species, and *Pseudomonas aeruginosa* may be the etiologic agents.

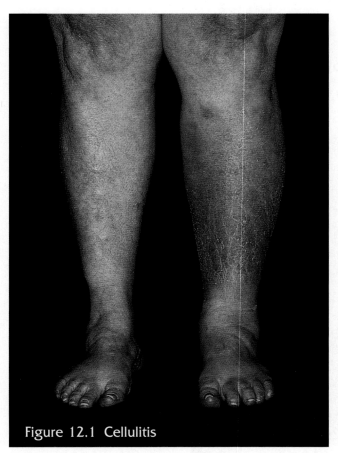

Figure 12.1 Cellulitis

Cellulitis of the left leg characterized by erythema and mild swelling. (Courtesy of Frank Birinyi, MD.)

Differential Diagnosis

Deep venous thrombosis of the lower extremities, erythema nodosum, septic or inflammatory arthritis, osteomyelitis, herpes zoster, allergic reactions, arthropod envenomation, and burns are included in the differential diagnosis of cellulitis.

Emergency Department Treatment and Disposition

Treatment of minor cases commonly consists of immobilization, elevation, analgesia, and oral antibiotics with reevaluation in 48 h. Admission and parenteral administration of antibiotics may be necessary for immunocompromised or toxic-appearing patients or those who do not initially respond to outpatient therapy.

Clinical Pearls

1. Aggressive treatment of cellulitis with broad-spectrum parenteral antibiotics in immunocompromised patients (e.g., diabetes mellitus) is warranted.
2. Fever is uncommon and often associated with bacteremia.
3. Radiography for the presence of foreign body or gas in the tissue should be considered.
4. Leading-edge aspirates are of low yield but may be of help in a toxic-appearing patient.
5. The incidence of *Haemophilus influenzae* cellulitis in children has decreased significantly with HIB vaccination.

Associated Clinical Features

A felon is a pyogenic infection of the distal pulp space often caused by staphylococci or streptococci. A felon cannot decompress itself because the collection of pus is trapped between septa that attach the skin to the distal phalanx. This condition is characterized by severe pain, exquisite tenderness, and tense swelling of the distal pulp with erythema (Fig. 12.2). There may be a visible collection of pus or palpable fluctuance. Complications include deep ischemic necrosis, osteomyelitis, septic arthritis, and septic tenosynovitis.

Differential Diagnosis

Hematoma following traumatic injury, paronychia, and herpetic whitlow should be considered.

Emergency Department Treatment and Disposition

Several incision and drainage techniques are employed in the treatment of a felon, and there is controversy surrounding which technique is the best to use. Incision and drainage utilizing a midlateral approach along the nondominant side of the finger or over the area of greatest fluctuance is commonly used to drain a felon. An alternative technique is to make a longitudinal volar incision directly through the finger pad into the pulp space and pus collection. To ensure complete drainage of the abscess cavity, all compartments should be entered. The packing of the abscess space is made with a small, loose-fitting wick to facilitate drainage. Oral antibiotics directed against gram-positive organisms should be used for 10 days and the packing removed or replaced after 24 to 48 h.

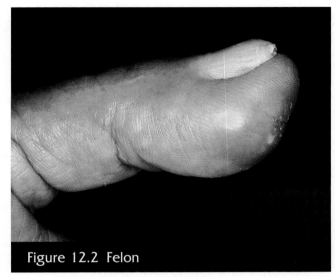

Figure 12.2 Felon

Note the area of purulence at the center of the palmar pad in this thumb with a felon. There is also swelling and erythema. (Courtesy of Daniel L. Savitt, MD.)

Clinical Pearls

1. Do not extend the incision proximal to the distal flexion crease.
2. Incisions should be made dorsal to the neurovascular bundle; the pincer surfaces (radial aspects of the index and long fingers and ulnar aspect of the thumb and small finger) should be avoided when possible.
3. "Hockey stick" and "fish mouth" incisions are associated with increased occurrence of unnecessary sequelae and are not recommended.
4. If there is radiographic evidence of osteomyelitis, bone debridement as well as antibiotic coverage is required.

Associated Clinical Features

Gangrene denotes tissue that has lost its blood supply and is undergoing necrosis. The term *dry gangrene* (Figs. 12.3, 12.4) is used for tissues undergoing sterile ischemic coagulative necrosis, whereas *wet gangrene* is associated with bacteria proteolytic decomposition. *Streptococcus pyogenes* is often implicated in rapidly developing (6 h to 2 days) gangrene in traumatic and surgical wounds. Clostridia, anaerobic streptococci, and mixed aerobic and anaerobic flora can also be seen in wounds caused by trauma, surgery, or diabetic ulcers.

Differential Diagnosis

Gas gangrene, frostbite, cyanosis, traumatic ecchymosis, deep venous thrombosis (DVT), and subungual hematoma are some conditions that should be included in the differential diagnosis of gangrene.

Emergency Department Treatment and Disposition

The treatment consists of amputation, debridement, and antibiotic therapy as needed. Underlying vascular pathology must be evaluated by arteriography and corrected surgically. Hospitalization is usually required; patients who present with systemic toxicity may require resuscitation in the ED.

Clinical Pearls

1. Obtain radiographs to help rule out clostridial myonecrosis and osteomyelitis.
2. Soft-tissue infection may complicate this condition.

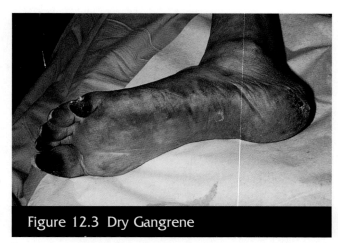

Figure 12.3 Dry Gangrene

Dry gangrene of the toes showing the areas of total tissue death, appearing as black and lighter shades of discoloration of the skin demarcating areas of impending gangrene. (Courtesy of Lawrence B. Stack, MD.)

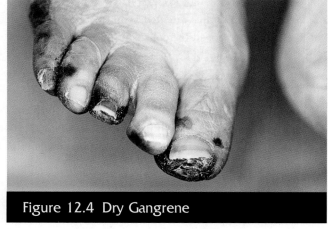

Figure 12.4 Dry Gangrene

Dry gangrene of the toes as a result of vascular disease. (Courtesy of Selim Suner, MD, MS.)

Associated Clinical Features

Also called clostridial myonecrosis, this infection causes rapid necrosis and liquefaction of fascia, muscle, and tendon. The vast majority of cases involve *Clostridium perfringens,* which produces a lethal necrotizing hemolytic alpha exotoxin. Myonecrosis is classically associated with trauma and diabetes. The inoculation of bacteria occurs either directly into the wound or by hematogenous spread. There is edematous bronze or purple discoloration, flaccid bullae with watery brown nonpurulent fluid (Fig. 12.5), and a foul odor. The most important clinical presentation is pain due to edema and the rapid production of gas in the infected tissue (Fig. 12.6). Pain out of proportion to the appearance of the injury is classic. Low-grade fever, which is an unreliable index of the severity of the infection, and tachycardia out of proportion to the fever are often present.

Crepitance and appearance of gross pockets of air in the tissue may be appreciated but may not be present early in the course of the illness. The incubation period for clostridia ranges between 1 and 4 days, but it can be as early as 6 h. Decreased tissue oxygen tension along with wound contamination are required for the infection to progress. Factors favoring decreased tissue oxygen tension include decreased blood supply, foreign body, tissue necrosis, or wound bacteria, which consume oxygen.

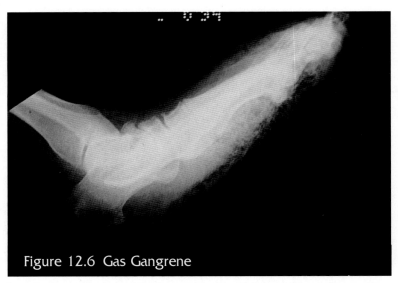

Figure 12.6 Gas Gangrene

Lateral view radiograph of the foot seen in Fig. 12.5. In addition to the swelling, there is air within the soft tissues, best seen in the plantar portion of the foot. (Courtesy of Selim Suner, MD, MS.)

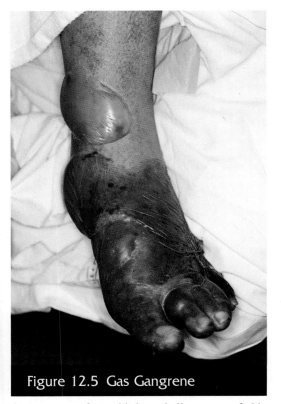

Figure 12.5 Gas Gangrene

A gangrenous foot with large bullae, areas of skin that are sloughing, and necrotic skin. There is also significant swelling. (Courtesy of Selim Suner, MD, MS.)

Differential Diagnosis

Crepitant cellulitis, synergistic necrotizing cellulitis, acute streptococcal hemolytic gangrene, and streptococcal myositis are some conditions that may be mistaken for clostridial myositis. Aspiration and Gram's stain showing gram-positive rods and few leukocytes may help, but often surgical exploration of the fascia and muscle is required to make the correct diagnosis.

Emergency Department Treatment and Disposition

Aggressive resuscitation with intravenous fluids is initiated, and consideration is given to packed red blood cell transfusion. Broad-spectrum antibiotics in conjunction with penicillin G, in the non-penicillin-allergic patient, is given in the ED. Tetanus prophylaxis must not be overlooked. Surgical debridement or amputation, the mainstays of therapy, must be initiated promptly. Hyperbaric oxygen, in conjunction with surgical and antibiotic therapy, has been suggested to have a synergistic effect in preventing the progression of infection and production of toxin.

Clinical Pearls

1. Clostridial infection should be considered in patients presenting with low-grade fever, tachycardia out of proportion to the fever, and pain out of proportion to physical findings.
2. Mortality is 80 to 90% if untreated, 10 to 25% when treated appropriately.
3. Mixed gram-negative rods and enterococci are found in nonclostridial gas gangrene, which is exclusively seen in diabetics and carries a mortality of only 4% when treated.
4. Gram's stain yielding gram-positive bacilli with a relative lack of leukocytes can rapidly confirm clinically suspected clostridial myonecrosis.

Associated Clinical Features

This uncommon, severe infection involves the subcutaneous soft tissues, including the superficial and deep fascial layers, with early sparing of the skin and late involvement of the muscle. It is most commonly seen in the lower extremities, abdominal wall, perianal and groin area, and postoperative wounds but can manifest in any body part. The infection is spread most commonly from a site of trauma or surgical wound, abscess, decubitus ulcer, or intestinal perforation. Alcohol, parenteral drug abuse, and diabetes mellitus are predisposing factors. Omphalitis may progress to necrotizing fasciitis in the newborn. Pain, tenderness, erythema, swelling, warmth, shiny skin, lymphangitis, and lymphadenitis are early clinical findings. Later, there is rapid progression with changes in skin color, formation of bullae with clear pink or purple fluid (Fig. 12.7), and cutaneous necrosis (Fig. 12.8), within 48 h. The skin becomes anesthetic and subcutaneous gas may be present. Systemic toxicity may be manifest by fever, dehydration, leukocytosis, and frequently positive blood cultures. Fournier's gangrene is a form of necrotizing fasciitis occurring in the groin and genitalia (see Figs. 8.9, 8.10). It is rapidly progressive and is associated with a high mortality rate, particularly in diabetics. The infection can pass through Buck's fascia of the penis, dartos fascia of the scrotum and penis, Colles' fascia of the perineum, and Scarpa's fascia of the abdominal wall. Two groups of organisms are implicated in necrotizing fasciitis. Type I includes anaerobic species (*Bacteroides* and *Peptostreptococcus*) and type II group A streptococci alone or with *Staphylococcus aureus*.

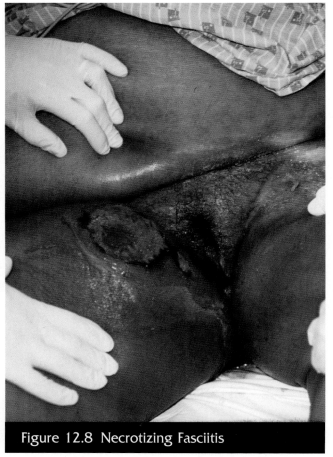

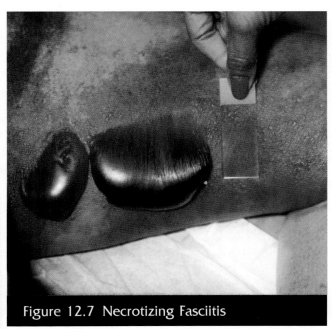

Figure 12.7 Necrotizing Fasciitis

Large cutaneous bullae are seen on the leg of this patient with necrotizing fasciitis. Note the dark purple fluid in the bullae. (Courtesy of Lawrence B. Stack, MD.)

Figure 12.8 Necrotizing Fasciitis

Necrotizing fasciitis with cutaneous necrosis can be seen in the inner thigh of this patient. (Courtesy of Lawrence B. Stack, MD.)

Differential Diagnosis

Cellulitis, osteomyelitis, gas gangrene, streptococcal myonecrosis, infected vascular gangrene, and trauma should all be considered.

Emergency Department Treatment and Disposition

Prompt diagnosis is critical in the treatment of this condition. If the diagnosis is made within 4 days from the onset of symptoms, the mortality rate is reduced from 50 to 12%. The initial treatment involves resuscitation with volume expansion. One recommended initial antibiotic regimen includes a combination of ampicillin, gentamicin, and clindamycin. Prompt surgical excision is essential.

Clinical Pearls

1. Intravenous calcium replacement may be necessary to reverse hypocalcemia from subcutaneous fat necrosis.
2. Radiographs may be used to detect subcutaneous gas that is not palpable.
3. Hemolysis and disseminated intravascular coagulation (DIC) may be seen in association with necrotizing fasciitis.
4. Necrotizing fasciitis does not involve muscle, whereas gas gangrene has extensive muscle involvement.

Associated Clinical Features

Gout is an inflammatory disease characterized by deposition of sodium urate monohydrate crystals in cartilage, subchondral bone, and periarticular structures. Gout is most frequently associated with inborn errors of metabolism, myeloproliferative disorders, leukemia, hemolytic anemia, glycogen storage disease, hypertension, diabetes mellitus, obesity, heavy alcohol consumption, and worsening renal function (gouty nephropathy). An acute attack is characterized by sudden onset of monarticular arthritis, most commonly in the metatarsophalangeal (MTP) joint of the great toe (named after the bad-tempered virgin foot goddess "Podagra") (Fig. 12.9). While the great toe MTP is the most common site, gout can occur in other joints (Figs. 12.10, 12.11). The deposits of crystals in the tissues about the joint in gout produce a chronic inflammatory response termed a *tophus*. Swelling, erythema, and tenderness are common.

In pseudogout, calcium pyrophosphate dihydrate (rod- or rhombus-shaped, weakly birefringent) crystals are deposited. Pseudogout is most frequently seen in association with hyperparathyroidism, hemochromatosis, hypophosphatasia, hypomagnesemia, myxedematous hypothyroidism, and ochronosis. Although any joint may be involved, knees and wrists are the most common sites. After joint deposition, the crystals are phagocytized by leukocytes that release proteolytic enzymes. The acute presenting signs and symptoms are identical with those of gout, but formation of tophi is not seen with pseudogout. Fever, pain, and erythema are common to both entities.

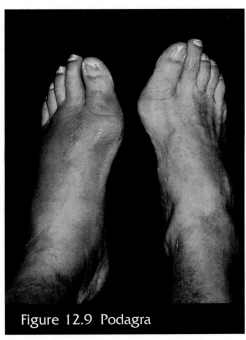

Figure 12.9 Podagra

Podagra denotes gouty inflammation of the first MTP joint. Note the swelling and erythema of the left first MTP. (Courtesy of Kevin J. Knoop, MD, MS.)

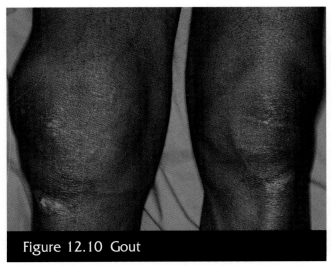

Figure 12.10 Gout

Large tophi of gout located in and around the right knee. (Courtesy of Daniel L. Savitt, MD.)

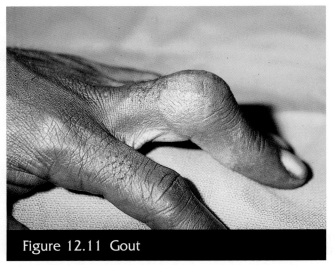

Figure 12.11 Gout

The finger is an unusual site for gouty arthritis. Examination of the synovial fluid confirmed the diagnosis. (Courtesy of Alan B. Storrow, MD.)

Differential Diagnosis

Cellulitis and septic arthritis must be excluded. In the cell count of the synovial fluid obtained from an inflamed joint, 2,000 to 50,000 WBCs with polymophonuclear neutrophil leukocyte (PMN) predominance is expected. Rheumatoid arthritis, sarcoidosis, hyperparathyroidism, cellulitis, septic arthritis, and traumatic injury may present much like crystalline-induced synovitis. The diagnosis is made by seeing negatively birefringent urate crystals or rod (or rhombus)-shaped, weakly birefringent calcium pyrophosphate dihydrate crystals on polarized microscopy (see Fig. 21.6A–C) with negative Gram's stain and cultures. Punched out lesions on subchondral bone may be seen on radiography in chronic tophaceous gout. Chondrocalcinosis may be seen in pseudogout.

Emergency Department Treatment and Disposition

Nonsteroidal anti-inflammatory medications are used with excellent results in the acute setting (e.g., indomethacin, 50 mg PO tid if renal function is normal), along with joint immobilization and rest. Colchicine is a reasonable alternative, but it often has side effects such as nausea, vomiting, and diarrhea. It is also associated with serious toxicity, including bone marrow suppression, neuropathy, myopathy, and death (particularly when given intravenously). Intramuscular injection of adrenocorticotropic hormone (ACTH, 40 to 80 U IM or SC) or steroids may be used in patients with contraindications to colchicine and nonsteroidal anti-inflammatory medications. Intraarticular injection of steroids will alleviate symptoms rapidly without systemic side effects. Allopurinol or probenecid are used in the chronic management of gout and play no role in acute treatment.

Clinical Pearls

1. Most (90%) of patients with crystalline-induced synovitis are male and older than 40 years.
2. Serum urate may be elevated or normal during acute episode.
3. Polyarticular presentation becomes increasingly more common with long-standing disease.
4. Acute gouty arthritis attacks may be triggered by minor trauma, diuretic or salicylate use, alcohol abuse, or dietary indiscretion.

Associated Clinical Features

This painful condition is the result of impingement and puncture of the medial or lateral nail fold epithelium by the nail plate. Tenderness and swelling of the nail fold is followed by granulation tissue growth causing sharp pain, erythema, and further swelling (Fig. 12.12). If not promptly treated, the granulation tissue becomes epithelialized, preventing elevation of the nail above the medial or lateral nail groove. Often there is secondary bacterial or fungal infection.

Differential Diagnosis

Paronychia, felon, and benign or malignant mass should be considered in the differential diagnosis of an ingrown toenail.

Emergency Department Treatment and Disposition

Early: Elevation of the nail out of nail fold and placement of gauze under nail to prevent contact, in conjunction with warm soaks, is the initial mode of therapy. *Late*: Surgical management involves removal of part of the nail and the inflamed tissue and sometimes destruction of the involved nail matrix. In the ED, the lateral portion of the affected nail is removed after digital block followed by packing of the paronychial fold with petroleum gauze or other nonadherent dressing. Dressing changes should be done daily, with follow-up by a podiatrist until growth of the nail plate is complete. The destruction of the nail matrix is required only in patients with recurrent infected ingrown toenails and is not part of ED routine management.

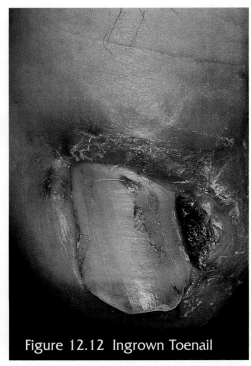

Figure 12.12 Ingrown Toenail

An ingrown toenail on the medial aspect of the left great toe. (Courtesy of Frank Birinyi, MD.)

Clinical Pearls

1. Ingrown toenail is most common in the great toe, is associated with tight-fitting footwear, and may result from improper nail trimming (i.e., cutting the nail too short).
2. Antibiotics are indicated only if cellulitis is suspected, the patient is diabetic, or there is significant peripheral vascular disease.
3. Use of antibiotics is not a substitute for surgical excision and will result in only transient improvement of symptoms.

Associated Clinical Features

Inflammation of lymphatic channels in the subcutaneous tissues is commonly caused by the spread of local bacterial infection. Group A streptococcus is the most frequently implicated agent. Lymphangitis is characterized by red linear streaks (Figs. 12.13 and 12.14) extending from the site of infection (e.g., finger, toe) to regional lymph nodes (e.g., axilla, groin). The lymph nodes are often enlarged and tender. There may be associated peripheral edema of the involved extremity. Lymphangitis may develop within 24 to 48 h of the initial infection.

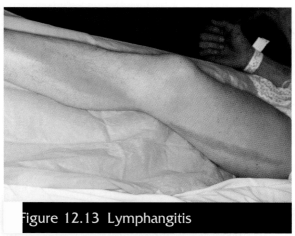

Figure 12.13 Lymphangitis

Severe lymphangitis is seen in the lower extremity. The red streak extends from the ankle to the groin and follows lymphatic channels. In this case, the site of infection was the great toe. (Courtesy of Liudvikas Jagminas, MD.)

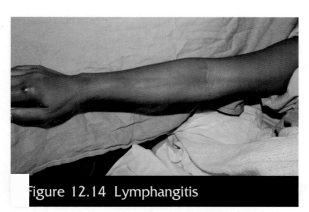

Figure 12.14 Lymphangitis

The lymphangitis extends from the wrist to the upper arm. Lymphangitis in the upper extremity commonly arises from nail biting. (Courtesy of Daniel L. Savitt, MD.)

Differential Diagnosis

Cellulitis, trauma, and superficial thrombophlebitis are in the differential diagnosis of lymphangitis.

Emergency Department Treatment and Disposition

Rest, elevation, and immobilization in addition to antibiotics are the mainstays of treatment. Lymphangitis may be treated with oral antibiotics in afebrile patients who are not immunocompromised. Coverage for *Streptococcus* and *Staphylococcus* is appropriate. Toxic-appearing patients require admission for parenteral antibiotics. Any patient sent home with oral antibiotics should be followed up in 24 to 48 h. Patients who subsequently do not show improvement require admission for parenteral antibiotic therapy.

Clinical Pearls

1. Consider *Pasteurella multocida* with cat bites, *Spirillum minus* with rat bites, and *Mycobacterium marinum* in association with swimming pools and aquaria.
2. Chronic lymphangitis may be associated with mycotic, mycobacterial, and filarial infection.
3. In Africa and Southeast Asia, filariasis (*Wuchereria bancrofti*) is the most common etiologic agent.

Associated Clinical Features

Lymphedema occurs from obstruction of lymphatic channels and is associated with malignancy, radiation, trauma, surgery, inflammation, infection, parasitic invasion, paralysis, renal insufficiency, congestive heart failure, cirrhosis, and malnutrition. Lymphedema is characterized by painless pitting edema (Fig. 12.15), fatigue, increase in limb size—particularly during the day, and presence of lymph vesicles. The skin becomes thickened and brown in the late stages.

Differential Diagnosis

Cellulitis, deep venous thrombosis (DVT), lymphangitis, traumatic hematoma, right heart failure, tuberculosis, and lymphogranuloma venereum should be considered when the diagnosis of lymphedema is made. Subcutaneous dye injection, radiographic lymphography, and radionuclide lymph clearance may be used to aid in the diagnosis.

Emergency Department Treatment and Disposition

Control of edema with elevation, pneumatic compression boots and firm elastic stockings, maintenance of healthy skin, and avoidance of cellulitis and lymphangitis are the mainstays of symptomatic treatment. Treatment of the underlying disease may be curative.

Clinical Pearls

1. Swelling usually starts distally and progresses proximally.
2. The dorsum of the toes and feet is always involved in lymphedema, unlike other causes of edema.
3. Careful examination for right heart failure and screening for renal insufficiency should be completed for all patients with lymphedema.

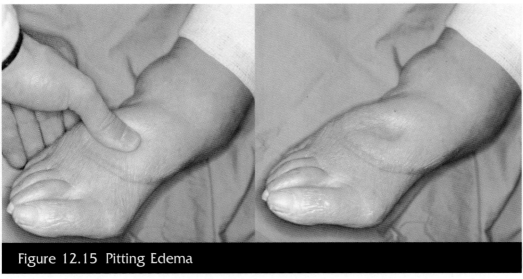

Figure 12.15 Pitting Edema

Pitting edema is seen in a woman with lymphedema of the lower extremities. Note how the impression of the thumb remains on the foot. (Courtesy of Selim Suner, MD, MS.)

Associated Clinical Features

Bursitis is a reaction in a fluid-filled synovial sac, commonly over the subacromial (Fig. 12.16), prepatellar (Fig. 12.17), olecranon, or hip trochanteric bursa. It is associated with repetitive motion, trauma, or infection. The fluid collection may be bacterial (septic bursitis, Fig. 12.18), gouty, or, most commonly, inflammatory. Bursitis is characterized by pain, tenderness, and swelling. There may be erythema, warmth, and limited range of motion. It is critical to differentiate septic from benign inflammation as well as bursal from intraarticular involvement. Typically, intraarticular arthritis is associated with pain on minor range of motion, while bursitis discomfort occurs with the stretching of the skin and synovial sac at the more extreme ranges of joint movement. The prepatellar bursa is anterior to the infrapatellar tendon. Bursitis in this area is often the result of repetitive kneeling ("housemaid's knee").

Differential Diagnosis

Septic arthritis, crystal synovitis, fracture, contusion, and traumatic effusion may mimic this condition. Since bursitis does not involve the intraarticular space, signs and symptoms should be isolated to the bursal area. When this differentiation is difficult by history and examination, fluid aspiration and analysis of the bursa or joint for cell count, Gram stain, protein, glucose, and polarized microscopy (see "Crystal-Induced Synovitis," above) may be helpful. Fluid with > 50,000 cells per cubic millimeter, polymorphonuclear neutrophil predominance, increased protein, reduced glucose, and a positive Gram's stain are associated with bacterial infection.

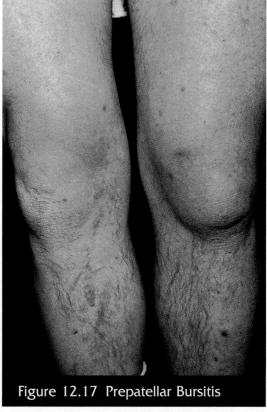

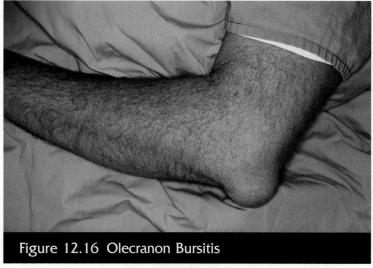

Figure 12.16 Olecranon Bursitis

Olecranon bursitis is evident in this flexed elbow. (Courtesy of Selim Suner, MD, MS.)

Figure 12.17 Prepatellar Bursitis

Local bursal swelling is evident over the left knee. (Courtesy of Kevin J. Knoop, MD, MS.)

Emergency Department Treatment and Disposition

Rest, bulky compression dressings, and nonsteroidal anti-inflammatory medications are used for inflammatory bursitis. Bursal injection of local anesthetics (e.g., 2 to 3 mL of lidocaine or bupivacaine) mixed with corticosteroids (e.g., 1 mL of betamethasone or methylprednisolone) can also be considered. Reducing the volume of the inflammatory effusion by aspiration may provide temporary relief, although the effusion has a propensity to recur. Septic bursitis requires aspiration, gram-positive antibiotic coverage, and consideration of open incision and drainage. Most patients can be treated as outpatients with close follow-up.

In contrast, an intraarticular infection requires aspiration, antibiotics, and admission for consideration of open drainage. Aspiration and blood cultures prior to antibiotic administration are helpful to guide therapy toward specific organisms. Inflammatory arthritis may be treated with anti-inflammatories, and intraarticular anesthetics and steroids may be considered.

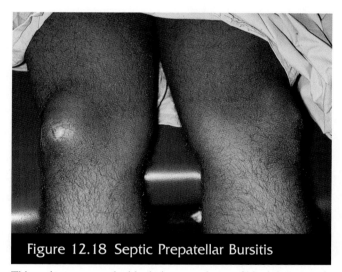

Clinical Pearls

1. The most important diagnostic issue is differentiation between bursitis and a septic joint.
2. Septic joint infections in patients with cancer, who are taking corticosteroids, or who are intravenous drug users may have lower synovial fluid leukocyte counts ($< 30,000/mm^3$) then usual ($> 50,000/mm^3$).
3. Incision and drainage are not recommended for routine inflammatory bursitis.

Figure 12.18 Septic Prepatellar Bursitis

This patient presented with obvious purulence of his right prepatellar bursal sac. Aspiration confirmed septic bursitis. (Courtesy of Alan B. Storrow, MD.)

Associated Clinical Features

Palmar space infections occur within the deep soft-tissue planes of the hand and involve the mid-palmar space, the web spaces (collar button abscess), and the thenar (Fig. 12.19) or hypothenar spaces. These infections commonly arise from callus, fissures, puncture wounds to the palm, and rupture of flexor tenosynovitis of the digits. The palm loses its concavity, and there is dorsal swelling. In addition, tenderness, erythema, warmth, and fluctuance are evident in the palm. A *thenar space* infection is characterized by swelling over the thenar eminence and pain with abduction of the thumb. With a *midpalmar space* infection, motion is limited and painful for the middle and ring fingers. *Hypothenar space* infections are extremely rare. A high morbidity is associated with these infections.

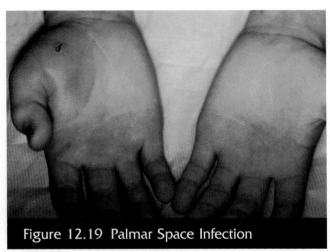

Figure 12.19 Palmar Space Infection

Thenar space infection following injury to the thumb. In this palmar view, erythema and swelling in the right thenar area and abduction of the thumb are evident. (Courtesy of Richard Zienowicz, MD.)

Differential Diagnosis

Cellulitis, local traumatic injury, fractures, and soft tissue mass are included in the differential diagnosis of palmar space infections.

Emergency Department Treatment and Disposition

All deep space infections of the hand should be managed by a hand surgeon. Prompt incision and drainage in the operating room is necessary for the best outcome. Frequently, both palmar and dorsal incisions are necessary. Loose packing and antibiotic treatment follow surgery. Parenteral antibiotics against *Staphylococcus aureus* as well as anaerobes should be started in the ED.

Clinical Pearls

1. Palmar space infections may cause swelling on the dorsal hand.
2. In general, erythema, fluctuance, or tenderness are seen on the palmar aspect with very little seen dorsally.

Associated Clinical Features

Tenosynovitis, an inflammation of the tendon and the surrounding synovial sheath, is characterized by pain and tenderness. Pyogenic flexor tenosynovitis is infection of the tendon sheath from hematogenous origin, puncture wounds, or local extension. Tenosynovitis is characterized by the four signs of Kanavel (described for a finger flexor tendon): mild flexion contracture; fusiform swelling along the volar finger surface; tenderness along the entire tendon sheath, especially at the palmar surface of the metacarpophalangeal (MCP) joint; and severe pain with passive extension (Fig. 12.20). Tenosynovitis may be complicated by fibrosis and adhesions leading to stiffness, loss of function, and tendon necrosis from destruction of the blood supply.

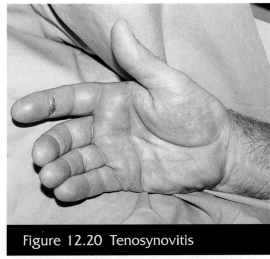

Figure 12.20 Tenosynovitis

This patient presented with flexor tenosynovitis of the index finger after a laceration at the level of the palmar DIP joint. Note the fusiform swelling and redness extending to the thenar eminence. (Courtesy of Selim Suner, MD, MS.)

Differential Diagnosis

Cellulitis, traumatic injury, lymphangitis, osteomyelitis, septic arthritis, carpometacarpal arthritis, and allergic reactions may mimic some of the signs and symptoms of tenosynovitis.

Emergency Department Treatment and Disposition

It is difficult to distinguish infectious and noninfectious etiologies early in the course of this illness. Early (24 to 48 h) management of tenosynovitis thought to be noninfectious is accomplished with immobilization and nonsteroidal anti-inflammatory medications. Parenteral antibiotics, rest, immobilization, elevation, compressive dressing, and early consultation with a hand surgeon for incision and drainage within 24 to 48 h are mandated with pyogenic flexor tenosynovitis.

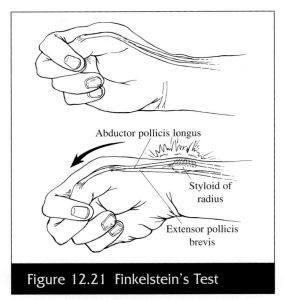

Figure 12.21 Finkelstein's Test

Pain over the radial styloid is elicited with ulnar deviation of the wrist as shown.

Clinical Pearls

1. *Staphylococcus aureus* is the most common organism, but *Streptococcus* as well as gram-negative and anaerobic organisms may also be responsible.
2. The most specific sign of tenosynovitis is pain with passive extension of the digit.
3. The abductor pollicis longus (APL), the extensor pollicis brevis (EPB), and the wrist are the most common sites for tenosynovitis.
4. Finkelstein's test is used to support the diagnosis of de Quervain's tenosynovitis (Fig. 12.21). The patient is instructed to make a fist with the thumb tucked inside the other fingers. The wrist is passively deviated to the ulnar side. Sharp pain along the APL and EPB tendons denotes a positive Finkelstein's test and is strong evidence of de Quervain's tenosynovitis.

Associated Clinical Features

Thrombophlebitis is superficial thrombosis and inflammation of veins or varicosities characterized by redness, tenderness, and palpable, indurated, cordlike venous segments (Fig. 12.22). Common causes of thrombophlebitis are intravenous catheter insertion, irritant solutions through the intravenous line, and trauma. There is little risk of embolism when this condition is associated with varicose veins or superficial veins distal to the popliteal fossa; however, pulmonary embolism can occur secondary to propagation of the thrombus of more proximal veins into the deep venous system.

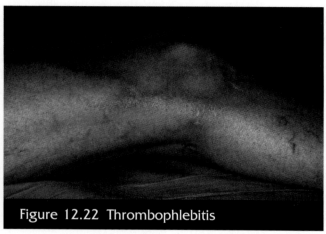

Figure 12.22 Thrombophlebitis

This photograph shows thrombophlebitis of the superficial veins in the leg. The thrombosed veins are erythematous, close to the surface, and palpable. (Courtesy of Lawrence B. Stack, MD.)

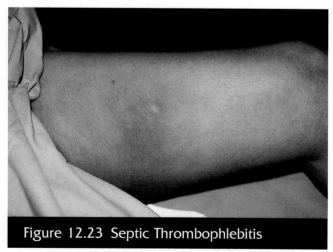

Figure 12.23 Septic Thrombophlebitis

Thrombophlebitis may be complicated by bacterial infection. Note the purulence associated with the erythematous thrombosed veins. (Courtesy of Lawrence B. Stack, MD.)

Differential Diagnosis

Septic superficial thrombophlebitis (Fig. 12.23), lymphangitis, deep venous thrombosis (DVT), and cellulitis should be included in the differential diagnosis of thrombophlebitis. The patient must be evaluated for the possibility of deep venous thrombosis if no underlying cause of superficial thrombosis is elucidated.

Emergency Department Treatment and Disposition

Elevation with warm compresses, rest, and analgesia is sufficient treatment for uncomplicated superficial thrombophlebitis. Superficial thrombophlebitis and involvement of the saphenofemoral or iliofemoral system requires admission to the hospital with anticoagulation and treatment as a DVT. Also, admission to the hospital is warranted if there is extensive involvement, septic signs, progression of symptoms despite treatment, or severe inflammatory reactions.

Clinical Pearls

1. Thrombophlebitis of the greater saphenous vein may be confused with lymphangitis, since the lymphatic drainage from the leg runs along the vein.
2. This condition is frequently associated with malignancy—an association is known as Trousseau's syndrome.
3. Since lymphatic drainage follows the greater saphenous vein, Doppler studies or venography may be needed to distinguish superficial thrombophlebitis from lymphangitis in this area.

PARONYCHIA

Associated Clinical Features

Paronychia is the most common infection seen in the hand and is characterized by infection and pus accumulation along a lateral nail fold. Paronychia may spread to involve the eponychium (Fig. 12.24) at the base of the nail and the opposite nail fold if untreated. *Staphylococcus aureus* is the most frequently implicated organism.

Differential Diagnosis

Felon, dactylitis, herpetic whitlow, hydrofluoric acid burn, and traumatic injury should be considered in making the diagnosis of paronychia.

Emergency Department Treatment and Disposition

If paronychia is recognized early, warm soaks with or without oral antibiotics may be sufficient. After 2 to 3 days, there may be sufficient pus accumulation along the eponychial fold to warrant incision and drainage. After digital block, a longitudinal incision is made along the eponychial fold. If the affected portion begins under the nail, removal of the proximal nail may be necessary. Another technique is elevation of the infected eponychium and lateral nail fold with a number 11 scalpel blade. Incisions should be packed open with gauze (removed in 24 to 48 h). Oral antibiotics should be prescribed, and the finger should be reevaluated in 2 to 3 days.

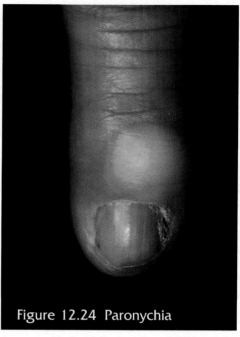

Figure 12.24 Paronychia

A paronychia involving one lateral fold and the eponychium. There is swelling, erythema, and tenderness on the dorsum of the distal phalanx. (Courtesy of Frank Birinyi, MD.)

Clinical Pearls

1. Paronychia is typically associated with nail biting, manicure trauma, and small foreign bodies.
2. Superinfection with fungal agents may occur with immunocompromised patients or neglected paronychia.
3. Damage to the germinal matrix during excision of the nail plate results in nail deformity.
4. It is important to distinguish a paronychia from herpetic whitlow, where incision and drainage is contraindicated.

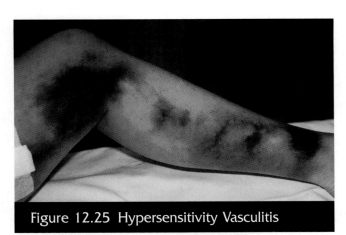

Figure 12.25 Hypersensitivity Vasculitis

The palpable purpura of a patient with hypersensitivity vasculitis secondary to new use of a nonsteroidal anti-inflammatory medication. (Courtesy of Lawrence B. Stack, MD.)

Associated Clinical Features

This patient presented with discrete palpable purpuric lesions with central necrosis (Fig. 12.25) surrounded by a rim of erythema. Biopsies of the lesions demonstrated leukocytoclastic vasculitis consistent with hypersensitivity vasculitis.

The eruption typically begins in or is limited to the lower extremities. The palpable, nonblanching purpura or petechiae are usually secondary to a primary vasculitis or an embolic event which activates complement proteins. These proteins cause small blood vessel wall segmental inflammation, necrosis, and fibrin deposition, much as in Henoch-Schönlein purpura (HSP). Features typical of this problem include self-limited palpable purpura, adult age, equal sexual incidence, and lack of other examination or laboratory abnormalities. There may be systemic involvement of the muscles, joints, GI tract, or kidney as well as pruritus and pain. The duration can be acute (especially drug-induced), subacute, or chronic.

Hypersensitivity vasculitis is more likely if the patient has recently received a new drug, or one known to cause purpura (Fig. 12.25). It can also be caused by sensitivity to infectious antigens. The cause is idiopathic in approximately 40 to 60% of patients.

Differential Diagnosis

The differential of purpura must include infections (bacterial and viral), hematologic abnormalities (e.g., thrombotic thrombocytopenic purpura, idiopathic thrombocytopenic purpura, disseminated intravascular coagulation), collagen-vascular diseases (e.g., systemic lupus erythematosus, rheumatoid arthritis, Sjögren's syndrome), and neoplasm. The primary vasculitides—such as HSP, polyarteritis nodosa, Wegener's granulomatosis, and temporal arteritis—must also be considered.

The diagnostic criteria for hypersensitivity vasculitis includes at least three of the following: age >16 years, related medication, palpable purpura, maculopapular rash, and appropriate biopsy.

Emergency Department Treatment and Disposition

Since the differentiation of hypersensitivity vasculitis with a vasculitis of bacterial origin is often difficult, initial antibiotic therapy, blood cultures, and admission are usually indicated. Multiple episodes, especially if idiopathic, can occur. The suspected medication should be discontinued immediately, and the use of steroids can be considered. Other treatment modalities include the use of immunosuppressive medications and plasmapheresis.

Clinical Pearls

1. Diagnosis of the primary vasculitides is almost always made histopathologically.
2. There may be overlap between the causes of purpura.
3. Self-limited or irreversible damage may occur to the kidneys.
4. Synonyms for this entity include *necrotizing vasculitis* and *allergic vasculitis*.

Associated Clinical Features

Thrombosis of the subclavian vein (Paget–Von Schroetter syndrome) is an uncommon condition usually of iatrogenic origin. It may also be seen in young patients following exercise and results from compression injury to the subclavian or axillary vein from a narrow thoracic outlet (effort thrombosis). Symptoms of pain, discomfort, and tightness or swelling in the arm are manifest within a day of the thrombosis (Fig. 12.26). Pitting edema develops in the fingers, hand, and forearm. There is no arterial insufficiency, and the pulses are palpable. There is a 15% risk of developing pulmonary embolism from thrombosis of veins in the upper extremity; however, large or fatal emboli from this source are very rare. Ascending venography is the gold standard for diagnosis. Duplex scan, impedance plethysmography, and Doppler studies are also used, but their accuracy has not been studied in the upper extremity.

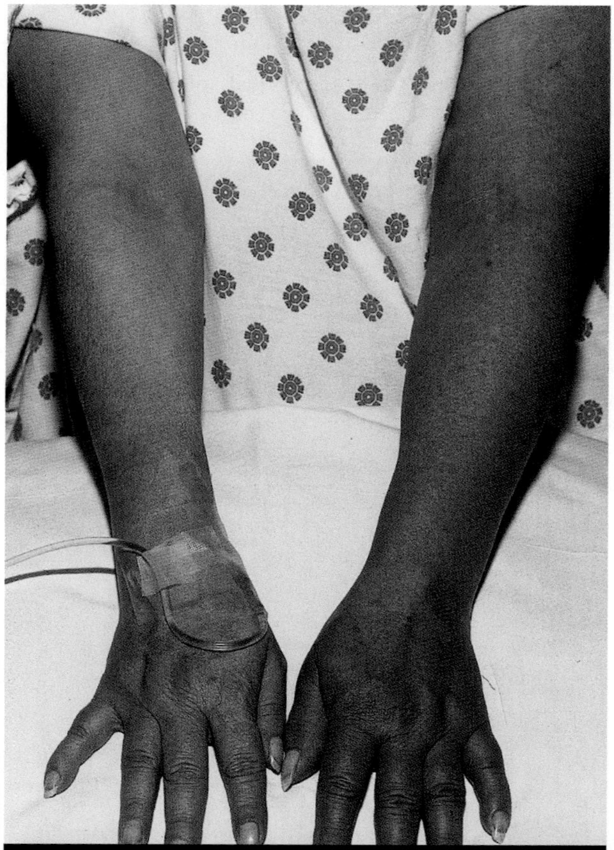

Differential Diagnosis

Superior vena cava syndrome, trauma to the upper extremity, congestive heart failure, angioedema, and lymphatic obstruction must be considered in the differential diagnosis.

Emergency Department Treatment and Disposition

Treatment consists of elevation, local heat, analgesia, and anticoagulation with intravenous heparin for patients presenting with long-term thrombosis. Patients should be admitted to the hospital. In cases of acute thrombosis (within 5 days of symptom onset), the treatment is thrombolysis with direct catheter infusion of urokinase or streptokinase. Surgical thrombectomy has also been employed. Operative correction of anatomic abnormalities should be accomplished to prevent long-term morbidity.

Figure 12.26 Subclavian Vein Thrombosis

Left subclavian vein thrombosis is manifest in this patient by swelling of the left upper extremity. (Courtesy of Frank Birinyi, MD.)

Clinical Pearls

1. Swelling of the neck and face signifies thrombosis of the superior vena cava.
2. The superficial veins in the upper extremity are often distended and do not collapse when the arm is elevated.
3. There is a greater incidence of subclavian vein thrombosis in men and in the right arm.
4. There may be late sequelae related to the thrombus, such as pain, recurrent swelling, and early fatigue of the upper extremity.
5. Balloon angioplasty has been used to correct stenosis of the subclavian vein.

Associated Clinical Features

Cervical radiculopathy is often caused by compression of a nerve root by a laterally bulging or herniated intervertebral disk. Osteoarthritis and spondylosis may also cause radiculopathy in the cervical spine. Pain results from injury to the nerve roots and nerves innervating the dura, ligaments, facet joints, and bone. Common clinical features associated with cervical radiculopathy include pain, paresthesia, and root signs (sensory loss, lower motor neuron muscle weakness, impaired reflexes, and trophic changes). The pain is sharp and stabbing and worse with cough, and it radiates over the shoulder down the arm. There is often numbness and tingling following a dermatomal distribution. Root signs may be found corresponding to anatomic distribution of nerves (e.g., triceps muscle weakness, pinprick deficit along the middle finger, and atrophy with loss of triceps jerk associated with C-7 radiculopathy). Magnetic resonance imaging (MRI) and computed tomography (CT) myelography are the commonly used modalities to distinguish cervical radiculopathy from disk and bone disease. Electromyelography studies may also be helpful in ruling out other disease processes.

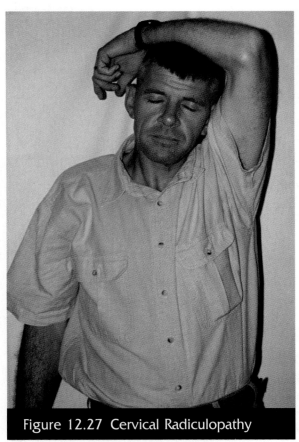

Figure 12.27 Cervical Radiculopathy

This is the classic position of relief for cervical radicular pain. This patient presented with severe pain in the neck with radiation to the extremity. The only way the patient was able to get relief was by holding his arm over his head in the position shown. This patient has a C5–C6 herniated nucleus pulposus. (Courtesy of Kevin J. Knoop, MD, MS.)

Differential Diagnosis

Trauma, myelopathy, plexopathy, neurofibromatosis, metastatic tumor infiltration of nerve roots, neoplasm, shingles, and central cord syndrome should be considered in the differential diagnosis of cervical radiculopathy.

Emergency Department Treatment and Disposition

The mainstay of ED treatment is pain control and referral to an orthopedic surgeon or neurosurgeon. Since prolonged nerve root compression can lead to permanent neurologic deficits, immediate referral is necessary for progressive neurologic signs. Patients with intractable pain, progressive weakness in the upper extremities, and myelopathy should be admitted to the hospital.

Clinical Pearls

1. Most radiculopathies resulting from cervical disk disease is seen in the 30 to 60 year age group and in the C-5 to C-7 region.
2. Risk factors for cervical radiculopathy include heavy lifting, cigarette smoking, frequent diving from a board, and prior trauma to the neck.
3. Patients with acute cervical radiculopathy may present with their upper extremity supported by their head to counteract the cervical root distraction caused by the weight of their dependent extremity (Fig. 12.27).

Associated Clinical Features

Digital clubbing results from increased soft tissue density at the tips of the fingers, particularly on the dorsum. Associated with the increased tissue mass is enhanced blood flow, excessive curvature of the fingernails, and hyperemic and swollen skin folds around the fingernail (Fig. 12.28). Clubbing may also be seen in the toes. The mechanism underlying clubbing is not known, but it is postulated that the end result is dilatation of the distal digital blood vessels with soft tissue hypertrophy. Clubbing may be hereditary, idiopathic, or acquired and is associated with multiple medical conditions including carcinoma, intrathoracic sepsis, bacterial endocarditis, cyanotic congenital heart disease, esophageal disorders, cirrhosis, inflammatory bowel disease, pulmonary disorders, atrial myxoma, repeated pregnancies, and pachydermoperiostosis. The incidence of clubbing with each of these conditions is variable. Digital clubbing may be reversible in certain disease processes.

Differential Diagnosis

Hypertrophic osteoarthropathy, infection, and trauma should be considered in the differential diagnosis of clubbing.

Emergency Department Treatment and Disposition

Treatment of the underlying condition is indicated. The disposition depends on the underlying diagnosis and condition of the patient.

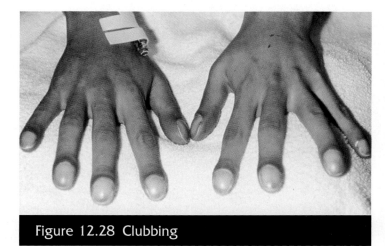

Figure 12.28 Clubbing

Marked digital clubbing can be seen in this patient. Note the hyperemia in the skin folds around the nail. (Courtesy of Alan B. Storrow, MD.)

Clinical Pearls

1. Bone radiographs can be used to diagnose hypertrophic osteoarthropathy. Subperiosteal formation of bone is seen in the distal diaphyses of long bones.
2. Patients rarely recognize clubbing in their own fingers even if the condition is marked.

Associated Clinical Features

Phlegmasia alba dolens (painful white leg, or milk leg) is caused by extensive thrombosis of the iliofemoral veins and characterized by pitting edema of the entire lower extremity, tenderness in the inguinal area, and a pale extremity due to reflex spasm of the femoral artery. Phlegmasia cerulea dolens (painful blue leg, Fig. 12.29) arises from thrombosis of the veins in the lower extremity including the perforating and collateral veins resulting in a cool, painful, swollen, tense, and cyanotic lower extremity, occasionally with bullae formation. Compartment syndrome and gangrene may follow.

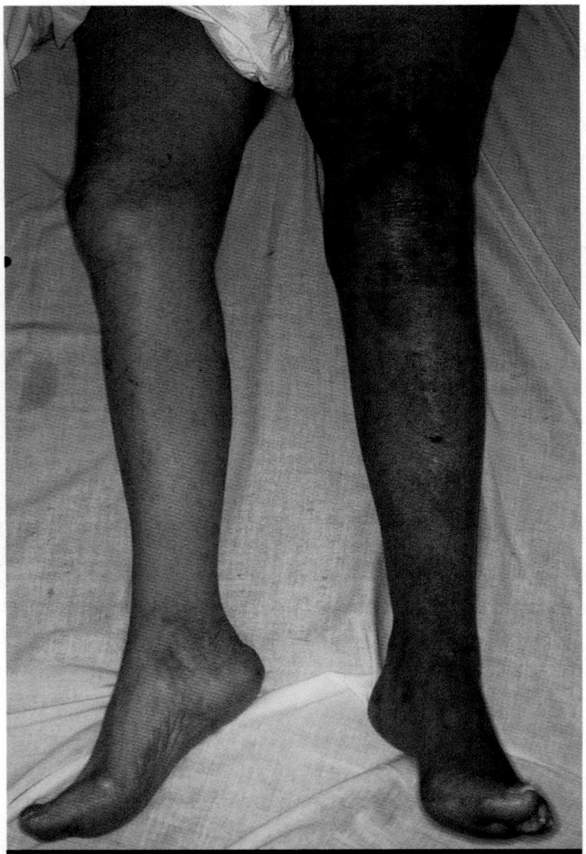

Figure 12.29 Phlegmasia Dolens

Phlegmasia cerulea dolens of the left lower extremity. Note the bluish discoloration and swelling. (Courtesy of Daniel L. Savitt, MD.)

Differential Diagnosis

Arterial insufficiency or thrombosis, aortic dissection, abdominal aortic aneurysm, deep venous thrombosis, cellulitis, and lymphedema may mimic these conditions. Doppler ultrasound, impedance plethysmography, and venography (most accurate for determining extent) are used in the diagnosis.

Emergency Department Treatment and Disposition

Systemic anticoagulation with intravenous heparin is indicated for this condition. If there is no improvement in 12 to 24 h, then iliofemoral venous thrombosis should be suspected. The role of intravenous thrombolytic therapy is controversial.

Clinical Pearls

1. Pregnancy is one risk factor for phlegmasia alba dolens.
2. Forty-four percent of patients with phlegmasia cerulea dolens have an underlying malignancy.
3. Phlegmasia dolens is seen in fewer than 10% of patients with venous thrombosis.
4. Hypotension may result from venous pooling of blood in the lower extremity and diminished venous return to the heart.
5. Petechiae on the skin of the lower extremity may be present.

Associated Clinical Features

Porphyrias are problems associated with enzymatic defects in heme biosynthesis. Porphyria cutanea tarda (PCT) presents as a condition of fragile skin and vesicles found on the dorsum of the hands, especially after trauma. The classic symptoms are easily traumatized skin, leading to blisters in sun-exposed areas, erosions, milia, and hypertrichosis (Fig. 12.30). It may be induced by ethanol, estrogens, oral contraceptives, iron overload, and certain environmental exposures. The typical bullae and erosions may also occur in other areas, especially the feet and nose. In contrast to other porphyrias, PCT is not associated with life-threatening respiratory failure, abdominal pain, or peripheral autonomic neuropathies. Confirmation of the diagnosis requires 24-h urine testing for various porphyrins.

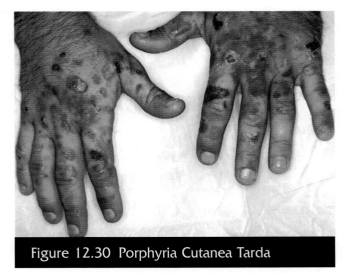

Figure 12.30 Porphyria Cutanea Tarda

Blisters and erosions of porphyria cutanea tarda. (Courtesy of Selim Suner, MD, MS.)

Differential Diagnosis

Other forms of porphyria, other bullous diseases, systemic lupus erythematosus (SLE), sarcoidosis, and Sjögren's syndrome must be considered.

Emergency Department Treatment and Disposition

Laboratory examination may begin in the ED with blood chemistries, porphyrin studies, and consideration of appropriate biopsies. Treatment includes discontinuation of any drugs that might initiate PCT. Phlebotomy and the use of chloroquine can be considered.

Clinical Pearls

1. PCT is the most common type of porphyria.
2. Examination of the urine may reveal orange-red fluorescence with a Wood's lamp.
3. This condition is sometimes termed *fragile skin*.

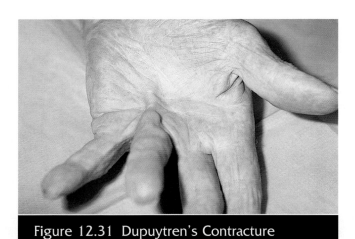

Figure 12.31 Dupuytren's Contracture

This chronic problem is seen at the most common site: the ring finger. (Courtesy of Alan B. Storrow, MD.)

Associated Clinical Features

Dupuytren's contracture results from shortening and fibrotic changes of the subcutaneous tissues of the palm and longitudinal bands of the palmar aponeurosis. It may begin as a nodule and then progress to contracture of a finger or fingers (Fig. 12.31). Usually, this is noted at the metacarpophalangeal (MCP) joint, but the proximal interphalangeal (PIP) or distal interphalangeal (DIP) joint, may be involved.

Emergency Department Treatment and Disposition

The only effective treatment is surgery. Recurrence and development of a contracture in other areas may occur.

Clinical Pearls

1. The flexor tendons are not involved.
2. The ring and small fingers are the most commonly involved.

Associated Clinical Features

Thrombosis in the venous system results from a disruption of normal hemostasis. As described by Virchow, blood vessel endothelial injury, coagulopathy, and venous stasis contribute to formation of clots in the venous system. Deep venous thrombosis (DVT) is often encountered in patients with intrinsic coagulopathy or impaired fibrinolysis or those who have had recent (within 3 months) surgery or trauma. Other associated conditions include immobilization (e.g., long car or plane trips, bed rest for more than 3 days), increased estrogen (pregnancy, oral contraceptive pills, with tobacco smoking), cancer, a history of prior DVT, inflammatory disease processes, or coronary artery disease. Intravenous catheters are also a major cause of DVT, particularly in the upper extremity.

It is clinically difficult to tell superficial thrombophlebitis from DVT without diagnostic studies. Unilateral swelling and tenderness, classically in the calf and thigh, characterize DVT (Fig. 12.32). Associated erythema, redness and warmth may lead to a misdiagnosis of cellulitis. Homans' sign—pain elicited with dorsiflexion of the foot—is not reliable. Even though venography is considered to be the gold standard test, venous Doppler ultrasonography is commonly used as the test of choice. Venography is painful, uses a dye load, and itself may cause DVT. Magnetic resonance imaging (MRI) is highly sensitive and specific but is costly and not readily available.

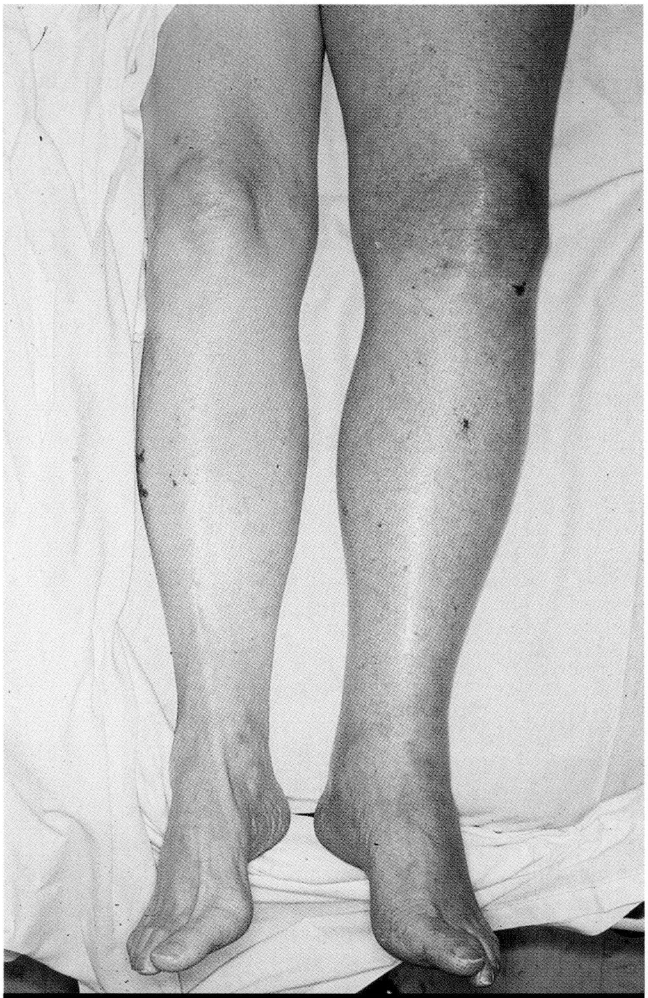

Differential Diagnosis

Cellulitis is an important differential diagnosis. Fracture, lymphedema, heart failure, compartment syndrome, myositis, arthritis, and superficial phlebitis should also be considered when DVT is diagnosed. A Baker's cyst is a herniation of the synovial membrane through the posterior knee capsule. While the acute clinical presentation is swelling behind the knee, rupture of a Baker's cyst may present with unilateral swelling similar to DVT (Fig. 12.33).

Figure 12.32 Deep Venous Thrombosis

This patient has some classic findings of left lower extremity DVT: swelling, erythema, pain, and tenderness. (Courtesy of Kevin J. Knoop, MD, MS.)

Emergency Department Treatment and Disposition

Classic treatment of DVT has been heparin anticoagulation and admission for warfarin loading. With the development of low-molecular-weight heparins (LMWH), one may consider a subgroup for LMWH administration and outpatient treatment. Careful risk stratification, preexisting protocols, and close medical follow-up are necessary for successful outpatient treatment. Thrombolysis should be reserved for severe cases, where the viability of the extremity is threatened. Although DVT in the calf and superficial veins of the lower extremity do not typically embolize, these thrombi can propagate into the deep venous system and may eventually lead to emboli. Serial diagnostic studies are performed to follow the course of untreated DVT of the distal calf.

Clinical Pearls

1. Weight-based heparin is 80 U/kg followed by 18 U/kg/h.
2. Patients with unexplained DVT should be screened for occult malignancy.
3. Measurement of the calf or Homans' sign should not be used in isolation to rule out DVT.
4. Patients with an unclear diagnosis of cellulitis should have an objective study to rule out DVT.

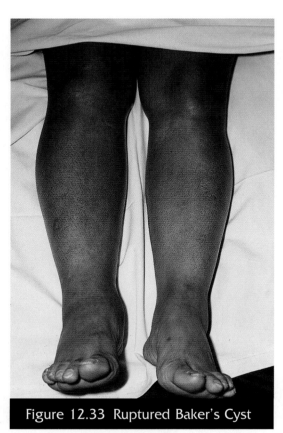

Figure 12.33 Ruptured Baker's Cyst

Comparison of this patient's ankles reveals circumferential swelling around the right side. MRI revealed a ruptured Baker's cyst in the right popliteal fossa. Such a presentation may mimic acute lower extremity DVT. (Courtesy of Lawrence B. Stack, MD.)

Associated Clinical Features

Inorganic arsenic compounds as well as sodium and potassium arsenite and arsenate are found in insecticides and wood preservatives as well as in glass manufacturing. Arsine gas is produced with metal refining, galvanizing, etching, lead plating, and in the silicone microchip industry. Acute arsenic poisoning, the most common cause of acute heavy metal poisoning, is encountered in accidental ingestion, industrial accidents, suicide, and homicide attempts. Low-dose exposure in industry or from contaminated water and food products may lead to chronic poisoning. Arsenic poisoning produces a syndrome involving the skin, hair, nails, GI system, bone marrow, liver, peripheral and central nervous systems, and kidneys. Acute symptoms of arsenic poisoning include violent gastroenteritis, hypotension, prolonged QT interval, seizures, and coma. Other symptoms such as hair loss (Fig. 12.34), raindrop hyperpigmentation, characteristic Mees' lines on the nails (Fig. 12.35), anemia and leukopenia, jaundice, subacute sensorimotor polyneuropathy, paralysis, hematuria, and renal failure are characteristic of chronic arsenic poisoning. Arsine gas exposure results in hemolysis and secondary renal failure. Arsenic binds with tissue sulfhydryl groups, causes direct capillary injury, has direct toxic effects on large organs, and causes uncoupling of oxidative phosphorylation.

Differential Diagnosis

Similar symptoms may be seen with other heavy metal ingestions including thallium toxicity, food-borne toxins, bacterial diarrhea, renal failure, malaria, psoriasis, and Hodgkin's disease.

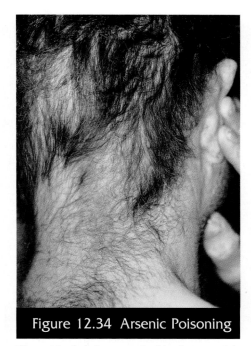

Figure 12.34 Arsenic Poisoning

The patchy hair loss seen in this photograph is from chronic arsenic poisoning. (Courtesy of Selim Suner, MD, MS.)

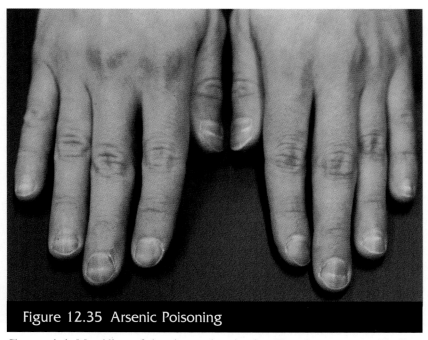

Figure 12.35 Arsenic Poisoning

Characteristic Mees' lines of chronic arsenic poisoning. Note the transverse white lines on all the nails of both hands. Mees' lines are often seen in conjunction with polyneuropathy of arsenic poisoning. (Courtesy of Robert Hoffman, MD.)

Emergency Department Treatment and Disposition

In the setting of acute arsenic poisoning, the first priority is to institute advanced life support measures to stabilize vital signs. Acute ingestion commonly requires resuscitation with intravenous fluids. Attention is directed to hydration status, cardiac monitoring, and gathering routine laboratory data. Standard gastric decontamination techniques, including gastric lavage and administration of activated charcoal, have been recommended. Although activated charcoal adsorbs arsenic poorly, it may be effective against coingestions. Toxicologic consultation should be obtained to determine the choice of chelating agents, which include dimercaprol (BAL), dimercaptosuccinic acid (DMSA), and D-penicillamine. Hemodialysis is indicated in the setting of renal failure. Diagnosis is based on clinical findings and 24-h urine arsenic level greater than 100 μg. CBC, liver function tests, electrolytes, BUN, creatinine, and urinalysis may be helpful in the diagnosis. The level of care is determined by the presentation, but most patients require admission and observation for a minimum of 24 h. A 24-h urine collection should be initiated on all admitted patients.

Clinical Pearls

1. Consider the diagnosis of acute arsenic poisoning in any patient with unexplained hypotension accompanied or preceded by severe gastroenteritis.
2. Consider the diagnosis of chronic arsenic poisoning in any patient with a peripheral neuropathy, typical skin or hair manifestations, or recurrent gastroenteritis.
3. Remote arsenic exposure can be elucidated by obtaining levels in scalp and pubic hair.
4. There is a garlic odor on the breath or skin with arsenic poisoning. 5-Arsenic is absorbed through the skin, lungs, and GI tract and it crosses the placenta.

CHAPTER 13

CUTANEOUS CONDITIONS

Sean P. Collins*

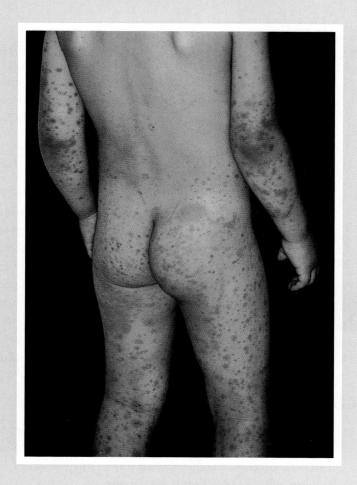

*The author acknowledges Christopher R. Sartori, MD, and Michael B. Brooks, MD, for portions of this chapter written for the first edition of this book.

Associated Clinical Features

Considered a hypersensitivity syndrome, erythema multiforme (EM) presents with characteristic target or iris-shaped papules and vesicobullous plaques (Fig. 13.1). These lesions are frequently cutaneous manifestations of a drug reaction, viral infection, *Mycoplasma,* or malignancy. These plaques are usually symmetric, pruritic, and painful, often involving the mucous membranes and extremities, including the palms and soles. The milder form of the disease has minimal mucosal involvement, no bullae, and no systemic symptoms. Fever, malaise, extensive mucosal involvement, and other constitutional symptoms are noted in the severe form of EM, known as Stevens-Johnson syndrome (see next diagnosis).

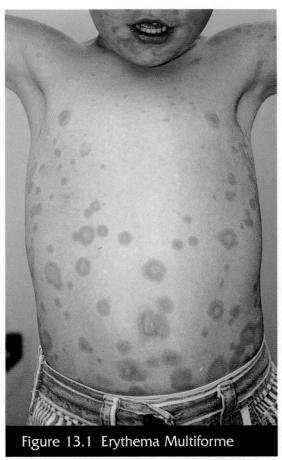

Figure 13.1 Erythema Multiforme

Note the symmetric distribution of the target macules. (Courtesy of Michael Redman, PA-C.)

Differential Diagnosis

The maculopapular presentation may be confused with urticaria or fixed drug eruption, whereas the oral vesicobullous plaques resemble herpetic gingivostomatitis. However, the cutaneous target lesions and their symmetry are typical of EM.

Emergency Department Treatment and Disposition

Elimination of any possible etiology (idiopathic cause noted approximately 50%) and supportive measures to allay the burning and itching are basic to treating this disorder. Milder forms of the disease usually resolve spontaneously within 2 to 3 weeks. Corticosteroids are reserved for the severest presentations. EM minor can be treated on an outpatient basis. However, patients with significant systemic illness and additional eruptions involving the mucosal surfaces (Stevens-Johnson syndrome) may require admission and supportive care.

Clinical Pearls

1. Symmetrically distributed target lesions on the extensor surfaces of the extremities and a lack of significant systemic manifestations are classified as EM minor.
2. Drug-associated EM usually begins within 2 to 3 weeks of initiating therapy. Sulfonamides and penicillins are most often the culprits.
3. Many clinicians treat idiopathic cases empirically with a trial of acyclovir therapy owing to the high incidence of subclinical herpes simplex infection as the cause of the EM.

Associated Clinical Features

Stevens-Johnson syndrome is a severe, rarely fatal variety of erythema multiforme. An abrupt onset of constitutional symptoms precedes the hemorrhagic bullae found on multiple mucosal surfaces and the edematous, erythematous cutaneous plaques (Fig. 13.2). The bullae erode, producing stomatitis, conjunctivitis, vulvovaginitis, or balanitis. Patients appear extremely ill and may develop pneumonia, arthritis, seizures, coma, and hepatic dysfunction. Death, when it occurs, is usually due to overwhelming sepsis.

Differential Diagnosis

Meningococcemia must be considered in the differential diagnosis. The severe involvement of mucous membranes is characteristic of Stevens-Johnson syndrome.

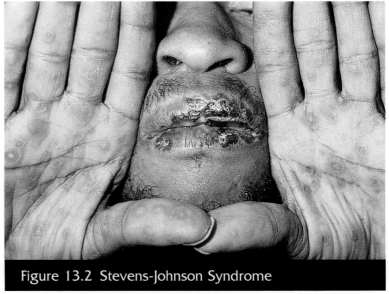

Figure 13.2 Stevens-Johnson Syndrome

Note the target lesions on the hands of this patient, as well as the mucosal involvement on the lips. (Courtesy of Alan B. Storrow, MD.)

Emergency Department Treatment and Disposition

Patients presenting with significant evidence of toxicity should be admitted to the hospital. Supportive measures and selective use of systemic corticosteroids are the cornerstone of therapy.

Clinical Pearls

1. Stevens-Johnson syndrome is self-limited and usually resolves in approximately 1 month.
2. Sulfonamides, penicillins, and anticonvulsants are common causes of Stevens-Johnson syndrome.

Associated Clinical Features

Toxic epidermal necrolysis (TEN) is characterized by the formation of erythematous (scalded) skin followed by widespread bullae (Fig. 13.3), usually a cutaneous manifestation of a drug reaction. The epidermis eventually becomes necrotic, leading to extensive exfoliation and exposure of the raw dermis (Fig. 13.4). A prodrome of fever, fatigue, myalgias, and skin tenderness occurs in the majority of patients. The mortality rate approaches 25%, with death usually due to sepsis or gram-negative pneumonia. TEN is generally considered to be the most severe form of erythema multiforme.

Differential Diagnosis

Early in its course, TEN may resemble scarlet fever, toxic shock syndrome, or erythema multiforme. In children, staphylococcal scalded-skin syndrome closely mimics TEN; however, it involves only the superficial epidermis without extension to the dermis.

Emergency Department Treatment and Disposition

Supportive care includes debridement of necrotic tissue, pain control, aggressive hydration, appropriate antibiotic therapy, and covering exposed dermis, even with cadaver allografts, to avoid infection and reduce pain. These patients are best managed in burn treatment centers.

Clinical Pearls

1. Slight pressure causing the skin to slide laterally and separate from the dermis is a positive Nikolsky's sign.
2. The initial bullae coalesce, leading to exfoliation of the entire epidermis.

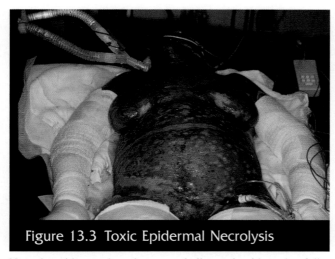

Figure 13.3 Toxic Epidermal Necrolysis

Note the widespread erythematous bullae and epidermal exfoliation. (Courtesy of James J. Nordlund, MD.)

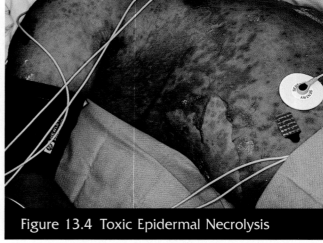

Figure 13.4 Toxic Epidermal Necrolysis

The initial bullae have coalesced, leading to extensive exfoliation of the epidermis. (Courtesy of Keith Batts, MD.)

Associated Clinical Features

Necrotizing vasculitis is a hypersensitivity vasculitis in adults associated with infectious agents, connective tissue diseases, malignancy, and drugs. Symptoms may be confined to the skin in the form of symmetric petechiae and palpable purpura over the distal third of the extremities. Systemic vascular involvement occurs in the kidneys (glomerulonephritis), muscles, joints, gastrointestinal tract (abdominal pain and bleeding), and peripheral nerves (neuritis). Henoch-Schönlein purpura (HSP) (Fig. 13.5) is the classic example of vasculitis in children, consisting of a clinical triad of palpable purpura, arthritis, and abdominal pain. It is usually a benign, self-limited disease that occurs in children most commonly after a bacterial or viral infection.

Differential Diagnosis

Idiopathic thrombocytopenic purpura (ITP), disseminated intravascular coagulation (DIC), meningococcemia, gonococcemia, Rocky Mountain spotted fever, staphylococcal septicemia, and embolic endocarditis must all be considered in the differential diagnosis; however, patients with septic vasculitis are generally more severely ill, with rapidly progressive symptoms. Also, the purpura of septic vasculitis tend to be fewer in number, asymmetric, and distal in location. Biopsy of the purpura is helpful in distinguishing necrotizing vasculitis from septic vasculitis, DIC, and embolic endocarditis.

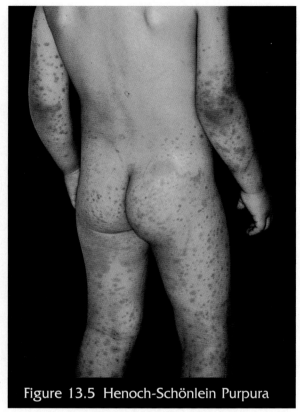

Figure 13.5 Henoch-Schönlein Purpura

Note the classic acral distribution of HSP. It is immunoglobulin A (IgA)–mediated and most commonly occurs in children after a streptococcal or viral infection. (Courtesy of Kevin J. Knoop, MD, MS.)

Emergency Department Treatment and Disposition

A majority of cases are self-limited and require only rest, elevation, and analgesics. Severe cases with systemic manifestations may require admission for supportive care, corticosteroids, and cytotoxic immunosuppressive therapy. Antibiotics should be utilized if the vasculitis follows an infection.

Clinical Pearls

1. The petechiae and purpura of necrotizing vasculitis are usually localized to the lower third of the extremities.
2. A patient presenting with purpura and the signs and symptoms of serum sickness should lead the examiner to consider necrotizing vasculitis.

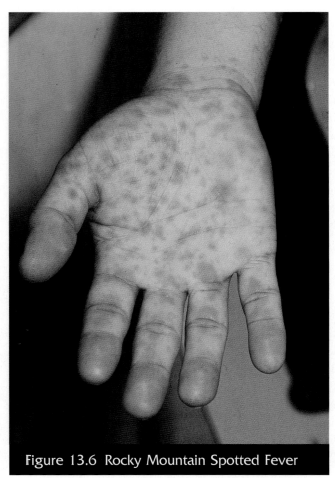

Figure 13.6 Rocky Mountain Spotted Fever

These erythematous macular lesions will evolve into a petechial rash that will spread centrally. (Courtesy of Daniel Noltkamper, MD.)

Associated Clinical Features

Rickettsia rickettsii is transmitted by the bite of an infected tick. Fever, rigors, headache, myalgias, and weakness occur 7 to 10 days after inoculation. The initially blanching macular eruption begins at approximately 4 days on the distal extremities and somewhat later on the palms and soles (Fig. 13.6). It soon becomes petechial as it spreads centrally to involve the trunk and abdomen. However, it can also present without obvious cutaneous manifestations.

Differential Diagnosis

Viral exanthems, drug eruptions, necrotizing vasculitis, purpuric bacteremia, and meningococcemia may all resemble this potentially fatal illness.

Emergency Department Treatment and Disposition

Doxycycline or chloramphenicol is required for this potentially fatal illness. Doxycycline is the drug of choice, yet it should be avoided in pregnant or lactating women and children younger than 8 years of age. Mildly ill patients may be treated with oral antibiotics on an outpatient basis as long as close follow-up can be arranged. More severely ill patients should be admitted because their care can be complicated by circulatory collapse and coma. Approximately 20% of untreated patients will die; overall mortality is 3 to 7%.

Clinical Pearls

1. Palmar and plantar petechiae in a severely ill patient should be treated as Rocky Mountain spotted fever until proved otherwise.
2. Most cases occur between April and October, with the highest incidence occurring in the Southeast and South-Central states.

Associated Clinical Features

Disseminated gonococcus (GC) is a systemic infection, with septic vasculitis following the hematogenous dissemination of the organism *Neisseria gonorrhoeae*. The spectrum of disease varies from skin lesions alone to skin lesions with tenosynovitis or septic arthritis. The initial lesion is an erythematous macule that evolves into a necrotic, purpuric vesicopustule (Fig. 13.7). These purpura are few in number, asymmetric, and predominantly distal in location.

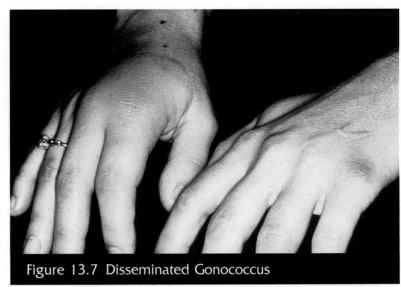

Figure 13.7 Disseminated Gonococcus

A classic presentation of the asymmetric purpuric rash, vesicopustule, and polyarthritis in the hands of an individual with disseminated GC. (Courtesy of Glaxo Wellcome Pharmaceuticals.)

Differential Diagnosis

The purpura may resemble meningococcemia, staphylococcal septicemia, necrotizing vasculitis, or endocarditis with emboli. Infectious arthritis or tenosynovitis must be considered when the patient presents with joint complaints. It is important to obtain Gram's stain of the contents of the vesicopustule, as well as all other body sites and fluids.

Emergency Department Treatment and Disposition

Therapy consists of intravenous or intramuscular ceftriaxone or cefotaxime until symptoms either improve or resolve, followed by an additional 7 days of orally administered ciprofloxacin or cefuroxime. Hospitalization is recommended for noncompliant patients or cases noted to have an associated septic arthritis.

Clinical Pearls

1. The most common symptom of disseminated GC is arthralgia of one or more joints, primarily involving the hands or knees.
2. Skin lesions develop in up to 70% of cases and will resolve within 4 days regardless of antibiotics.
3. Less than one-third of patients will have urethritis.
4. The purpura of septic vasculitis (of whatever bacterial etiology) tend to be fewer in number, asymmetric, and distal in location.

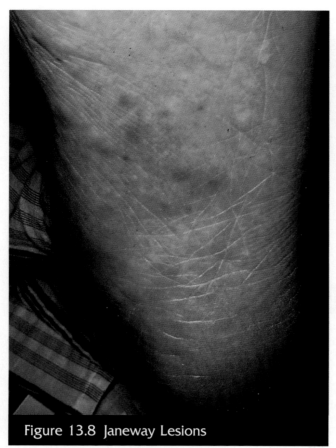

Figure 13.8 Janeway Lesions

Peripheral embolization to the sole, resulting in a cluster of erythematous macules known as Janeway lesions. (Courtesy of the Department of Dermatology, Wilford Hall USAF Medical Center and Brooke Army Medical Center, San Antonio, TX.)

Associated Clinical Features

Infective endocarditis is an illness characterized by fever, valve destruction, and peripheral embolization manifested by rare, usually distal purpura. *Streptococcus viridans* is the most common causative organism. Janeway lesions (Fig. 13.8) occur in 5% of cases and consist of nontender, small, erythematous macules on the palms or soles. Osler's nodes (Fig. 13.9) occur in 10% of cases and consist of transient, tender, purplish nodules on the pulp of the fingers and toes. Splinter hemorrhages are black, linear discolorations beneath the nail plate (Fig. 13.10). They are present in 20% of cases and are more suggestive of subacute bacterial endocarditis (SBE) if present at the proximal or middle nail plate. Murmurs, retinal hemorrhages, septic arthritis, and significant embolic episodes such as pulmonary embolism or stroke may also be present.

Differential Diagnosis

Meningococcemia, gonococcemia, staphylococcal septicemia, and necrotizing vasculitis must all be considered in the differential diagnosis. Echocardiography can aid in the diagnosis.

Emergency Department Treatment and Disposition

Antibiotics must be appropriate for the infectious agent; however, therapy is often required before the diagnosis is

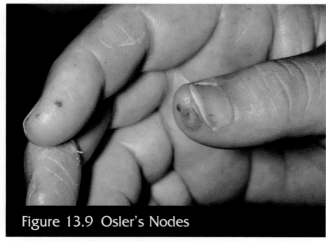

Figure 13.9 Osler's Nodes

Subcutaneous, purplish, tender nodules in the pulp of the fingers known as Osler's nodes. (Courtesy of the Armed Forces Institute of Pathology, Bethesda, MD.)

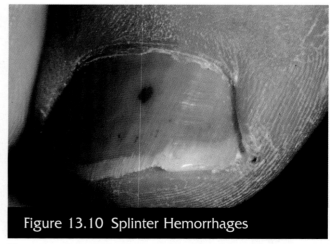

Figure 13.10 Splinter Hemorrhages

Note the splinter hemorrhages along the distal aspect of the nail plate, due to emboli from subacute bacterial endocarditis. (Courtesy of the Armed Forces Institute of Pathology, Bethesda, MD.)

confirmed or the infecting organism is known. All toxic patients require admission, as do all febrile patients who have prosthetic valves or who are intravenous drug abusers. These patients should receive gentamicin with nafcillin or vancomycin empirically pending the blood culture results. Patients with rheumatic or congenital valve abnormalities may receive streptomycin with penicillin or vancomycin.

Clinical Pearls

1. Janeway lesions, Osler's nodes, and splinter hemorrhages in a febrile patient with a murmur are virtually diagnostic of infective endocarditis.
2. Rheumatic heart disease is the most common predisposing factor, with the mitral valve being the most common site of damage.
3. Congenital heart disease, intravenous drug abuse, and prosthetic heart valves are additional predisposing factors to the development of infective endocarditis.

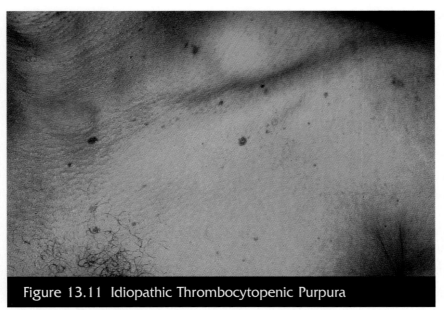

Figure 13.11 Idiopathic Thrombocytopenic Purpura

This thrombocytopenic patient with splenomegaly has pinpoint, nonblanching, nonpalpable petechiae. (Courtesy of the Department of Dermatology, Wilford Hall USAF Medical Center and Brooke Army Medical Center, San Antonio, TX.)

Associated Clinical Features

Idiopathic thrombocytopenic purpura (ITP) occurs as the result of platelet injury and destruction. Pinpoint, red, nonblanching petechiae or nonpalpable purpura and ecchymoses are found on the skin (Fig. 13.11) and mucous membranes, either spontaneously (platelets $<10,000/mm^3$) or at the site of minimal trauma (platelets $<40,000/mm^3$). Melena, hematochezia, menorrhagia, and severe intracranial hemorrhages may also occur in conjunction with the purpura. The acute form affects children 1 to 2 weeks after a viral illness; the chronic form occurs most often in adults, with women outnumbering men 3:1, and may present with an associated splenomegaly.

Differential Diagnosis

Nonhemorrhagic vascular dilatations like telangiectasia or true petechiae and purpura, as found in scurvy or posttraumatic purpura, must be differentiated from this potentially debilitating illness. Assessment of the platelet count aids in making the diagnosis.

Emergency Department Treatment and Disposition

Hospitalization at the time of diagnosis is recommended because the differential diagnosis is extensive and the bleeding risks are significant. Platelets are transfused only if there is life-threatening bleeding or the total count is $<10,000/mm^3$. Immunosuppressive drugs, steroids, and intravenous immunoglobulin are of benefit in the acute cases; splenectomy is utilized in chronic cases.

Clinical Pearls

1. Petechiae and purpura in a thrombocytopenic patient with splenomegaly make the diagnosis.
2. The acute form of ITP has an excellent prognosis (90% spontaneous remission), whereas the course of chronic ITP is one of varying severity with little hope of remission.

Associated Clinical Features

The diagnosis of thrombotic thrombocytopenic purpura (TTP) is characterized by the following pentad of symptoms:

1. Microangiopathic hemolytic anemia, with characteristic schistocytes on the peripheral blood smear and a reticulocytosis.
2. Thrombocytopenia with platelet counts ranging from 5000 to 100,000/μL (Fig. 13.12).
3. Renal abnormalities including renal insufficiency, azotemia, proteinuria, or hematuria.
4. Fever.
5. Neurologic abnormalities including headache, confusion, cranial nerve palsies, seizures, or coma.

The disease affects women more than men and can affect any age group, but it occurs most commonly in ages 10 to 60.

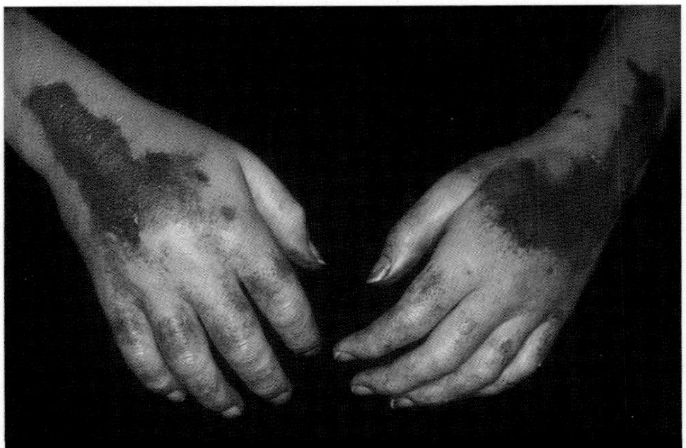

Figure 13.12 Thrombic Thrombocytopenic Purpura

Bleeding at initial presentation is seen in about 30 to 40% of patients with TTP. (Courtesy of James J. Nordlund, MD.)

Differential Diagnosis

Hemolytic uremic syndrome (HUS), disseminated intravascular coagulation, and the pregnancy-associated HELLP (Hemolysis, Elevated Liver enzymes, Low Platelet count) syndrome can all present like TTP. HUS and TTP appear to be closely related and may represent variants of a single disease.

Emergency Department Treatment and Disposition

The cornerstone of therapy is plasma exchange transfusion. Some patients can be treated with plasma infusions alone. It is thought that the transfusions provide a missing substrate and the exchange may remove some unknown toxic substance. Prednisone and antiplatelet therapy with aspirin may be helpful. Patients recalcitrant to standard therapy may be treated with immunosuppressives (vincristine, azathioprine, cyclophosphamide) and even splenectomy. All patients should be admitted.

Clinical Pearls

1. Platelet transfusions should be avoided unless there is life-threatening hemorrhage; they can worsen the thrombotic process.
2. Typically TTP is acute and fulminant, but it can become a chronic, relapsing form.
3. Hemoglobin less than 6 g/dL, platelet count less than 20,000, elevated indirect bilirubin and LDH, and a negative Coombs test are typically found.

Associated Clinical Features

Livedo reticularis presents as a macular, reticulated (lace-like) patch of nonpalpable cutaneous vasodilatation (Fig. 13.13) in response to a variety of vascular occlusive processes. This pattern predominates in the peripheral or acral areas and may or may not be associated with purpura. In time, the overlying epidermis and dermis may infarct and form ulcerations or develop palpable dermal papules or nodules. Livedo reticularis is usually representative of a severe underlying systemic disease. Inflammatory vascular diseases (livedo vasculitis, polyarteritis nodosa, lupus erythematosus), septic emboli (meningococcemia), tumors (pheochromocytoma), and systemic illnesses associated with mechanical vessel blockage (anticardiolipin antibody syndrome, polycythemia vera, sickle cell anemia, cholesterol embolus) are a few diseases associated with or responsible for livedo reticularis. It can also occur independent of any disease association.

Differential Diagnosis

The most important consideration in making this diagnosis is to rule out an associated vascular occlusion of whatever etiology.

Emergency Department Treatment and Disposition

The treatment of livedo reticularis is treatment of the underlying disorder and avoiding exposure to cold.

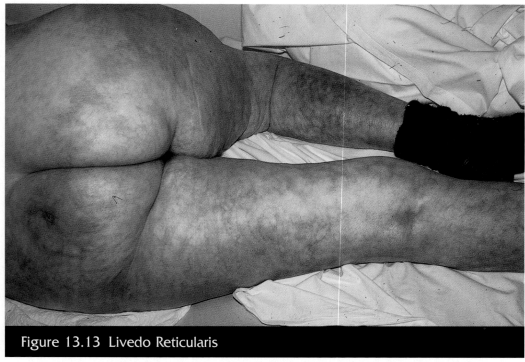

Figure 13.13 Livedo Reticularis

Note the reticulated (lace-like) blanching erythema symmetrically distributed over the lower extremities. (Courtesy of James J. Nordlund, MD.)

Clinical Pearls

1. Livedo vasculitis is an inflammatory vascular disease usually found symmetrically on the ankles and dorsum of the feet. It consists of painful stellate-shaped ulcerations surrounded by an erythematous livedo pattern.
2. Cholesterol emboli usually occur after an intraarterial procedure. Pain often precedes the livedo pattern of purpura on the distal extremities.
3. Patients with anticardiolipin antibody syndrome have extensive livedo reticularis and recurrent arterial and venous thromboses involving multiple organ systems.

Associated Clinical Features

Herpes zoster is a dermatomal, unilateral reactivation of the varicella zoster virus. Pain, tenderness, and dysesthesias may present 4 to 5 days prior to an eruption composed of umbilicated, grouped vesicles on an erythematous, edematous base (Fig. 13.14). The vesicles may become purulent or hemorrhagic. Nerve involvement may actually occur without cutaneous involvement. Ophthalmic zoster involves the nasociliary branch of the fifth cranial nerve and presents with vesicles on the nose and cornea (Hutchinson's sign). Ramsay-Hunt syndrome is a herpes zoster infection of the geniculate ganglion that presents with decreased hearing, facial palsy, and vesicles on the tympanic membrane, pinna, and ear canal.

Differential Diagnosis

The most likely differential diagnosis is herpes simplex infection, which is usually recurrent. Herpes zoster recurs in fewer than 5% of immunocompetent patients. The eruption may resemble contact dermatitis, localized cellulitis, or grouped insect bites. The prodromal pain must be differentiated from potential pleural, cardiac, or abdominal origin. Tzank smear of the floor of a vesicle demonstrating multinucleated giant cells makes the diagnosis of a herpes family infection (Fig. 13.15). Cultures may be necessary to distinguish herpes zoster forms.

Emergency Department Treatment and Disposition

Uncomplicated cases of herpes zoster can be managed with supportive care, especially pain control. Admission to the hospital for intravenous acyclovir is usually reserved for complicated cases involving multiple dermatomal distribution or the ophthalmic branch of the trigeminal nerve, disseminated disease, or immunocompromised patients. Acyclovir or famciclovir hasten the healing

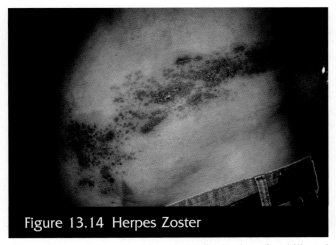

Figure 13.14 Herpes Zoster

This eruption consists of a dermatomal distribution of umbilicated vesicles on an erythematous base. Note the occasional cluster of hemorrhagic vesicles. Tzank smear is positive. (Courtesy of the Department of Dermatology, Wilford Hall USAF Medical Center and Brooke Army Medical Center, San Antonio, TX.)

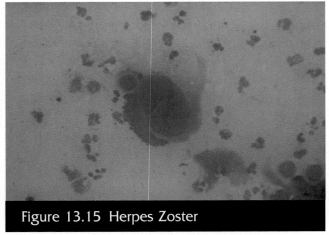

Figure 13.15 Herpes Zoster

A Tzank smear of both the roof and floor of a herpetic vesicle demonstrating a multinucleated giant cell. (Courtesy of the Department of Dermatology, Wilford Hall USAF Medical Center and Brooke Army Medical Center, San Antonio, TX.)

and decreases the pain if started within 72 h of appearance of the vesicles. These agents have also been shown to reduce the duration of postherpetic neuralgia. Prednisone may also prove useful. Herpes zoster keratitis requires immediate ophthalmologic consultation to avoid any potential vision loss.

Clinical Pearls

1. Dermatomally grouped, umbilicated vesicles on an erythematous base are diagnostic of herpes zoster.
2. The thorax is the most common area involved, followed by the face (trigeminal nerve).
3. The nonimmune or immunocompromised should avoid lesional contact from prodrome until reepithelialization, since the crusts can contain the varicella zoster virus.
4. Typically, an infected patient may transmit chickenpox to a nonimmune individual.
5. Zoster during pregnancy seems to have no deleterious effects on the mother or baby.

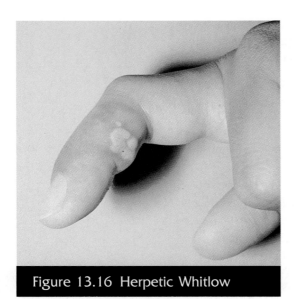

Figure 13.16 Herpetic Whitlow

Note the cluster of vesicles on an erythematous base located at the distal finger. Tzank smear is positive. (Courtesy of Lawrence B. Stack, MD.)

Associated Clinical Features

Herpetic whitlow is a painful herpes simplex infection of the distal finger characterized by edema, erythema, vesicles, and/or pustules grouped on an erythematous base (Fig. 13.16). Fever, lymphangitis, and regional adenopathy often accompany the lesion.

Differential Diagnosis

Paronychia, felon, and contact dermatitis must be differentiated from this contagious illness. A Tzank smear of the floor of the vesicle demonstrating multinucleated giant cells makes the diagnosis.

Emergency Department Treatment and Disposition

Acyclovir in addition to analgesics and antipyretics are useful. To be most effective, acyclovir must be started within 72 h of the appearance of the eruption. Topical antibiotic ointments help prevent secondary infection and may speed healing.

Clinical Pearls

1. Grouped, umbilicated vesicles on an erythematous base are diagnostic of a herpes family infection.
2. Wear protective gloves; herpetic whitlow is an occupational hazard in the medical and dental professions.

Associated Clinical Features

Erysipelas is a group A streptococcal cellulitis involving the skin to the level of the dermis. The plaque is typically erythematous, edematous, and painful, with an elevated, well-demarcated border (Fig. 13.17). The associated edema tends to make the plaque appear shiny. Erysipelas frequently occurs on the face and lower extremities.

Differential Diagnosis

Other significant illnesses—such as deep venous thrombosis, thrombophlebitis, and necrotizing fasciitis—must be ruled out.

Emergency Department Treatment and Disposition

All infections require rest, elevation, heat, and antibiotics. Mild presentations may be treated on an outpatient basis with oral dicloxacillin or erythromycin in penicillin-allergic patients. More severe illness or toxicity requires hospitalization and intravenous antibiotics.

Clinical Pearls

1. The well-demarcated, tender, shiny, erythematous plaque is diagnostic of erysipelas.
2. This same shiny, erythematous plaque on the face of a febrile child may be caused by *Haemophilus influenzae,* necessitating intravenous chloramphenicol or a cephalosporin.
3. Lymphatic streaking is more common in erysipelas than cellulitis.

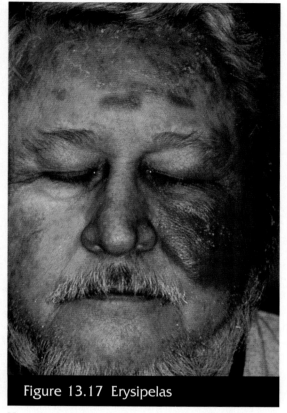

Figure 13.17 Erysipelas

Note the well-demarcated, edematous, erythematous, shiny plaque. (Courtesy of the Department of Dermatology, Wilford Hall USAF Medical Center and Brooke Army Medical Center, San Antonio, TX.)

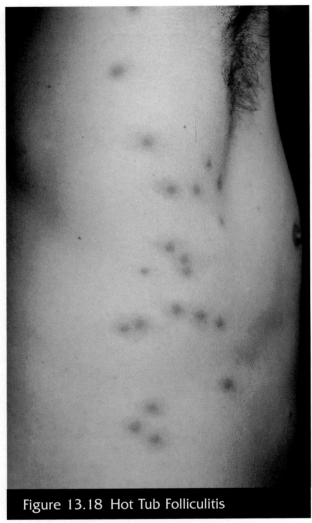

Figure 13.18 Hot Tub Folliculitis

Note the pustules localized to the hair follicles of the trunk and proximal extremity. (Courtesy of Jeffrey S. Gibson, MD.)

Associated Clinical Features

Hot-tub folliculitis is a pruritic, follicular, pustular eruption confined to the hair follicle and is secondary to a cutaneous infection with *Pseudomonas aeruginosa* (Fig. 13.18). Headache, sore throat, earache, and fever may accompany the pustules, which usually localize to the trunk and proximal extremities.

Differential Diagnosis

Other forms of folliculitis (including those caused by *Staphylococcus aureus*), acne, and miliaria rubra are usually considered in the differential diagnosis.

Emergency Department Treatment and Disposition

The folliculitis usually involutes in 7 to 10 days without treatment. Acetic acid compresses and local wound cleansing may speed recovery. In addition, the hot tub or source of exposure must be decontaminated to avoid reexposure.

Clinical Pearls

1. Pruritic pustules confined to the hair follicles of the trunk and proximal extremities is diagnostic of folliculitis.
2. This most commonly occurs in individuals who use hot tubs, whirlpools, or saunas.
3. This may also result from contact with chemicals (exfoliative beauty aids) or repetitive physical trauma (friction from tight clothing).

Associated Clinical Features

Ecthyma gangrenosum is a *Pseudomonas aerug-inosa* infection that usually occurs in the septic, immunocompromised, or neutropenic patient. The initially erythematous macules develop bullae or pustules (Fig. 13.19) surrounded by violaceous halos. The pustules become hemorrhagic and rupture, forming painless ulcers with necrotic, black centers.

Differential Diagnosis

Necrotizing vasculitis, fixed drug eruptions, pyoderma gangrenosum, and brown recluse spider bites must all be considered in the differential diagnosis.

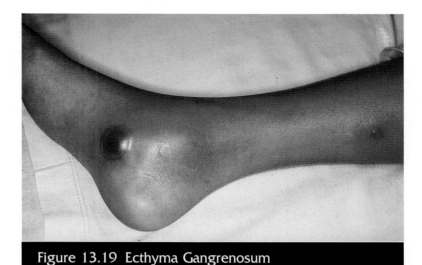

Figure 13.19 Ecthyma Gangrenosum

A typical hemorrhagic bulla of ecthyma gangrenosum secondary to pseudomonal sepsis. (Courtesy of James Mensching, MD.)

Emergency Department Treatment and Disposition

These patients are usually septic and immunocompromised. Admission is usually required for the patient to receive antipseudomonal antibiotics and general supportive care.

Clinical Pearls

1. Consider ecthyma gangrenosum when examining a septic patient who presents with bullae or pustules that rupture and form painless, necrotic ulcers.
2. It is important to consider underlying immunodeficiency when making this diagnosis.

Associated Clinical Features

Pityriasis rosea is a mild inflammatory, exanthematous, papulosquamous eruption. The pathognomonic finding is an oval salmon-colored papule with a central collarette of scale. It primarily occurs on the trunk with the long axis of the oval papule following the lines of cleavage in a Christmas tree–like distribution (Fig. 13.20). A herald patch, consisting of a much larger plaque with central clearing and scales, frequently precedes the exanthematous phase by 1 to 2 weeks (Fig. 13.21). The eruption usually lasts 4 to 6 weeks and is frequently pruritic.

Differential Diagnosis

This must be differentiated from the secondary lesions of syphilis, tinea versicolor, and some drug eruptions.

Emergency Department Treatment and Disposition

Symptomatic treatment is usually all that can be offered to the patient. Antihistamines may alleviate the associated pruritus. Ultraviolet light has also been used with some success.

Clinical Pearls

1. A salmon-colored papule with central scale, negative KOH examination for hyphae, and negative serologic testing for syphilis makes the diagnosis of pityriasis rosea.
2. It frequently appears in very atypical form in dark-skinned individuals (acral, face, and genital location).

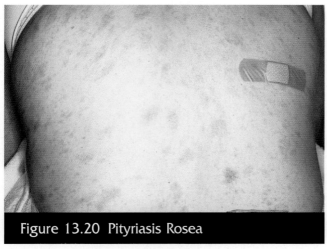

Figure 13.20 Pityriasis Rosea

An exanthematous, papulosquamous eruption, with the long axis of the oval papules following the lines of cleavage in a Christmas tree–like eruption. (Courtesy of James J. Nordlund, MD.)

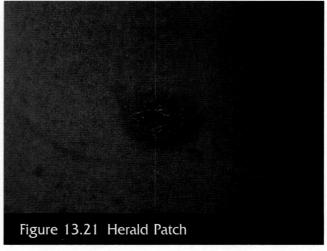

Figure 13.21 Herald Patch

A herald patch precedes the exanthematous phase: a larger, oval, salmon-colored patch with a central collarette of scale. (Courtesy of the Department of Dermatology, Wilford Hall USAF Medical Center and Brooke Army Medical Center, San Antonio, TX.)

Associated Clinical Features

The initial papules of secondary syphilis are usually asymptomatic, although they may be painful or pruritic; they appear 2 to 10 weeks after the primary chancre. Headache, sore throat, fever, arthralgias, myalgias, and a generalized lymphadenopathy may also be present. These exanthematous papules are symmetric and nondestructive, usually forming a pityriasis rosea–like pattern on the trunk, palms, and soles (Figs. 13.22, 13.23). Later lesions are firm, pigmented papules with a coppery tint and adherent scales (Fig. 13.24). Macerated papules may form on the mucous membranes; "motheaten" alopecia may occur on the scalp; and condylomata lata may occur in the intertriginous areas.

Differential Diagnosis

Syphilis is "the great imitator." It may resemble psoriasis, drug eruptions, pityriasis rosea, viral exanthems, tinea cor-

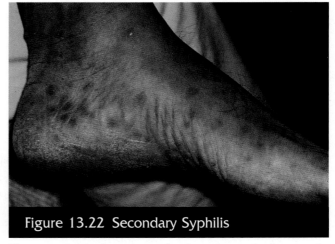

Figure 13.22 Secondary Syphilis

These eruptive, scaly, copper-colored papules on the foot may be the initial presentation of secondary syphilis. They are usually symmetric, asymptomatic, and nondestructive. (Courtesy of the Department of Dermatology, Wilford Hall USAF Medical Center and Brooke Army Medical Center, San Antonio, TX.)

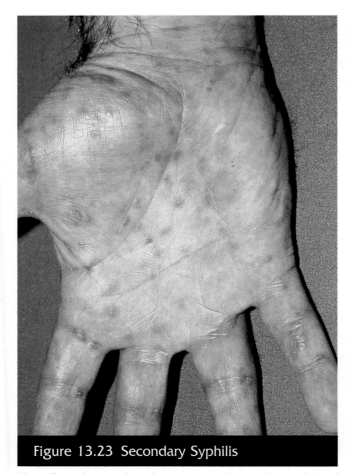

Figure 13.23 Secondary Syphilis

These firm, pigmented, erythematous papules are characteristic of secondary syphilis. (Courtesy of Lynn Utecht, MD.)

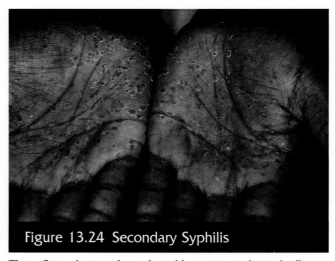

Figure 13.24 Secondary Syphilis

These firm, pigmented papules with a coppery tint and adherent scale are characteristic. (Courtesy of the Department of Dermatology, Wilford Hall USAF Medical Center and Brooke Army Medical Center, San Antonio, TX.)

397

poris, tinea versicolor, and condyloma acuminata. A positive serologic test for syphilis makes the diagnosis.

Emergency Department Treatment and Disposition

Penicillin is the agent of choice for treatment, with tetracycline or erythromycin used in cases of penicillin allergy. A Jarisch-Herxheimer reaction may occur several hours after treatment with antibiotics, correlating with the clearance of spirochetes from the bloodstream. This reaction lasts approximately 24 h, yet it may be more threatening than the disease itself. Increasing fever, rigors, myalgias, headache, tachycardia, hypotension, and a drop in the leukocyte and platelet count may be encountered. Fluid resuscitation to maintain the blood pressure and supportive care may be needed.

Clinical Pearls

1. Scaly palmar and plantar papules are strongly suggestive of secondary syphilis, the incidence of which is rising.
2. These scaling red-brown papules appear 2 to 10 weeks after the spontaneous resolution of the initial painless chancre.
3. The latent stage follows the resolution of the papules; it is characterized by a positive serology and an absence of signs and symptoms.
4. Tertiary syphilis occurs in untreated or poorly treated patients and may manifest itself as general paresis, tabes dorsalis, optic atrophy, and aortitis with aneurysms.
5. It is important to consider the prozone phenomenon (falsely negative agglutination in undiluted serum) in an AIDS patient with presumed syphilis in whom the serologic test is negative.

Associated Clinical Features

Borrelia burgdorferi is the tick-borne spirochete responsible for Lyme borreliosis, and erythema chronicum migrans (ECM) is the pathognomonic rash of Lyme disease occuring early in the infection. The initial prodromal symptoms of fever, myalgias, arthralgias, and headache are followed by a macule or papule progressing to a plaque at the site of the bite. This plaque expands its red, raised border as it clears centrally, leading to an annular appearance (Fig. 13.25). The plaque may burn and is rarely pruritic. On average, there are 9 days between the time of the bite and the appearance of the rash.

Differential Diagnosis

This annular plaque may resemble a fixed drug eruption, tinea corporis, urticaria, or the herald patch of pityriasis rosea. The multiple secondary annular papules and plaques that may rarely form can resemble secondary syphilis. However, the Lyme-related eruption spares the palms and soles.

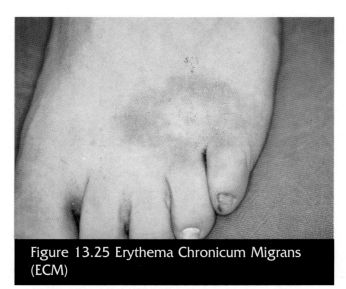

Figure 13.25 Erythema Chronicum Migrans (ECM)

This pathognomonic eruption of Lyme disease forms at the site of the tick bite. The initial papule forms into a slowly enlarging oval area of erythema while clearing centrally. (Courtesy of Timothy Hinman, MD.)

Emergency Department Treatment and Disposition

The duration of antibiotic treatment (10 to 30 days) depends on the severity of the symptoms. Tetracycline or doxycycline are the drugs of choice. Pregnant or lactating females and children younger than 8 years of age should be treated with penicillin or amoxicillin. Erythromycin is a suitable alternative. Patients with minimal symptoms may be treated on an outpatient basis. Those patients with significant toxicity and complications require admission, supportive care, and parenteral antibiotics.

Clinical Pearls

1. An annular plaque arising at the site of a tick bite in a patient with systemic symptoms should be treated as Lyme disease until proved otherwise.
2. Stage I of Lyme disease consists of constitutional symptoms and the characteristic rash of ECM.
3. Stage II of Lyme disease consists of neurologic (aseptic meningitis, encephalitis, bilateral Bell's palsy) and cardiac (myocarditis, conduction blocks) manifestations.
4. Stage III of Lyme disease consists of an asymmetric, episodic, oligoarticular arthritis.

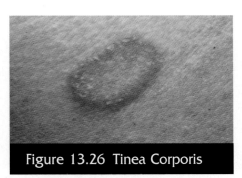

Figure 13.26 Tinea Corporis

This dermatophytosis is known as ringworm, a well-defined, pruritic, scaly plaque with a raised border and central clearing (annular). KOH preparation is positive. (Courtesy of the Department of Dermatology, Wilford Hall USAF Medical Center and Brooke Army Medical Center, San Antonio, TX.)

Associated Clinical Features

Tinea corporis includes all dermatophyte infections excluding the scalp, face, hands, feet, and groin. The dermatophytosis is pruritic and consists of well circumscribed scaly plaque with a slightly elevated border and central clearing (Fig. 13.26). This annular configuration is most commonly found on the trunk and neck. Skin scrapings viewed with a KOH preparation exhibit septate hyphae.

Tinea faciale is a dermatophyte infection of the facial skin. It commonly appears as a well circumscribed erythematous patch (Fig. 13.27). Tinea manus is a dermatophyte infection of the hands (Fig. 13.28).

Differential Diagnosis

Pityriasis rosea, secondary syphilis, psoriasis, seborrheic dermatitis, and tinea versicolor are all usually considered in the differential diagnosis. A KOH examination of the scale demonstrating hyphae confirms the diagnosis.

Emergency Department Treatment and Disposition

Small, localized plaques may be treated with a topical antifungal cream. Extensive or resistant infection requires systemic griseofulvin or ketoconazole. It is important to treat for 2 weeks beyond the point of clinical cure to ensure successful eradication of the fungus.

Clinical Pearls

1. The scale is usually located at the leading edge of erythema and provides the best yield for scraping as part of the KOH examination.
2. The recurrence rate is high, especially for tinea manus.

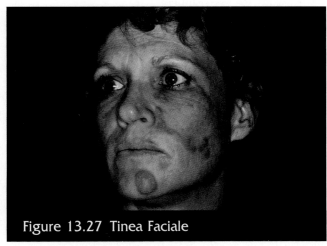

Figure 13.27 Tinea Faciale

Note the sharply marginated, polycyclic, scaly plaque with central clearing localized to the face. KOH preparation is positive. (Courtesy of the Department of Dermatology, Wilford Hall USAF Medical Center and Brooke Army Medical Center, San Antonio, TX.)

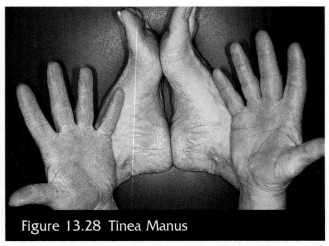

Figure 13.28 Tinea Manus

This dermatophytosis is usually unilateral when it involves the hands. Note the diffuse hyperkeratosis of the left hand as well as involvement of both feet (tinea pedis). (Courtesy of James J. Nordlund, MD.)

Associated Clinical Features

Tinea cruris, or "jock itch," is a pruritic dermatophytosis of the intertriginous areas, usually excluding the penis and scrotum. The scaly, erythematous plaque spreads peripherally, with central clearing (Fig. 13.29). The borders of the plaque are well defined.

Differential Diagnosis

Erythrasma, *Candida albicans,* seborrheic dermatitis, and psoriasis are usually considered in the differential diagnosis. A KOH examination of the scale demonstrating hyphae confirms the diagnosis.

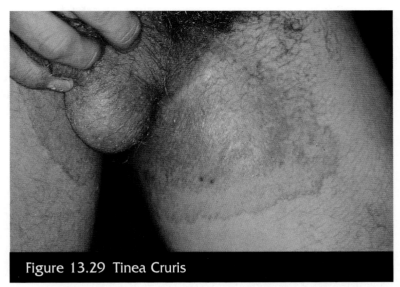

Figure 13.29 Tinea Cruris

This dermatophytosis is commonly called "jock itch." Note the erythematous, scaly plaque with its well-defined border. It characteristically does not involve the scrotum or penis. KOH preparation is positive. (Courtesy of James J. Nordlund, MD.)

Emergency Department Treatment and Disposition

Initial treatment consists of topical antifungal medications. Griseofulvin or ketoconazole are reserved for resistant cases. It is important to treat for 1 week beyond the point of clinical cure to ensure successful eradication of the fungus. Decreasing the amount of perspiration by using topical powders may help prevent recurrences.

Clinical Pearls

1. A less well defined, pruritic, intertriginous plaque that typically involves the scrotum is usually erythrasma. It is caused by *Nocarelia minutissimus* and is treated with topical erythromycin.
2. Warmth and moisture are predisposing factors.

Associated Clinical Features

Tinea pedis, or "athlete's foot," is a pruritic dermatophytosis. It consists of erythema and scaling of the sole (see Fig. 13.28), maceration, occasional vesiculation, and fissure formation between and under the toes (Fig. 13.30). These pruritic, painful fissures may become secondarily infected with gram-negative organisms. Frequently the toenails are also affected.

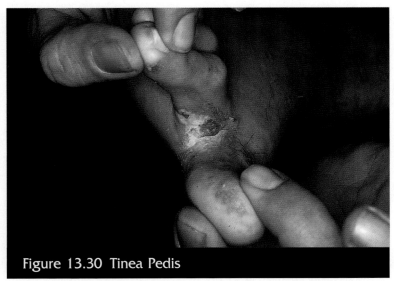

Figure 13.30 Tinea Pedis

A pruritic, scaling hyperkeratotic rash involving the soles of the feet and extending to the interdigital spaces is pathognomonic for tinea pedis. (Courtesy of James J. Nordlund, MD.)

Differential Diagnosis

Foot eczema, psoriasis, and Reiter's syndrome are considered in the differential diagnosis. A KOH examination of the scale demonstrating hyphae confirms the diagnosis.

Emergency Department Treatment and Disposition

Topical antifungal creams are the initial treatment of choice. Antibiotics may be used to treat secondary infection. Griseofulvin, then ketoconazole, are used for chronic or resistant cases. It is important to treat for 1 week beyond the point of clinical cure to ensure successful eradication of the fungus.

Clinical Pearls

1. If it scales, scrape it and look for hyphae.
2. Macerated areas may become secondarily infected by bacteria.

Associated Clinical Features

Tinea capitis is scalp ringworm, or a dermatophytosis of the scalp. It presents as a pruritic, erythematous, scaly plaque with broken or missing hairs frequently referred to as "gray patch" or "black dot" ringworm (Fig. 13.31). This may develop into a kerion. A kerion is a delayed-type hypersensitivity reaction to the fungus, where the initial erythematous, scaly plaque becomes boggy with inflamed, purulent nodules and plaques (Fig. 13.32). The hair follicle is frequently destroyed by the inflammatory process in a kerion, leading to a scarring alopecia.

Differential Diagnosis

Various inflammatory follicular conditions—such as folliculitis, impetigo, psoriasis, alopecia areata, and seborrheic dermatitis—may resemble tinea capitis. The diagnosis is made by a KOH examination of a scraping of the area, revealing hyphae and spores.

Emergency Department Treatment Disposition

Systemic griseofulvin is usually required for several weeks to treat tinea capitis successfully. Systemic antibiotics and corticosteroids are usually added when treating a kerion. Selenium sulfide lotion used as

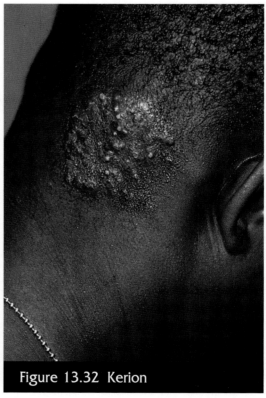

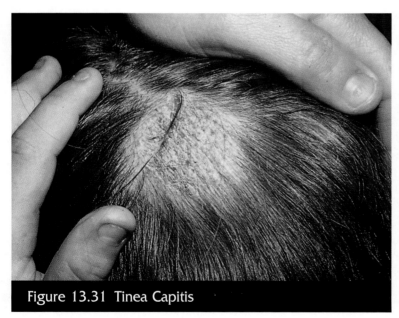

Figure 13.31 Tinea Capitis

This dermatophytosis is characterized by a pruritic, circular area of hair loss covered by adherent scales. KOH preparation is positive. (Courtesy of the Department of Dermatology, Wilford Hall USAF Medical Center and Brooke Army Medical Center, San Antonio, TX.)

Figure 13.32 Kerion

This collection of boggy, inflamed, purulent nodules and papules is the result of a delayed-type hypersensitivity reaction to the fungus. Scarring alopecia will follow as a result of the actual destruction of the hair follicle. (Courtesy of the Department of Dermatology, Wilford Hall USAF Medical Center and Brooke Army Medical Center, San Antonio, TX.)

a shampoo may actually decrease the duration of the infection. It is important to treat for 2 weeks beyond the point of clinical cure to ensure successful eradication of the fungus. Ketoconazole is reserved for resistant cases.

Clinical Pearls

1. Tinea capitis is a disease of childhood; it is rare in immunocompetent adults.
2. It is epidemic in many African American communities.
3. The KOH scrape is aided by using a disposable urethral brush or similar device.

Associated Clinical Features

Onychomycosis is an invasion of the nails by any fungus. Four clinical subtypes are noted. *Distal subungual* presents as discolorations of the free edge of the nail with hyperkeratosis leading to a subungual accumulation of friable keratinaceous debris (Fig. 13.33). *White superficial* consists of sharply outlined white areas on the nail plate which leave the surface friable. *Proximal subungual* presents as discolorations which start proximally at the nail fold. *Candidal onychomycosis* encompasses the entire nail plate, leaving the surface rough and friable.

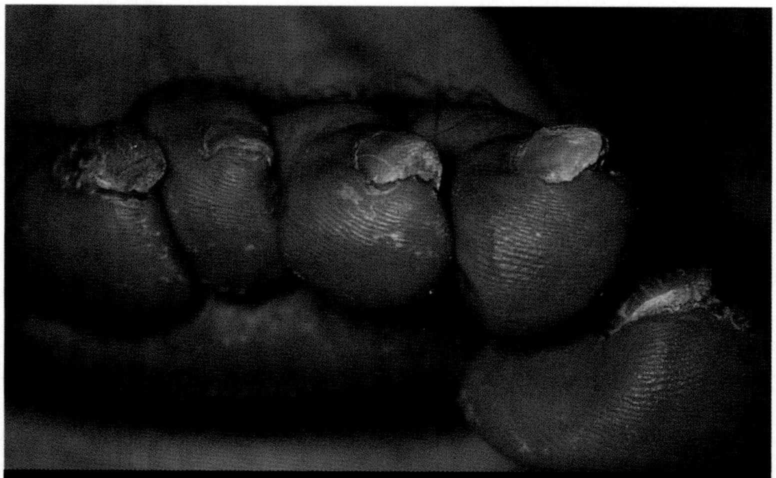

Figure 13.33 Onychomycosis

Differential Diagnosis

Psoriasis and various other nail dystrophies, such as distal onycholysis caused by excessive water exposure or drugs, must be differentiated

Note that multiple nail beds have been invaded by the fungus, leading to chronic hyperkeratosis and subungual accumulation of friable keratinaceous debris. (Courtesy of the Department of Dermatology, Wilford Hall USAF Medical Center and Brooke Army Medical Center, San Antonio, TX.)

from this fungal infection. Pseudomonal nail infection is characterized by the subungual accumulation of green debris. A KOH examination of the keratinaceous debris demonstrating hyphae confirms onychomycosis.

Emergency Department Treatment and Disposition

The most common treatment consists of oral griseofulvin, fluconazole, lucenazole, or terbinafine. Candidal infections require oral ketoconazole. Toenail onychomycosis is very difficult to eradicate.

Clinical Pearls

1. All that causes the nail plate to separate from the nail bed is not necessarily fungus.
2. Distal subungual is the most common type of onychomycosis.

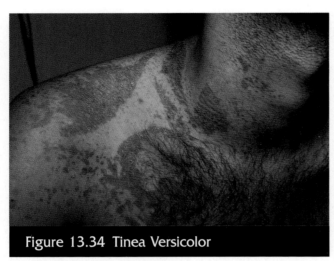

Figure 13.34 Tinea Versicolor

This chronic superficial fungal infection leads to the formation of multiple well-defined, scaly brown macules on the trunk and extremities. (Courtesy of the Department of Dermatology, Wilford Hall USAF Medical Center and Brooke Army Medical Center, San Antonio, TX.)

Associated Clinical Features

Tinea versicolor is a chronic, superficial fungal infection that involves the trunk and extremities with little or no involvement of the face. The fungus is part of normal skin flora. Finely scaling brown macules are present in fair-skinned patients (Fig. 13.34), whereas scaly hypopigmented macules are often noted in the dark-skinned (Fig. 13.35). These sharply demarcated macules are intermittently pruritic.

Differential Diagnosis

Pityriasis rosea, secondary syphilis, and some drug eruptions must all be considered in the differential diagnosis. A KOH examination of a scraping of the area revealing hyphae and spores makes the diagnosis (see Fig. 21.16).

Emergency Department Treatment and Disposition

Treatment consists of short applications of selenium sulfide lotion, topical antifungal creams, or topical ketoconazole. Resistant cases require oral ketoconazole. Ultraviolet exposure is required to regain any lost pigment.

Clinical Pearls

1. Tinea versicolor is more common in adolescents and young adults.
2. Clinically active areas or areas colonized with the fungus may be identified by orange fluorescence noted on Wood's light examination.

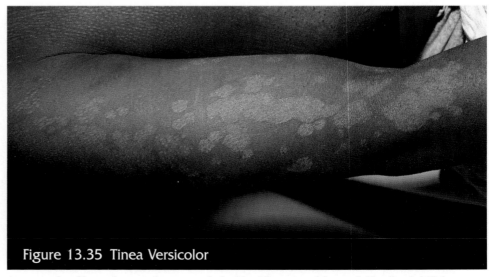

Figure 13.35 Tinea Versicolor

An example of hypopigmented areas on dark skin. (Courtesy of James J. Nordlund, MD.)

Associated Clinical Features

Basal cell carcinoma is a malignancy of the basal cell layer of the epidermis, presenting as a translucent, pearly papule with central ulceration and rolled borders with fine superficial telangi-ectasias (Fig. 13.36). It is most frequently located on the head, neck, and upper trunk. The patient frequently notes easy bleeding of the papule with poor to nonhealing. There are several variants of basal cell carcinomas. Pigmented basal cell carcinoma consists of a brownish-black, firm nodule with irregular surface and central ulceration (Fig. 13.37). Superficial multicentric basal cell carcinoma is psoriasiform in nature, consisting of a flat, erythematous, scaly translucent plaque without central ulceration or raised border (Fig. 13.38).

Differential Diagnosis

Pigmented basal cell carcinoma resembles nodular melanoma. Superficial multicentric basal cell carcinoma resembles psoriasis, tinea corporis, and squamous cell carcinoma in situ.

Emergency Department Treatment and Disposition

Excisional surgery, cryosurgery, or electrosurgery are recommended forms of treatment. If there is a potential for disfigurement, radiation therapy is usually instituted instead of surgery. Prompt

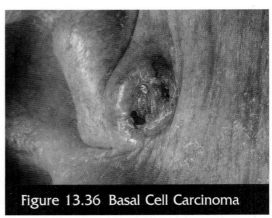

Figure 13.36 Basal Cell Carcinoma

Nodular basal cell carcinoma consists of a firm, centrally ulcerated (rodent ulcer) nodule with a raised, rolled, pearly, telangiectatic border. (Courtesy of the Department of Dermatology, Wilford Hall USAF Medical Center and Brooke Army Medical Center, San Antonio, TX.)

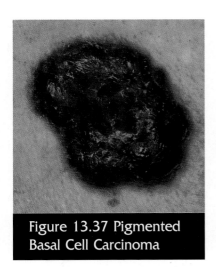

Figure 13.37 Pigmented Basal Cell Carcinoma

This pigmented basal cell carcinoma consists of a firm, translucent, brownish-black ulcerated nodule with an irregular surface and asymmetry of its border. (Courtesy of the Department of Dermatology, Wilford Hall USAF Medical Center and Brooke Army Medical Center, San Antonio, TX.)

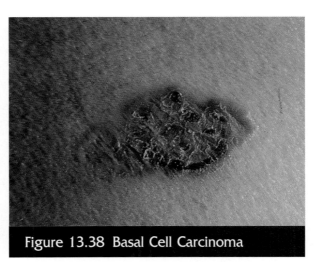

Figure 13.38 Basal Cell Carcinoma

A superficial multicentric basal cell carcinoma is frequently psoriasiform in nature. Note the flat, erythematous, scaly plaque with its elevated, irregular border. (Courtesy of the Department of Dermatology, Wilford Hall USAF Medical Center and Brooke Army Medical Center, San Antonio, TX.)

dermatologic consultation must be arranged when evaluating any suspicious lesion. Up to half of patients will develop a recurrence.

Clinical Pearls

1. Basal cell carcinoma is the most common form of skin cancer.
2. This malignancy forms in the epidermis that has developing hair follicles; therefore, it is not found on the vermilion border of the lips or the genital mucosal membranes.
3. The pearly, rolled, telangiectatic border with central ulceration is diagnostic of basal cell carcinoma.
4. Despite being locally invasive, basal cell carcinoma does not metastasize.

Associated Clinical Features

Squamous cell carcinoma varies from erythematous, hyperkeratotic, sharply demarcated plaques to elevated, ulcerative nodules (Fig. 13.39). It may be sun-induced or related to ionizing radiation or industrial carcinogens. Invasive squamous cell carcinoma is characterized by a discrete elevated plaque or nodule with thick keratotic scale and ulceration.

Differential Diagnosis

Squamous cell carcinoma must be differentiated from a benign lesion such as tinea corporis, psoriasis, impetigo, wart, seborrheic keratosis, or keratoacanthoma (Fig. 13.40).

Emergency Department Treatment and Disposition

Excisional surgery is required, with radiation therapy utilized in potentially disfiguring cases. All suspicious lesions require prompt dermatologic consultation.

Clinical Pearls

1. Squamous cell carcinoma is the second most common type of skin cancer.
2. This malignancy develops more commonly in fair-skinned people with a significant history of sun exposure.
3. Most lesions are found on the lips or other sun-exposed areas.
4. A rapidly evolving (2 to 4 weeks) nodule or plaque with a dense hyperkeratotic core is a keratoacanthoma. It is closely related to squamous cell carcinoma and frequently occurs at a site of trauma. Treatment is the same.
5. Risk of metastasis is related to size, location, and histology.

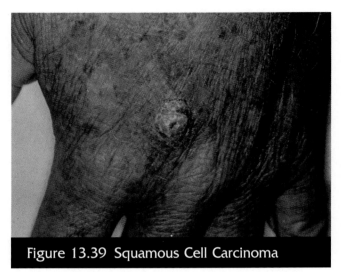

Figure 13.39 Squamous Cell Carcinoma

Note the single erythematous, scaly plaque on the dorsal aspect of this sun-exposed hand. (Courtesy of the Department of Dermatology, Wilford Hall USAF Medical Center and Brooke Army Medical Center, San Antonio, TX.)

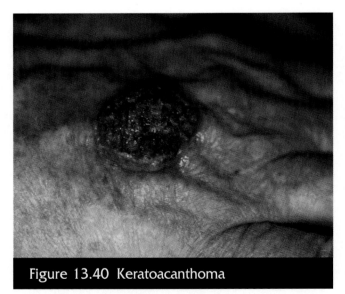

Figure 13.40 Keratoacanthoma

This rapidly evolving neoplasm consists of an erythematous nodule with a hyperkeratotic core. It most closely resembles a squamous cell carcinoma although it is a benign epithelial neoplasm. Biopsy serves to differentiate these two conditions. (Courtesy of the Department of Dermatology, Wilford Hall USAF Medical Center and Brooke Army Medical Center, San Antonio, TX.)

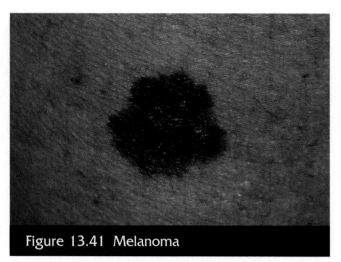

Figure 13.41 Melanoma

Note the asymmetry, irregular border, and focal hyperpigmentation in this melanoma. (Courtesy of the Department of Dermatology, Wilford Hall USAF Medical Center and Brooke Army Medical Center, San Antonio, TX.)

Associated Clinical Features

Melanoma is a malignancy involving the melanocytes of the epidermis. Asymmetry, an irregular border, a mottled display of color, a diameter greater than 5 to 6 mm, and an elevation or distortion of the surface are five signs that a lesion may be a melanoma (Fig. 13.41). Melanoma may or may not occur in sun-exposed areas.

Differential Diagnosis

Lentigo maligna is characterized by a single, flat, freckle-like macule with an irregular border, usually on the face (Fig. 13.42). This melanoma in situ is often confused with a solar lentigo or a seborrheic keratosis and has about a 5% risk of being malignant. Superficially spreading melanoma is the most common form of melanoma. It usually presents as a brown macule with irregular borders and variegation in color. Nodular melanoma usually starts as a papule which becomes an elevated nodule with irregular borders and variegation in color (Fig. 13.43). It must be differentiated from a hemangioma, angiokeratoma, or pigmented basal cell carcinoma. Acral lentiginous melanomas, which are agressive and metastasize easily, are often mistaken for plantar warts or subungual hematomas; they are flat, pigmented, irregularly bordered macules of the palms, soles, and subungual areas (Fig. 13.44).

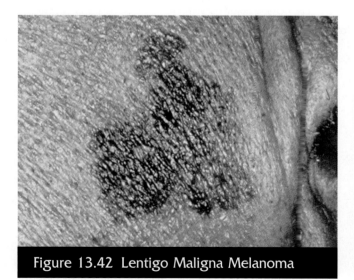

Figure 13.42 Lentigo Maligna Melanoma

This long-lived melanoma in situ has now invaded the dermis, forming a black nodule classified as lentigo maligna melanoma. (Courtesy of the Department of Dermatology, Wilford Hall USAF Medical Center and Brooke Army Medical Center, San Antonio, TX.)

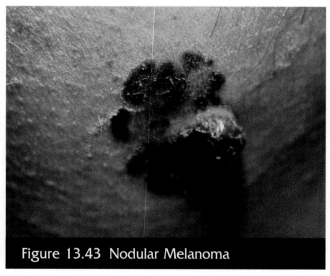

Figure 13.43 Nodular Melanoma

This melanoma has progressed to an exophytic tumor, which was deeply invasive histopathologically. (Courtesy of the Department of Dermatology, Wilford Hall USAF Medical Center and Brooke Army Medical Center, San Antonio, TX.)

410

Emergency Department Treatment and Disposition

A melanoma must be surgically excised with adequate margins. Prompt dermatologic consultation is required of all suspicious lesions, because the prognosis of melanoma correlates directly with early detection and treatment.

Clinical Pearls

1. Prognosis of melanoma is most dependent on the depth of invasion, therefore, early detection and treatment are essential.
2. Only 20% of melanomas arise from preexisting moles, so the appearance of a new mole, especially after the age of 30, is particularly significant.
3. Most benign moles have symmetry, one color, and are less than 7 mm in diameter.

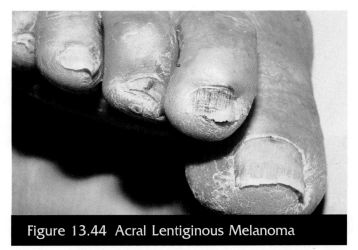

Figure 13.44 Acral Lentiginous Melanoma

The finding of a pigmented, irregularly bordered macule involving the proximal nail fold is called Hutchinson's sign. It represents melanoma of the nail matrix and is therefore classified as an acral lentiginous melanoma. (Courtesy of the Department of Dermatology, Wilford Hall USAF Medical Center and Brooke Army Medical Center, San Antonio, TX.)

Associated Clinical Features

Pyogenic granuloma is characterized by a solitary, violaceous, pedunculated or sessile vascular nodule which usually forms at the site of cutaneous injury (Fig. 13.45). The well demarcated nodule consists of exuberant granulation tissue ("proud flesh") which may be erosive and encrusted. Pyogenic granuloma commonly occurs on the digits and is particularly common in pregnancy.

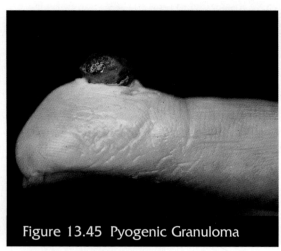

Figure 13.45 Pyogenic Granuloma

This solitary, violaceous, pedunculated, vascular nodule formed at the site of an injury. Note that the nodule is well demarcated by a thin rim of epidermis. (Courtesy of the Department of Dermatology, Wilford Hall USAF Medical Center and Brooke Army Medical Center, San Antonio, TX.)

Differential Diagnosis

This benign vascular neoplasm resembles a hemangioma; however, it must be differentiated from amelanotic melanoma, squamous cell carcinoma, and metastatic renal cell carcinoma.

Emergency Department Treatment and Disposition

Since this neoplasm usually does not resolve spontaneously, it may be shaved off with electrodessication of the base.

Clinical Pearls

1. A fine collarette of scale surrounding an exophytic vascular neoplasm is diagnostic.
2. The lesion may exhibit recurrent bleeding episodes.
3. Nearly 25 to 33% of these benign lesions follow some form of minor trauma.

Associated Clinical Features

A fixed drug eruption is a cutaneous reaction to an ingested drug, usually an over-the-counter laxative, barbiturate, tetracycline, or sulfa drug. The reaction occurs at the identical site with repeated exposure to the same drug, usually on the genital skin or proximal extremity. It presents as a round, pruritic, erythematous, sharply demarcated plaque that may evolve into a painful bulla with secondary erosion (Fig. 13.46). Residual hyperpigmentation frequently follows healing.

Differential Diagnosis

Early cellulitis, erythema multiforme, arthropod assault, and genital herpes are usually considered in the differential diagnosis.

Emergency Department Treatment and Disposition

The etiology must be identified and removed before the plaque will resolve. Symptomatic treatment includes antihistamines and analgesics.

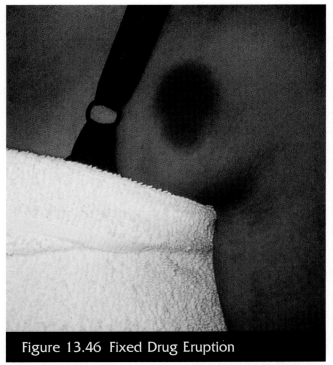

Figure 13.46 Fixed Drug Eruption

This red to violaceous, pruritic, sharply demarcated patch is a cutaneous reaction to a drug. Repeated exposure will cause a similar reaction in the same location. (Courtesy of the Department of Dermatology, Wilford Hall USAF Medical Center and Brooke Army Medical Center, San Antonio, TX.)

Clinical Pearls

1. The identical recurrence of a painful, pruritic, well-demarcated violaceous plaque makes the diagnosis.
2. This reaction occurs with repeated exposure to the same drug.
3. Some patients have a refractory period following exposure.

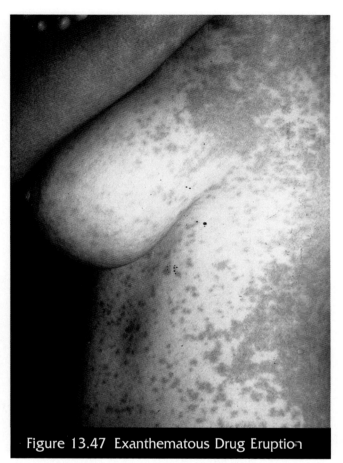

Figure 13.47 Exanthematous Drug Eruption

This symmetric, morbilliform, blanching eruption may eventually become confluent, leading to an exfoliative dermatitis. (Courtesy of GlaxoWellcome Pharmaceuticals.)

Associated Clinical Features

Exanthematous drug eruptions are an adverse hypersensitivity reaction to a drug. This symmetric, pruritic, morbilliform, blanching, erythematous eruption is the most frequent of cutaneous drug eruptions (Fig. 13.47). The initially pruritic macules or papules usually become confluent and may progress to an exfoliative dermatitis.

Differential Diagnosis

Viral exanthem, secondary syphilis, atypical pityriasis rosea, and scarlet fever must all be considered in the differential diagnosis. A serologic test for syphilis, antistreptolysin O titer, and a good history are usually sufficient to make the diagnosis. Severe drug eruptions may be accompanied by eosinophilia, lymphadenopathy, and liver function abnormalities.

Emergency Department Treatment and Disposition

The eruption may resolve despite the drug's continued use. The drug should be discontinued if considered to be the cause of the rash. It may take as long as 2 weeks for the eruption to fade after discontinuation of the causative drug. Symptomatic management includes antihistamines and topical corticosteroids.

Clinical Pearls

1. Drug eruptions are usually symmetric and pruritic as opposed to viral eruptions, which are usually asymmetric and asymptomatic.
2. Mononucleosis patients taking amoxicillin or AIDS patients taking sulfa drugs frequently experience this reaction.

Associated Clinical Features

Erythema nodosum is a delayed hypersensitivity reaction, usually to certain drugs, infections, or systemic illnesses. This panniculitis (inflammation of the fat) consists of painful, nonulcerated, poorly marginated nodules with overlying erythematous, warm, shiny skin. (Fig. 13.48). The lower legs are the most common site; the face is rarely involved. Fever, malaise, and arthralgias often accompany the cutaneous manifestations.

Differential Diagnosis

Erythema induratum, syphilitic gummas, and nodular vasculitis are considered in the differential diagnosis.

Emergency Department Treatment and Disposition

Identify and treat the underlying etiology. Oral contraceptives, sulfa drugs, tuberculosis, sarcoidosis, fungal infections, and inflammatory bowel disease are common predisposing factors. Symptomatic treatment includes nonsteroidal anti-inflamatory drugs (NSAIDs), bed rest, and compressive dressings.

Clinical Pearls

1. Erythema nodosum most commonly presents in young women secondary to oral contraceptives or sulfa drugs.
2. Its appearance in association with systemic fungal infections (coccidioidomycosis) indicates a likely recovery from the disease.

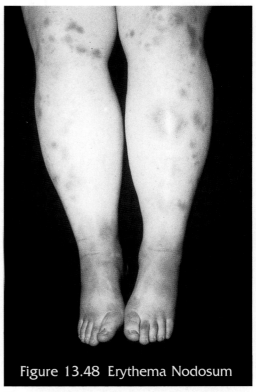

Figure 13.48 Erythema Nodosum

These multiple painful nodules with overlying erythematous, warm and shiny skin were associated with coccidioidomycosis and are typical of erythema nodosum. (Courtesy of GlaxoWellcome Pharmaceuticals.)

415

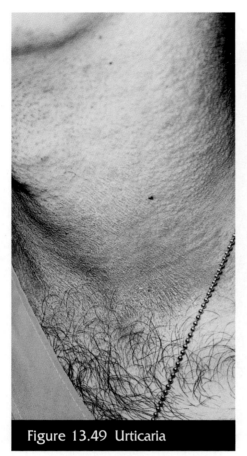

Figure 13.49 Urticaria

Note the edematous papules and wheals covering the skin of the neck. (Courtesy of Alan B. Storrow, MD.)

Associated Clinical Features

Urticaria, a vascular reaction localized to the skin, is composed of transient, erythematous, edematous, pruritic papules or plaquelike wheals (Figs. 13.49, 13.50). It tends to favor the covered areas (back, chest, buttocks). Angioedema comprises thicker plaques that result from fluid shift into the dermis and subcutaneous tissues. It generally affects the distensible tissues (lips, eyelids, earlobes, Fig. 13.51) and is usually nonpruritic. There are countless causes of urticaria; the most common being food, medications, and underlying infection. Cholinergic urticaria involves micropapular lesions induced by exercise or heat. Dermatographism presents as linear hives at the site of skin stroking. Cold urticaria (Fig. 13.52) can be diagnosed with the ice cube test, and solar urticaria occurs in areas exposed to sunlight. Urticaria may also occur as a result of exposure to pressure, heat, and water. Hereditary angioedema is an autosomal dominant disorder with systemic manifestations secondary to edema of the subcutaneous and mucosal tissues of the respiratory and gastrointestinal tract in addition to the face and extremities. Mortality rates approach 30%, usually from airway obstruction. There is also an acquired form of angioedema secondary to an underlying malignancy, usually lymphoreticular. The use of angiotensin converting enzyme (ACE) inhibitors is a frequent cause of angioedema.

Differential Diagnosis

Bacterial or viral exanthems, erythema multiforme, and drug eruptions must be considered in the differential diagnosis of urticaria. Edema of any etiology (congestive heart failure, glomerulonephritis, chronic liver disease) must be differentiated from the soft tissue swelling associated with angioedema.

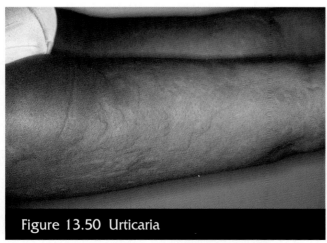

Figure 13.50 Urticaria

Note the classic raised plaques on the lower extremity of this patient with urticaria. (Courtesy of James J. Nordlund, MD.)

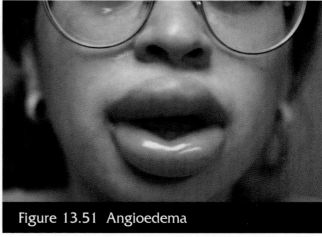

Figure 13.51 Angioedema

Prominent lip involvement in a young woman with ACE inhibitor–induced angioedema. (Courtesy of Alan B. Storrow, MD.)

Emergency Department Treatment and Disposition

This involves the identification and elimination of any potential etiology. Antihistamines can be effective for urticaria, often requiring both H_1 and H_2 blockers and steroids for stubborn cases. Life-threatening attacks of hereditary angioedema do not respond well to antihistamines, epinephrine, or steroids. Admission for supportive care and active airway management is the mainstay of treatment. Danazol may be utilized for prophylactic management.

Clinical Pearls

1. Both urticaria and angioedema are acute and evanescent.
2. Urticaria is pruritic and responsive to antihistamines, epinephrine, and steroids.
3. Angioedema is only rarely pruritic and minimally responsive to epinephrine; it may require danazol for long-term treatment.
4. Doxepin may be considered for refractory cases due to its potent H_1 and H_2 blocking effect.

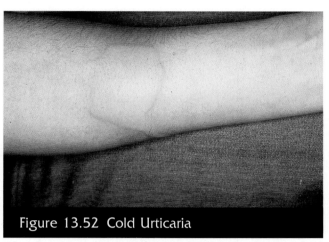

Figure 13.52 Cold Urticaria

Plaque formation after placement of an ice cube on the skin confirms cold urticaria. (Courtesy of James J. Nordlund, MD.)

Associated Clinical Features

Dyshidrotic eczema is a papulovesicular plaque involving the epidermis of the fingers, palms, and soles. The dermatosis initially consists of pruritic, deep-seated vesicles grouped in clusters (Fig. 13.53). Scaling and painful fissure formation are late complications, as is secondary bacterial infection. Spontaneous remissions and recurrent attacks are usually the rule. The bullous form is called *pompholyx*.

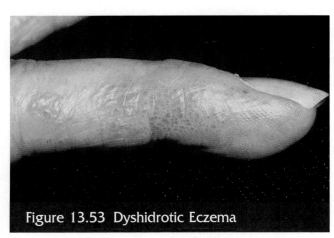

Figure 13.53 Dyshidrotic Eczema

Note the cluster of deep-seated vesicles along the sides of the fingers. Scaling and painful fissure formation may also occur. No overlying erythema is present. (Courtesy of the Department of Dermatology, Wilford Hall USAF Medical Center and Brooke Army Medical Center, San Antonio, TX.)

Differential Diagnosis

Acute contact dermatitis must be considered in the differential diagnosis of the acute eruption. Psoriasis and dermatophytosis are considered in the differential diagnosis of the chronic eruption.

Emergency Department Treatment and Disposition

Burow's wet dressings should be utilized during the early vesicular stage. High-potency topical steroids are used in all stages of the eruption. Systemic corticosteroids should be avoided except for the most severe cases. Antihistamines treat the pruritus. Dicloxacillin or erythromycin are used to treat secondary bacterial infections. Minimal exposure to water and generous emolliation also hasten healing.

Clinical Pearls

1. Deep-seated, tapioca-like vesicles on the sides of the digits, followed by scaling and fissure formation, are typically seen in this disease.
2. Dyshidrotic eczema is frequently associated with psychosocial stressors.
3. The "id reaction," due to fungal infections and drug eruptions, may have similar clinical presentations.

Associated Clinical Features

Atopic dermatitis is a broadly defined pruritic inflammation of the epidermis and dermis, with approximately 60% of the cases occurring during the first year of life. The characteristic pattern is erythema, papules, and lichenified plaques with excoriation and exudation of wet crusts (Fig. 13.54). Its distribution is the face (sparing of the mouth), the antecubital and popliteal fossae, and the dorsal surfaces of the forearms, hands, and feet. This is generally considered a life-long condition with gradual improvement toward adulthood.

Differential Diagnosis

Nummular eczema, allergic contact dermatitis, impetigo, dermatophytosis, and psoriasis are usually considered in the differential diagnosis. A KOH examination of the scale rules out dermatophytosis. A biopsy may help differentiate this condition from nummular eczema and contact dermatitis.

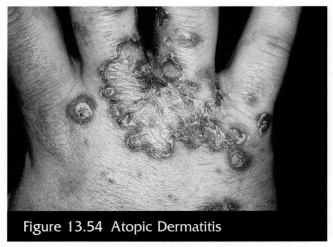

Figure 13.54 Atopic Dermatitis

Emergency Department Treatment and Disposition

Antihistamines treat the pruritus. Unscented emollients prevent xerosis (dry skin). Topical corticosteroids treat the underlying inflammation. Systemic corticosteroids should be avoided except for the most severe cases. Since these patients are frequently colonized with *Staphylococcus aureus,* antistaphylococcal antibiotics are also used during flares of the condition.

Lichenfied plaques, erosions, and fissures are characteristic of atopic dermatitis. (Courtesy of James J. Nordlund, MD.)

Clinical Pearls

1. Scaly plaques on the flexural surface with excoriation and exudation of crusts is diagnostic of atopic dermatitis.
2. Asthma and allergic rhinitis may develop as the atopic dermatitis improves.

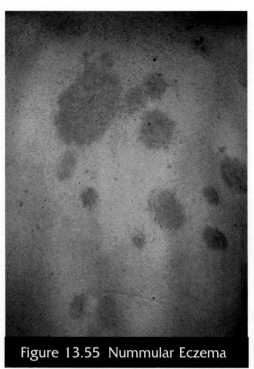

Figure 13.55 Nummular Eczema

An example of multiple erythematous, coin-shaped plaques with fine scales, representative of this pruritic, eczematous dermatitis. (Courtesy of the Department of Dermatology, Wilford Hall USAF Medical Center and Brooke Army Medical Center, San Antonio, TX.)

Associated Clinical Features

Nummular eczema is a pruritic, eczematous dermatitis consisting of closely grouped vesicles that coalesce into coin-shaped, erythematous plaques with poorly defined borders (Fig. 13.55). These plaques may become encrusted or dry and scaly. They are usually found on the trunk and extremities (especially the hand) of a middle-aged or elderly patient.

Differential Diagnosis

Allergic contact dermatitis, impetigo, dermatophytosis, and psoriasis must all be considered in the differential diagnosis. If it scales, scrape it and look for hyphae to differentiate a dermatophytosis. A biopsy may help differentiate contact dermatitis from nummular eczema.

Emergency Department Treatment and Disposition

Antihistamines treat the pruritus. Unscented emollients prevent xerosis. Topical corticosteroids treat the underlying inflammation. Systemic corticosteroids should be avoided except for the most severe cases.

Clinical Pearls

1. Coin-shaped, pruritic, eczematous plaques not responsive to antibiotics are diagnostic of nummular eczema.
2. Recurrences tend to appear in previously involved sites.

Associated Clinical Features

Allergic contact dermatitis is an acute or chronic delayed-type hypersensitivity reaction caused by contact exposure to a variety of agents. The acute form is characterized by multiple, closely grouped vesicles with exudative erosions and crust formation on a well defined erythematous, edematous base (Fig. 13.56). Subacute contact dermatitis consists of dry, scaly patches with areas of desquamation, whereas the chronic form consists of hyperkeratosis and pigmentation. All forms of allergic contact dermatitis are pruritic.

Differential Diagnosis

Atopic dermatitis, nummular eczema, impetigo, and dermatophytosis are included in the differential diagnosis. If it scales, scrape it and look for hyphae to differentiate a dermatophytosis. A positive patch test is diagnostic of an allergic contact dermatitis. Contact exposure of the skin to the allergen leading to erythema and vesicle formation is considered a positive test.

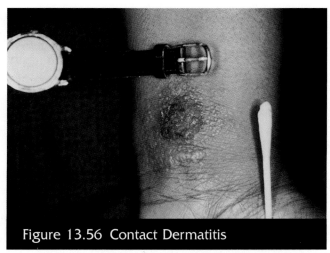

Figure 13.56 Contact Dermatitis

Note that the erythematous, edematous base of the eruption corresponds to the posterior surface of the watch. Superimposed on the erythematous base are multiple vesicles with exudate and crust. (Courtesy of the Department of Dermatology, Wilford Hall USAF Medical Center and Brooke Army Medical Center, San Antonio, TX.)

Emergency Department Treatment and Disposition

Identify and remove any potential allergen. Antihistamines relieve the pruritus. Topical corticosteroids treat the underlying inflammation. Systemic corticosteroids should be avoided except for the most severe cases.

Clinical Pearls

1. Well-defined, pruritic areas of erythema superimposed on exudative vesicles and a recent history of exposure to a specific allergen are diagnostic of allergic contact dermatitis.
2. Poison ivy and oak are the most common causes of allergic contact dermatitis.
3. In treating dermatitis with topical ointments, worsening may signify an allergic reaction to the medication.

Associated Clinical Features

Phytophotodermatitis is a pruritic, linear dermatitis that occurs when skin exposed to certain plants becomes exposed to sunlight. Bizarre patterns of pruritic erythema convert into vesicles and bullae that undergo involution, leaving behind a residual intense hyperpigmentation (Fig. 13.57).

Drug-induced photosensitivity is an adverse skin reaction due to simultaneous exposure to certain drugs and ultraviolet radiation. The rash is erythematous and edematous, much like sunburn (Fig. 13.58).

Differential Diagnosis

Rhus dermatitis is most often mistaken for this eruption. Photosensitivity can be caused by other diseases.

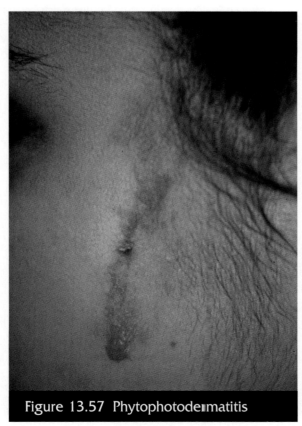

Figure 13.57 Phytophotodermatitis

This linear, photodistributed, eczematous plaque resulted from contact with a plant-derived photosensitizer (lime juice). This frequently resolves with hyperpigmentation. (Courtesy of the Department of Dermatology, Wilford Hall USAF Medical Center and Brooke Army Medical Center, San Antonio, TX.)

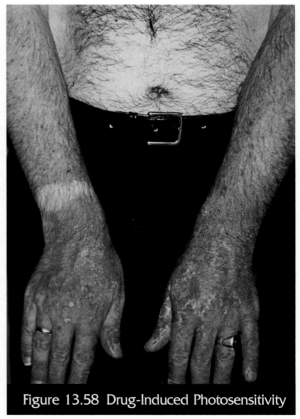

Figure 13.58 Drug-Induced Photosensitivity

Erythematous reaction to ultraviolet radiation associated with carbamazepine use. (Courtesy of the Department of Dermatology, Naval Medical Center, Portsmouth, VA.)

Emergency Department Treatment and Disposition

Symptomatic treatment includes wet dressings, antihistamines, calamine lotion, and corticosteroid creams. For drug-induced photosensitivity, the offending drug should be discontinued. Counsel patients about the use of sunscreens and sun avoidance to prevent recurrences.

Clinical Pearls

1. Linearly distributed, pruritic vesicles in a photodistribution with a history of plant exposure make the diagnosis.
2. The distribution of the rash is limited to sun-exposed areas.
3. Common drugs causing drug-induced photosensitivity are carbamazepine, amiodarone, doxycycline, furosemide, phenothiazines, and sulfonamides.

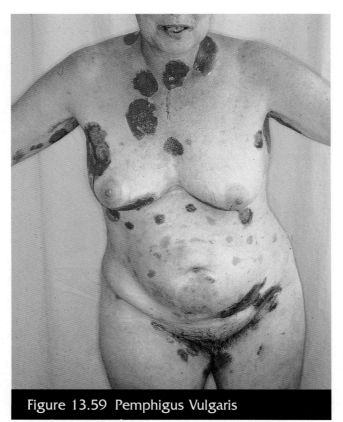

Figure 13.59 Pemphigus Vulgaris

Classic vesiculobullous lesions of pemphigus vulgaris throughout the chest and abdomen. (Courtesy of James J. Nordlurd, MD.)

Associated Clinical Features

Pemphigus vulgaris is a bullous autoimmune disease of the skin and mucous membranes caused by IgG autoantibodies. Previously, mortality was high, but now it only occurs in 10% of cases, usually secondary to steroid complications. This disease typically affects middle-aged adults. Vesicles and bullae arise on the skin of the scalp, chest, umbilicus, and intertriginous areas (Fig. 13.59).

Differential Diagnosis

Pemphigus vulgaris must be distinguished from all other bullous diseases by a skin biopsy.

Emergency Department Treatment and Disposition

High-dose steroids are the mainstay of therapy. Other immunosuppressives—such as azathioprine, methotrexate, and cyclophosphamide—can be helpful. Plasmapheresis is used in cases resistant to standard treatment.

Clinical Pearls

1. Nikolsky's sign can be seen—dislodging of the epidermis with lateral finger pressure on the edge of the bulla.
2. Ulcers and erosions of the oral mucosa are the presenting sign in up to 90% of patients.

Associated Clinical Features

Vitiligo is an acquired loss of pigmentation that commonly involves the backs of the hands, the face, and body folds (Fig. 13.60). There is a positive family history in 30% of the cases. Initially the disease is limited, but it then slowly progresses over years. Vitiligo is secondary to absence of epidermal melanocytes, which may be due to an autoimmune phenomenon against melanocytes. Approximately half of these cases begin in patients less than 20 years of age.

Differential Diagnosis

Vitiligo must be differentiated from tinea versicolor (which has scale and a positive KOH scraping), postinflammatory hypopigmentation, leprosy, and pityriasis alba.

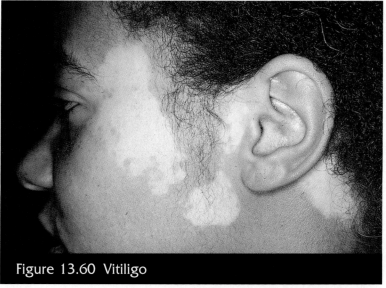

Figure 13.60 Vitiligo

Note the hypopigmented areas characteristic of vitiligo. (Courtesy of James J. Nordlund, MD.)

Emergency Department Treatment and Disposition

Vitiligo requires referral to a dermatologist for PUVA (psoralen plus ultraviolet A), topical therapy, or skin grafting. The best results from therapy occur on the face and neck.

Clinical Pearls

1. Vitiligo occurs at sites of trauma (Koebner's phenomenon).
2. Wood's lamp examination helps identify hypopigmented areas in patients with light complexions.
3. Tinea versicolor has a scale and positive KOH prep.

Associated Clinical Features

Transmission of scabies occurs after direct skin contact with an infected individual and possibly from clothing and bedding infested with the mite. The female mite burrows into the individual's skin and deposits two to three eggs daily. Fecal pellets (scybala) are also deposited in the burrow and may be responsible for the localized pruritus. Nocturnal pruritus is characteristic of scabies. The pink-white, slightly elevated burrows (Fig. 13.61) are typically found in the web spaces of the hands and feet, penis, buttocks, scrotum, and extensor surfaces of the elbows and knees. Norwegian scabies (Fig. 13.62) tends to cause asymptomatic crusting—rather than the typical inflammatory papules and vesicles—as well as nail dystrophy and keratosis.

Differential Diagnosis

Infestation by lice, eczema, and insect bites can be confused with scabies.

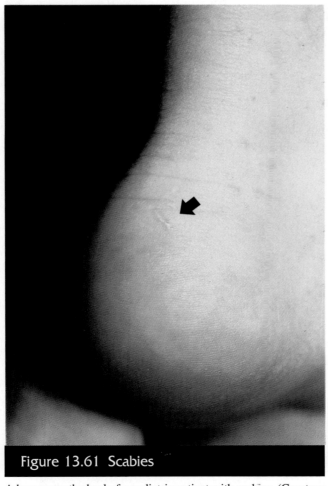

Figure 13.61 Scabies

A burrow on the heel of a pediatric patient with scabies. (Courtesy of Briana Hill, MD.)

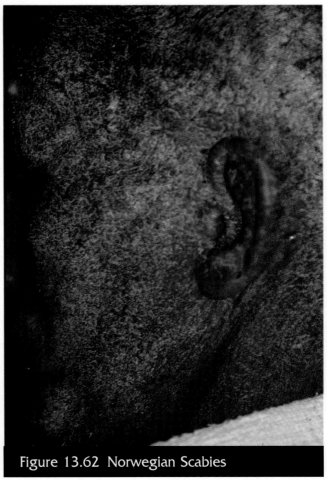

Figure 13.62 Norwegian Scabies

Gray scales and crusting consistent with Norwegian scabies. In these patients, many thousands (versus a few dozen) mites are present. (Courtesy of Lynn Utecht, MD.)

Emergency Department Management and Disposition

Topical permethrin or lindane are commonly used to treat scabies. Each of these products should be applied thoroughly and then, after 8 to 12 h washed from the skin. Lindane should be avoided during infancy and pregnancy because of reports of infant neurotoxicity following systemic absorption through the skin.

Clinical Pearls

1. Ivermectin given as a single 200-μg/kg dose or a 5% sulfur ointment can also be used for treatment.
2. Oral antipruritic therapy and analgesics will help alleviate discomfort.
3. Intimate contacts and all family members in the same household should be treated.

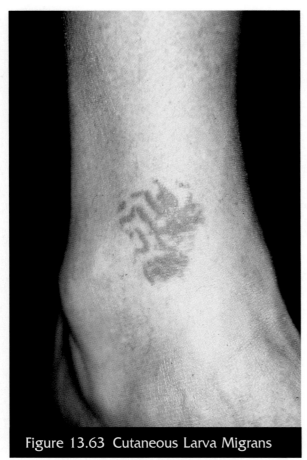

Figure 13.63 Cutaneous Larva Migrans

Note the elevated tracks caused by migration of the larva through the epidermis. (Courtesy of the Department of Dermatology, National Naval Medical Center, Bethesda, MD.)

Associated Clinical Features

Cutaneous larva migrans (CLM) presents as a serpiginous, red, raised, wavy rash that is approximately 3 mm wide (Fig. 13.63). The lacy rash is moderately to severely pruritic as a result of larval secretion of proteolytic enzymes. Infection is most frequent in warmer climates and occurs when the ova of adult hookworms penetrate the skin of a person walking in contaminated soil. Symptoms begin days to weeks after infestation. The nematodes prefer to infect cats or dogs; humans are infected accidentally. The goal of the larva is to eventually penetrate the intestines of its prey. However, owing to physiologic limitations in humans, penetration deeper than the basal layer of the epidermis is prevented.

Differential Diagnosis

The appearance of CLM and its associated pruritus can resemble an allergic reaction, but the lacy border usually distinguishes it.

Emergency Department Treatment and Disposition

Topical application of thiabendazole is the treatment of choice. It is applied two or three times per day for a total of 5 days. Thiabendazole is also available in an oral form; however, it is less effective. Albendazole is an alternative. Symptoms should improve in 48 h. Untreated CLM will usually resolve in 2 to 8 weeks.

Clinical Pearls

1. Löffler's syndrome can occur in patients with severe CLM infestation. In this condition, larval invasion of the bloodstream is manifest as a patchy infiltrate of the lung and eosinophilia of the blood and sputum.
2. The larval track represents an allergic reaction; the larva itself stays slightly ahead of the track.
3. Freezing the skin with ethyl chloride is a simple, effective treatment used in endemic areas.

Associated Clinical Features

Uremic frost is a classic manifestation of chronic renal failure; it is rarely seen today. It develops as a result of accumulation of urea in sweat. In advanced uremia, the accumulation of urea in sweat may reach such a critical level that, upon its evaporation, a fine white powder is left on the skin surface (Fig. 13.64). Associated hyperkalemia may also be present owing to renal failure.

Differential Diagnosis

Dried sweat from a patient with cystic fibrosis forms fern-like crystals that may resemble this condition. In an individual without known renal disease, uremic frost may be mistaken for a dermatologic problem or chemical exposure. However, in a patient with known end-stage renal disease, the differential of a white precipitate on the skin surface is limited.

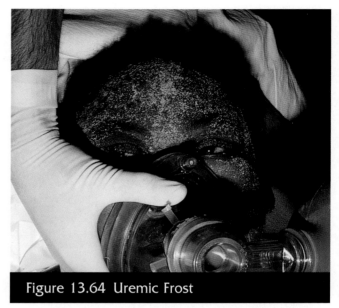

Figure 13.64 Uremic Frost

Note the fine white powder on the skin of this patient with end-stage renal disease. (Courtesy of Richard C. Levy, MD.)

Emergency Department Management and Disposition

Treatment of the underlying condition that resulted in the patient's uremia may prevent further accumulation of uremic frost. Typically, urgent dialysis is indicated.

Clinical Pearls

1. Although rare today, this condition may be seen in patients without adequate air conditioning who are poorly controlled on dialysis.
2. For patients presenting with altered mental status, attention to the airway, oxygenation, and rapid assessment and treatment of associated metabolic disorders such as hyperkalemia are indicated.

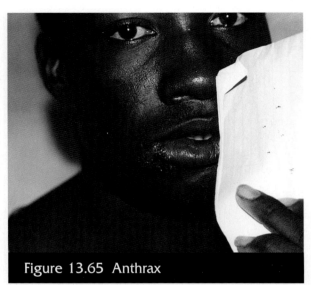

Figure 13.65 Anthrax

Note the early ulcer of cutaneous anthrax on the right of the lower lip. (Courtesy of Thea James, MD.)

Associated Clinical Features

Anthrax is usually a disease of herbivores; humans are infected when they come into contact with infected animals or contaminated animal products. Recently, anthrax has received increased international attention as a potential biological warfare agent. There are three distinct clinical manifestations of anthrax.

Cutaneous anthrax accounts for about 95% of human cases. After direct contact on exposed skin, the infection begins as a pruritic papule. It enlarges into an ulcer surrounded by vesicles in 1 to 2 days and then eventually becomes a characteristic black, necrotic central eschar surrounded by nonpitting edema (Fig. 13.65). Systemic manifestations (fever, hypotension, tachycardia) may accompany cutaneous involvement.

Respiratory anthrax (woolsorters' disease) occurs after exposure to anthrax spores and presents as an upper respiratory infection. Within 1 to 4 days, the disease progresses to severe respiratory distress, hypoxia and hypotension. Death uniformly occurs within 24 h after the onset of the fulminant phases of the infection.

Gastrointestinal anthrax is rare and occurs 3 to 7 days after exposure to contaminated animal meat. Initially it presents as a nonspecific gastroenteritis with fever, vomiting, diarrhea, and malaise. The disease then progresses to hematemesis, bloody diarrhea, sepsis and shock. Death usually occurs 2 to 5 days after symptom onset.

Differential Diagnosis

Cutaneous anthrax resembles staphylococcal infection, tularemia, and plague. Inhalation and gastrointestinal anthrax may initially be similar to a viral upper respiratory infection or gastroenteritis, respectively.

Emergency Department Treatment and Disposition

Admission is indicated for patients with anthrax. Intravenous penicillin is the primary treatment for all forms. Ciprofloxacin or doxycycline are alternatives. Oral ciprofloxacin is recommended for postexposure prophylaxis.

Clinical Pearls

1. Gastrointestinal and inhalation anthrax are almost uniformly fatal, even with antibiotic therapy.
2. Human killed vaccine is available and recommended for mill workers and veterinarians at high risk for exposure.
3. The virulence of anthrax is derived from its edema toxin, lethal toxin, and capsular material.
4. A classic pathologic finding for inhalation anthrax is hemorrhagic mediastinitis; this may be manifested on chest radiography as a widened mediastinum.
5. Decontamination of suspected anthrax spore exposure consists of removal of exposed clothing (place in a sealed plastic bag) and washing of the exposed area with soap and water.

PART 2

SPECIALTY AREAS

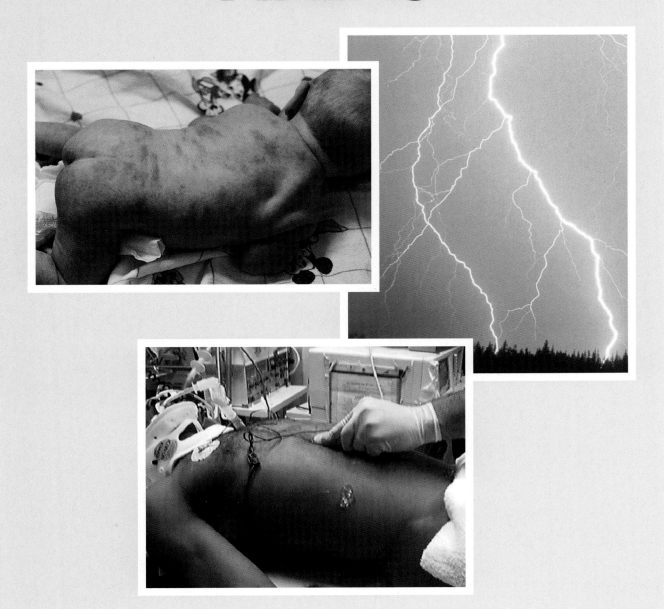

HEAD

CHAPTER 14

PEDIATRIC CONDITIONS

Javier A. Gonzalez del Rey
Richard M. Ruddy

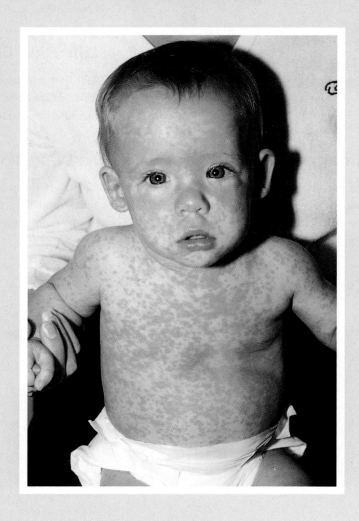

Newborn Conditions

ERYTHEMA TOXICUM

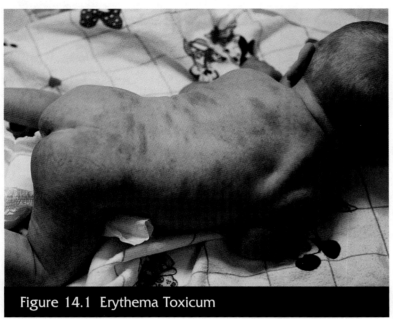

Figure 14.1 Erythema Toxicum

Newborn infant with diffuse macular rash of erythema toxicum. (Courtesy of Kevin J. Knoop, MD, MS.)

Associated Clinical Features

This benign, self-limited eruption of unknown etiology in newborns is characterized by small, erythematous macules 2 to 3 cm in diameter (Fig. 14.1) with 1- to 3-mm firm pale yellow or white papules or pustules in the center. This rash usually presents within the first 2 to 3 days of life. Each individual lesion usually disappears within 4 or 5 days. New lesions may occur during the first 2 weeks of life. Wright-stained slide preparations of the scraping from the center of the lesion demonstrate numerous eosinophils.

Differential Diagnosis

Transient neonatal pustular melanosis, newborn milia, miliaria, herpes simplex, and impetigo of the newborn should be considered.

Emergency Department Treatment and Disposition

As this condition is self-limiting, no therapy is indicated in the setting of a well-appearing newborn with normal activity and appetite. In cases where impetigo, *Candida,* or herpes infections are suspected, a smear from the center of the lesion and culture may be necessary to make a final diagnosis.

Clinical Pearl

1. Erythema toxicum is the most common rash of the newborn (up to 50% of full terms). The lesions may be present anywhere on the body but tend to spare the palms and soles.

Associated Clinical Features

Nevus simplex (salmon patches) is the most common vascular lesion in infancy, present in about 40% of newborns. It is described as a slightly red, flat, macular lesion on the nape of the neck, the glabella, forehead, or upper eyelids (Figs. 14.2 and 14.3). In general, the eyelid lesions fade within a year and the glabellar within 5 to 6 years. The lesions on the neck often persist.

Differential Diagnosis

Nevus flammeus (port-wine stain) can have a similar appearance.

Emergency Department Treatment and Disposition

Parental education and reassurance can be helpful, but no treatment is indicated.

Clinical Pearls

1. In general, flat, vascular birthmarks tend to persist through life. Raised vascular birthmarks usually disappear with time.
2. When this lesion is seen on the nape of the neck, it is frequently referred to as a *stork bite*.

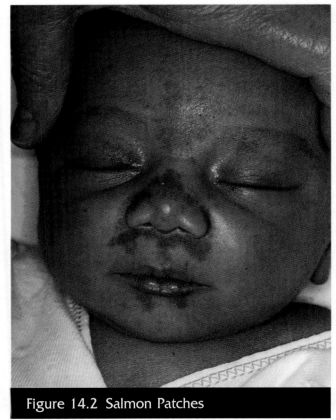

Figure 14.2 Salmon Patches

Newborn with characteristic salmon patches over his face. (Courtesy of Anne W. Lucky, MD.)

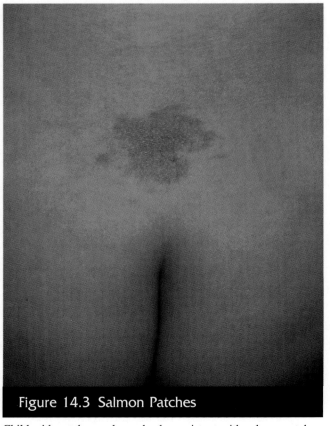

Figure 14.3 Salmon Patches

Child with patch over lower back consistent with salmon patches. (Courtesy of Anne W. Lucky, MD.

435

Associated Clinical Features

Physiologic jaundice (Fig. 14.4) is observed in 25 to 50% of term newborns. Most cases are self-limited and generally without sequelae. The physiologic (<12 mg/dL) jaundice of the newborn usually peaks between the second and fourth day. In preterm infants, this peak occurs later. Physiologic jaundice is believed to be due to a combination of factors including an increase of bilirubin production following a breakdown of fetal red blood cells associated with a temporary decrease in conjugation of these by-products by the immature newborn liver. Risk factors for unconjugated hyperbilirubinemia include maternal diabetes, prematurity, drugs, polycythemia, traumatic delivery with cutaneous bruising or hematoma, and breast-feeding. Most infants with jaundice have no disease, but a careful history and organized approach is necessary to identify pathologic causes when these patients present to the ED.

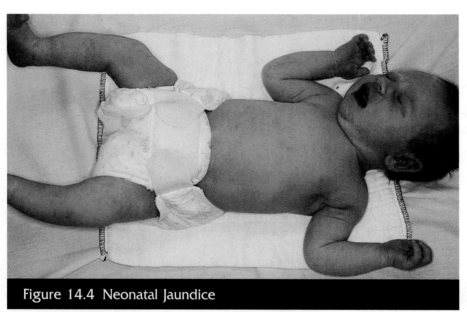

Figure 14.4 Neonatal Jaundice

Newborn with yellowish hue to skin consistent with jaundice. (Courtesy of Kevin J. Knoop, MD, MS.)

Kernicterus is a condition resulting from a severe form of unconjugated hyperbilirubinemia and is associated with mental retardation, deafness, seizures, choreoathetosis, and a multitude of other irreversible neurologic abnormalities.

Differential Diagnosis

Jaundice within the first 24 h of life is usually associated with sepsis, erythroblastosis fetalis, and bleeding disorders or hemorrhage (traumatic delivery with cutaneous bleeding or hematomas). Physiologic jaundice first appears on the second or third day. Any patient presenting with jaundice after the third day of life should be carefully evaluated for the possibility of sepsis. Late-onset jaundice could be suggestive of septicemia, breast milk jaundice, galactosemia, hemolytic anemias, drug-induced hyperbilirubinemia, pyloric stenosis or duodenal atresia, Crigler-Najjar syndrome, or Gilber's disease.

Emergency Department Treatment and Disposition

Initial laboratory workup should include blood type and Coombs' test, complete blood count with smear for red cell morphology and reticulocyte count, and indirect and direct bilirubin. Other studies may be ordered according to the clinical presentation and history. Initial management should ensure adequate hydration and treatment of the underlying condition. Acidosis should be corrected, since bilirubin precipitates in acid media. In cases of physiologic jaundice, the level of serum bilirubin at which to start phototherapy is not clearly defined. The traditional approach is to initiate phototherapy to maintain bilirubin level below 20 mg/dL. Exchange transfusion is considered if the serum level remains elevated (22 to 28 mg/dL) despite appropriate phototherapy.

Clinical Pearls

1. Physiologic jaundice in the presence of a good hemoglobin level is orange in color. It is often visible when the bilirubin level exceeds 8 mg/dL. Jaundice associated with anemia is usually lemon in color.

2. Bilirubin levels should be modified for prematurity, sepsis, low birth weight, and other risk factors when phototherapy or exchange transfusion is considered.

Associated Clinical Features

Because of transplacenta hormonal effects (maternal estrogens and possibly endogenous prolactin), both sexes are equally liable to develop enlarged breasts. This phenomenon occurs with or without galactorrhea in 60% of normal newborns. After the first 48 h, the hypertrophied breasts may become engorged, and a form of lactation occurs (Fig. 14.5). The engorgement and edema begin to subside after the second week of life. The hypertrophy and galactorrhea may persist up to 6 months in girls. These infants are occasionally predisposed to infections (mastitis or abscess).

Differential Diagnosis

Early mastitis with purulent discharge may resemble normal neonatal milk production.

Emergency Department Treatment and Disposition

Treatment is not necessary; reassurance for parents is very important.

Clinical Pearl

1. Newborns with hypertrophied mammary tissue and evidence of clear colostrum-like secretion in the absence of erythema, tenderness, and/or fluctuation usually do not present with neonatal mastitis.

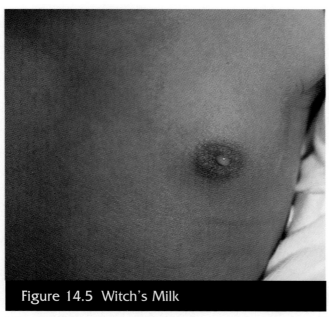

Figure 14.5 Witch's Milk

Milky fluid draining from the nipple in a newborn. (Courtesy of Michael J. Nowicki, MD.)

NEONATAL MASTITIS

Associated Clinical Features

Neonatal mastitis is most common in full-term females, particularly in their second or third week of life. Clinically it manifests as swelling, induration, and tenderness of the affected breast with or without erythema or warmth (Fig. 14.6). In some cases purulent discharge may be obtained from the nipple. Bacteremia and fever are rare. This infection is usually caused by *Staphylococcus* aureus, coliform bacteria, or group B streptococcus. If treatment is delayed, mastitis may progress rapidly with involvement of subcutaneous tissues and subsequent toxicity and systemic findings.

Differential Diagnosis

In the initial stages, neonatal mastitis may mimic mammary tissue hypertrophy owing to maternal passive hormonal stimulation. Minor trauma, cutaneous infections, and duct blockage may precede this infection.

Emergency Department Treatment and Disposition

Institution of treatment is important to avoid cellulitic spread and breast tissue damage. In cases of mild cellulitis and no fluctuation, culture of nipple discharge and antibiotic coverage (semisynthetic penicillin or first-generation cephalosporins) completes the treatment. Adjustment of coverage may be done once results of cultures or Gram's stain are available, espe-

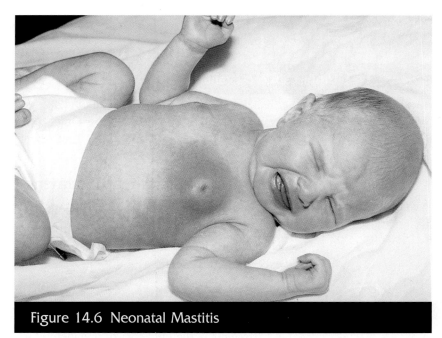

Figure 14.6 Neonatal Mastitis

Neonate with left-sided breast swelling, erythema, and purulent discharge. (Courtesy of Raymond C. Baker, MD.)

cially in the presence of gram-negative bacilli. If no organism is seen initially, semisynthetic penicillin and an aminoglycoside or cefotaxime should be used. In case of toxicity or subcutaneous spreading, a complete sepsis workup should be performed, and hospitalization is usually indicated. In cases of palpable fluctuation, prompt surgical incision and drainage should be performed by a surgeon to avoid further damage of the mammary tissue. Recovery is usually in 5 to 7 days.

Clinical Pearl

1. Consider mastitis in the neonate with edema, induration, and tenderness of the breast tissue. Erythema and fluctuation to palpation ensue if treatment is delayed.

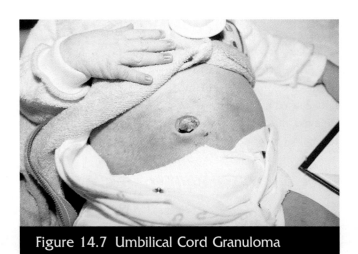

Figure 14.7 Umbilical Cord Granuloma

Newborn infant with umbilical cord demonstrating granuloma on base of umbilical cord. (Courtesy of Michael J. Nowicki, MD.)

Associated Clinical Features

Umbilical cord granuloma develops in response to a mild infection at the base of the umbilical cord caused by saprophytic organisms. Usually parents describe a persistent discharge from the base of the cord. The granuloma is soft, pink, and vascular (Fig. 14.7) and is the result of persistence of exuberant granulation tissue.

Differential Diagnosis

An umbilical polyp is a rare anomaly resulting from the persistence of the omphalomesenteric duct (Figs. 14.8, 14.9) or the urachus and may have a similar appearance. This polyp is usually firm and resistant, with a mucoid secretion. Omphalitis, an infection secondary to gram-negative organisms, should be considered.

Emergency Department Treatment and Disposition

Cleaning and drying of the umbilical cord base with alcohol several times a day may prevent granuloma formation. Cauterization of the granuloma with silver nitrate is the treatment of choice. It is important to protect the surrounding skin to avoid chemical burns produced by the excess of silver nitrate.

Clinical Pearls

1. Commonly the only sign of granuloma formation is the presence of nonpurulent discharge noted in the diaper area in contact with the umbilicus.
2. Omphalitis presents with redness on the abdominal wall and often with a purulent discharge from the umbilicus.

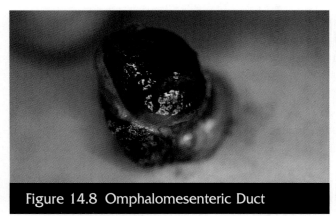

Figure 14.8 Omphalomesenteric Duct

This red mass resembling a granuloma was found to be an omphalomesenteric duct. (Courtesy of Kevin J. Knoop, MD, MS.)

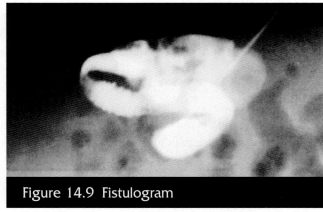

Figure 14.9 Fistulogram

A fistulogram confirms the diagnosis of persistent omphalomesenteric duct. (Courtesy of Kevin J. Knoop, MD, MS.)

Associated Clinical Features

HPS is characterized by postprandial, nonbilious vomiting due to hypertrophy and hyperplasia of the pyloric musculature, producing gastric outlet obstruction. It is usually diagnosed in infants from birth to 5 months, most commonly at 2 to 8 weeks of life. The vomiting progresses to forceful and is described as projectile (although this pattern is not always present). There is a familial incidence, and white males are more frequently affected. During the physical examination, peristaltic waves may be observed traveling from the left upper to right upper quadrants (Fig. 14.10). The hypertrophy and hyperplasia of the antral and pyloric musculature produces the "olive" to palpation (best palpated after emptying the stomach with a nasogastric tube). Because of persistent vomiting, hypochloremic alkalosis with various degrees of dehydration and failure to thrive may occur when this is not diagnosed early. The finding of the pyloric olive is pathognomonic. Ultrasound and fluoroscopy are useful diagnostic tools to confirm the diagnosis when the olive is not evident.

Differential Diagnosis

Intestinal obstruction, atresia, malrotation with volvulus, hiatal hernia, gastroenteritis, adrenogenital syndrome, increased intracranial pressure, esophagitis, sepsis, gastroesophageal reflux, and poor feeding technique should be considered.

Emergency Department Treatment and Disposition

Once the diagnosis is considered, treatment includes correction of fluids and electrolyte imbalance followed by surgical referral for curative pylorotomy. Patients benefit from a nasogastric tube on low intermittent suction.

Clinical Pearls

1. Any infant in the first 2 months of life who presents with postprandial vomiting, some evidence of failure to gain weight, easy refeeding, hunger after vomiting, and infrequent bowel movements should be carefully evaluated to rule out the possibility of HPS.
2. Clinical suspicion can be heightened with serial examinations and observation of the child after oral fluid challenges for persistent projectile vomiting.
3. Correction of any electrolyte imbalance should occur prior to surgery.

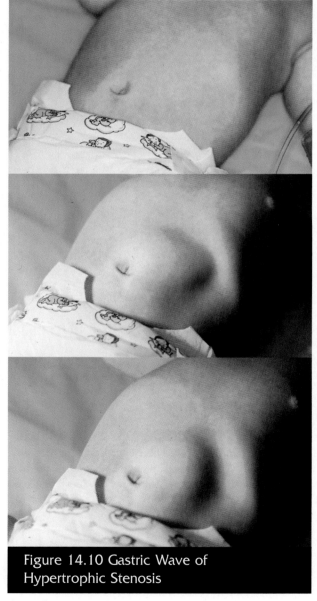

Figure 14.10 Gastric Wave of Hypertrophic Stenosis

A gastric wave can be seen traversing the abdomen in this series of photographs of a patient with HPS. (Courtesy of Kevin J. Knoop, MD, MS.)

Rashes and Lesions

ERYTHEMA INFECTIOSUM (FIFTH DISEASE)

Associated Clinical Features

Erythema infectiosum is a viral infection caused by parvovirus B19. It is characterized by an eruption that presents initially as an erythematous malar blush followed by an erythematous maculopapular eruption on the extensor surfaces of extremities that evolves into a reticulated, lacy, mottled appearance (Fig. 14.11). It may present with low-grade fever, malaise, general aches, arthritis, or arthralgias.

Differential Diagnosis

Morbilliform eruptions may be caused by viruses such as measles, rubella, roseola, and infectious mononucleosis. Bacterial infections (i.e., scarlet fever), drug reactions, and other skin conditions such as guttate psoriasis, papular urticaria, and erythema multiforme are included in the differential.

Emergency Department Treatment and Disposition

There is no specific treatment. Once the rash appears, the patient is no longer contagious. It is important to educate the patient and family about the possible risk of B19 virus as a cause of hydrops fetalis or fetal deaths early in pregnancy and the issue of an aplastic crisis in patients with hematologic problems such as sickle cell disease, hereditary spherocytosis, other hemolytic anemias, or immunosuppressed host.

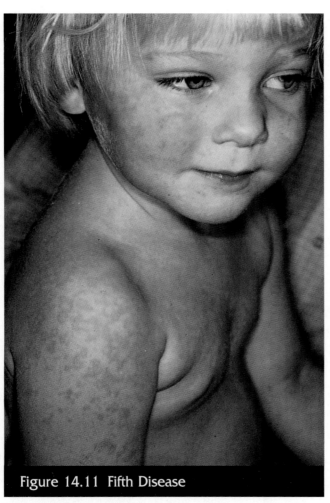

Figure 14.11 Fifth Disease

Toddler with the classic slapped-cheek appearance of fifth disease caused by parvovirus B19. Also note the lacy reticular macular rash on the shoulder and upper extremity. (Courtesy of Anne W. Lucky, MD.)

Clinical Pearl

1. Classically this infection begins with the intense redness of both cheeks ("slapped-cheek appearance"). Although the eruption tends to disappear within 5 days of the initial presentation, recrudescences may occur with exercise, overheating, and sunburns as a result of cutaneous vasodilatation.

Associated Clinical Features

The typical presentation of roseola infantum is that of a child with a 2- or 3-day history of fever and irritability. This is followed by rapid defervescence and the appearance of an erythematous morbilliform eruption (Fig. 14.12). It has been associated with various viral agents such as parvovirus, echovirus, and other enteroviruses. Most recently it has been associated with herpesvirus 6.

Differential Diagnosis

Morbilliform eruptions may be caused by common viruses such as measles, rubella, parvovirus B19, or infectious mononucleosis. Bacterial infections (e.g., scarlet fever), drug reactions, and other skin conditions such as guttate psoriasis, papular urticaria, and erythema multiforme may be included in the differential.

Emergency Department Treatment and Disposition

As with most viral infections, only supportive therapy is necessary. Special attention should be paid in maintaining fluid intake, fever control for the patient's comfort, and parental education about the benign, self-limiting characteristics of this illness.

Clinical Pearls

1. The presence of mild eyelid edema with posterior cervical adenopathy in the febrile child without a source may be early indicators for the diagnosis of roseola. Once the fever ends and the rash appears, the diagnosis is clinically confirmed.
2. Rashes *during* the febrile course of an illness are not roseola.

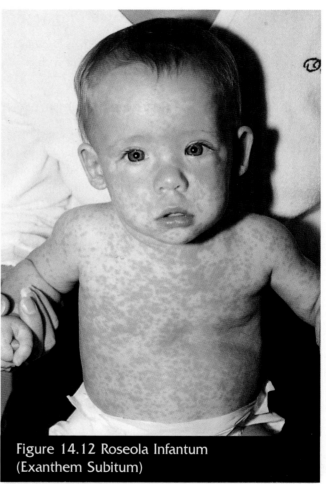

Figure 14.12 Roseola Infantum (Exanthem Subitum)

Toddler with maculopapular eruption of roseola. (Courtesy of Raymond C. Baker, MD.)

Associated Clinical Features

Impetigo is a bacterial infection of the skin produced by *Streptococcus pyogenes* and *Staphylococcus aureus*. It begins as small vesicles or pustules with very thin roofs that rupture easily with the release of a cloudy fluid and the subsequent formation of a honey-colored crust (Figs. 14.13, 14.14). Often the lesions spread rapidly and coalesce to form larger ones.

Differential Diagnosis

Second-degree burns, cutaneous diphtheria, herpes simplex infections, nummular dermatitis, and kerion may present with crusts and be confused with impetigo.

Emergency Department Treatment and Disposition

Since these lesions are contagious, good hand washing and personal hygiene should be discussed with the patient and family. Antibiotic coverage should be directed against the organisms mentioned above. Effective oral agents include erythromycin, first-generation cephalosporins, cloxacillin, or amoxicillin with clavulanic acid. Topical agents such as mupirocin ointment have proved to be as effective as oral antibiotics.

Clinical Pearls

1. A red, weeping surface and the presence of moist, thin vesicles with honey-colored crusts makes the diagnosis of impetigo.
2. Inflicted cigarette burns may resemble the lesions of impetigo.

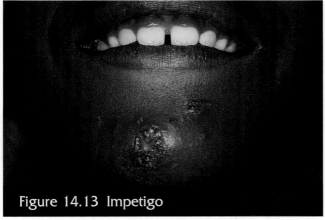

Figure 14.13 Impetigo

Young girl with crusting impetiginous lesions or her chin. (Courtesy of Michael J. Nowicki, MD.)

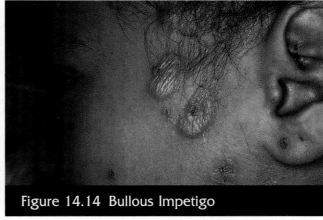

Figure 14.14 Bullous Impetigo

A child with impetiginous lesions on the face. Note the formation of bullae. (Courtesy of Anne W. Lucky, MD.)

Associated Clinical Features

A kerion consists of inflammatory boggy nodules with pustules caused by an exaggerated host delayed hypersensitivity response to infections with either *Microsporum canis* or *Trichophyton tonsurans*. These lesions usually remain localized to one area (Fig. 14.15). It appears 2 to 8 weeks after the initial fungal infection and resolves over 4 to 6 weeks. If untreated, scarring and hair loss may occur.

Differential Diagnosis

Bacterial pyoderma is commonly mistaken for kerion but yields a purulent discharge when aspirated. The diagnosis should be made on clinical appearance.

Emergency Department Treatment and Disposition

Topical agents have no role in the treatment of tinea capitis or kerion. Griseofulvin for 4 to 6 weeks is the treatment of choice. Ketoconazole has also been used. Viable spores can be eradicated by adding selenium sulfide shampoo (2.5%) to this therapy. In cases of severe inflammatory reaction, prednisone combined with griseofulvin ensures a rapid resolution of the infection and immunogenic reaction. Incision should be avoided to prevent scar tissue.

Clinical Pearl

1. If a kerion happens to be aspirated or incised, only serosanguineous fluid is obtained.

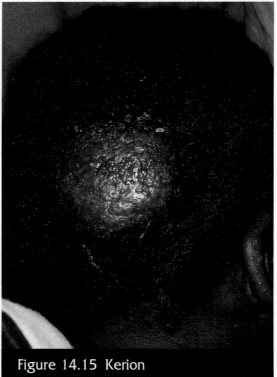

Figure 14.15 Kerion

Occipital boggy swelling with hair loss consistent with kerion. (Courtesy of Anne W. Lucky, MD.)

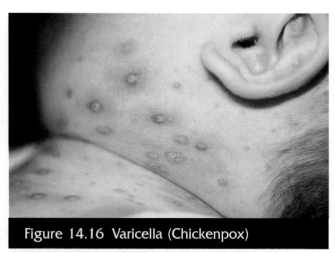

Figure 14.16 Varicella (Chickenpox)

Multiple umbilicated cloudy vesicles of varicella. (Courtesy of Lawrence B. Stack, MD.)

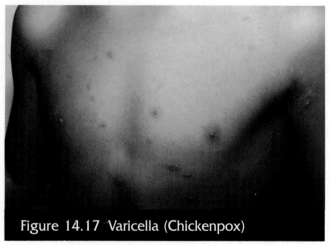

Figure 14.17 Varicella (Chickenpox)

Vesicles in different stages of maturation. Note the clear vesicle on an erythematous base ("dewdrop in a rose petal") in the center of the chest. (Courtesy of Judith C. Bausher, MD.)

Associated Clinical Features

Chickenpox results from a primary infection with varicella virus and is characterized by a generalized pruritic vesicular rash (Fig. 14.16), fever, and mild systemic symptoms. The skin lesions have an abrupt onset, develop in crops, and evolve from papules to vesicles (rarely bullae) and finally to crusted lesions within 48 h. The classic lesions are teardrop vesicles surrounded by an erythematous ring (dewdrop on a rose petal) (Fig. 14.17). Secondary bacterial infection of these lesions can occur, causing cellulitis, which may be severe. Other complications from varicella include encephalitis, pancreatitis, hepatitis, pneumonia, arthritis, or meningitis. Cerebritis (ataxia) may develop and is usually self-limiting.

Differential Diagnosis

Although several illnesses can present with vesiculobullous lesions, the typical case of varicella is seldom confused with other problems. Common viral infections that manifest with vesicular rashes include herpes simplex, herpes zoster, coxsackie, influenza, and echovirus infections or vaccinia. On occasion varicella can be confused with papular urticaria.

Emergency Department Treatment and Disposition

Most patients do not develop any complications. Treatment should be symptomatic and directed to pruritus and fever control (avoid salicylates because of their association with Reye's syndrome). Oral acyclovir given within 24 h of the onset of the illness may result in a modest decrease in the duration of symptoms and in the number and duration of skin lesions. Acyclovir is not recommended routinely for treatment of uncomplicated varicella in an otherwise healthy child. In the immunocompromised host, VZIG (varicella zoster immunoglobulin) and intravenous acyclovir are effectively used.

Clinical Pearl

1. Skin lesions in varicella present in successive crops, so that papules, vesicles, and crusted lesions may all be present at the same time. The earliest lesions may begin at the hairline on the nape of the neck.

Associated Clinical Features

Measles presents as an acute febrile illness with a 3- to 4-day prodromal period characterized by cough, coryza, and conjunctivitis associated with fever (101° to 104°F), chills, and malaise. Koplik's spots, the pathognomonic sign of measles, appear as 1- to 3-mm white elevations on the buccal mucosa (Fig. 14.18). They usually present 1 to 2 days before the development of the characteristic erythematous maculopapular rash. This rash appears during the third or fourth day of the illness. It usually begins around the hairline, behind the earlobes, and spreads downward (Fig. 14.19). It tends to fade in the same order it appears. Most cases recover without complications; others may develop otitis media, croup, pneumonia, encephalitis, and rarely subacute sclerosing panencephalitis (SSPE), a very late complication.

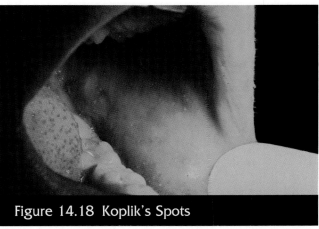

Figure 14.18 Koplik's Spots

Tiny white dots (Koplik's spots) are seen on the buccal mucosa. (Courtesy of Lawrence B. Stack, MD.)

Differential Diagnosis

The differential diagnosis of the characteristic rash is vast and includes exanthem subitum; rubella; infections caused by echovirus, coxsackie and adenoviruses; toxoplasmosis; infectious mononucleosis; scarlet fever; Kawasaki disease; drug reactions; Rocky Mountain spotted fever; and meningococcemia.

Emergency Department Treatment and Disposition

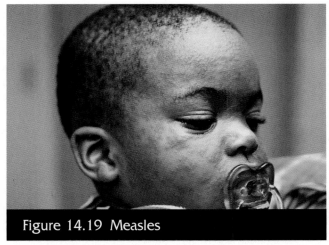

Figure 14.19 Measles

School-age child with a morbilliform rash on his face consistent with measles. (Courtesy of Javier A. Gonzalez del Rey, MD.)

Supportive therapy includes bed rest, antipyretics, and adequate fluid balance. Complications should be treated according to the presentation. Current available antiviral compounds are not effective. The use of gamma globulins and steroids in SSPE is limited. Passive immunization is effective for prevention and attenuation of measles if given within 5 days of the initial exposure. During outbreaks, measles-mumps-rubella (MMR) vaccine is given earlier than 15 months and may need to be repeated. A second dose is recommended after the primary series for those born after 1956. This is given at age 11 or 12 years or by entry to junior high school.

Clinical Pearls

1. The classic presentation includes a prodromal phase (fever, hacking cough, coryza, and conjunctivitis), Koplik's spots followed by an abrupt temperature rise, and a rash spreading in a caudal distribution.
2. Examination of the oral mucosa to identify Koplik's spots may diagnose measles early if performed in all children with an acute febrile illness.

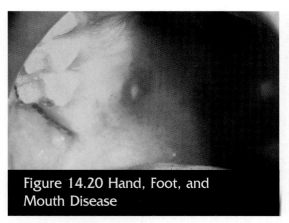

Figure 14.20 Hand, Foot, and Mouth Disease

Discrete vesicular erosions on the posterior oropharynx and soft palate secondary to coxsackievirus. (Courtesy of James F. Steiner, DDS.)

Associated Clinical Features

Hand, foot, and mouth disease is a seasonal (summer–fall) viral infection caused by coxsackievirus A16. It is characterized by fever, malaise, and anorexia over 1 to 2 days, followed by oral lesions (small, red macules that evolve into small vesicles 1 to 3 mm in diameter) in the posterior oropharynx (Fig. 14.20). This enanthem is then followed by a superficial, nonloculated vesicular eruption on the hands and feet (3 to 7 mm) (Figs. 14.21 and 14.22). These may also be present on the buttocks, face, and legs.

Differential Diagnosis

Herpes simplex, varicella, varicella zoster, influenza, echovirus infections, vaccinia, and other coxsackieviruses should all be considered.

Emergency Department Treatment and Disposition

Supportive therapy, especially fluid maintenance and fever control for the patient's comfort, is the mainstay of treatment. The duration and characteristics of the illness should be discussed with the parents. In the majority of cases, the course is self-limited and the prognosis excellent. On rare occasions, secondary complications such as myocarditis, pneumonia, and meningoencephalitis may occur

Clinical Pearl

1. The individual lesions are usually seen on the palms, fingertips, and soles. Oral cavity lesions appear as discrete oval erosions and most are classically seen in the posterior oropharynx and soft palate.

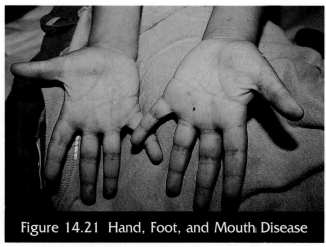

Figure 14.21 Hand, Foot, and Mouth Disease

Erythematous vesicular rash scattered on the palms, consistent with coxsackievirus. (Courtesy of Michael J. Nowicki, MD.)

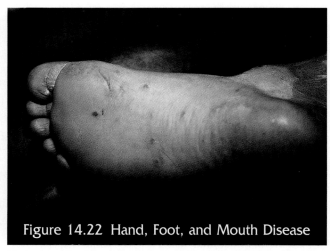

Figure 14.22 Hand, Foot, and Mouth Disease

Vesicular rash of the feet consistent with coxsackievirus. (Courtesy of Raymond C. Baker, MD.)

Associated Clinical Features

Cold panniculitis is an acute cold injury to the fat of the cheeks in infants. It manifests as red, indurated nodules and plaques on exposed skin, especially the face (Fig. 14.23). These lesions appear 1 to 3 days after exposure and gradually soften and return to normal over 1 or more weeks. This phenomenon is caused by subcutaneous fat solidification when exposed to low temperature. It is more frequent in children than in adults.

Differential Diagnosis

Facial cellulitis, trauma, pressure erythema, giant urticaria, and contact dermatitis may have a similar presentation.

Emergency Department Treatment and Disposition

Treatment is not necessary; parental reassurance is very important.

Clinical Pearl

1. Because these lesions may also be painful, the differentiation of cold panniculitis from cellulitis may be difficult on occasion. The absence of systemic symptoms, especially fever, and the history of cold exposure are very suggestive of cold panniculitis.

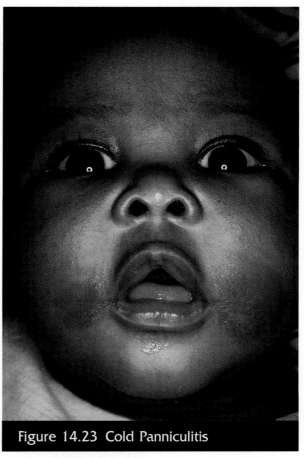

Figure 14.23 Cold Panniculitis

Infant with cheek erythema, swelling, and discoloration consistent with popsicle panniculitis or cold injury. (Courtesy of Anne W. Lucky, MD.)

Associated Clinical Features

Herpetic gingivostomatitis is a viral infection commonly seen in infants and children; it is caused by herpes simplex. Patients usually present with fever, malaise, cervical adenopathy, and pain in the mouth and throat on attempting to swallow. Vesicular and ulcerative lesions appear throughout the oral cavity. The gingiva becomes very friable and inflamed, especially around the alveolar rim. Increased salivation with foul breath may be present. Although fever disappears in 3 to 5 days, children may have difficulty eating for 7 to 14 days. Sometimes, autoinoculation produces vesicular lesions on the fingers (herpetic whitlow) (Fig. 14.24).

Differential Diagnosis

Vincent's angina, aphthous stomatitis, erythema multiforme, Behçet's disease, and other viral infections such as herpangina and hand, foot, and mouth disease (coxsackieviruses) should be considered.

Emergency Department Treatment and Disposition

No specific treatment is available. In immunocompromised patients, acyclovir should be considered. In the normal host, fluid balance should be maintained throughout the illness. Because of ulcerative lesions, avoidance of citrus juices or spicy food prevents pain on swallowing. Clear fluids, ice pops, and ice cream may be used in small children. Not infrequently, admission for

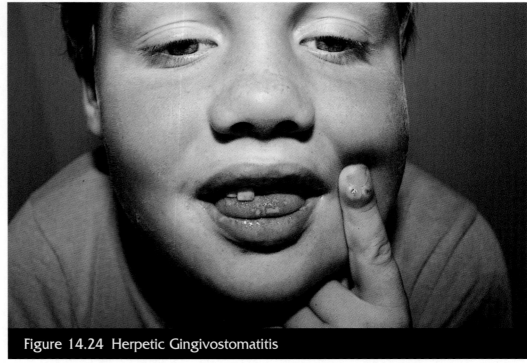

Figure 14.24 Herpetic Gingivostomatitis

Multiple oral vesicular lesions consistent with herpes gingivostomatitis. Vesicular lesions from autoinoculation are present on the finger (herpetic whitlow). (Courtesy of Michael J. Nowicki, MD.)

intravenous hydration is necessary. Adequate fever control is also necessary for patient comfort and to avoid an increase in fluid losses. Pain control may be achieved by using mixtures of antihistamine (diphenhydramine elixir) and antacids (1:1) applied to lesion with Q-tips. In small children, local application of viscous lidocaine (Xylocaine) should be avoided, since patients may develop toxic plasma levels due to an altered absorption from an inflamed oral mucosa.

Clinical Pearl

1. Most of these lesions are in the anterior two-thirds of the oral cavity. Posterior lesions sparing the gingiva are most commonly seen in coxsackievirus infections.

Associated Clinical Features

Urticaria is a localized, edematous skin reaction from histamine release that usually follows an infection, insect sting or bite, ingestion of certain foods, or medications. It is characterized by a sudden onset of pruritic, transient, well-circumscribed wheals scattered over the body. These are flat-topped and may vary from pinpoint size to several centimeters in diameter. They usually have a central clearing and peripheral extension and can have tense edema (Fig. 14.25). Most urticarial reactions last 24 to 48 h; on rare occasions, they may take weeks to resolve. Rarely, there may be systemic reactions such as wheezing, stridor, or angioedema.

Differential Diagnosis

Erythema multiforme, arthropod bites, dermatographism, contact dermatitis, reactive erythemas, allergic vasculitis, juvenile rheumatoid arthritis, mastocytosis, and pityriasis rosea can all present with a similar-appearing rash.

Emergency Department Treatment and Disposition

Treatment is symptomatic. Oral antihistamines are useful in the control of pruritus. If a systemic reaction is also part of the initial presentation, epinephrine and steroids should be added to the therapy. In most cases it is very difficult to identify the etiologic factor. Unless there is evidence of acute angioedema, most cases can be discharged home on oral antihistamines.

Clinical Pearl

1. Erythema multiforme can be commonly mistaken for polycyclic urticaria (multiple red wheals of different sizes). Clinicially these two entities can be differentiated by the duration and color of the lesions. In urticaria, the center is clear and each lesion usually lasts a few hours. In erythema multiforme, the center is dusky and the lesion remains in the same place for several days to weeks.

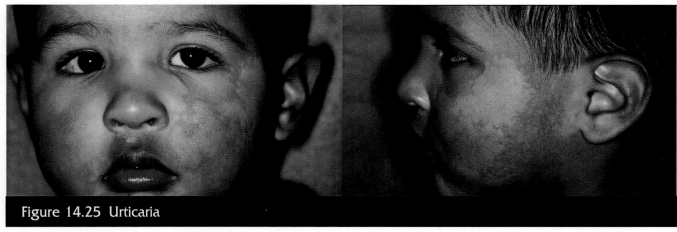

Figure 14.25 Urticaria

Preschool child with annular, raised pruritic lesions with the central clearing and tense edema of polycyclic urticaria. The lesions had completely disappeared after about 5 min. (Courtesy of Kevin J. Knoop, MD, MS.)

Associated Clinical Features

Staphylococcal scalded skin syndrome is caused by a staphylococcal toxin-producing strain. It may present with fever, malaise, and irritability following an upper respiratory infection. Patients develop a diffuse faint erythematous rash that becomes tender to touch. Crusting around the mouth, eyes, and neck is not uncommon. Within 2 to 3 days, the upper layers of dermis may be easily removed; finally a flaccid bulla develops with subsequent exfoliation of the skin (Fig. 14.26). In young patients, this exfoliation may involve a large surface area with significant fluid and electrolyte losses.

Differential Diagnosis

Toxic epidermal necrolysis, exfoliative erythroderma, bullous erythema multiforme, bullous pemphigoid, bullous impetigo, sunburn, acute mercury poisoning, toxic shock syndrome, and scarlet fever should be considered.

Emergency Department Treatment and Disposition

Treatment is directed at the eradication of *Staphylococcus,* thus terminating the production of toxin. Synthetic penicillins should be used intravenously. Admission is usually necessary, especially in young infants. This age group requires careful attention to fluid and electrolyte losses and the prevention of secondary infection of the affected skin.

Clinical Pearl

1. The wrinkling or peeling of the upper layer of the epidermis (pressure applied with a Q-tip or gloved finger) that occurs within 2 or 3 days of the onset of this illness is known as Nikolsky's sign.

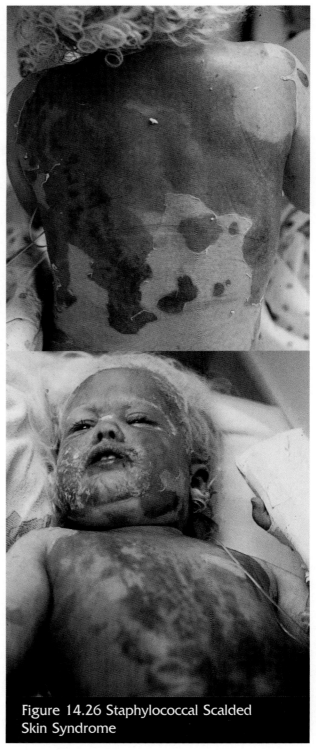

Figure 14.26 Staphylococcal Scalded Skin Syndrome

Toddler with diffuse macular peeling eruption consistent with scalded skin syndrome from *Staphylococcus aureus.* (Courtesy of Judith C. Bausher, MD.)

Associated Clinical Features

Meningococcemia is an acute febrile illness with generally rapid onset of marked toxicity, purpura, and petechiae (Fig 14.27). It progresses rapidly to hypotension with multisystem failure. In cases of fulminant disease, this shock stage is accompanied by disseminated intravascular coagulation and massive mucosal hemorrhages. Occasionally there may be a specific prodrome with upper respiratory infection and malaise.

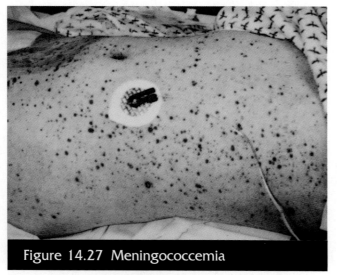

Figure 14.27 Meningococcemia

Diffuse petechiae in a patient with meningococcemia. (Courtesy of Richard Straight, MD.)

Differential Diagnosis

Gonococcemia, *Haemophilus influenzae* infection, pneumococcemia, Rocky Mountain spotted fever, sepsis with thrombocytopenia or disseminated intravascular coagulation (DIC), endocarditis, Henoch-Schönlein purpura, typhoid fever, leukemia, hemorrhagic measles, or hemorrhagic varicella may have a similar appearance.

Emergency Department Treatment and Disposition

In stable patients in whom the diagnosis of meningococcemia is entertained, cultures of blood, spinal fluid, nasopharynx, complete blood count, platelet count, and coagulation studies should be obtained. Consider arterial blood gas, liver function tests, and other studies as indicated. These patients should be admitted for close monitoring to institutions capable of delivering critical care services. Broad-spectrum parenteral antibiotics should be used in the initial coverage until the organism is identified and sensitivities are available. In the unstable septic patient, adequate ventilation and cardiac function must be ensured in addition to performing the above tests and treatment. Hemodynamic monitoring and support (fluids and vasoactive drugs) are of paramount importance in the management. Peripheral and central venous catheters and urinary and arterial catheters are usually necessary for optimal care of these patients.

Clinical Pearls

1. Skin scrapings of the purpuric lesion can be microscopically examined for the presence of gram-negative diplococci and may be cultured for organisms.
2. A child with a fever and a petechial rash must be presumed to have meningococcemia.

Associated Clinical Features

Scarlet fever manifests itself as erythematous macules and papules that result from an erythrogenic toxin produced by a group A streptococcus. The most common site for invasion by this organism is the pharynx and occasionally skin or perianal areas. The disease usually occurs in children (2 to 10 years of age) and less commonly in adults. The typical presentation of scarlet fever includes fever, headache, sore throat, and malaise followed by the scarlatiniform rash (Fig. 14.28). The rash is typically erythematous; it blanches (in severe cases may include petechiae), and—owing to the grouping of the fine papules—gives to the skin a rough, sandpaper-like texture (Fig. 14.29). On the tongue, a thick, white coat and swollen papillae give the appearance of a strawberry ("strawberry tongue").

Differential Diagnosis

A similar syndrome is caused by staphylococci producing an exfoliative exotoxin, which can be differentiated from the streptococcal infection because of the absence of pharyngitis, strawberry tongue, and negative cultures. Enteroviral infections, viral hepatitis, infectious mononucleosis, toxic shock syndrome, drug eruptions, rubella, mercury intoxication, and mucocutaneous lymph node syndrome should be considered.

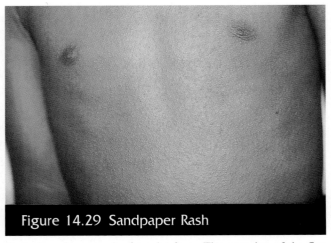

Figure 14.29 Sandpaper Rash

Typical sandpaper rash of scarlet fever. The grouping of the fine papules gives the skin a rough, sandpaper-like texture. (Courtesy of Jeffery S. Gibson, MD.)

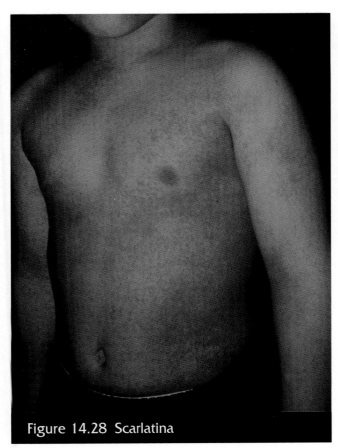

Figure 14.28 Scarlatina

Erythematous scarlatiniform rash of scarlet fever. (Courtesy of Lawrence B. Stack, MD.)

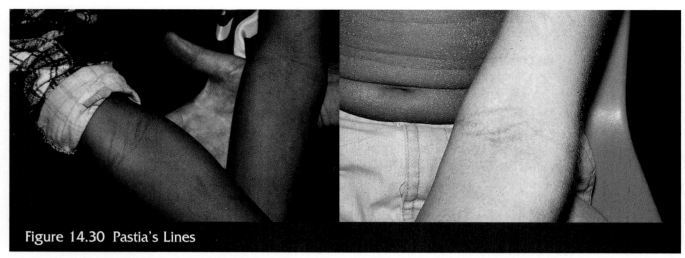

Figure 14.30 Pastia's Lines

Confluent petechia in a linear pattern in the antecubital fossa consistent with Pastia's lines are seen in these patients with scarlet fever. Left: The forearm on the right belongs to the patient's sister and does not show Pastia's lines. Right: Pastia's lines in a Caucasian patient. A classic sandpaper rash is also evident on the arm and trunk. (Courtesy of Stephen Corbett, MD.)

Emergency Department Treatment and Disposition

Penicillin, either benzathine penicillin G or oral penicillin, to maintain levels for 10 days is the key to therapy. Alternatives include erythromycin or clindamycin in penicillin-allergic patients.

Clinical Pearls

1. Petechiae (commonly found as part of the scarlatiniform eruption) in a linear pattern seen along the major skin folds in the axillae and antecubital fossa are known as "Pastia's lines" (Fig. 14.30).
2. In black skin, the rash may be difficult to differentiate and may consist only of punctate papular elevations called "goose flesh."

Associated Clinical Features

Blistering distal dactylitis is a cellulitis of the fingertips (Fig. 14.31) caused by beta-hemolytic streptococcal and, in rare occasions, by *Staphylococcus aureus* infections. The typical lesion is a fluid-filled, tense blister with surrounding erythema located over the volar fat pad on the distal portion of the fingers. Polymorphonuclear leukocytes and gram-positive cocci can be found in the Gram's stain of the purulent exudate from the lesion.

Differential Diagnosis

Bullous impetigo, burns, friction blisters, and herpetic whitlow should be considered.

Emergency Department Treatment and Disposition

There is usually a rapid response to incision and drainage of the blister and a 10-day course of antibiotic therapy (dicloxacillin, cephalexin, or erythromycin).

Clinical Pearl

1. This diagnosis should be entertained in any child presenting with a tender, cloudy, fluid-filled blister of the fingertips or toes.

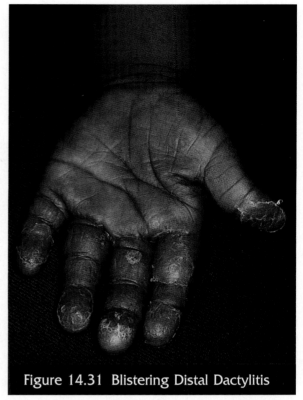

Figure 14.31 Blistering Distal Dactylitis

Blistering rash of the distal fingers with surrounding erythema typically caused by *Streptococcus*. Note the location of the rash over the volar finger pad. (Courtesy of Anne W. Lucky, MD.)

Associated Clinical Features

Strawberry hemangioma often appears as small telangiectatic papules or a patch surrounded by an area of pallor. These lesions grow and become vascularized during the first 2 months of life. The classic lesion is a raised gray to reddish nodule with defined borders (Fig. 14.32). It commonly regresses in almost all patients by 2 to 3 years of age. In a few cases, very large vascular lesions can cause platelet trapping or high-output cardiac failure. Localized hemangiomas can affect the airway, eyes, or other areas where they occur.

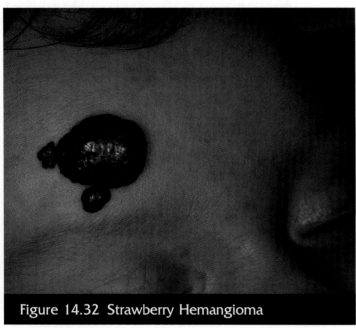

Figure 14.32 Strawberry Hemangioma

Raised umbilicated vascular lesion on the right forehead consistent with strawberry hemangioma. (Courtesy of Anne W. Lucky, MD.)

Differential Diagnosis

Malignant vascular tumors, pyogenic granulomas, and giant melanocytic birthmarks should be considered.

Emergency Department Treatment and Disposition

Most cases require no therapy because strawberry hemangiomas usually regress without residua. Treatment is indicated when there is an obstruction of a vital orifice (i.e., airway, mouth, or nares) or vision (eyelids) or if hematologic or cardiovascular complications are present. Parental reassurance is important because there is great pressure to treat for cosmetic reasons. Steroids, liquid nitrogen, grenz-ray therapy, and pulse dye laser are some of the different therapeutic modalities used in its treatment. In complex cases, dermatologic consultation is recommended.

Clinical Pearl

1. The diagnosis of strawberry hemangioma should always be considered in the presence of any purplish, red, raised, tumorlike lesion not present at birth that appears in the first month of life.

Associated Clinical Features

Orbital cellulitis is a serious bacterial infection characterized by painful purple-red swelling of the eyelids, restriction of eye movement (Fig. 14.33), proptosis, and a variable degree of decreased visual acuity. It may begin with eye pain and low-grade temperature. In general it is caused by *Staphylococcus aureus, Haemophilus influenzae, Streptococcus,* or *Pneumococcus.* It usually follows an upper respiratory tract infection or sinusitis but can occur from local trauma. If not treated promptly, it can lead to abscess formation, blindness, or meningitis. Periorbital (preseptal) cellulitis usually presents with edema and erythema of the eyelids (Fig. 14.34), minimal pain of the affected area, and fever. Proptosis or ophthalmoplegia are not characteristic. Common organisms are *H. influenzae* type B or *Pneumococcus.* In cases of eyelid trauma, *S. aureus* and group A streptococcus are the most common pathogens.

Differential Diagnosis

Erysipelas, allergic reactions, trauma, sunburn, frostbite, chemical burns, subperiosteal abscess, and cavernous sinus thrombosis should be considered.

Emergency Department Treatment and Disposition

Parenteral antibiotic coverage with broad-spectrum antistaphylococcal coverage, ophthalmologic consultation, and admission are indicated in cases of orbital cellulitis. Computed tomography of the orbit is necessary in certain cases to rule out the possibility of an abscess requiring surgical drainage. In febrile or ill-appearing patients with periorbital cellulitis, admission with broad-spectrum antibiotic therapy is indicated. This coverage can be adjusted once results of cultures are available. Mild cases of preseptal cellulitis (especially those with history of trauma, e.g., abrasion, insect sting) can be treated as outpatients with close follow-up. Adequate coverage for *Staphylococcus* and *Streptococcus* is necessary.

Clinical Pearls

1. Periorbital cellulitis presents with circumferential redness, edema, and tenderness in the febrile toddler. Orbital cellulitis must be considered if there is eye pain or limitation of globe motion.
2. The conjunctiva is typically clear with periorbital cellulitis.

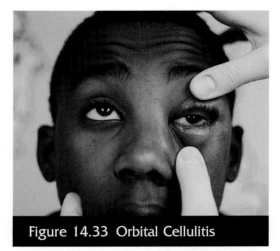

Figure 14.33 Orbital Cellulitis

Left orbital cellulitis with decreased range of motion secondary to edema. Note the infected conjunctiva. (Courtesy of Javier A. Gonzalez del Rey, MD.)

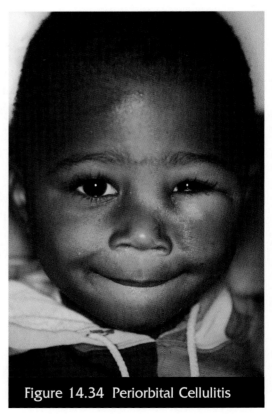

Figure 14.34 Periorbital Cellulitis

Left periorbital cellulitis with edema and erythema of the eyelids. Note that the conjunctiva is clear and not infected. (Courtesy of Kevin J. Knoop, MD, MS.)

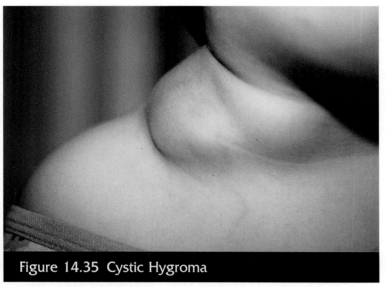

Figure 14.35 Cystic Hygroma

A bright, supraclavicular, soft, boggy, compressible mass consistent with cystic hygroma. (Courtesy of Richard M. Ruddy, MD.)

Associated Clinical Features

Cystic hygromas are lymphatic tumors found in the head and neck region (Fig. 14.35). They present as nontender or nonpainful, compressible, unilocular or multilocular masses with thin, transparent walls and are filled with straw-colored fluid. Unlike hemangiomas, these lesions rarely undergo spontaneous regression. The vast majority tend to grow and infiltrate adjacent structures. In cases where the tongue is involved, they may produce tracheal compression and respiratory difficulty.

Differential Diagnosis

Cavernous hemangiomas and cavernous lymphangiomas should be considered.

Emergency Department Treatment and Disposition

Surgery is the treatment of choice in the vast majority of cases, since these lesions do not regress and may affect local tissues. Extent of the lesion should be evaluated prior to its removal (x-rays and computed tomography). The earlier these lesions can be removed, the better the cosmetic results.

Clinical Pearls

1. The diagnosis of cystic hygroma should be considered in all cases of spongy, soft, tumor-like masses in the neck that are filled with fluid. Such a lesion may appear spontaneously during a coughing episode or after Valsalva as a mass in the neck.
2. This "benign" tumor can locally invade adjacent tissues and become life-threatening.

Associated Clinical Features

Cat-scratch disease is a benign, self-limited condition that manifests with regional lymphadenopathy (Fig. 14.36), which usually follows (1 to 2 weeks) a skin papule at the presumed site of bacterial inoculation. A history of contact with or scratch from a cat (Fig. 14.37) is usually present. Lymphadenopathy may persist for months and in rare cases patients may develop complications such as encephalitis, osteolytic lesion, hepatitis, weight loss, fever, and fatigue. A skin test using cat-scratch antigen can identify the etiology in suspected patients when confirmation of the diagnosis is needed.

Differential Diagnosis

Lymphogranuloma venereum, bacterial adenitis, sarcoidosis, infectious mononucleosis, tumors (benign or malignant), tuberculosis, tularemia, brucellosis, and histoplasmosis should be considered.

Emergency Department Treatment and Disposition

The disease is usually self-limited and management is primarily symptomatic. Parents and patients should be reassured that the nodes are benign and frequently resolve within 2 to 4 months. In cases of painful, fluctuant nodes, needle aspiration may be necessary for relief of symptoms. Antibiotic therapy should be considered for acutely or severely ill patients. Several anecdotal reports have suggested that oral antibiotics such as rifampin, trimethoprim-sulfamethoxazole, and ciprofloxacin or intravenous gentamicin, cefotaxime, and mezlocillin may be effective. Surgical excision of the affected nodes is generally unnecessary.

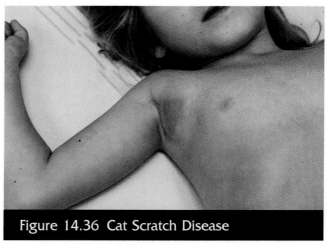

Figure 14.36 Cat Scratch Disease

An erythematous, tender, suppurative node is seen in a young febrile patient with a history of cat scratch on the extremity. The node required drainage 2 days later. (Courtesy of Kevin J. Knoop, MD, MS.)

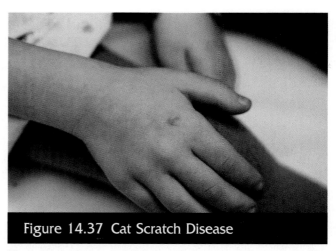

Figure 14.37 Cat Scratch Disease

The precipitating wound that caused the suppurative node in Fig. 14.36. (Courtesy of Kevin J. Knoop, MD, MS.)

Clinical Pearl

1. Cat-scratch disease is the most common cause of regional adenitis and should be considered in all children or adolescents with persistent lymphadenopathy.

General Conditions

Associated Clinical Features

Epiglottitis is a life-threatening condition characterized by sudden onset of fever, toxicity, moderate to severe respiratory distress with stridor, and variable degrees of drooling. The patient prefers a sitting position, leaning forward in a sniffing position with an open mouth. This symptomatology is the result of a direct infection and subsequent swelling of the epiglottis and aryepiglottic folds (Figs. 14.38 and 14.39) from *Haemophilus influenzae* type B (HIB). However, since the release of the vaccine in 1985, there has been a dramatic decrease in the incidence of this disease. Adults have a more indolent course and are infrequently protected by the vaccine. Other infectious causes include staphylococcal or streptococcal disease, thermal epiglottitis, and *Candida* in the immunocompromised host. Direct thermal injuries have been reported as a noninfectious cause of epiglottitis. On x-ray, the epiglottis is seen as rounded and blurred (thumbprint) (Fig. 14.40). Epiglottitis frequently worsens to complete obstruction if not treated with endotracheal intubation and antibiotics.

Differential Diagnosis

Acute infectious laryngitis, acute laryngotracheobronchitis, acute spasmodic laryngitis, membranous tracheitis, diphtheritic croup, aspiration of foreign body, retropharyngeal abscess, and extrinsic or intrinsic compression of the airway (tumors, trauma, cysts) should be considered.

Emergency Department Treatment and Disposition

Immediate intervention is required. An artificial endotracheal airway must be established. If time and clinical status permit, this should be done in the operating room or designated area where

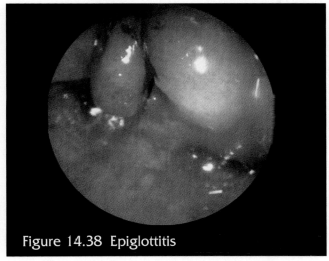

Figure 14.38 Epiglottitis

Endoscopic view of almost complete airway obstruction secondary to epiglottitis. Note the slit-like opening of the airway. (Courtesy of Department of Otolaryngology, Childrens Hospital Medical Center, Cincinnati, OH.)

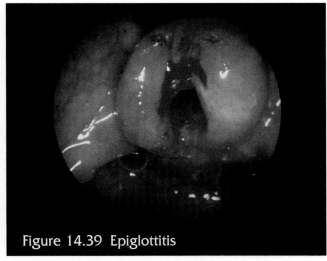

Figure 14.39 Epiglottitis

Endoscopic view of the same patient immediately after extubation. Although erythema and some edema persist, the airway is widely patent. (Courtesy of Department of Otolaryngology, Childrens Hospital Medical Center, Cincinnati, OH.)

advanced airway management with sedation but not neuromuscular paralysis can be implemented. An experienced anesthesiologist and surgeon should be available in case a surgical airway is needed. Once the airway has been protected, the patient should be sedated to avoid accidental extubation and adequate antibiotic therapy should be immediately instituted (second- or third-generation cephalosporins or ampicillin/chloramphenicol).

Clinical Pearls

1. Children with epiglottitis usually present with respiratory distress of sudden onset and high fever. Because of the inflammation of the epiglottis, they commonly refuse to drink fluids secondary to pain.
2. Every effort should be made to allow the child to remain undisturbed (in mother's lap) in a position of comfort while urgent preparations are made for airway management. An agitated child is at risk for suddenly losing the airway.

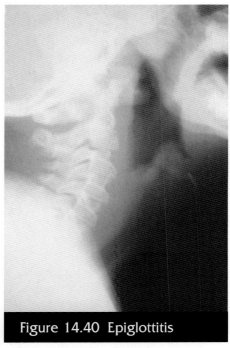

Figure 14.40 Epiglottitis

Lateral soft-tissue x-ray of the neck demonstrating thickening of aryepiglottic folds and thumbprint sign of epiglottis. (Courtesy of Richard M. Ruddy, MD.)

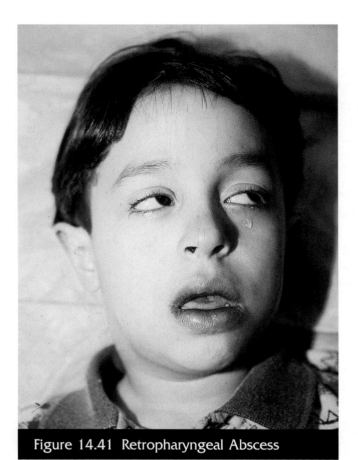

Figure 14.41 Retropharyngeal Abscess

This ill-appearing 6-year-old child presented with a several-day history of fever, neck pain, sore throat, cough, and headache. Soft tissue lateral radiography of the neck showed thickened prevertebral tissues opposite C2-4. Computed tomography (CT) showed the airway narrowed to a width of 5 mm within the oropharynx. (Courtesy of Mark Ralston, MD.)

Associated Clinical Features

Patients with a retropharyngeal abscess usually present with fever, difficulty in swallowing, excessive drooling, sore throat, changes in voice, or neck stiffness (Fig. 14.41). The resultant edema (Fig. 14.42) is the result of a cellulitis and suppurative adenitis of the lymph nodes located in the prevertebral fascia and is seen on a soft tissue lateral x-ray of the neck as prevertebral thickening (Fig. 14.43). The initial insult may be the result of pharyngitis, otitis media, or a wound infection following a penetrating injury into the posterior pharynx. [It is helpful for the examiner to be familiar with the normal laryngeal structures (Fig. 14.44)].

Differential Diagnosis

Acute laryngotracheobronchitis, epiglottitis, membranous tracheitis, acute bacterial laryngitis, infectious mononucleosis, peritonsillar abscess, aspiration of foreign body, and diphtheria should be considered. These patients may present with stiff neck mimicking meningitis.

Emergency Department Treatment and Disposition

This illness requires immediate intervention to prevent respiratory obstruction. The first step is to evaluate the airway and establish an artificial one if necessary. Antibiotic coverage should be initiated immediately (semisynthetic penicillin or equivalent). Analgesia should be given as

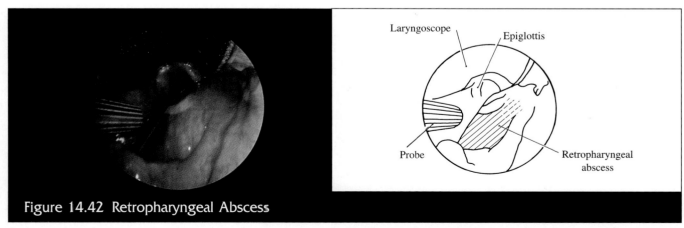

Figure 14.42 Retropharyngeal Abscess

Endoscopic view of a retropharyngeal abscess. Note the massive swelling posteriorly. (Courtesy of Department of Otolaryngology, Childrens Hospital Medical Center, Cincinnati, OH.)

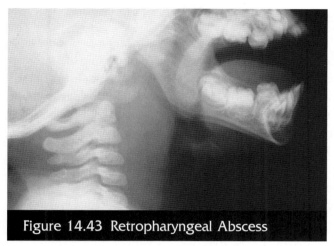

Figure 14.43 Retropharyngeal Abscess

Lateral soft tissue neck x-ray demonstrating prevertebral soft tissue density consistent with retropharyngeal abscess. (Courtesy of Richard M. Ruddy, MD.)

needed. If obstruction is present or there is evidence of abscess, immediate incision and drain-age should be performed in the operating room. These patients require hospitalization and immediate otolaryngologic or surgical consultation.

Clinical Pearls

1. If the diagnosis of retropharyngeal abscess is considered in a patient with the above presentation, a lateral soft tissue neck x-ray may help to confirm the diagnosis. In these cases, the retropharyngeal soft tissue at the level of C-3 is > 5 mm, or more than 40% of the diameter of the body of C-4 at that level.
2. Computed tomography of the neck is a useful tool to evaluate the extent of the lesion.

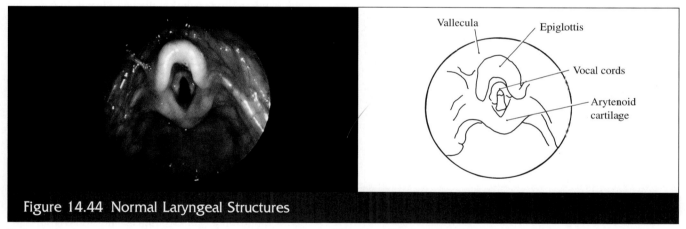

Figure 14.44 Normal Laryngeal Structures

Endoscopic view of a normal epiglottis and surrounding structures. (Courtesy of Department of Otolaryngology, Childrens Hospital Medical Center, Cincinnati, OH.)

Associated Clinical Features

Membranous tracheitis is an acute bacterial infection (*Staphylococcus aureus, Haemophilus influenzae,* streptococci, and pneumococci) of the upper airway capable of causing life-threatening airway obstruction. It is considered a bacterial complication because it almost always follows an apparent viral infection of the upper respiratory tract. The infection produces marked swelling and thick, purulent secretions of the tracheal mucosa below the vocal cords. The secretions form a thick plug that, if dislodged, may ultimately lead to an acute tracheal obstruction. Patients appear toxic, with fever and a croup-like syndrome that can progress rapidly. The usual treatment for croup is ineffective in these patients. The characteristic "membranes" may be seen on x-rays of the airway as edema with an irregular border of the subglottic tracheal mucosa. On direct laryngoscopy, copious purulent secretions can be found in the presence of a normal epiglottis.

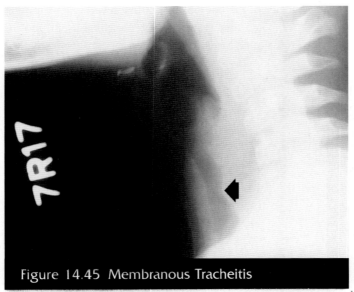

Figure 14.45 Membranous Tracheitis

Lateral soft tissue x-ray of the neck reveals mild subglottic narrowing (*arrow*) and membrane consistent with bacterial tracheitis. (Courtesy of Alan S. Brodie, MD.)

Differential Diagnosis

Acute laryngotracheobronchitis, retropharyngeal abscess, peritonsillar abscess, foreign-body aspiration, and acute diphtheric laryngitis can present in a similar manner.

Emergency Department Treatment and Disposition

Otolaryngologic consultation should be obtained as soon as the diagnosis is considered. Aggressive airway management, including endotracheal intubation, may be needed to protect the airway and allow for repeated suctioning to prevent acute airway obstruction. The patient should be admitted to the intensive care unit for close monitoring and sedation needs. Appropriate antibiotic coverage against suspected organisms should be instituted immediately.

Clinical Pearls

1. Bacterial tracheitis often presents with acute, severe airway obstruction after a short prodrome. It should be suspected in all patients with an atypical croup-like presentation: unusual age group, toxicity, not improving with routine croup therapy, and unusual roentgenographic changes.
2. Up to 50% of soft tissue films may delineate a subglottic membrane (Fig. 14.45).

Associated Clinical Features

There are several fractures unique to children. These include physeal fractures, torus fracture, greenstick fractures, avulsion fractures, and bowing fractures or deformities. Physis fractures (growth plate fractures) are relatively common because of weakness of the germinal growth plate. The Salter-Harris (SH) classification was designed to describe each type of physeal fracture, its prognosis, and its treatment (Fig. 14.46).

Differential Diagnosis

SH type I: Fracture that extends through the physis. It is a very difficult radiologic diagnosis since the fracture may not be displaced. It is usually a clinical diagnosis, but occasionally a physeal widening is observed on the x-ray.

SH type II: Oblique fracture extending through the metaphysis into the physis. It is the most common type and the prognosis is good.

SH type III: This rare type of fracture goes along the growth plate, then extends through the epiphysis, ossification center, and articular cartilage into the joint.

SH type IV: Fracture that extends from the metaphysis, across the growth plate and into the joint.

SH type V: Crushing injury to the growth plate.

Emergency Department Treatment and Disposition

Immobilization by splinting is the treatment of choice in types I and II (minimum of 3 weeks). In these cases, reduction is easy to achieve and maintain. Growth is unimpaired. Types III and IV may require open reduction to avoid later traumatic arthritis and, in some cases, growth arrest. Type V fractures are rare and require very close follow-up because of arrest of growth caused by the death of the germinal cells. Types III, IV, and V require immediate orthopedic consultation.

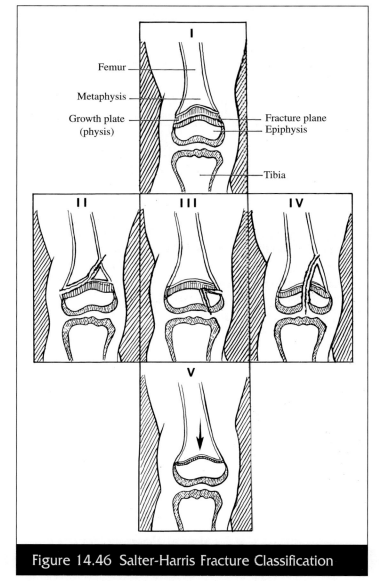

Figure 14.46 Salter-Harris Fracture Classification

Salter-Harris classification for epiphyseal plate fractures.

Clinical Pearl

1. After initial assessment and evaluation, always suspect SH type I if there is evidence of tenderness around the growth plate area despite negative x-rays.

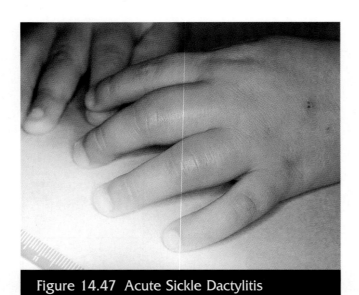

Figure 14.47 Acute Sickle Dactylitis

Bilateral cylindrical swelling of soft tissue of the hands in sickle cell disease consistent with vasoocclusive crisis or dactylitis. (Courtesy of Donald L. Rucknagel, MD, PhD.)

Associated Clinical Features

This painful condition is commonly the first clinical manifestation of sickle cell disease. It usually presents in children younger than 5 years of age. The pain and abnormalities are the result of ischemic necrosis of the small bones caused by the decreased blood supply as the bone marrow rapidly expands. These children present acutely ill, with fever, refusal to bear weight, and puffy hands and feet (Fig. 14.47). They may have a marked leukocytosis, and the initial x-rays may be normal. It is not until 1 to 2 weeks later that subperiosteal new bone, cortical thickening, and even complete bone destruction can be seen.

Differential Diagnosis

Osteomyelitis, trauma, cold injuries, acute rheumatic fever, juvenile rheumatoid arthritis, and leukemias should be considered.

Emergency Department Treatment and Disposition

The most important aspects in the treatment of vasoocclusive crisis in sickle cell disease (hemoglobin SS) include an adequate fluid balance, oxygenation, and analgesia. Therapy should be individualized. Codeine, hydromorphone, morphine, and ketorolac are analgesic agents commonly used in the treatment of children with painful sickle crisis. In cases of dactylitis, very close follow-up is necessary not only for the management of sickle cell disease but to reevaluate the radiologic changes in small bones. In most instances, the previously described changes disappear; however, in rare cases, shortening of the fingers and toes has been described as the result of severe bone infarcts.

Clinical Pearl

1. Most clinical manifestations of sickle cell disease occur after the first 5 to 6 months of life. The hemolytic anemia gradually develops over the first 2 to 4 months (changes that follow the replacement of fetal hemoglobin by hemoglobin S) and leads to the clinical syndromes associated with an increased SS hemoglobin.

Associated Clinical Features

A single strand of hair or thread may encircle a finger, a toe, or the penis, leading to constriction (Fig. 14.48). Children in their first year of life are particularly at risk from inadvertent attachment of a parent's hair or loose thread. The digit appears edematous, erythematous, and painful. If not corrected vascular compromise or infection can ensue.

Differential Diagnosis

Insect bites, trauma, or cellulitis of the digit may have a similar appearance.

Emergency Department Treatment and Disposition

Visualization of the constricting material may be difficult. Edema, erythema, and periarticular skin folds may hide the hair or thread. It is imperative to carefully retract the skin around the proximal aspect of the edema. A magnifying lens may be helpful in identifying the band. Since the removal can be painful, consider local digital block prior to removal. Using a small hemostat, grasp a portion of the material, and then cut it with a surgical blade. On occasions, depilatory agents have been used to remove hair fibers. Elevation of the involved digit after removal of the constricting agent provides resolution of the edema and erythema within 2 to 3 days. In some cases the digit's blood supply may have been irreversibly compromised. Subspecialty consultation should be considered whenever neurovascular integrity is in question.

Clinical Pearl

1. In the vast majority of cases, a clear line of demarcation can be identified between the normal tissue and the affected area.

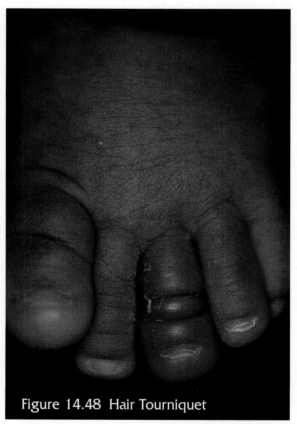

Figure 14.48 Hair Tourniquet

A strand of hair has encircled the middle toe in two places, causing erythema and swelling. (Courtesy of Kevin J. Knoop, MD, MS.)

Associated Clinical Features

Failure to thrive (FTT) is a chronic pattern of inability to maintain a normal growth pattern in weight, stature, and occasionally in head growth (Fig. 14.49). It is most common in infancy, and the condition is nonorganic (50%), organic (25%), or mixed (25%) in etiology. The diagnosis is made after complete history and physical examination with comparison of the measurements of length (supine in children <3 years of age), weight, and head circumference (maximal occipital-frontal circumference) to standard measurements. In cases of deficient caloric intake or malabsorption, the patient's head circumference is normal and the weight is reduced out of proportion to height. Subnormal head circumferences with weight reduced in proportion to height and normal or increased head circumferences with weight moderately reduced are usually indicative of an organic problem.

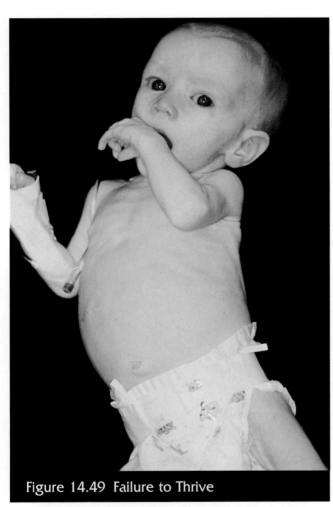

Figure 14.49 Failure to Thrive

This infant has not been able to maintain a normal growth pattern and appears cachectic. (Courtesy of Kevin J. Knoop, MD, MS.)

Differential Diagnosis

The differential diagnosis of failure to thrive is lengthy. Nonorganic disorders include poor feeding technique, disturbed maternal-child interaction, emotional deprivation, inadequate caloric intake, and child neglect. Organic causes are numerous.

Emergency Department Treatment and Disposition

Depending on history, physical findings, and the social situation, some cases can be managed as outpatients. The primary care provider can determine whether outpatient management is indicated. For the vast majority of cases, if the diagnosis of failure to thrive is made in the ED, admission is suggested to complete the evaluation. This could be the only indication of a poor social environment or inadequate access to medical care. Initial laboratory investigations should include a complete blood count, electrolytes, BUN and creatinine urinalysis, and stool examination if the stool pattern is abnormal. More specific testing should be used only if clinically indicated and targeted to the possible underlying cause. Early involvement of social services may facilitate the evaluation and follow-up. Treatment will vary according to the underlying disorder.

Clinical Pearl

1. Failure to thrive in neglected children is accompanied by signs of developmental delays, emotional deprivation, apathy, poor hygiene, withdrawing behavior, and poor eye contact.

Associated Clinical Features

Nursemaid's elbow is a condition that occurs commonly in children younger than 5 years of age who are usually picked up or pulled by the arm while the arm is pronated. The children present unwilling to supinate or pronate the affected elbow (Fig. 14.50). Generally they keep the arm in a passive pronation and develop pain over the head of the radius. Radiographic studies should be considered only in patients with an unusual mechanism of injury or those who do not become rapidly asymptomatic after the reduction maneuvers.

Differential Diagnosis

Radial head fracture or complete dislocation, posterior elbow dislocation, condylar and supracondylar fractures of the distal humerus, or buckle fracture of radius or ulna should be considered.

Emergency Department Treatment and Disposition

Carefully palpate for tenderness at all points of the affected arm. (No tenderness is found when not rotating the involved arm.) Orthopedic consultation is generally not indicated unless an underlying fracture is diagnosed. Reduction is usually achieved by one of two maneuvers: (1) while supinating the forearm, pressure is applied over the radial head and the elbow is flexed, or (2) while holding the elbow in extension, hyperpronation of the forearm is maintained until reduc-

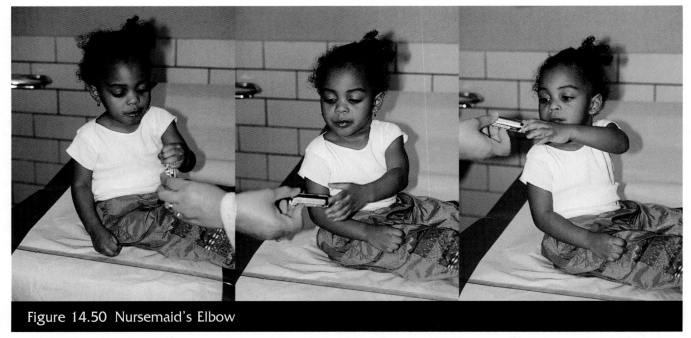

Figure 14.50 Nursemaid's Elbow

This child presents with pseudoparalysis of the right arm after a pulling injury. Note how she avoids use of the affected arm and preferentially uses the other arm. (Courtesy of Kevin J. Knoop, MD, MS.)

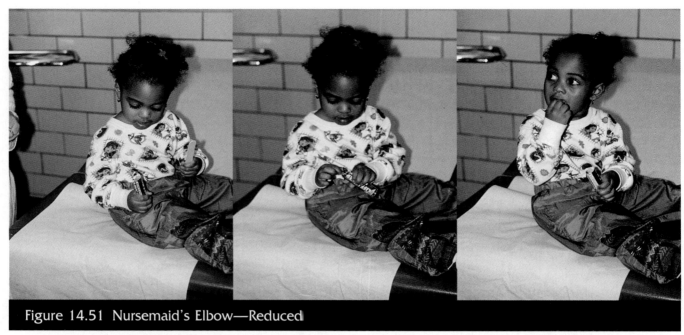

Figure 14.51 Nursemaid's Elbow—Reduced

After reduction, there is initial reluctance to use the injured arm. With distraction and encouragement, the patient demonstrates successful use of the extremity. (Courtesy of Kevin J. Knoop, MD, MS.)

tion is achieved. The patient usually becomes asymptomatic after a few minutes (Fig. 14.51). When the injury has been present for several hours, reduction may be difficult, and it may take several hours to recover full function of the elbow.

Clinical Pearls

1. In any child (usually between 1 to 5 years of age) who presents with sudden onset of elbow pain and immobility following a traction injury, the diagnosis of nursemaid's elbow should be strongly considered.
2. Nonjudgmental parental education about the mechanism should be an integral part of the visit.

Associated Clinical Features

This extensive form of tooth decay (generally in the necks of the teeth near the gingiva) is the result of sleeping with a bottle containing milk or sugar-containing juices. The condition generally occurs before 18 months of age and is more prevalent in medically underserved children. Upper central incisors are most commonly involved (Fig. 14.52).

Differential Diagnosis

Less extensive tooth decay (caries) may be seen in some infants who do not sleep with a bottle. Caries can also result from tooth trauma. Dental referral is indicated.

Emergency Department Treatment and Disposition

Parental education and immediate referral to a dentist is necessary to prevent complications. If untreated, the caries may destroy the teeth and spread to contiguous tissues. These patients have a high risk for microbial invasion of the pulp and the alveolar bone, with the subsequent development of a dental abscess and facial cellulitis. In these cases, aggressive treatment with antibiotics (penicillin) and pain control, with prompt dental referral for definitive care, is necessary.

Clinical Pearl

1. The role of the ED physician is to recognize this pattern of dental decay (upper incisors most commonly) and immediately initiate dental referral and parental education.

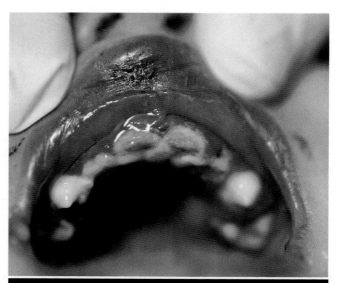

Figure 14.52 Nursing Bottle Caries

Extensive tooth decay from sleeping with a bottle containing milk or sugar-containing juices. (Courtesy of Lawrence B. Stack, MD.)

473

Associated Clinical Features

Enterobius vermicularis is a 0.5-in. threadlike white worm that infects the colon and causes intense pruritus of the perianal region, where the adult gravid female migrates to deposit eggs (Fig. 14.53). On rare occasions it can cause vulvovaginitis. The diagnosis can be made by direct visualization of the nematode by the parents or by using a transparent adhesive tape and touching it to the perianal lesion (at night). This tape is then applied to a glass slide for microscopic examination under low power.

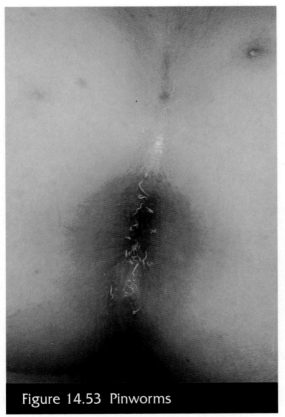

Figure 14.53 Pinworms

Multiple tiny pearly-white worms are seen at the anus. (Courtesy of Timothy D. McGuirk, DO.)

Differential Diagnosis

Perianal irritation, fissures, hemorrhoids, and contact dermatitis should be considered.

Emergency Department Treatment and Disposition

The treatment of choice is pyrantel pamoate or mebendazole. Either of these drugs is given as a single dose and repeated in 1 to 2 weeks (to treat secondary hatchings of the organism). Because of the high frequency of reinfection, families should be treated as a group.

Clinical Pearls

1. Reinfection from other infected individuals or autoinfection is necessary to maintain enterobiasis in the individual, since these nematodes usually die after depositing their eggs in the perianal region. Good personal hygiene may reduce chances of infection.
2. If there is evidence of cellulitis, antibiotic coverage primarily against *Staphylococcus* is indicated.
3. If infection and point tenderness (in the absence of cellulitis) persist, antipseudomonal coverage should be considered.
4. Pinworms are the most common cause of pruritus in children.

Associated Clinical Features

Oculogyric crisis (OGC) is the most common of the ocular dystonic reactions. It includes blepharospasm, periorbital twitches, and protracted staring episodes. Usually it occurs as a side effect of neuroleptic drug treatment. OGC represents approximately 5% of the dystonic reactions. The onset of a crisis may be paroxysmal or stuttering over several hours. Initial symptoms include restlessness, agitation, malaise, or a fixed stare followed by the more characteristically described maximal upward deviation of the eyes in a sustained fashion. The eyes may also converge, deviate upward and laterally, or deviate downward. The most frequently reported associated findings are backward and lateral flexion of the neck, widely opened mouth, tongue protrusion, and ocular pain (Fig. 14.54). A wave of exhaustion follows some episodes. Other features noted during attacks include eye blinking, lacrimation, pupil dilation, drooling, facial flushing, vertigo, anxiety, and agitation.

Differential Diagnosis

Several medications have been associated with the occurrence of OGC: neuroleptics, amantadine, benzodiazepines, carbamazepine, chloroquine, levodopa, lithium, metoclopramide, and nifedipine. Careful history and physical examination should exclude the possibility of focal seizures, encephalitis, head injury, conversion reaction, and other types of movement disorders.

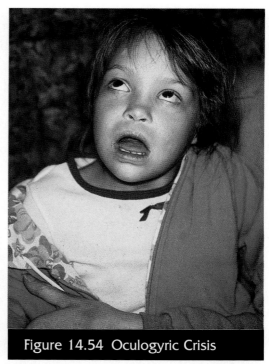

Figure 14.54 Oculogyric Crisis

This 6-year-old boy developed extrapyramidal symptoms, including opisthotonos and oculogyric crisis, after his dosage of risperidone was increased. Benadryl 12.5 mg PO given at home resolved the opisthotonos. Persistent oculogyric crisis (vertical gaze deviation) and hypertonia resolved completely after Benadryl 25 mg IM. (Courtesy of Mark Ralston, MD.)

Emergency Department Treatment and Disposition

Treatment in the acute phase in children involves reassurance and diphenhydramine at a dosage of 1 mg/kg initially; this may be repeated if there is no effect. Occasionally, doses up to 5 mg/kg are required. Benztropine and/or diazepam or lorazepam can also be used; however, benztropine is not approved for children below 3 years of age, and this agent has been noted to cause dystonic reactions. Close monitoring of these drug side effects is important during treatment and for a few hours thereafter because dystonic reactions are occasionally accompanied by fluctuations in blood pressure and disturbances of cardiac rhythm.

Clinical Pearls

1. The abrupt termination of the psychiatric symptoms at the conclusion of the crisis, after the use of diphenhydramine, is diagnostic and most striking.

2. In infants presenting with "seizures" and unusual behavior, eye deviation and history of reflux treated with metoclopramide, the possibility of OGC should always be included in the differential. Although the overall incidence of extrapyramidal effects associated with this drug is 0.2%, very old and very young patients are affected more commonly, with an incidence as high as 10%. These side effects usually occur within a few days after initiation of the medication, as in this case, and are more common at higher doses.

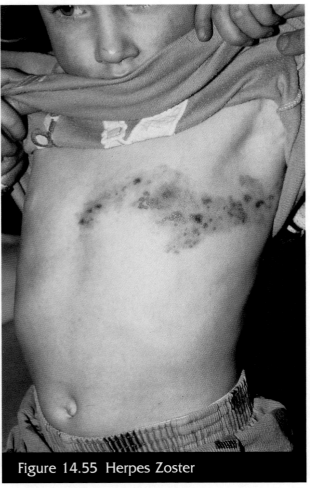

Figure 14.55 Herpes Zoster

Vesicles in a classic dermatomal distribution are seen in this child. (Courtesy of Frank Birinyi, MD.)

Associated Clinical Features

Herpes zoster virus (HZV) has been noted as early as the first week of life (in infants born to mothers who contracted varicella during pregnancy). These lesions can present in the distribution of one to three sensory dermatomes (Fig. 14.55). Pain is intense and in certain cases can persist beyond 1 month after the lesions have disappeared (postherpetic neuralgia). The diagnosis is usually made clinically; however, tissue cultures, direct fluorescent antibodies, and Tzanck smears (see Fig. 13.15) can be done from vesicle scraping to confirm the diagnosis.

Differential Diagnosis

The diagnosis is usually clinically apparent but not always straightforward. Impetigo and cutaneous burns (cigarette) may mimic the appearance of herpetic vesicles. Varicella is more diffusely spread, although a small crop of lesions may mimic zoster. Zoster may mimic herpes simplex virus (HSV), although a close examination should reveal a dermatomal distribution in zoster.

Emergency Department Treatment and Disposition

The management of HZV in children is limited to symptomatic treatment and prevention of secondary infections. Oral acyclovir is not recommended for routine use in otherwise healthy children with zoster or varicella. However, acyclovir therapy should be considered in older children with severe cases, chronic cutaneous or pulmonary disorders, and patients receiving salicylates or corticosteroids therapy. Intravenous antiviral therapy is recommended for immunocompromised patients. There is no pediatric formulation of famciclovir and valacyclovir or sufficient data on their use in children.

Clinical Pearls

1. HZV can occur in children of all ages.
2. A vesicular rash with a dermatomal distribution is diagnostic of HZV.
3. Reports are that acyclovir is of benefit only if used within 24 h of the initial presentation (modest decrease of symptoms).
4. An infected patient can transmit chickenpox (varicella) to a nonimmune child.

Associated Clinical Features

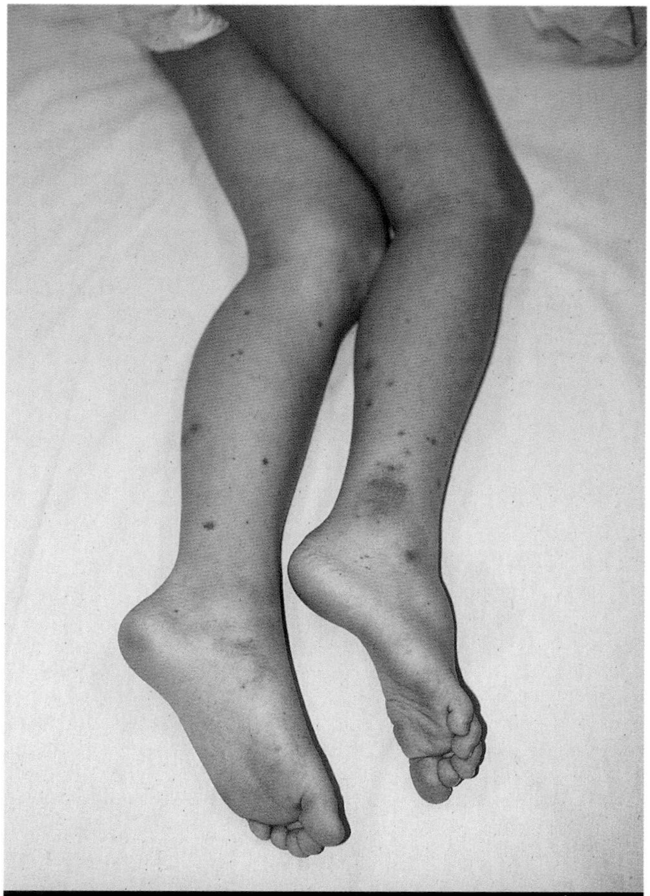

Also known as "anaphylactoid purpura," HSP is a systemic vasculitis of small vessels characterized by 2- to 10-mm erythematous hemorrhagic papules in a symmetric acral distribution, over the buttocks, and extremities (Fig. 14.56; see Fig. 15.19). Lesions occur in crops, fade after 5 days, and are followed by purpura ("palpable purpura"), abdominal pain (caused by edema and hemorrhage of the intestinal wall), and joint symptoms. HSP is a disease of children (commonly aged 3 to 12 years) and young adults. Mucosal involvement is rare; however, edema of the scalp, hands, scrotum, and periorbital tissue is not uncommon. Gastrointestinal symptoms (abdominal pain, occult and gross bleeding, and intussusception) may precede the rash. Renal involvement is the most frequent and serious complication and usually occurs during the first month. It commonly manifests itself as acute glomerulonephritis. Hypertension is uncommon. The diagnosis is made by history and clinical examination. Laboratory tests are usually normal (platelets, complement level, and antinuclear antibodies) except for the urinalysis, which may be positive for blood or protein in 50% of the patients. The prognosis is excellent, with full recovery in most instances. The course of HSP is marked by relapses and remissions in 50% of patients (rash seems to recur within the first 6 weeks). Prognosis is dictated by the renal involvement. Overall, 1 to 4% of patients progress to end-stage renal disease.

Figure 14.56 Henoch-Schönlein Purpura

These erythematous, hemorrhagic papules and petechiae in a symmetric acral distribution are classic findings in HSP. This child presented with no other symptons. (Courtesy of Kevin J. Knoop, MD, MS.)

Differential Diagnosis

During the initial phases of the disease, the diagnosis may be difficult. Rash may be confused with drug reactions, erythema multiforme, urticaria, and even physical abuse. Other causes of purpura, bleeding disorders, and/or infection (meningococcemia) should always be included in the differential diagnosis.

Emergency Department Treatment and Disposition

Treatment is empiric, symptomatic, and supportive. Corticosteroids are used acutely to treat severe abdominal pain or arthritis. In cases where intussusception is suspected, prompt surgical consultation and diagnostic ultrasonography or air-contrast enema fluoroscopy (diagnostic and therapeutic) is indicated. Patients with HSP limited to the skin and joints can be managed as outpatients. Severe abdominal pain, gastrointestinal hemorrhage, intussusception, and severe renal involvement are indications for admission.

Clinical Pearls

1. All children presenting to the ED with suspected HSP and gastrointestinal symptoms should have a stool guaiac test performed and a urinalysis to monitor for nephritis.
2. Intussusception associated with HSP is seen in 2% of patients, most commonly in boys, particularly those about 6 years of age.

CHAPTER 15
CHILD ABUSE

Robert A. Shapiro
Charles J Schubert

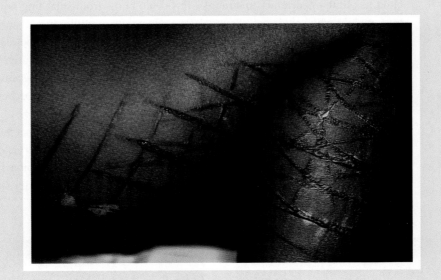

Physical Abuse

Associated Clinical Features

Burns in children are frequently the result of child abuse. The most common types of pediatric burns from abuse are immersion burns and contact burns. Certain clues may assist the physician in differentiating accidental burns from inflicted burns, but often considerable doubt remains even after a careful evaluation.

In an *immersion burn,* a thoughtful assessment of the pattern and location of the burns, as well as of the unaffected areas, helps to differentiate between accidental and inflicted burns. Postulate possible mechanisms for the injury and correlate the assessment with the given history. A child who is held firmly and deliberately immersed has burn margins that are sharp and distinct. If the child has little opportunity to struggle, few or no burns from splashing liquid will occur. In contrast, a child who accidentally comes into contact with a hot liquid will move about in an attempt to escape further injury. This movement causes the burn margins to be less distinct and may result in additional small burns as hot liquid splashes onto the skin. Children who are "dipped" into a bath of hot water often show sparing of their feet and/or buttocks because they are held firmly against the tub's bottom (Fig. 15.1). A child who has had a hand dipped into hot water and held there may reflexively close the fingers, sparing the palm and fingertips.

Contact burns usually have a distinct and recognizable shape. Contact burn patterns most commonly associated with abuse include burns from curling irons, hair dryers, heater elements, and cigarettes (Figs. 15.2, 15.3, 15.4, 15.5). A child who has multiple contact burns or burns to areas that are unlikely to come in contact with the hot object accidentally should be evaluated for abuse.

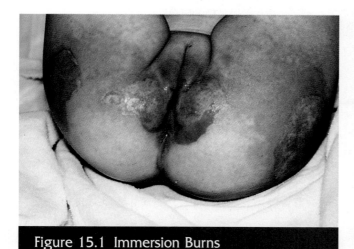

Figure 15.1 Immersion Burns

Immersion burns are often associated with toilet training accidents. This girl was plunged into hot water after soiling herself. She shows sparing of the buttocks, which contacted the surface of the bathtub and avoided being burned. (Courtesy of *The Visual Diagnosis of Child Physical Abuse.* American Academy of Pediatrics, 1994.)

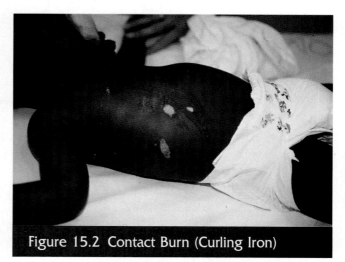

Figure 15.2 Contact Burn (Curling Iron)

Burns on the chest and abdomen from a curling iron. The burn pattern on the injured skin indicates multiple contact burns from an object the size and shape of a curling iron. Accidental curling iron burns occur, but because this infant has so many burns, the injury is suspicious for abuse. Child abuse should be suspected and reported unless the historian can provide a plausible explanation of how these burns occurred accidentally. (Courtesy of Robert A. Shapiro, MD.)

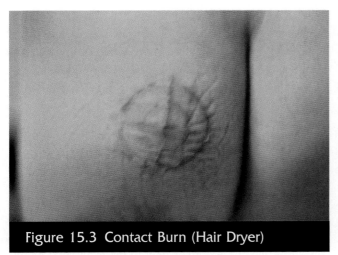

Figure 15.3 Contact Burn (Hair Dryer)

The heated grid from the end of a hair dryer caused this child's burns. The burn size and pattern marks of the burn matched exactly the hair dryer grid that was found in the child's home. The history of accidental injury was thought to be unlikely, and child abuse was suspected. (Courtesy of Robert A. Shapiro, MD.)

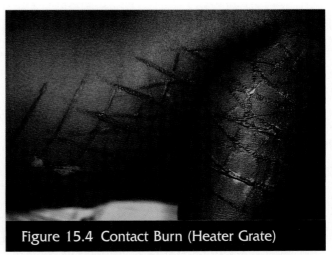

Figure 15.4 Contact Burn (Heater Grate)

This child was held against a heater grate. The pattern became more obvious with the child's knee flexed—the position of the leg at the time of the injury. (Courtesy of David W. Munter, MD.)

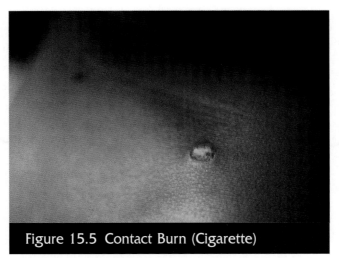

Figure 15.5 Contact Burn (Cigarette)

Cigarette burns are circular injuries with a diameter of about 8 mm. It can be difficult for the clinician to determine if the burn is from an accidental injury or from abuse. Children who accidentally run into a lit cigarette often have burns to the face or distal extremities. Accidental burns may be less distinct and deep compared with inflicted burns. A report of alleged child abuse should be made if there are multiple cigarette burns, burns to locations unlikely to come into contact with a cigarette accidentally, or other signs that suggest abuse. (Courtesy of Robert A. Shapiro, MD.)

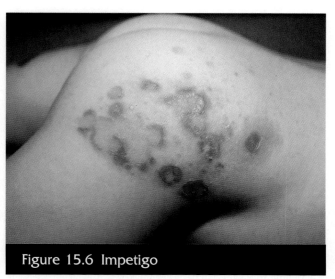

Figure 15.6 Impetigo

These circular lesions of impetigo resemble healing cigarette burns. (Courtesy of Michael J. Nowicki, MD.)

Differential Diagnosis

Some burn look-alikes may be confused with child abuse. Impetigo (Fig. 15.6) may be mistaken for healing cigarette burns, and bullous impetigo can resemble second-degree burns. Contact dermatitis and cellulitis may resemble first-degree burns.

Emergency Department Treatment and Disposition

Document thoroughly all burns that may be due to abuse. Draw sketches and take photographs of the injuries. Obtain a skeletal survey in children under the age of 2 years. Report any suspected abuse immediately to the local child protective agency before discharge from the ED. Provide standard burn therapy.

Clinical Pearls

1. Evaluate the alleged history carefully and obtain sufficient details before making any judgment. Assess whether the explanation and history that are given of the alleged episode are inconsistent with the injuries and/or with the child's developmental abilities. Suspect abuse if, without convincing explanation, the historian alters the initial history.
2. Maintain a high index of suspicion whenever caring for a pediatric burn patient. Look carefully for other signs of abuse, such as bruising, fractures, or signs of neglect.
3. Accidental burns from a cigarette are usually single, superficial, and not completely round. Common sites of accidental cigarette burns are the face, trunk, and hands.
4. Report suspicions to the mandated child protection agency whenever a burn may have been deliberately inflicted.
5. Injuries due to suspected child abuse may be photographed without parental consent in most states.

Associated Clinical Features

Bruises are the most common manifestation of physical child abuse. Child abuse should be suspected whenever bruises are (1) over soft body areas, such as the thighs, buttocks (Fig. 15.7), cheeks, abdomen, and genitalia, since common childhood activities do not commonly cause trauma to these areas; (2) more numerous than usual; (3) of different ages (suggests repeated episodes of abuse); (4) the shape of objects such as belts, cords, or hands (demonstrates that the injuries were inflicted) (Figs. 15.8, 15.9, 15.10); or (5) noted in young, nonambulating children (infants are not capable of getting into accidents).

The color of the ecchymosis will change as healing progresses. New injuries are usually red and purple. They may also be tender and swollen. Within a few days, the bruise may turn blue, then green, then yellow, and finally brown. The shape and margins of the bruise become less distinct as it heals. The time period in which these color changes occur is variable. Some bruises resolve within a few days, whereas others resolve over weeks. The amount of time until resolution depends on factors such as the location, size, and depth of the injury.

Bite marks (Figs. 15.11, 15.12, 15.13) have special forensic characteristics that should be recorded. The size, shape, and pattern of the injury can identify a specific perpetrator. Most human bite injuries are caused by children, not adults, but recognition of an adult bite is important because the injury represents abuse. Compared with an adult's, the shape of a child's bite is rounder. If the impressions from the canines are visible in the bite, the perpetrator's age can be estimated. Most children under 8 years of age have less than 3 cm between their canines. Some bites have saliva within the center of the bite, which can also be used to identify

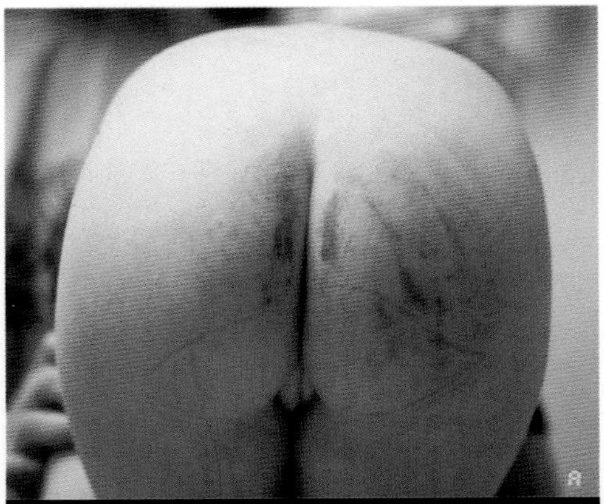

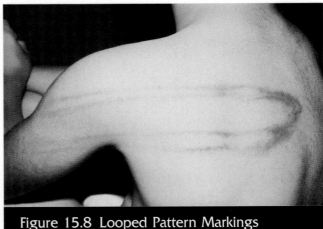

Figure 15.7 Gluteal Fold Bruises

This injury to the buttocks demonstrates linear, parallel bruises near the gluteal folds. Forceful spanking causes gluteal fold bruises. They do not indicate a separate trauma in addition to the spanking. (Courtesy of Robert A. Shapiro, MD.)

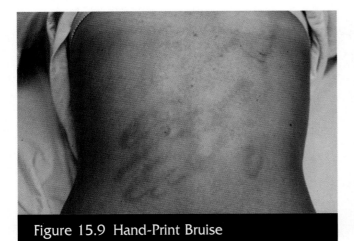

Figure 15.9 Hand-Print Bruise

Bruise from a slap showing the outline of her father's hand is clearly seen on the back of this adolescent. (Courtesy of Robert A. Shapiro, MD.)

Figure 15.8 Looped Pattern Markings

Loop marks are clearly seen within the bruising on this child's back. The loop marks indicate that an extension cord, belt, or some similar object was used to punish him. The color of the bruise is red, which indicates that the injury is only a few days old. (Courtesy of Robert A. Shapiro, MD.)

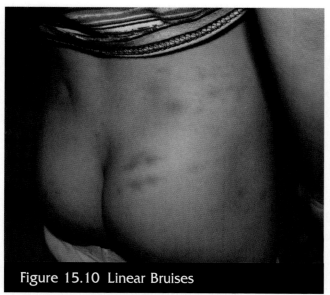

Figure 15.10 Linear Bruises

These linear, parallel bruises on the buttocks with unaffected skin between them are indicative of an injury caused by an object. The width of the object can be determined by measuring the space between the parallel lines. Common objects that cause injuries like these, include belts, fingers, cords, and rulers. (Courtesy of Robert A. Shapiro, MD.)

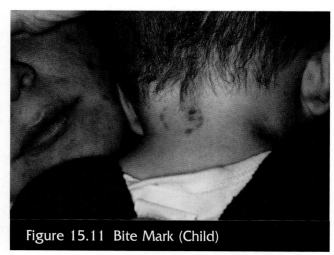

Figure 15.11 Bite Mark (Child)

Distinct impressions of teeth are seen in this injury. The shape of the injury outlines the upper and lower oral arches. Note the size of the mother's mouth in relation to the size of the bite on the neck, making an adult mouth an unlikely source. (Courtesy of Kevin J. Knoop, MD, MS.)

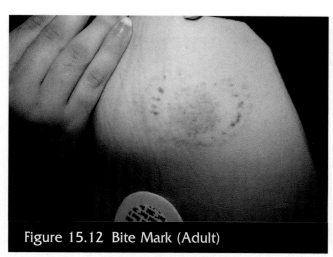

Figure 15.12 Bite Mark (Adult)

This bite mark is on a young girl's breast. Note the larger size of the wound, which is more consistent with an adult bite. (Courtesy of Robert A. Shapiro, MD.)

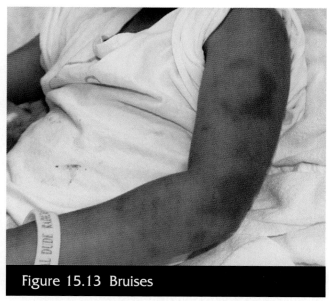

Figure 15.13 Bruises

Bruises cover this child's left arm. The circular bruise on the upper arm is a human bite. Saliva from the perpetrator will usually be present within the center of the bite if the injury is acute and the skin has not yet been washed. Moistened swabs should be used to transfer the saliva from the skin onto the gauze. This gauze must be saved for DNA analysis. As with all trace evidence, the chain of evidence must be documented. (Courtesy of Robert A. Shapiro, MD.)

the perpetrator. Although some bite marks are immediately obvious during the initial inspection, others can be difficult to recognize. If an adult bite is suspected but unprovable because distinct impressions of the teeth are absent, reexamination of the injury a few days later may facilitate recognition and documentation.

The bites of animals are usually easy to distinguish from human bites. The size is usually smaller and the shape of the arch mark is narrower than a human's. Sharp animal canines often cause tearing of the skin instead of the crushing seen in human bites.

Differential Diagnosis

Bleeding disorders—such as idiopathic thrombocytopenic purpura (ITP), Henoch-Schönlein purpura, and leukemia—can mimic child abuse. Folk remedies, such as cupping and coining, may result in soft tissue findings that are not reportable as abuse (see "Lesions Mistaken for Abuse," below).

Emergency Department Treatment and Disposition

Completely undress the child and look for additional signs of abuse (Figs. 15.14 and 15.15). Obtain a complete history of all injuries. Sketch and photograph the injuries. Obtain a platelet count and bleeding studies [prothrombin time and partial thromboplastin time (PT and PTT)] to rule out a bleeding diathesis as the cause of the findings. For children under 2 or 3 years of age who have extensive injuries, obtain a skeletal survey, alanine transferase (ALT), aspartate aminotransferase (AST), amylase, and urinalysis.

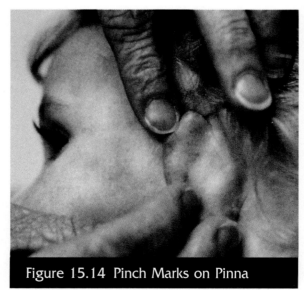

Figure 15.14 Pinch Marks on Pinna

Children may be pulled up or along by their ears, causing this injury. A child's ears should be inspected for this injury whenever abuse is suspected. (Courtesy of Robert A. Shapiro, MD.)

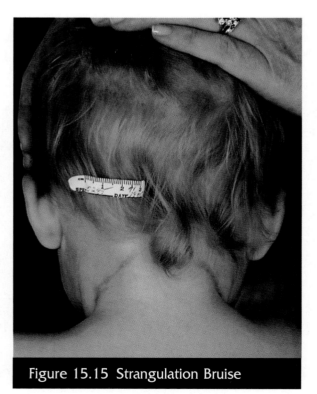

Figure 15.15 Strangulation Bruise

This child was beaten while at the sitter's and suffered circumferential linear neck abrasions consistent with attempted strangulation. There is also occipital ecchymosis from the abuse. (Courtesy of Barbara R. Craig, MD.)

If human bites are found or suspected, consider consultation with a forensic dentist. If appropriate, collect swabs for DNA forensic analysis from the center of unwashed, fresh bites, which may contain saliva from the perpetrator.

Report suspected abuse to the legally mandated child protection agency before the child is discharged from the ED.

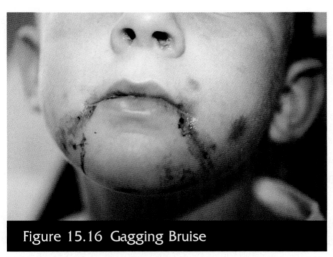

Figure 15.16 Gagging Bruise

This child had a sock stuffed into his mouth and tied around his head. The bruises in the corners of the child's mouth are indicative of gagging. Additionally, there are circular bruises on his left and right cheeks caused from the perpetrator's fingers while holding the child still to insert the sock. Pattern markings within the bruises match the fabric pattern of the sock. Photographs of these patterns should be obtained and provided to the police. The red color of the bruises and the fresh facial excoriations indicate that the injuries are recent. (Courtesy of Robert A. Shapiro, MD.)

Clinical Pearls

1. Determination of the age of a bruise is imprecise. Bruises that are "fresh" (< 48 h) are usually recognizable because they are tender, red, and swollen. Occasionally, bruises may not be visible for up to 48 h after an injury.

2. Children may deny abuse when questioned because of threats made to them. The child in Fig. 15.16 initially denied that he had been gagged. He told the examining physician that he had spilled some cleaning fluid onto his lips.

3. When a parent or caretaker inflicts an injury while disciplining a child, the incident must be reported to the local child protection agency. Even if corporal punishment is lawful in a given state, the infliction of an injury is never lawful.

4. Place a millimeter ruler or coin next to a pattern injury before taking photographs so that measurements can be made.

5. Consent is not required in most states to photograph injuries suspicious for child abuse.

Associated Clinical Features

Whenever bruising is excessive, is not associated with a compatible history, or occurs in an unusual distribution, seek a specific etiology. It may be appropriate to suspect and report child abuse when these conditions exist but also consider other diagnoses.

Common Childhood Bruising

Accidental trauma can result in a bruise to any part of the body, but the forehead and the extensor surfaces of the tibia, elbow, and knee are the most common locations. When other areas of the body are bruised, etiologies other than accidental bruising should be considered.

Mongolian Spots

Mongolian spots are bluish sacral or truncal lesions, most often seen in non-Caucasian infants and young children. They may be mistaken for bruises. Mongolian spots may be limited to only a few lesions, or they may extend up the back and shoulders of the child (Fig. 15.17).

Cupping, Coining, and Moxibustion

Asian families sometimes practice traditional cures with their children, such as cupping, coining, and moxibustion. Each of these practices leaves markings on the child's skin, which may be interpreted as child abuse. In cupping, a flammable object is ignited and placed into a cup. After the flames have extinguished, the cup is inverted and placed onto the child's skin. As the warm air within the cup cools, a vacuum is produced. This "cure" leaves circular suction markings on the child's skin but should not be painful to the child. Coining (Fig. 15.18) is done by rubbing a coin up and down the child's back, just lateral to the spine. This results in petechiae and chronic skin changes on the back. Coining should also not be painful to the child. Neither of these practices should be reported as child abuse. In moxibustion, a flammable object, such as a thread, is ignited on or near the child's skin. Moxibustion may cause superficial burns. Whether moxibustion is reported as child abuse would depend on the physical findings and the judgment of the physician.

Henoch-Schönlein Purpura

Henoch-Schönlein purpura (HSP) is a vasculitis of the small blood vessels. The skin lesions are usually small, symmetric, palpable purpuras. They may appear in a linear pattern and are often confined to the lower extremities (Fig. 15.19). Associated symptoms may include joint and abdominal pain.

Idiopathic Thrombocytopenic Purpura

Idiopathic thrombocytopenic purpura (ITP) is an acquired platelet disorder that results in abnormal bleeding. It is most common in

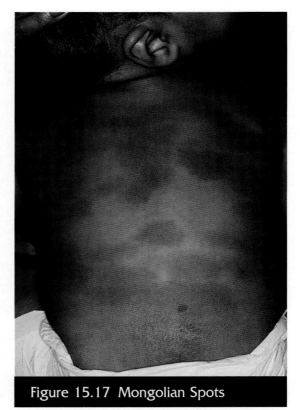

Figure 15.17 Mongolian Spots

Numerous mongolian spots on this youngster extend up the back and shoulders. (Courtesy of Douglas R. Landry, MD.)

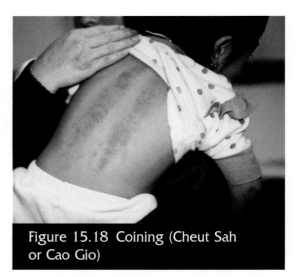

Figure 15.18 Coining (Cheut Sah or Cao Gio)

This child has petechiae and bruising along her spine. Her parents were practicing the Southeast Asian practice of coining, a healing remedy, in which a coin is rubbed along the spine to heal an illness. Coining should not be painful and is not considered abusive. (Courtesy of Charles Schubert, MD.)

487

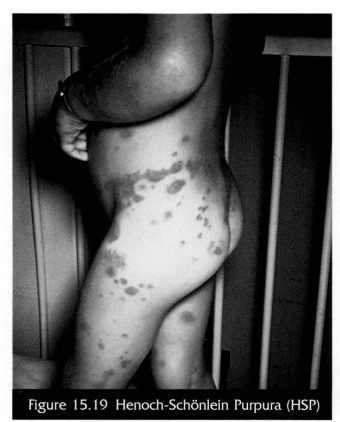

Figure 15.19 Henoch-Schönlein Purpura (HSP)

This child has palpable purpura on the extensor surfaces of the legs. HSP should be considered whenever there is symmetric ecchymosis along the extensor surfaces of the extremities and buttocks. The illness is most often seen in school-age children. Migratory arthritis and abdominal pain may be present. (Courtesy of Ralph A. Gruppo, MD.)

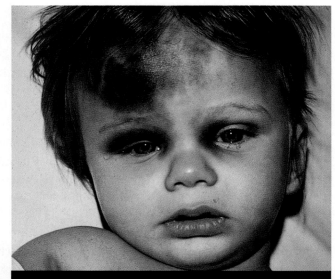

Figure 15.20 Hemophiliac with Bruising

This child's bruising is due to factor VIII deficiency. The degree of bleeding within the ecchymosis is more extensive than that seen in children without coagulopathies. A history of other abnormal bleeding episodes or a history that the child suffers from a coagulopathy is most often obtained at the time of presentation. (Courtesy of Ralph A. Gruppo, MD.)

1- to 4-year-old children. The presenting complaint is most often abnormal bruising. The bruises can appear anywhere on the body and are numerous, mimicking child abuse. The child may also have epistaxis, hematuria, or other bleeding.

Hemophilia

Hemophilia is usually diagnosed soon after birth because of abnormal bleeding. The ecchymosis and soft-tissue swelling are greater than would be expected given the history of trauma (Figs. 15.20, 15.21).

Differential Diagnosis

Diagnostic suspicion and awareness of the above conditions is the most important step leading to the correct diagnosis. HSP, mongolian spots, and cultural practices such as moxibustion and cupping are diagnosed clinically. If ITP or other thrombocytopenic disorders are suspected, a platelet count is diagnostic. Newborns and infants with significant bleeding should have PT and PTT tests to rule out a coagulopathy.

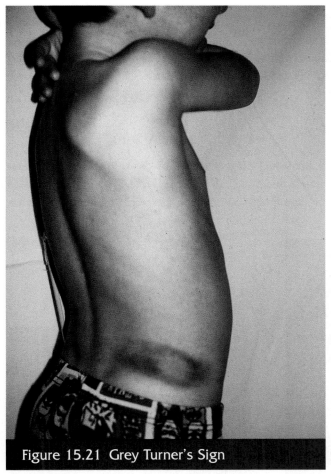

Figure 15.21 Grey Turner's Sign

This child presented after a minor fall. This pattern of bruising (flank ecchymosis) should alert the examiner to the possibility of retroperitoneal bleeding, which was found on CT scan in this hemophiliac patient. (Courtesy of Louis LaVopa, MD.)

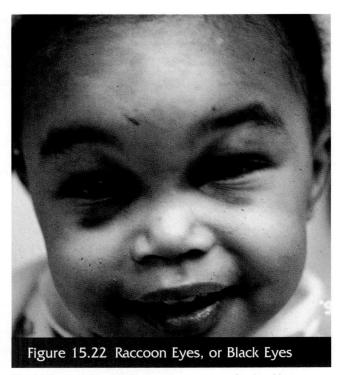

Figure 15.22 Raccoon Eyes, or Black Eyes

The etiology of this child's raccoon eyes was a forehead hematoma. He fell onto his forehead a few days earlier and developed a hematoma, a common accidental injury. As the hematoma healed, blood from the hematoma tracked down along the facial soft tissues and settled under his eyes. The resulting ecchymosis suggests that he was punched, leaving him with two black eyes. The absence of other trauma about the eyes—such as lacerations, abrasions, soft tissue swelling, or eye injury—should cause the examiner to consider a diagnosis other than direct trauma. Observation or palpation of forehead soft tissue swelling results in the correct diagnosis. (Courtesy of Robert A. Shapiro, MD.)

Emergency Department Treatment and Disposition

A hematologist should be consulted for children with platelet disorders and coagulopathies. HSP requires supportive care and close follow-up. The most serious complication of HSP is bowel obstruction from intussusception.

Clinical Pearls

1. Mongolian spots are noted first in the newborn period.
2. Consider HSP in school-age children with purpura of the lower extremities.
3. Consider ITP in preschool children who have multiple ecchymosis and petechiae without other signs or indications of abuse.
4. Vitamin K deficiency is a cause of bleeding in infancy.
5. Trauma to the forehead may cause bilateral eye ecchymosis (Fig. 15.22) within a few days and can be mistaken for eye trauma.

Associated Clinical Features

Certain fractures should always raise a suspicion of child abuse, such as metaphyseal corner fractures, rib fractures, fractures in a nonambulating child, and untreated healing fractures. Fractures incompatible with the history and those for which no explanation is available are also suspicious of child abuse (Figs. 15.23 to 15.29).

Differential Diagnosis

Normal pediatric radiographic variants, periosteal changes caused by conditions other than healing fractures, and illnesses that cause fragile bones may all be mistaken for fractures due to child abuse. A pediatric radiologist should be consulted if any doubt exists about the radiographic in-

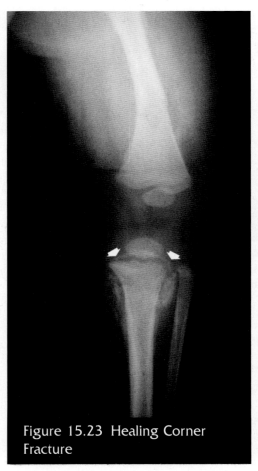

Figure 15.23 Healing Corner Fracture

This radiograph shows a healing metaphyseal corner fracture of the proximal tibia, sometimes referred to as a bucket-handle fracture. Arrows point to the impressive periosteal elevation, causing the bucket-handle appearance. This fracture is most often seen in children who have been the victims of child abuse, the result of shaking or pulling. (Courtesy of Alan E. Oestreich, MD.)

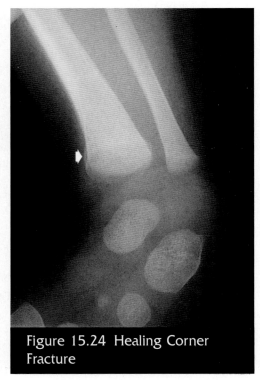

Figure 15.24 Healing Corner Fracture

Periosteal reaction (*arrow*) of the distal tibia from a corner fracture. (Courtesy of Alan E. Oestreich, MD.)

This radiograph shows a displaced spiral femur fracture with faint callus formation. The age of the fracture is just over 10 days. There is also periosteal reaction of the proximal tibia, which is more solid and therefore older than the femur fracture. Spiral femur fractures are caused by trauma that includes a twisting, rotational force to the bone. Accidental falls can result in spiral fractures if the child's foot is fixed while his or her body is rotating. Spiral fractures from abuse are often caused by an angry adult who twists the leg of the child. The radiographic finding in this photograph is almost certainly indicative of child abuse because there are two injuries which occurred at different times and no treatment was obtained when the injuries occurred. (Courtesy of Alan E. Oestreich, MD.)

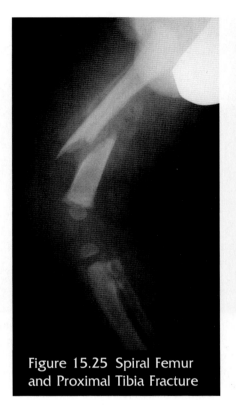

Figure 15.25 Spiral Femur and Proximal Tibia Fracture

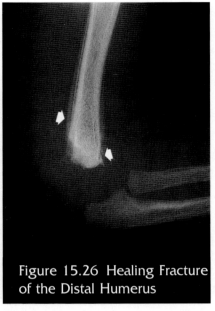

Figure 15.26 Healing Fracture of the Distal Humerus

The periosteal reaction along the distal humerus dates this fracture as older than 10 days. No treatment was obtained for the acute injury. (Courtesy of Alan E. Oestreich, MD.)

There are healing rib fractures of the right posterior fifth, sixth, and seventh ribs, the right lateral sixth rib, the left posterior fourth rib, and the right proximal humerus. The surrounding callus indicates the fractures are older than 10 days. Rib fractures must always raise a suspicion of child abuse since accidental rib fractures are unusual. Rib fractures are usually due to very firm squeezing and may be seen with shaken baby syndrome. Normal handling of infants or playful activities do not cause rib fractures. (Courtesy of Alan E. Oestreich, MD.)

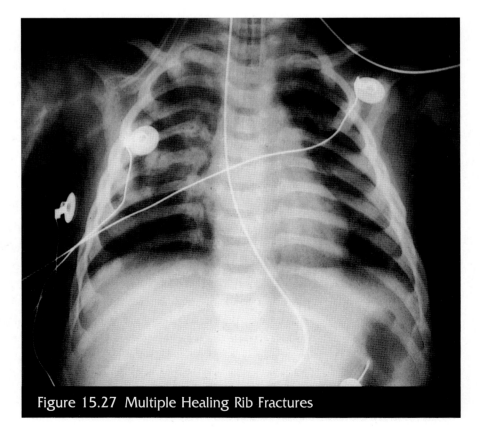

Figure 15.27 Multiple Healing Rib Fractures

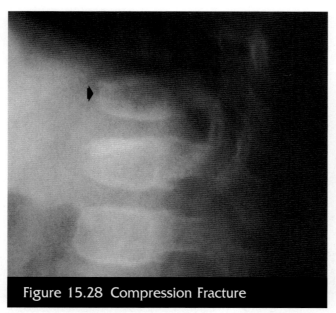

Figure 15.28 Compression Fracture

The wedging of T-12 (*arrow*) and probably L-1 indicates vertebral compression fractures. These fractures are the result of significant forces applied to the spinal column and are often indicative of child abuse. (Courtesy of Alan E. Oestreich, MD.)

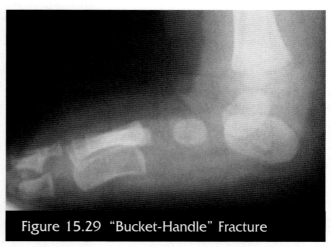

Figure 15.29 "Bucket-Handle" Fracture

Metaphyseal fractures may appear as in this photograph. When captured at this angle, the fracture is frequently described as a bucket-handle fracture. (Courtesy of Michael P. Poirier, MD.)

terpretation. Specific disorders that can be mistaken for child abuse include osteogenesis imperfecta, copper deficiency, osteopetrosis, rickets, scurvy, hypervitaminosis A, osteomyelitis, tumors, leukemia, prostaglandin E overdose, and Caffey's infantile cortical hyperostosis.

Conditions that cause "brittle bones" must be considered when unexpected fractures are discovered, even though such cases are rare. The most frequently discussed brittle bone disorder is osteogenesis imperfecta (OI), a rare inherited connective-tissue disorder. Associated features seen in some children with OI include blue sclerae, wormian bones (seen on the skull x-ray), and osteopenia. A family history of bone fragility, hearing loss, and short stature is often present. In rare instances, children with OI lack these associated features.

Emergency Department Treatment and Disposition

If abuse is suspected in a child under 2 or 3 years of age, obtain a skeletal survey. The skeletal survey should include a minimum of 19 films (Table 15.1), including frontal views of the appendicular skeleton and frontal and lateral views of the axial skeleton. Coned down views over a joint may be needed for best visualization of metaphyseal injuries. Oblique views are useful for hand, rib, and nondisplaced lone bone-shaft fractures. All images obtained (including those of the chest) should use bone technique. Ideally, all studies should be read by a radiologist while the patient is still in the ED. Consider computed tomography or magnetic resonance imaging of the head in infants with skull fractures when abuse is suspected. Suspected abuse must be reported immediately to the appropriate child protection agency. Fractures should be managed appropriately.

Table 15.1	
SKELETAL SURVEY FOR SUSPECTED CHILD ABUSE	

AP skull
Lateral skull
Lateral cervical spine
AP thorax
Lateral thorax
AP pelvis
Lateral lumbar spine
AP humeri (2)[a]
AP forearms (2)[a]
Oblique hands (15°–20°) (2)[a]
AP femurs (2)[a]
AP tibias (2)[a]
AP feet (2)[a]

[a] Each a separate exposure: can be combined on one film.
Source: Courtesy of Paul Kleinman, MD.

Clinical Pearls

1. Suspect abuse when a child has multiple fractures, fractures of different ages, unsuspected (occult) fractures, or fractures without a consistent trauma history.
2. Accidental trauma that includes rotational forces can result in a spiral fracture.
3. Obtain a skeletal survey in any child under 2 years of age who has injuries suspicious of abuse.
4. Radiographic signs of healing are typically first seen 10 days after a fracture.
5. Fractures that are not immobilized have a larger callus than immobilized fractures.

Associated Clinical Features

Infants who are violently shaken may suffer intracranial injury, commonly referred to as "shaken baby syndrome." Typically, the infant is held by the chest and violently shaken back and forth. This shaking results in subdural hemorrhages and cerebral contusions (Figs. 15.30 to 15.32). Most of the victims are under 1 year of age. Some investigators believe that shaking alone is insufficient to cause these injuries and that therefore some blunt head trauma must also occur. The name "shaken impact syndrome" has been suggested to include this mechanism. There are usually no external signs of trauma, although infants who are shaken may also have fractures, abdominal trauma, bruises, and other injuries. Neurologic symptoms such as apnea, seizures, irritability, or altered mental status are commonly seen but may be absent. Retinal hemorrhages (Figs. 15.33, 15.34) are seen in 80% of shaken babies. The hemorrhages may be unilateral or bilateral. Shaken baby syndrome should be strongly considered when retinal hemorrhages are found in any child under 2 years of age.

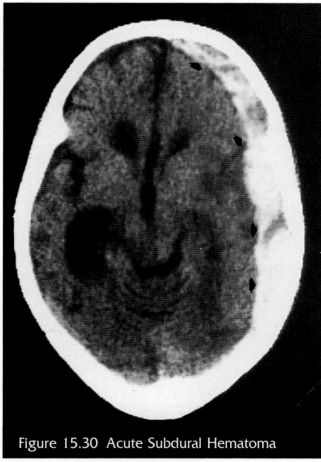

Figure 15.30 Acute Subdural Hematoma

There is a crescent-shaped, hyperdense collection, indicating an acute subdural hematoma over the left cerebral hemisphere (*arrows*). In addition, the brain demonstrates chronic injury from a previous insult, which left the child severely impaired. (Courtesy of William S. Ball, MD.)

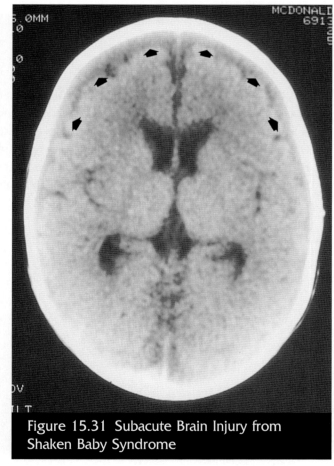

Figure 15.31 Subacute Brain Injury from Shaken Baby Syndrome

This noncontrast computed tomography scan demonstrates bilateral subdural collections over the frontal convexity (*arrows*). (Courtesy of William S. Ball, MD.)

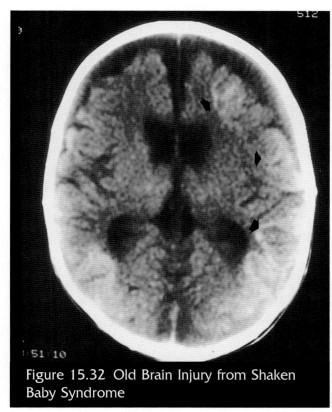

Figure 15.32 Old Brain Injury from Shaken Baby Syndrome

Three months later there is evidence of diffuse cerebral volume loss with multifocal areas of increased density (*arrows*), representing diffuse cortical and subcortical injury. (Courtesy of William S. Ball, MD.)

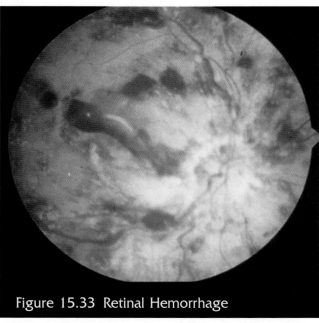

Figure 15.33 Retinal Hemorrhage

Multiple retinal hemorrhages are present. (Courtesy of Rees W. Shepherd, MD.)

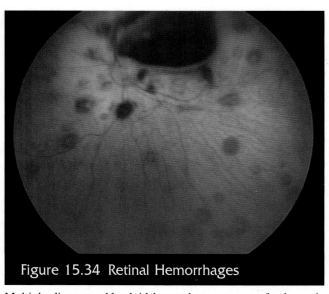

Figure 15.34 Retinal Hemorrhages

Multiple discreet subhyaloid hemorrhages seen on funduscopic examination in an infant with shaken baby syndrome. (Courtesy of John D. Baker, MD, and Massie Research Laboratories, Inc.)

Differential Diagnosis

Shaken baby syndrome is the most common cause of intracranial injury in infants. Relatively minor trauma, such as a fall off a couch or bed, should not cause intracranial damage unless there are predisposing conditions such as a bleeding disorder or a preexisting intracranial vascular disorder. Retinal hemorrhages in association with intracranial trauma is almost always indicative of shaken baby syndrome.

Findings on computed tomography (CT) or magnetic resonance imaging (MRI) that may mimic SBS include benign extraoral fluid collections, glutaric aciduria type, ruptured aneurysm, or arteriovenous malformation.

Retinal hemorrhages may be caused by birth trauma, blunt eye trauma, meningitis, severe hypertension, sepsis, and coagulopathies. The hemorrhages that result from birth usually resolve within 3 weeks. There have been reports of cardiopulmonary resuscitation (CPR) causing retinal hemorrhages. Retinal hemorrhages from CPR and mechanisms other than major trauma are typically less extensive than those seen in SBS.

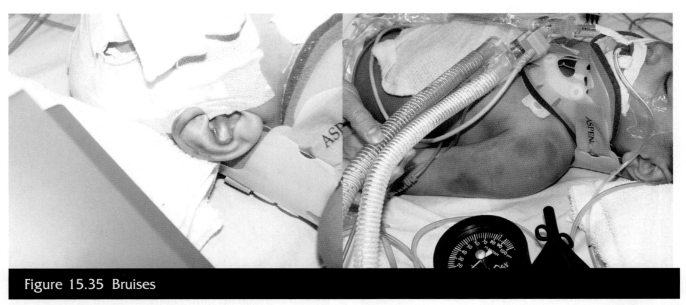

Figure 15.35 Bruises

This child was a victim of shaken baby syndrome (SBS). Unlike most victims of SBS, he also has signs of cutaneous injury. Bruises on his right pinna (A) and left upper arm (B) were noted on examination. (Courtesy of Robert A. Shapiro, MD.)

Emergency Department Treatment and Disposition

CT or MRI of the head should be obtained and the patient treated in the usual fashion. A report of suspected child abuse must be made to the child protective agency. A skeletal survey should also be obtained and other injuries noted (Fig. 15.35). An ophthalmologist should follow the patient's retinal injuries.

Clinical Pearls

1. Child abuse should be suspected in any infant with retinal hemorrhages or facial bruising.
2. Infants with SBS may have no external signs of trauma and minimal neurologic deficits.
3. When retinal hemorrhages are present, an ophthalmologist should be consulted to assist with the differential diagnosis and for medicolegal documentation.
4. SBS is most common in children under 1 year of age.

Associated Clinical Features

The genital examination of prepubertal girls is usually limited to inspection of the external genitalia and hymen for injury and infection. An internal inspection is rarely required. Children should first be examined in the "frog-leg" position. The child can lie on the examination table or sit on a parent's lap (Fig. 15.36), whichever makes her most comfortable. Position the patient in a supine position with her knees flexed and out. The soles of her feet should be opposed (Fig. 15.36). Alternatively, the child can be placed in a knee-chest position. The knee-chest position is particularly useful to visualize foreign bodies in the vagina as well as the posterior vaginal rim.

First, examine the perineum for trauma, condylomata, herpetic lesions, or discharge. Next examine the hymen. To visualize the hymen, hold the labia majora between the thumb and index fingers of each hand. Apply lateral and posterior traction to the labia while pulling them outward (Fig. 15.37). When done properly, this procedure is not painful and provides excellent visualization of the hymen

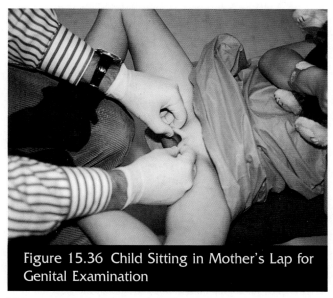

Figure 15.36 Child Sitting in Mother's Lap for Genital Examination

This young girl is being examined while she sits in her mother's lap. Many young children are less fearful of the examination if they are held by a parent during the examination. Her legs are held in the "frog-leg" position as labial traction is applied. (Courtesy of Robert A. Shapiro, MD.)

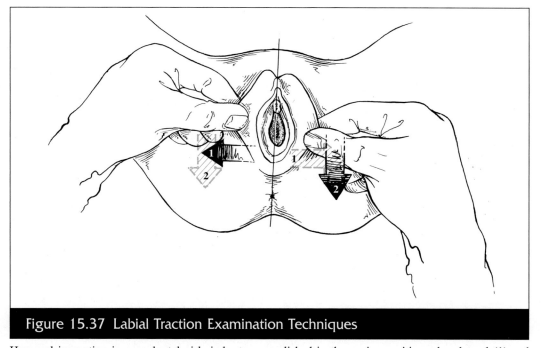

Figure 15.37 Labial Traction Examination Techniques

Hymenal inspection in prepubertal girls is best accomplished in the supine position when lateral (1) and posterior (2) traction to the labia is applied as shown here. (Adapted from Giandino AP et al: *A Practical Guide to the Evaluation of Sexual Abuse in the Prepubertal Child.* Sage Publications, 1992.)

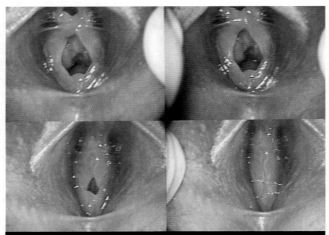

Figure 15.38 Effect of Labial Traction on the Appearance of the Prepubertal Introitus

These photographs demonstrate how the appearance of the introitus changes using different examination techniques in a prepubertal girl. Each photograph shows the introitus of the same child as different types of labial traction are used. *A. Bottom right*: Lateral labial traction only. The hymenal introitus is closed and the hymenal margins cannot be visualized. *B. Bottom left*: More aggressive lateral traction is applied. The introitus is now partially visible. *C. Top right and left*: Lateral, posterior, and caudal labial traction (as illustrated in 15.37). The introitus is now clearly seen, and the hymen can be adequately inspected for signs of injury. (Courtesy of Robert A. Shapiro, MD.)

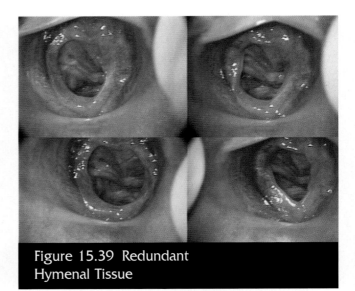

Figure 15.39 Redundant Hymenal Tissue

These photographs show the genitalia of the same patient. Because of redundant hymenal tissue, the introitus appears asymmetric in the top two photos as well as the bottom left. The text describes methods to handle redundant hymen. When the hymen is no longer adherent to itself, the introitus appears symmetric and normal. (Courtesy of Robert A. Shapiro, MD.)

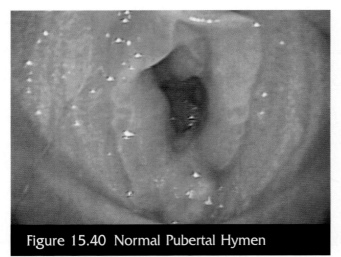

Figure 15.40 Normal Pubertal Hymen

The hymen is thicker and more redundant in this pubertal child compared to a prepubertal hymen. This redundancy is due to the effects of estrogen and begins during puberty. The hymen at 6 o'clock is not adequately documented by this photograph. Additional examinations—discussed in the above text—should be used to visualize the posterior hymen. (Courtesy of Robert A. Shapiro, MD.)

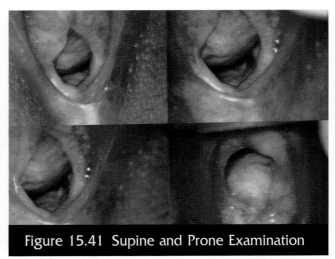

Figure 15.41 Supine and Prone Examination

Image (A) of this examination was obtained while the child was supine. The posterior hymen at 6 o'clock appears to be very narrow. When the child was examined in the prone (knee-chest) position (B), the 6 o'clock area, now at the top of the photo, is better seen and is completely normal in appearance. (Courtesy of Robert A. Shapiro, MD.)

(Figs. 15.38 to 15.40). If the hymen cannot be visualized in the supine frog-leg position, the knee-chest position should be attempted (Fig. 15.41). Examine the hymen for indications of trauma, such as swelling, ecchymoses or tears. In pubertal girls, a Foley catheter can help the examiner inspect the edges of the hymen for injury (Fig. 15.42). To perform this procedure, insert the deflated catheter into the vagina and inflate the catheter balloon with 10 mL of saline. Gentle traction can then be placed on the catheter by pulling until the balloon expands the hymenal edges. By moving the inflated balloon from side to side to different sections of the hymen can be exposed.

Techniques

Supine or "frog-leg" position:

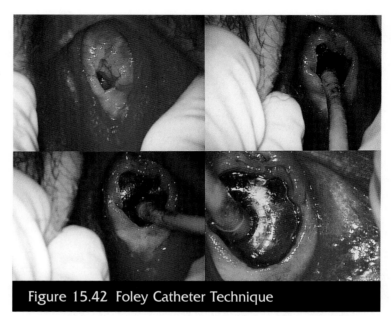

Figure 15.42 Foley Catheter Technique

A Foley catheter inserted into the vaginal subsequently filled with 10 cc saline is used to inspect the hymenal edges for injury. Gentle traction and movement of the inflated balloon from side to side exposes different sections of the hymen. The hymen shown in these photographs is normal. (Courtesy of Robert A. Shapiro, MD.)

1. The child can lie on an examination table or, if more comfortable, can sit on her parent's lap.
2. Position the child in a supine position with her knees out and soles together.
3. Apply traction, as demonstrated in Fig. 15.38.

Prone or knee-chest position:

1. On the examination table, position the child on her hands and knees. Her knees should be spread wider than her shoulders.
2. Have the child rest her chest to the examination table.
3. Maintain the knee placement with a swayed backbone.

Emergency Department Treatment and Disposition

If sexual abuse is suspected, a report of alleged sexual abuse must be made to the child protective agency. Suspicious or abnormal examination findings should be documented. The child should be referred for a definitive examination by an expert in child abuse.

Clinical Pearls

1. Allow the child to sit on her mother's lap during the examination if this makes her more cooperative and less afraid.
2. Speculum examinations are rarely indicated in prepubertal girls and are reserved for removal of an intravaginal foreign body or evaluation of intravaginal trauma. General anesthesia is often required before inserting a speculum into a prepubertal child.
3. Apply caudal traction to the labia during examination to prevent a superficial tear of the posterior fourchette.

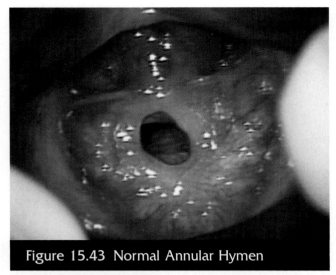

Figure 15.43 Normal Annular Hymen

The hymen in this prepubertal girl is annular in shape, extending completely around the vaginal opening. The inner hymenal ring (introitus) is smooth and free of any defects, such as lacerations or scars. The color of the hymen is more deeply red than seen in pubertal women and does not necessarily indicate infection or trauma. (Courtesy of Robert A. Shapiro, MD.)

4. If a portion of the hymen cannot be visualized because it is adherent to the adjacent labia or to itself, gently touch the adherent tissue with the contralateral labia to pull it free. A drop of saline placed onto the posterior hymen may also separate adherent tissues without causing discomfort to the child.

5. The inner hymenal ring is usually smooth and uninterrupted. Notches at 3 and 9 o'clock are normal.

6. The shape and appearance of the normal prepubertal hymen is variable. Annular (Fig. 15.43) and crescentic (Fig. 15.44) configurations are the most common. Normal hymens may also be septate (Fig. 15.45), imperforate (no central opening), or cribriform (multiple small openings).

7. A normal examination does not exclude sexual abuse. The majority of abused prepubertal girls have normal genital examinations. Examination findings specific for sexual abuse are found in approximately 10 to 20% of girls who allege abuse.

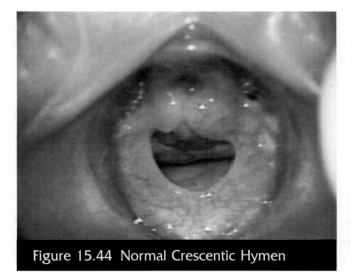

Figure 15.44 Normal Crescentic Hymen

The hymen in this prepubertal girl extends from 2 to 10 o'clock and is absent beneath the urethra between 10 and 2 o'clock. This annular shape is very common and should not be mistaken for trauma or rupture of the superior (2 to 10 o'clock) section. The inner hymenal ring (the introitus) is smooth and free of any defects, such as lacerations or scars. (Courtesy of Robert A. Shapiro, MD.)

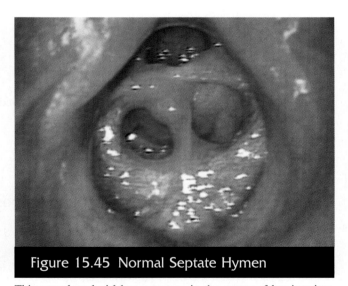

Figure 15.45 Normal Septate Hymen

This prepubertal girl has a septum in the center of her introitus. Hymenal septa are rarely seen after puberty. (Courtesy of Robert A. Shapiro, MD.)

Associated Clinical Features

Sexual abuse must be considered in any child with a genital or rectal injury, a sexually transmitted infection, a history of alleged abuse, or symptoms or behaviors seen in abused children.

Acute injuries include lacerations, bruises, abrasions and swelling (Figs. 15.46 to 15.49). Acute injuries heal quickly, often within a few days to a week. Nonacute findings of trauma secondary to sexual abuse can be more difficult to recognize and should be considered by a child abuse expert. Nonacute findings include scars, absent hymen, abnormal clefts (Fig. 15.50), and anal changes. Accurate interpretation of genital findings is dependent on examination technique (see preceding section for suggestions on examination technique).

Sexually transmitted infections diagnosed in a young person may indicate sexual abuse (Fig. 15.51). Children infected with *Neisseria gonorrhoeae, Chlamydia trachomatis, Trichomonas,* and syphilis (Fig. 15.52) who did not become infected through perinatal transmission have almost

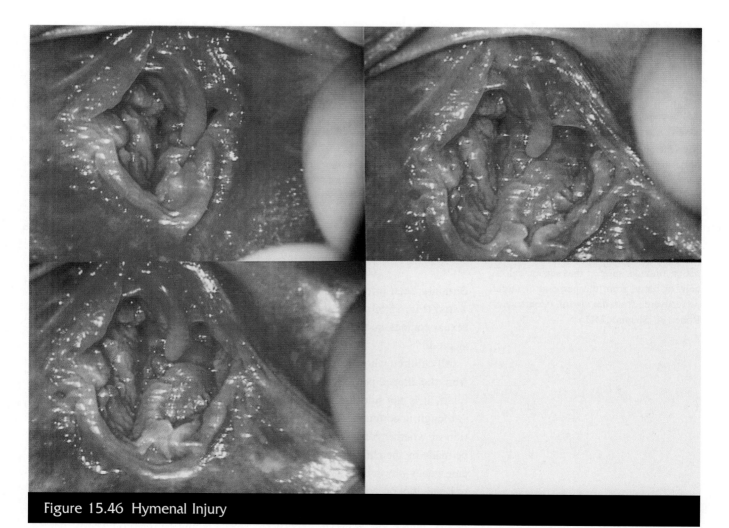

Figure 15.46 Hymenal Injury

Healed injuries to the vaginal introitus have caused significant distortion of the anatomy. The vaginal opening is gaping revealing multiple vaginal rugae. Only small remnants of the hymen remain.

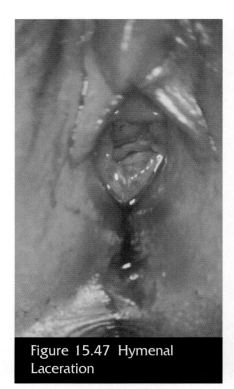

Figure 15.47 Hymenal Laceration

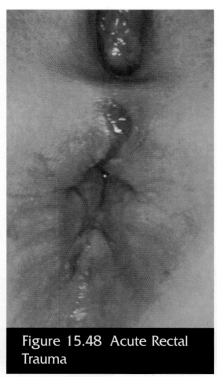

Figure 15.48 Acute Rectal Trauma

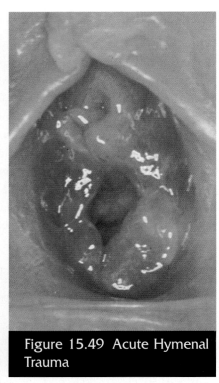

Figure 15.49 Acute Hymenal Trauma

An acute laceration with bruising of the posterior fourchette. The nearby hymen is edematous and ecchymotic. This injury is most likely less than 72 h old. Injuries to the hymen and posterior fourchette are usually indicative of sexual assault. Forensic specimens should be collected after acute sexual assault when the history or examination findings suggest that semen, saliva, hair, or blood from the perpetrator might be recovered from the victim. (Courtesy of Robert A. Shapiro, MD.)

An acute rectal injury is visible at 12 o'-clock. The perianal skin may normally be darker, with red or blue coloration, than the surrounding skin. (Courtesy of Robert A. Shapiro, MD.)

There is a deep laceration of the hymen at 7 o'clock and ecchymosis of the hymen at 6 o'clock after recent sexual assault. (Courtesy of Robert A. Shapiro, MD.)

certainly been infected through sexual contact. Condylomata acuminata (genital warts) (Fig. 15.53) and herpes simplex may be transmitted through sexual or nonsexual contact, so that sexual abuse as well as other mechanisms should be considered.

All children who allege sexual abuse should be evaluated, treated, and protected from the alleged perpetrator. Because of threats by family members or the perpetrator, it is not unusual for a child to recant initial allegations of sexual abuse. Although uncommon, some children falsely allege sexual abuse. The determination of whether allegations are false or of the significance of recantation should be made by the child protective services worker or by law enforcement, not by the emergency physician.

Behaviors or symptoms of abuse are frequently absent at the time of diagnosis but can include fear or avoidance of an individual, genital or rectal pain, sleep disorders, regression, enuresis, encopresis, sexual acting out or promiscuity, depression, declining in school performance, and perpetration of sexual abuse on younger victims.

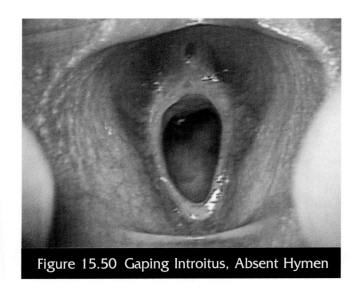

Figure 15.50 Gaping Introitus, Absent Hymen

The hymen is almost totally absent in this prepubertal girl. There may be a slight rim of hymen at 6 o'clock. The hymen in young girls is often very thin and may be totally destroyed after vaginal penetration. (Courtesy of Robert A. Shapiro, MD.)

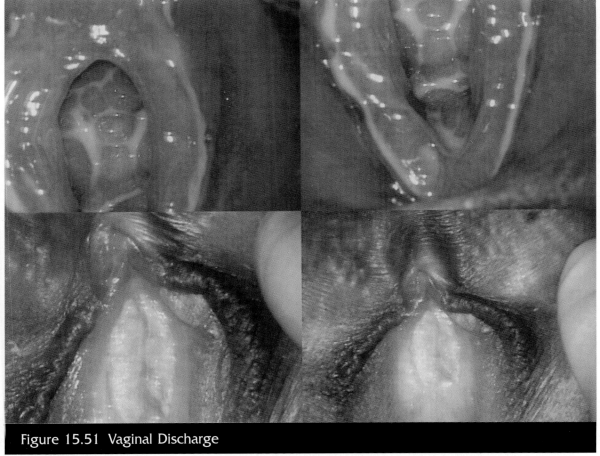

Figure 15.51 Vaginal Discharge

Copious white discharge is present in this photograph. Vaginal discharge in a prepubertal child may be an indication of an STD. All children with vaginal discharge should be cultured for *N. gonorrhoeae* and *Chlamydia.* (Courtesy of Robert A. Shapiro, MD.)

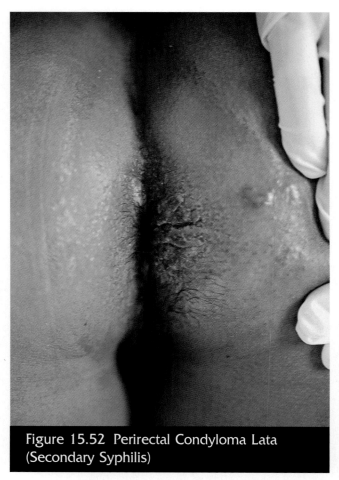

Figure 15.52 Perirectal Condyloma Lata (Secondary Syphilis)

Perirectal condyloma lata are visible around the rectum. (Courtesy of Robert A. Shapiro, MD.)

Differential Diagnosis

Injury to the hymen from an event other than sexual abuse is possible though unusual. Masturbation and self-exploration do not cause vaginal injury in the vast majority of children. Subtle findings of hymenal trauma are difficult to recognize. Normal hymenal anatomy may be misdiagnosed as trauma by inexperienced examiners. Other genital findings mistaken for sexual abuse are listed in the next section.

Emergency Department Treatment and Disposition

Report suspected or alleged sexual abuse to the appropriate child protection agency. Clearly document all examination findings. If injuries require repair, appropriate consultation with surgery or gynecology should be made. Culture for sexually transmitted infections if there is a vaginal or urethral discharge. If the history of abuse suggests a risk for infection, obtain cultures from the genitalia, rectum, and pharynx. Consider syphilis and HIV testing. Obtain forensic specimens if the alleged abuse occurred within the previous 72 h and the examination findings or history suggests that blood, semen, saliva, or hair of the perpetrator might be found on the victim's body. Offer sexually transmitted disease (STD) and pregnancy prophylaxes when indicated. Make discharge plans in consultation with the child protection worker so that the child is not returned to the abusive environment.

Clinical Pearls

1. It is not necessary to measure the vaginal opening of prepubertal girls. The size of the introitus is dependent on examination technique, degree of patient relaxation, patient age, and other variables. There is no consensus on normal introitus size among experts.
2. Hymenal notches at 3 and 9 o'clock can be a normal finding.
3. Changes to the posterior hymen, such as narrowing and notching, may be indicative of penetrating injury.
4. Rectal abuse often results in no visible trauma. When trauma does occur, healing may be complete within 1 to 2 weeks, leaving no visible indication of the injury.
5. The external anus is darker in color than the rest of the skin and should not be mistaken for erythema from abuse or infection.
6. Consider sexual abuse when significant anal fissures are present on examination.
7. Condyloma lata (syphilis) can be mistaken for condylomata acuminata (warts).

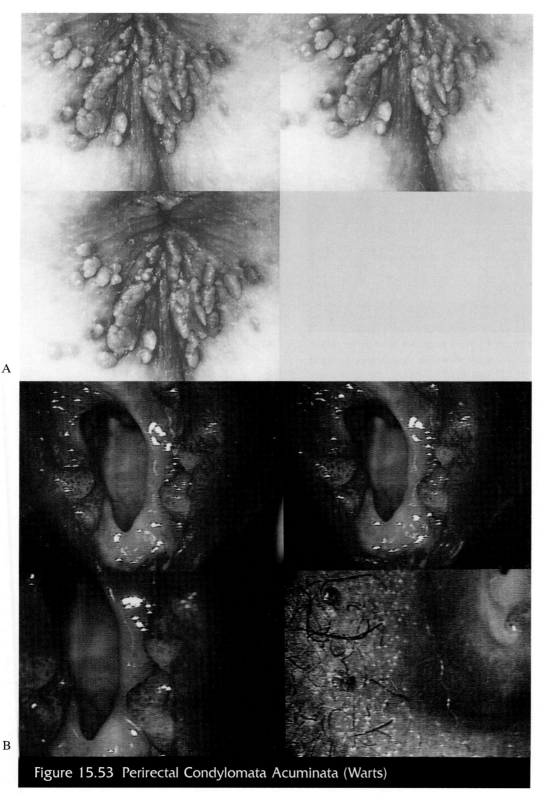

Figure 15.53 Perirectal Condylomata Acuminata (Warts)

Multiple perianal (A) and perihymenal (B) condyloma acuminata are visible in these photographs. Both individual and multidigitate lesions are seen. The hymen appears to be normal. (Courtesy of Charles J. Schubert, MD.)

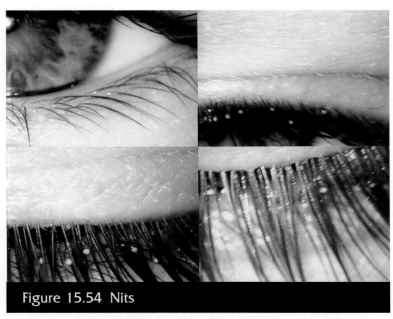

Figure 15.54 Nits

Nits (the larval form of the louse) from *Phthirus pubis* are seen firmly adherent to the eyelashes in this child. Sexual abuse should be considered. (Courtesy of Robert A. Shapiro, MD.)

8. Vaginal discharge in a prepubertal child should always be cultured for *Neisseria gonorrhoeae* and *Chlamydia.*

9. When nits are observed in the eyelashes of children (Fig. 15.54), the infecting louse is the pubic louse. The mode of transmission must be sought and sexual abuse must be suspected.

Findings Mistaken for Physical Abuse

Associated Clinical Features

Straddle injuries are a frequent cause of genital trauma and most often result in unilateral abrasions, bruising, and hematomas of the labia majora and clitoral hood (Fig. 15.55). A clear history describing the straddle injury should be given by the caretaker.

Differential Diagnosis

Sexual abuse must be considered in all children with genital injuries. Injuries involving the hymen are not typical of straddle injuries and are usually the result of sexual abuse or assault.

Emergency Department Treatment and Disposition

Check for urethral injury. Sitz baths and Polysporin ointment promote healing and minimize discomfort. If the child has difficulty voiding, she should be encouraged to void in a bath of warm water.

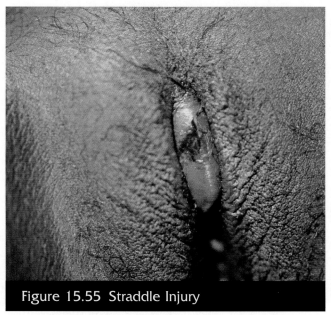

Figure 15.55 Straddle Injury

Laceration of the clitoral hood due to a fall onto the bar of a bicycle. (Courtesy of Robert A. Shapiro, MD.)

Clinical Pearls

1. Straddle injuries usually present with a clear mechanism of injury and a physical examination that supports the history.
2. Straddle injuries do not typically involve the hymen or internal vaginal mucosa.

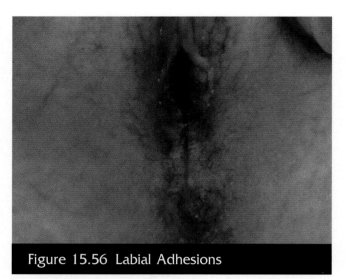

Figure 15.56 Labial Adhesions

Labial adhesions obscure the hymen in this prepubertal girl. (Courtesy of Robert A. Shapiro, MD.)

Associated Clinical Features

Adhesions of the labia minora occur in young girls and may persist until puberty. A thin translucent line is seen where the labia meet (Fig. 15.56). The extent of the adhesions varies from child to child. Involvement is often limited to the posterior portion of the labia, but some children have more extensive adhesions completely obscuring the introitus. It is postulated that vulvar irritation and poor hygiene contribute to the etiology of labial adhesions.

Differential Diagnosis

The hymen and introitus may be obscured by the adhesions. If the adhesions are unrecognized, a diagnosis of hymenal trauma and "gaping" introitus may be incorrectly made. Adhesions may be mistaken for vaginal scars.

Emergency Department Treatment and Disposition

Estrogen cream (Premarin) can be prescribed and applied gently over the adhesions twice daily for 2 to 4 weeks. Recurrence is not uncommon.

Clinical Pearls

1. Adhesions may be congenital or acquired.
2. It is postulated that vulvar irritation from sexual abuse may cause labial adhesions, but clear supporting evidence is lacking.

Associated Clinical Features

Prepubertal girls with urethral prolapse present with vaginal bleeding, vaginal mass, or urinary complaints. On examination, an annular, erythematous vaginal mass is seen (Fig. 15.57). Upon close examination, the mass can be seen to originate from the urethra. If necrotic, the mass is friable.

Differential Diagnosis

Urethral prolapse may be mistaken for vaginal injury, sexual abuse, or vaginal mass.

Emergency Department Treatment and Disposition

The prolapse may resolve within a few weeks with conservative medical management consisting of daily sitz baths and topical antibiotics. Topical estrogen cream and oral antibiotic therapy have also been used with some success. Surgical repair is usually not required but may be indicated if necrosis is present or conservative management fails.

Clinical Pearls

1. Urethral prolapse often presents with painless genital bleeding of unknown etiology.
2. Prolapse is more common in African American girls.

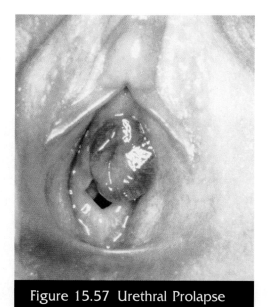

Figure 15.57 Urethral Prolapse

A round reddish-purple mass is seen in this child's introitus. Careful examination reveals that the mass originates from the urethra. (Courtesy of Michael P. Poirier, MD.)

Associated Clinical Features

Acute bruising to the glans and corona of the penis can occur if the toilet seat falls onto the penis during voiding, trapping the penis between the seat and toilet bowl (Fig. 15.58). This injury is not uncommon in boys of about 3 years of age who are both inexperienced at voiding while standing and are short enough for this injury to occur.

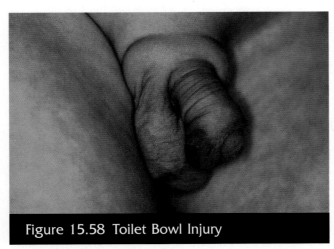

Figure 15.58 Toilet Bowl Injury

This toddler presented with a straightforward history of the toilet seat falling onto his penis during voiding. Despite the swelling and ecchymosis, he was able to void without difficulty. (Courtesy of Kevin J. Knoop, MD, MS.)

Differential Diagnosis

Genital trauma is always suspicious for sexual abuse. The mechanism of injury may be difficult to determine if the injury was unwitnessed.

Emergency Department Treatment and Disposition

No specific treatment is needed unless the child is unable to void. If the child cannot void, a retrograde urethrogram and urologic consult are indicated.

Clinical Pearl

1. Genital injuries are suspicious of sexual abuse if no appropriate history of accidental trauma is given.

Associated Clinical Features

Presenting complaints are often rectal pain, itching, bleeding, and rash. Symptoms may be present for months prior to the diagnosis. The child may be constipated because of stool retention and may have recently been given laxatives because of these symptoms. Systemic symptoms are absent. The perianal area is erythematous and tender (Fig. 15.59). The involved area is well demarcated from the uninfected skin. Anal fissures and bleeding may be seen.

Differential Diagnosis

Sexual abuse is often misdiagnosed because of the child's complaints of rectal pain and bleeding and the above findings on examination. This infection can also be mistaken for poor hygiene, dermatitis, nonspecific irritation, and constipation.

Emergency Department Treatment and Disposition

Culture or obtain direct antigen studies for group A beta-hemolytic streptococci. Treat with oral penicillin for 10 days. Substitute erythromycin for patients allergic to penicillin. Treatment failures should be treated with IM penicillin and/or oral clindamycin.

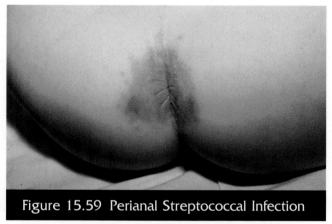

Figure 15.59 Perianal Streptococcal Infection

Intense erythema around the anus consistent with perianal streptococcal infection. (Courtesy of Raymond C. Baker, MD.)

Clinical Pearls

1. Direct antigen studies are sensitive (89%) and specific (100%) for perianal group A streptococcal infection.
2. Examine the pharynx for streptococcal infection when considering perianal strep infection.
3. Infection is unusual in children older than 10 years.

Associated Clinical Features

Lichen sclerosus atrophicus (LSA) is an unusual dermatitis that affects the anogenital area. The diagnosis should be suspected whenever an area of hypopigmentation in the shape of an hourglass is seen around the child's anus and genitalia. The hypopigmented area is caused by small white or yellowish papules which coalesce into large plaques. The affected skin is atrophic and bleeds easily after minor trauma. The hemorrhagic form of LSA includes subepithelial hemorrhagic lesions to the labia and affected skin, which can be mistaken for traumatic lesions (Fig. 15.60). Children may complain of pruritus and dysuria.

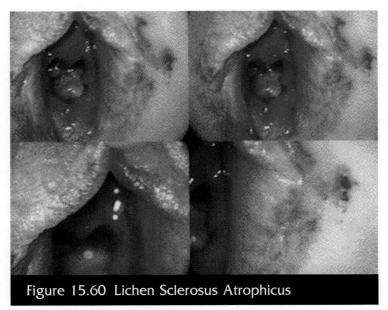

Figure 15.60 Lichen Sclerosus Atrophicus

The perineum surrounding the vagina has a bruised appearance. Atrophic skin is also evident. (Courtesy of Robert A. Shapiro, MD.)

Differential Diagnosis

The findings of hemorrhage around the genitalia and rectum are often mistaken for signs of sexual abuse.

Emergency Department Treatment and Disposition

Use symptomatic treatment if needed; 1% hydrocortisone cream can be prescribed. Refer to dermatologist for treatment.

Clinical Pearl

1. Lichen sclerosus atrophicus is the most common dermatitis mistaken for sexual abuse.

CHAPTER 16

ENVIRONMENTAL CONDITIONS*

Ken Zafren
R. Jason Thurman
Alan B. Storrow

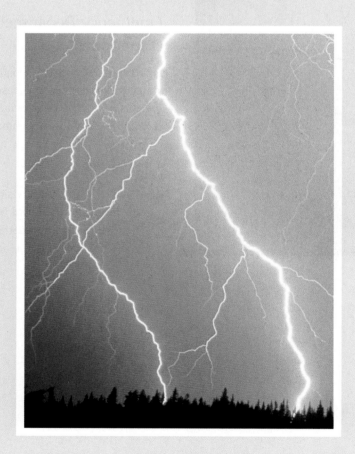

*The authors acknowledge the special contributions of Peter Hackett, MD, FACEP, St. Mary's Hospital, Grand Junction, Colorado; Edward Otten, MD, University of Cincinnati, Cincinnati, Ohio; James O'Malley, MD, Providence Alaska Medical Center, Anchorage, Alaska; and the Nova Scotia Museum of Natural History, Halifax, Nova Scotia, Canada. The authors thank Joseph C. Schmidt, MD, and Lawrence B. Stack, MD, for their contributions to the first edition.

Associated Clinical Features

Retinal hemorrhages (Fig. 16.1) are common above 5200 m and above these altitudes need not be associated with acute mountain sickness (AMS). Below 5200 m there is an association with altitude illness. High-altitude retinal hemorrhages (HARH) are rarely symptomatic, but if found over the macula, these hemorrhages may cause temporary blindness.

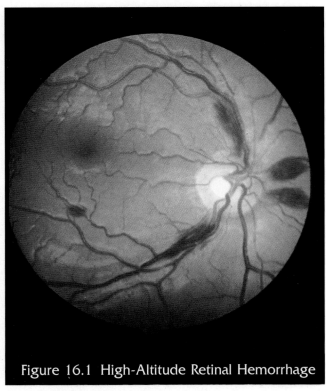

Figure 16.1 High-Altitude Retinal Hemorrhage

(Courtesy of Peter Hackett, MD.)

Differential Diagnosis

The diagnosis can be established by ophthalmoscopy. Without visualization of the lesion, the differential diagnosis of unilaterally decreased vision or blindness at high altitude would include high-altitude cerebrovascular accident as well as all conditions found at sea level.

Emergency Department Treatment and Disposition

HARH generally resolve spontaneously after descent to lower altitudes. No treatment is necessary for asymptomatic HARH. Patients with HARH associated with a decrease in vision should be referred to an ophthalmologist for follow-up.

Clinical Pearls

1. Patients with blurred vision and unilateral mydriasis at the high altitude should be asked about use of medications, including transdermal scopolamine patches.
2. As with almost all altitude-related problems, descent is the primary treatment.

Associated Clinical Features

High-altitude pulmonary edema (HAPE) is a noncardiogenic form of pulmonary edema (Fig. 16.2). It generally begins within the first 2 to 4 days after ascent above 2500 m. The earliest symptoms are fatigue, weakness, dyspnea on exertion, and decreased exercise performance. Symptoms of acute mountain sickness (AMS) such as headache, anorexia, and lassitude may also be present. If untreated, a persistent dry cough develops, followed by tachycardia and tachypnea at rest with cyanosis. HAPE generally begins and is worse at night. Eventually the victim develops dyspnea at rest and orthopnea with audible crackles in the chest. Pink frothy sputum is a grave sign. There may be mental status changes and ataxia due to hypoxemia or associated high-altitude cerebral edema (HACE).

Differential Diagnosis

Cardiogenic pulmonary edema is rare at high altitude. Respiratory infections may also be present; distinction is made difficult by the fact that fever up to 38.5°C is common with HAPE.

Emergency Department Treatment and Disposition

Mild cases (oxygen saturation in the 90s on low-flow oxygen) at moderate altitudes (below 3500 m) may be treated at altitude with bed rest and oxygen. If supplemental oxygen and a reliable person are available, the patient may be discharged with oxygen therapy and bed rest at home or, more often, in lodgings. More severe cases should descend immediately and may require admission to a hospital at a lower altitude. These patients may require intubation and mechanical ventilation. Nifedipine may be of some benefit but is not a substitute for altitude or descent. Hyperbaric therapy, especially with a portable hyperbaric chamber (Fig. 16.3), has an efficacy equal to that of supplemental oxygen and is mainly helpful in prehospital settings where oxygen availability is limited.

Clinical Pearls

1. Crackles may be unilateral or bilateral but usually start in the right middle lobe and are heard first in the right axilla.
2. HAPE limited to the left lung in association with a small right hemothorax without pulmonary markings is pathognomonic for unilateral absent pulmonary artery syndrome. These patients develop HAPE at relatively low altitudes, sometimes below 2500 m.

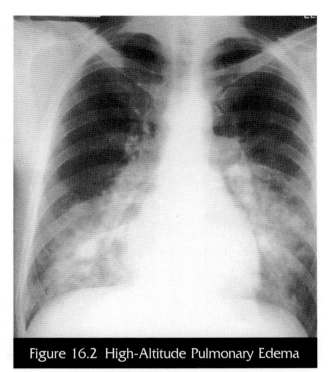

Figure 16.2 High-Altitude Pulmonary Edema

Chest x-ray in patient with HAPE. Note normal heart size with bilateral "patchy" pulmonary infiltrates. (Courtesy of Peter Hackett, MD.)

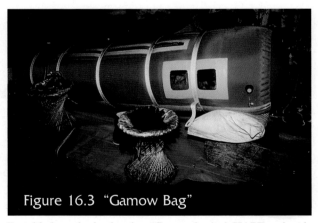

Figure 16.3 "Gamow Bag"

Portable hyperbaric chamber (Gamow bag). A HAPE patient is being treated at 4300 m at Pheriche, Nepal. Due to orthopnea, the patient was unable to tolerate lying flat, so the bag was propped up immediately after inflation. (Courtesy of Ken Zafren, MD.)

Associated Clinical Features

Accidental hypothermia is an unintentional decline in core temperature below 35°C. Presentation may be obvious or subtle, especially in urban settings. Symptoms vary from vague complaints to altered levels of consciousness, and physical findings include progressive abnormalities of every organ system. Following initial tachycardia, there is progressive bradycardia (50% decrease in heart rate at 28°C), with decline in blood pressure and cardiac output. ECG intervals may be prolonged; first the PR; then the QRS; and then especially the QTc. A J wave (Osborn wave; hypothermic "hump"; Fig. 16.4) may be seen, but is neither pathognomonic nor prognostic. The J wave is present at the junction of the QRS complex and the ST segment.

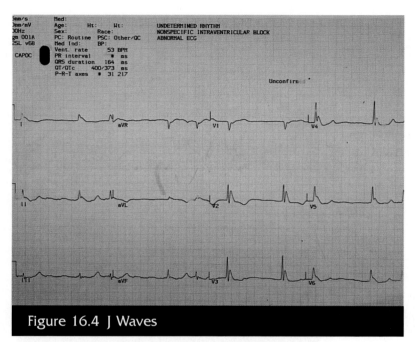

Figure 16.4 J Waves

J waves in a hypothermic patient with core temperature (rectal probe) of 25.5°C. J waves may be seen at any temperature below 32.2°C, most frequently in leads II and V_6. Below a core temperature of 25°C, they are most commonly found in the precordial leads (especially V_3 and V_4) and their size increases. J waves are usually upright in aVL, aVF, and the left precordial leads. (Courtesy of Alan B. Storrow, MD.)

Differential Diagnosis

J waves may also be associated with central nervous system lesions, focal cardiac ischemia, young age, and sepsis. In mildly hypothermic patients, invisible preshivering muscle tone may obscure P waves.

Emergency Department Treatment and Disposition

Core temperature measurement (using low-reading rectal or esophageal thermometers), gentle handling, and appropriate warming methods are the mainstays of ED treatment. Cardiovascular instability often complicates rewarming; Advanced Cardiac Life Support (ACLS) guidelines for hypothermia provide guidance. If not obvious, a cause should be sought (e.g., hypothyroidism, sepsis), as should associated pathology. Except for previously healthy patients with acute mild hypothermia, most patients require admission for observation or to treat associated injuries or comorbidities.

Clinical Pearls

1. The most common problems with the diagnosis of hypothermia in the ED stem from incomplete data on vital signs.
2. Low-reading thermometers, accurate core temperatures, averaging of respirations over several minutes, and Doppler location of pulses are crucial to appropriate management.

Associated Clinical Features

Frostbite is true tissue freezing resulting from heat loss sufficient to cause ice crystal formation in superficial or deep tissue. Frostbite may affect the extremities, nose, or ears (and the scrotum and penis in joggers). Severity of symptoms is usually proportional to the severity of the injury. A sensation of numbness with accompanying sensory loss is the most common initial complaint. Often, by the time the patient arrives in the ED, the frozen tissue has thawed. The initial appearance of the overlying skin may be deceptively benign (Fig. 16.5). Frozen tissue may appear mottled blue, violaceous, yellowish-white, or waxy. Following rapid rewarming, there is early hyperemia even in severe cases.

Favorable signs include return of normal sensation, color, and warmth. Edema should appear within 3 h of thawing; lack of edema is an unfavorable sign. Vesicles and bullae appear in 6 to 24 h. Early formation of large clear blebs that extend to the tips of affected digits is a good indicator. Small dark blebs that do not extend to the tips indicate damage to subdermal plexi and are a poor prognostic sign.

Differential Diagnosis

Seen early and after rewarming, frostbite may be indistinguishable from nonfreezing cold injury such as immersion foot. Mixed injuries are common.

Emergency Department Treatment and Disposition

If other injuries are ruled out by history and physical examination, rewarm frostbitten areas in a warm water bath (37 to 41°C). If associated with severe hypothermia, active core rewarming should precede frostbite rewarming. If swelling occurs, measure compartment pressures (including hands and feet) to determine the need for fasciotomy. Admit all patients with associated hypothermia or in whom swelling occurs. Superficial frostbite (minimal skin changes and erythema) may be treated by home care with nursing instructions. Deep superficial frostbite (clear, fluid-filled blebs, swelling, pain; Fig. 16.6) may be treated by home care in a reliable patient. Deep frostbite (proximal hemorrhagic blebs, no swelling, no pulses; Figs. 16.7 to 16.9) mandates hospital admission.

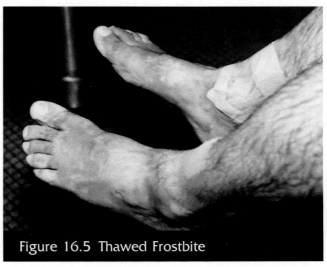

Figure 16.5 Thawed Frostbite

Typical appearance of frostbite soon after rewarming. Deep frostbite was caused by wearing mountaineering boots that were too tight in extreme cold at high altitude. Note deceptively benign appearance of this devastating injury. (Courtesy of James O'Malley, MD.)

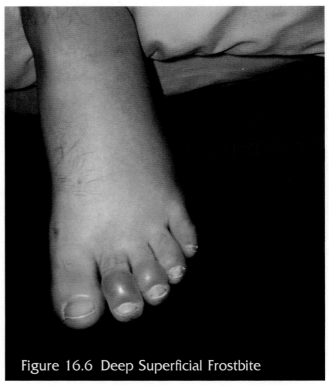

Figure 16.6 Deep Superficial Frostbite

Clear blebs extending distally are indicators for favorable outcome. (Courtesy of James O'Malley, MD.)

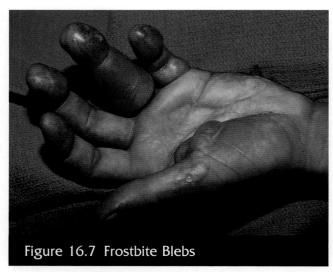

Figure 16.7 Frostbite Blebs

Proximal blebs, both clear and hemorrhagic. (Courtesy of Scott W. Zackowski, MD.)

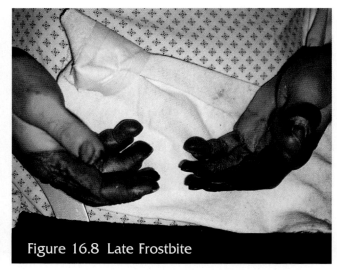

Figure 16.8 Late Frostbite

Late appearance of frostbite with demarcation starting to occur. Early surgery should be avoided in favor of autoamputation unless infection supervenes. (Courtesy of James O'Malley, MD.)

Clinical Pearls

1. Early transfer of the patient to a center experienced in the care of frostbite injuries (even if hundreds of miles away) should be considered. On the other hand, transfer of the patient to a major medical center that does not generally manage frostbite is seldom in the patient's best interest.
2. Treatment of clear versus hemorrhagic blisters is controversial; one approach is to debride clear blisters and use topical aloe vera while leaving hemorrhagic blisters intact.

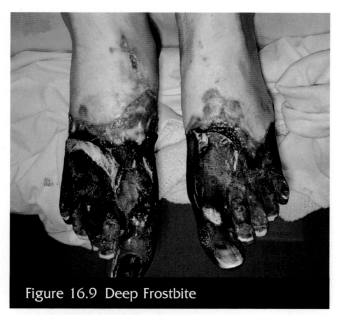

Figure 16.9 Deep Frostbite

Late appearance of deep frostbite with clear demarcation. (Courtesy of James O'Malley, MD.)

Associated Clinical Features

Pernio, also known as chilblain cold sores, is the result of nonfreezing cold exposure. Pernio appears within 24 h of cold exposure, most frequently on the face, ears, hands, feet, and pretibial areas. A large range of lesions may be seen, with localized edema, erythema, cyanosis, plaques, and blue nodules occasionally progressing to more severe lesions including vesicles, bullae, and ulcerations (Fig. 16.10). The lesions persist for up to 2 weeks and may become more chronic. They are typically very pruritic and associated with burning paresthesias. Following rewarming, pernio often takes the form of blue nodules, which are quite tender.

Differential Diagnosis

In the setting of recent cold exposure, pernio might be confused with the more severe syndrome of trench foot and its sequelae. If the history of cold exposure is not elicited, the differential diagnosis is potentially very broad.

Emergency Department Treatment and Disposition

Management is supportive. The skin should be warmed, washed, and dried. Affected extremities can be dressed in soft, dry, sterile dressings and elevated. Nifedipine (20 to 60 mg daily) may be helpful in chronic cases.

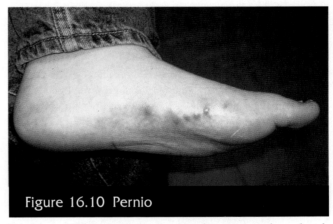

Figure 16.10 Pernio

Pernio or chilblains with localized erythema, cyanosis, and nodules. (Courtesy of Ken Zafren, MD.)

Clinical Pearls

1. Healing may be followed by hyperpigmentation.
2. Recurrences are possible following milder exposure.
3. Chilblains are said to be more frequent in young women, especially in association with Raynaud's phenomenon.

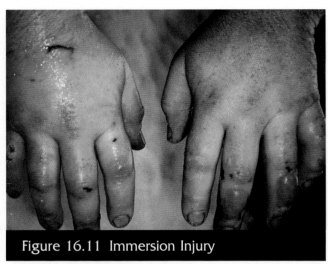

Figure 16.11 Immersion Injury

Immersion injury to hands (unusual location) several hours after rewarming. The patient spent 18 h bailing out a boat in waters just above freezing in Alaska. (Courtesy of James O'Malley, MD.)

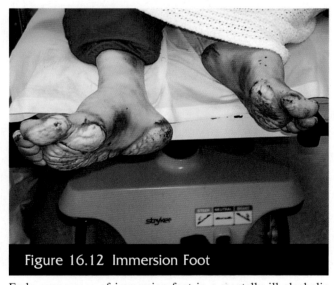

Figure 16.12 Immersion Foot

Early appearance of immersion foot in a mentally ill alcoholic homeless patient. (Courtesy of Ken Zafren, MD.)

Associated Clinical Features

Immersion injury is a peripheral nonfreezing cold injury resulting from exposure to water, usually at temperatures just above freezing. However, it can occur during prolonged exposure to any wet environment cooler than body temperature. Dependency and immobility predispose to immersion injury. The degree of injury seems to depend on time and temperature. The first symptoms appear in hours; tissue loss may require many days of exposure. Prior to rewarming, the distal extremities are numb and swollen. The skin is first red, then changes to pale, mottled, or black (Figs. 16.11 and 16.12). Cramping of the calves may occur.

Differential Diagnosis

Immersion injury is also known as trench foot, peripheral vasoneuropathy, shelter foot, sea boot foot, and foxhole foot. It is distinct from tropical immersion foot or warm-water immersion foot as seen in the Vietnam War. Tropical immersion foot was typically seen after 3 to 7 days of exposure to water at 22 to 32°C. Warm-water immersion foot was seen after 1 to 3 days at 15 to 32°C. These syndromes were characterized by burning in the feet, pain on walking, pitting edema, and erythema, with wrinkling and hyperhydration of the skin. They resolved completely after rest and removal from the wet environment.

Emergency Department Treatment and Disposition

Hypovolemia, hypothermia, and associated injuries are the rule and should be treated first. General treatment of immersion foot (or hand) is the same as that for frostbite that has been rewarmed. Swelling may produce compartment syndrome and require fasciotomy. Most patients require admission to the hospital.

Clinical Pearls

1. Pulses may be difficult to feel but may be found by Doppler.
2. Mixed injuries (frostbite and immersion) are common.

Associated Clinical Features

Ultraviolet (UV) radiation causes both acute and chronic skin changes. Sunburn is a partial-thickness burn (Fig. 16.13), which may become a full-thickness injury if infected. "Sun poisoning" is a severe systemic reaction to UV radiation. Patients complain of nausea, vomiting, headache, fever, chills, and prostration. Excessive UV radiation may cause injury to the cornea and conjunctiva, termed ultraviolet keratitis (photokeratitis, snow blindness). This painful condition may occur in skiers, welders, or tanning salon patrons who do not wear proper eye protection.

Photosensitivity reactions (photodermatoses) are of several types. Phototoxic reactions are an abnormal response to UV radiation caused by a substance that is ingested (e.g., prescription or over-the-counter medications) or applied to the skin (even seemingly innocuous perfumes or shampoos); there is a direct relation between the amount of UV exposure and severity. Photoallergic reactions are clinically similar to contact dermatitis and, like phototoxic reactions, may be precipitated by ingested or applied drugs. Unlike phototoxic reactions, photoallergies may be precipitated by a small amount of light. Phytophotodermatitis (Fig. 16.14, see also Fig. 13.57) is precipitated by skin contact with certain plants followed by exposure to UV radiation. It can resemble either phototoxic or photoallergic reactions.

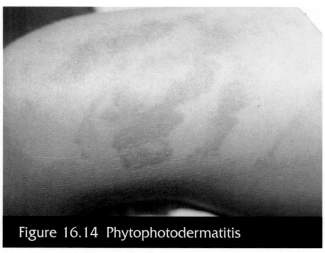

Figure 16.14 Phytophotodermatitis

This reaction may require aggressive systemic steroid therapy. The case illustrated is a mild one caused by exposure to limes and UVA. A clue to the diagnosis is the patchy distribution with linear edges. More severe reactions resemble rhus dermatitis. (Courtesy of Lee Kaplan, MD.)

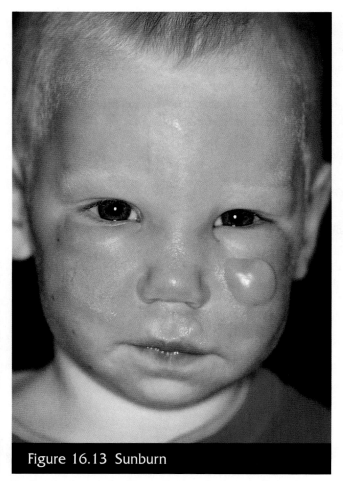

Figure 16.13 Sunburn

Sunburn is characterized by erythema, edema, warmth, tenderness, and blisters. (Courtesy of Kevin J. Knoop, MD, MS.)

Differential Diagnosis

Phototoxicity should be suspected in any patient with a severe or exaggerated sunburn. Photoallergy is easily misdiagnosed as allergic eczema or contact dermatitis, especially since onset is often delayed up to 2 days after exposure. Phytophotodermatitis may mimic severe sunburn or contact dermatitis, especially rhus (poison ivy, sumac, or oak; see "Toxicodendron Exposure," below) dermatitis. Endogenous photosensitizers (endogenous photodermatoses) include solar urticaria, porphyria cutanea tarda, polymorphous light eruption, and systemic lupus erythematosus. These may be provoked by visible light as well as by UV radiation. History is the key to the diagnosis of UV keratitis; the differential includes corneal abrasions, ocular foreign body, and conjunctivitis.

Emergency Department Treatment and Disposition

Treatment of sunburn and sun poisoning involves standard burn and supportive care. Sunburn is usually a self-limited problem. Cool compresses and nonsteroidal anti-inflammatory drugs may be beneficial. Steroids may be useful for sun poisoning. Ultraviolet keratitis is treated with mydriatic-cycloplegic eyedrops to decrease pain; initial examination is made easier with topical anesthetics. Severe cases may require bilateral eye patches for 12 to 24 h, antibiotic ointment, and narcotic analgesics. These patients require 24- to 48-h follow-up; ophthalmology referral is indicated to rule out retinal damage.

Treatment of photosensitivity reaction has two components: treatment of the sunburn and recognition of the sensitizing agent or endogenous medical condition. Topical steroids and oral analgesics and antipruritics may be helpful. Systemic steroids may be required. Patients with severe reactions should be referred to a dermatologist for possible photo patch testing.

Clinical Pearls

1. Even *para*-aminobenzoic acid (PABA) in sunscreens may be a photosensitizer and can cause a photoallergic reaction.
2. The unique properties of individual skin types produce marked differences in response to UV radiation.
3. Victims of UV keratitis typically present 2 to 12 h after exposure. Treatment should not include prolonged use of topical anesthetics or topical steroids.

Associated Clinical Features

Lightning produces injury from high voltage, heat production, and explosive shock waves. Direct injuries include cardiopulmonary arrest, other cardiac arrhythmias, and neurologic abnormalities such as seizures, deafness, confusion, amnesia, blindness, and paralysis. The patient may suffer contusions from the shock wave or from opisthotonic muscle contractions. Chest pain and muscle aches are common. One or both tympanic membranes rupture in more than 50% of victims. Cataracts are usually a delayed occurrence. Hematologic abnormalities including disseminated intravascular coagulation (DIC) have been described. Fetal demise may occur.

Burns may result from vaporization of sweat or moist clothing, heating of clothing and metal objects such as belt buckles, and direct effects of the strike. Linear burns and punctate burns (Figs. 16.15 and 16.16) are thermal burns. Feathering burns (Fig. 16.17) are not actually burns but are skin markings caused by electron showers. They are pathognomonic of lightning injury.

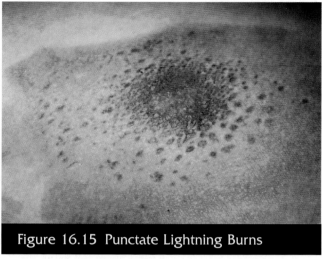

Figure 16.15 Punctate Lightning Burns

Punctate burns due to lightning are partial- or full-thickness thermal burns that range from a few millimeters to a centimeter in diameter. They are multiple and closely spaced. (Courtesy of Arthur Kahn, MD.)

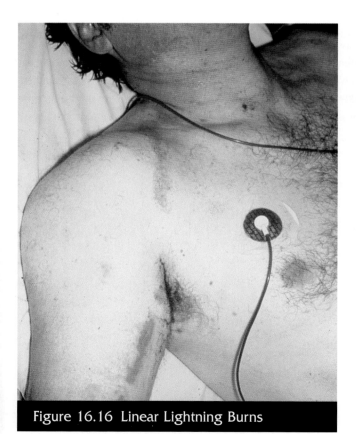

Figure 16.16 Linear Lightning Burns

Linear burns from lightning are due to thermal effects. (Courtesy of William Barsan, MD.)

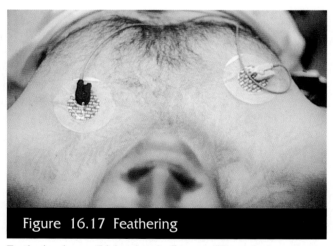

Figure 16.17 Feathering

Feathering burns (Lichtenberg's flowers, filigree burns, arborescent burns, ferning, or keraunographic markings) are pathognomonic of lightning injury. They are not true burns but are imprints on the skin of electron showers. Note the subtle but typical pattern in the clavicular areas. (Courtesy of Marco Coppola, DO., and Margaret J. Karnes, DO.)

Differential Diagnosis

Diagnosis is easy when there is a thunderstorm, when there are witnesses to the strike, or when there are typical physical findings. Lightning on relatively sunny days (without loud thunder) striking a lone victim may produce a confusing picture. The scattering of clothing and belongings may mimic an assault. Side flashes from metal objects and wiring may produce indoor victims during storms. Differential diagnosis of lightning injury includes cerebrovascular accident or intracranial hemorrhage, seizure disorder, spinal cord injury, closed head injury, hypertensive encephalopathy, cardiac arrhythmias, myocardial infarction, and toxic ingestions (especially heavy metals).

Emergency Department Treatment and Disposition

History and physical examination to rule out associated injuries and standard ED care for critical patients—including cardiac enzymes, urinalysis, and ECG—are necessary. All patients, even those apparently well, require admission for observation, since their condition may change over several hours following the lightning strike.

Clinical Pearls

1. The amount of damage to the exterior of the body does not predict the amount of internal injury.
2. Since lightning most commonly produces cardiac standstill by means of massive direct current countershock, prompt, spontaneous return of normal heart rhythm (by virtue of cardiac automaticity) is the rule. However, respiratory arrest is often more prolonged. In a triage situation, the normal rules do not apply, since victims breathing spontaneously are already recovering. The rule in lightning strikes is to resuscitate the "dead." Ventilatory support is often all that is required.

Associated Clinical Features

Ticks are blood-sucking parasites of people and animals. Ticks cause illness by acting as vectors for pathogens, or by secreting toxins or venoms.

Tick paralysis develops 5 to 6 days after an adult female tick attaches. Over the next 24 to 48 h, an ascending, symmetric, flaccid paralysis develops. Alternative presentations include ataxia and associated cerebellar findings without muscle weakness or isolated facial paralysis. Resolution of the paralysis after removal of the tick establishes the diagnosis.

Ticks carry more types of infectious pathogens than any other arthropods except mosquitoes. The most important of these include *Borrelia* (responsible for Lyme disease and relapsing fever), rickettsia (e.g., Rocky Mountain spotted fever), viral pathogens (e.g., Colorado tick fever), and babesiosis. Rashes are prominent in Lyme disease (see Fig. 13.25) and Rocky Mountain spotted fever (see Fig. 13.6), sometimes present in relapsing fever, uncommon in Colorado tick fever, and absent in babesiosis. The first two are covered in Chap. 13.

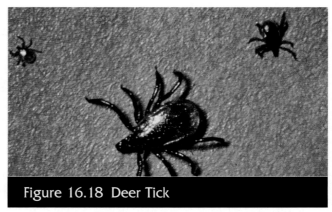

Figure 16.18 Deer Tick

Ixodes dammini, the deer tick, is a vector of Lyme disease and babesiosis. (Courtesy of the Centers for Disease Control and Prevention, Atlanta, GA.)

Clinically important ticks in North America include *Ixodes dammini,* the deer tick (Lyme disease and babesiosis; Fig. 16.18); *Dermacentor andersonii,* the wood tick (Rocky Mountain spotted fever and Colorado tick fever; Fig. 16.19); and *Amblyomma americanum,* the Lone Star tick (a very widespread tick implicated in the transmission of Lyme disease outside of the range of *I. dammini*; Fig. 16.20). More than 40 species of ticks can cause tick paralysis. In North America the most common cause is *D. andersonii,* but *A. americanum* and *Ixodes* species have also been associated with tick paralysis.

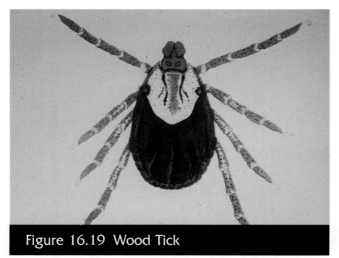

Figure 16.19 Wood Tick

Dermacentor andersonii, the wood tick, is a vector of Rocky Mountain spotted fever and Colorado tick fever. (Courtesy of the Centers for Disease Control and Prevention, Atlanta, GA.)

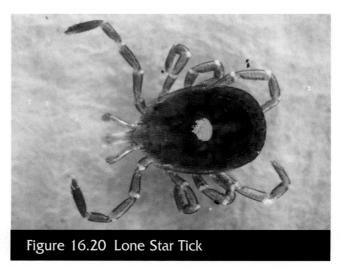

Figure 16.20 Lone Star Tick

Amblyomma americanum, the Lone Star tick, has been implicated as a vector in Lyme disease. (Courtesy of Sherman Minton, MD.)

Differential Diagnosis

Tick paralysis should be considered in any patient provisionally diagnosed with Guillian-Barré syndrome, Eaton-Lambert syndrome, myasthenia gravis, poliomyelitis, botulism, diphtheric polyneuropathy, or any disease producing ascending flaccid paralysis or acute ataxia. The main point of differential diagnosis of tick-borne illnesses is to consider these diseases in the differential of ill patients, especially those who have been outdoors in rural areas during seasons when ticks are active.

Emergency Department Treatment and Disposition

If still embedded, the tick should be removed promptly by grasping it as close to the skin surface as possible, using blunt curved forceps or tweezers. The tick should be pulled out with slow, gentle traction, taking care not to crush or squeeze the body, which may result in injection of contaminated tick fluids. Other methods of tick removal—such as application of fingernail polish, isopropyl alcohol, or a hot match head—have not been proven to effect detachment and may induce regurgitation of tick contents into the wound.

Patients with tick paralysis may require supportive care, including mechanical ventilation. Patients with tick-borne illnesses may require admission for supportive care or intensive antibiotic treatment.

Clinical Pearls

1. Prevention of tick bites includes the use of protective clothing containing N, N-diethylmetatoluamide (DEET).
2. A clear history of a tick bite is present in less than one-third of Lyme disease cases.
3. Unusual neurologic presentations, particularly bilateral peripheral seventh-nerve palsies, should prompt consideration of Lyme disease.

Associated Clinical Features

The pit vipers (Crotalidae family) indigenous to the United States comprise multiple rattlesnake species (Figs. 16.21, 16.22, 16.23), cottonmouths (Fig. 16.24), and copperheads (Fig. 16.25). Pit viper venom is complex and produces hematologic, cardiovascular, and neuromuscular effects. Clinically, snake bites can be divided into four categories. The category of no envenomation consists of only fang marks. Minimal envenomation (Fig. 16.26) consists of fang marks and local swelling but no systemic symptoms. Moderate envenomation (Figs. 16.27, 16.28) includes the above with the addition of nausea, vomiting, and mild changes in coagulation parameters. Severe envenomation (Fig. 16.29) includes all the above with marked local swelling and signs of significant coagulopathy (e.g., subcutaneous ecchymosis and/or hematuria).

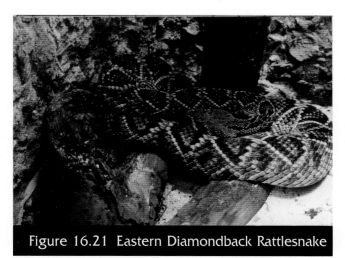

Figure 16.21 Eastern Diamondback Rattlesnake

The eastern diamondback is the largest U.S. rattlesnake and has a characteristic diamond-shaped pattern on its dorsal aspect. (Courtesy of R. Jason Thurman, MD.)

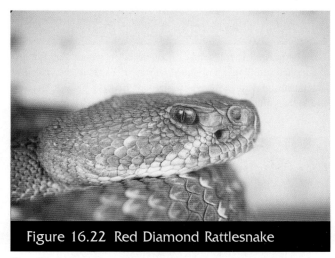

Figure 16.22 Red Diamond Rattlesnake

The elliptical pupils and heat-sensing pits in this red diamond rattlesnake are characteristic of pit vipers. (Courtesy of Sean P. Bush, MD.)

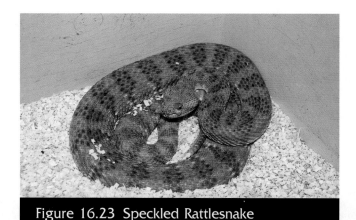

Figure 16.23 Speckled Rattlesnake

Note the triangular head, which is characteristic of pit vipers. (Courtesy of Sean P. Bush, MD.)

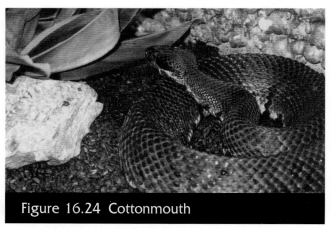

Figure 16.24 Cottonmouth

The cottonmouth is a semiaquatic venomous pit viper that may crawl or swim with its head raised at an angle of 45 degrees. When disturbed, it may open its mouth wide to reveal a white lining. (Courtesy of R. Jason Thurman, MD.)

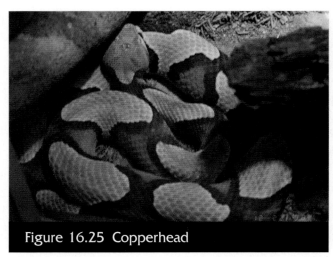

Figure 16.25 Copperhead

The copperhead is frequently encountered in wooded mountains, abandoned buildings, and damp, grassy areas. It is able to climb low bushes and trees in search of food. It is typically a bit more docile than other pit vipers. (Courtesy of R. Jason Thurman, MD.)

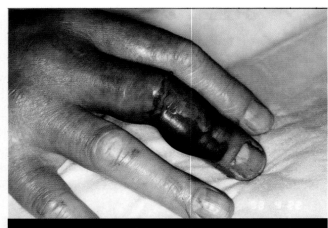

Figure 16.26 Rattlesnake Envenomation, Day 1

This rattlesnake bite shows local swelling, some edema beyond the initial bite site, and a hemorrhagic bleb at 6 h. It would be considered mild to moderate at this time. (Courtesy of Sean P. Bush, MD.)

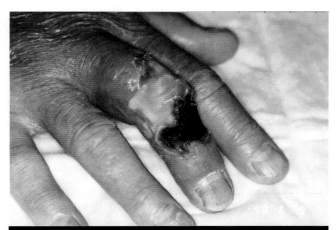

Figure 16.27 Progression of Rattlesnake Envenomation 7 Weeks

Seven weeks later, the patient shown in Fig. 16.26 has progressed to tissue loss, eschar formation, and mild changes in coagulation parameters. (Courtesy of Sean P. Bush, MD.)

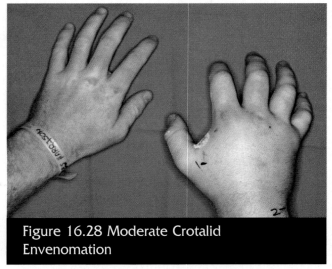

Figure 16.28 Moderate Crotalid Envenomation

Patient was bitten by a rattlesnake on the dorsal aspect of the right hand who presented with edema extending to the wrist as well as nausea and vomiting. (Courtesy of Edward J. Otten, MD.)

Differential Diagnosis

Bites by nonpoisonous snakes frequently present to the ED. However, unless clear identification of the snake is possible, all bites should be considered venomous. Physical characteristics of pit vipers include a triangular head, heat-sensing pits, elliptical pupils, and a single row of ventral scales (Figs. 16.22, 16.23, 16.30).

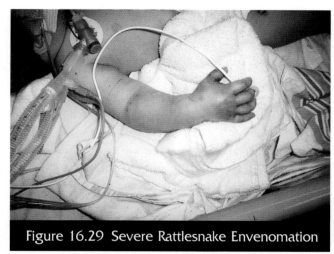

Figure 16.29 Severe Rattlesnake Envenomation

This patient sustained a rattlesnake bite to his hand and presented with marked and progressive swelling, subcutaneous ecchymosis, and a significant coagulopathy. (Courtesy of Sean P. Bush, MD.)

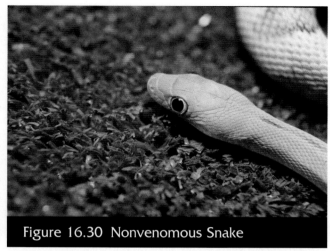

Figure 16.30 Nonvenomous Snake

In contrast to the elliptical pupils and triangular head characteristic of pit vipers, this nonvenomous rat snake has a rounded head and circular pupils. (Courtesy of Sean P. Bush, MD.)

Emergency Department Treatment and Disposition

Initial field management of pit viper bites should include immobilization and rapid transport. Application of lymphatic constriction bands and use of extractor devices may be helpful, but these steps are controversial. Tourniquets and local incision are most likely ineffective and may do more harm than good. Electric shock or cryotherapy are not recommended. ED management includes resuscitation, establishing a physiologic baseline, and determining the need for antivenin. Pit viper antivenin of horse serum derivation carries all the risks of any horse serum product. Recommendations for antivenin therapy vary for mild or moderate envenomation. The dose of antivenin increases with the severity of envenomation. The package insert details the current recommendations for antivenin administration and allergy testing. CroFab (Savage Labs), a new recombinant antivenin, eliminates the risk of horse serum allergy and should be used when available. Compartment syndrome is a possible complication; however, prophylactic fasciotomy is not recommended. Patients who do not develop evidence of envenomation after 6 h of observation may be safely discharged home with close follow-up.

Clinical Pearls

1. Approximately one-fourth of all pit viper bites are "dry" (without any injection of venom).
2. In cases of severe envenomation, antivenin should not be withheld, even in individuals with a history of horse serum allergy. Bedside vasopressors (e.g., epinephrine) and a separate intravenous line for their administration should be available.
3. Allergy testing should be performed only in patients who need antivenin therapy.
4. Subcutaneous epinephrine (0.3 mg) given prior to administration of horse serum antivenin may reduce the potential allergic response.

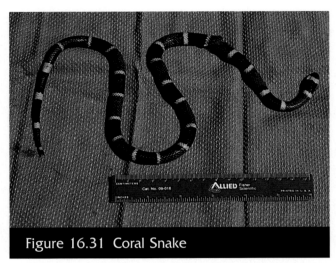

Figure 16.31 Coral Snake

United States coral snake with typical coloring and red-on-yellow bands. (Courtesy of Steven Holt, MD.)

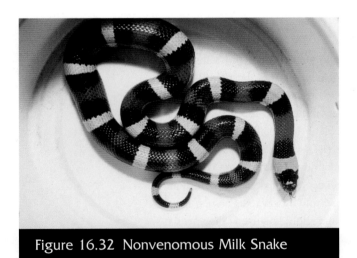

Figure 16.32 Nonvenomous Milk Snake

As opposed to the red-on-yellow rings seen in the venomous U.S. coral snake, these red-on-black rings indicate a nonvenomous snake. Unfortunately this applies only to animals native to the United States. (Courtesy of Sean P. Bush, MD.)

Associated Clinical Features

The United States is home to two members of the Elapidae, or coral snake, family (Fig. 16.31). Coral snakes have small mouths, and bites are usually limited to fingers, toes, or folds of skin. The bite typically produces minimal local inflammation and pain. Paresthesias and muscle fasciculations are common. Systemic symptoms can include tremors, drowsiness, euphoria, and marked salivation. Cranial nerve involvement, represented by slurred speech and diplopia, may be followed by bulbar paralysis with dysphagia and dyspnea. Deaths result from respiratory and cardiac arrest. Onset of severe symptoms may be delayed up to 12 h.

Differential Diagnosis

The identification of coral snake bites is more difficult than that of pit viper bites because the fang marks are small and hard to visualize. The identification of coral snakes is complicated because many nonpoisonous snakes mimic their markings. The adage "red on yellow, kill a fellow; red on black, venom lack" (Fig. 16.32) applies to all coral snakes found in the United States but does not hold true in other parts of the world.

Emergency Department Treatment and Disposition

Severe systemic symptoms following envenomation by Elapidae may be delayed and cannot be accurately predicted by local wound reactions. It is therefore recommended that four to six vials of antivenin be administered for all such suspected envenomations. Treatment of western coral snake bites is purely supportive because no antivenin is currently available.

Clinical Pearls

1. Treatment with antivenin should be initiated early in cases of eastern coral snake bites, since symptoms are often delayed and severe.
2. Coral snake venom is a potent neurotoxin, in contrast to venom from snakes of the Crotalidae family.

Associated Clinical Features

The brown recluse spider (*Loxosceles reclusa*) is the prototypical member of the genus *Loxosceles,* which as a group can produce the typical necrotic arachnidism following envenomation. These small spiders (approximately 1 cm in body length and 3 cm in leg length) have a worldwide distribution and are identified by the striking fiddle-shaped markings on their anterodorsal cephalothorax (Fig. 16.33). Initial envenomation may be painful, although patients often report no recollection of being bitten. Initial stinging gives way to aching and pruritus. The wound then becomes edematous, with an erythematous halo surrounding a violaceous center (Fig. 16.34). The erythematous margin often spreads in a pattern influenced by gravity, leaving the necrotic center near the top of the lesion (Fig. 16.35). Bullae may erupt, and—over a period of 2 to 5 weeks— the eschar sloughs, leaving a deep, poorly healing ulcer (Fig. 16.36). In unusual cases, systemic symptoms (loxoscelism) may present with hemolytic anemia as a predominant feature. Children are at higher risk of systemic disease. Other symptoms include fever, chills, nausea, vomiting, rash, arthralgia, and weakness. A leukocytosis may be seen.

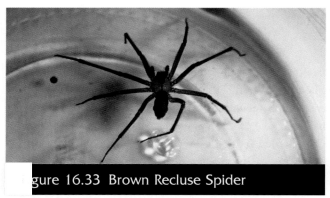

Figure 16.33 Brown Recluse Spider

Brown recluse spider with characteristic fiddle marking on the anterodorsal aspect of the cephalothorax. (Courtesy of Alan B. Storrow, MD.)

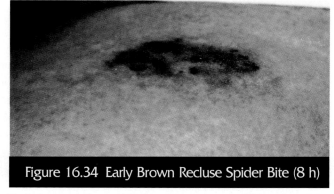

Figure 16.34 Early Brown Recluse Spider Bite (8 h)

Early brown recluse spider bite (approximately 8 h) with a violaceous center surrounded by faint spreading erythema. (Courtesy of Curtis Hunter, MD.)

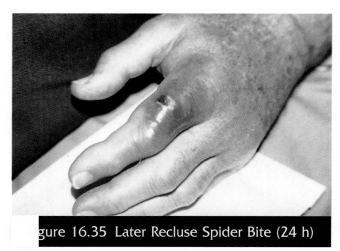

Figure 16.35 Later Recluse Spider Bite (24 h)

Brown recluse spider bite at approximately 24 h. Note asymmetric spread of erythema and early central ulcer formation. (Courtesy of Edward Eitzen, MD, MPH.)

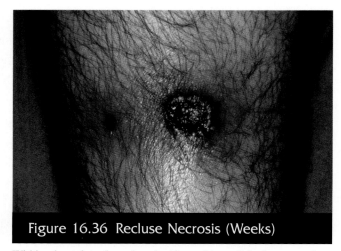

Figure 16.36 Recluse Necrosis (Weeks)

Within about 2 to 5 weeks, significant bites of the brown recluse spider may reveal a deep, poorly healing ulcer with necrosis. (Courtesy of Kevin J. Knoop, MD.)

Differential Diagnosis

The diagnosis of brown recluse spider envenomation is based on typical history, clinical features, and possible exposure to the offending species. The local wound can be confused with cellulitis, decubitus ulcer, burns, and pyoderma gangrenosum. Systemic involvement may present as an isolated hemolytic anemia, thrombocytopenia, jaundice, or hemoglobinuria.

Emergency Department Treatment and Disposition

Most cutaneous lesions secondary to brown recluse spider bites can be managed with cold compresses, elevation, loose immobilization, and attention to tetanus immunization. Severe lesions may require reconstructive plastic surgery several weeks after wound stabilization. The use of dapsone to prevent lesion progression is controversial. Any systemic reaction with evidence of hemolysis, hemoglobinuria, or coagulopathy should prompt admission. Hyperbaric oxygen (HBO) therapy and antivenin have been suggested as possible adjuncts, but no clear consensus of preferred treatment has been established.

Clinical Pearls

1. The asymmetric spread of erythema, due to the local effects of gravity on the toxin, may help to distinguish a brown recluse spider bite from other arthropod envenomations.
2. If dapsone therapy is to be administered, screening for glucose-6-phosphate dehydrogenase (G6PD) deficiency should be considered.
3. Prophylactic antibiotics have been suggested to lessen the chance of secondary infection.
4. Field use of suction devices, if done early, has been suggested to decrease the local reaction and may actually be successful in removing small amounts of venom.

Associated Clinical Features

The black widow spider (*Latrodectus mactans*) is the prototype for the genus *Latrodectus,* several members of which cause human disease (Fig. 16.37). Members of this genus are common worldwide. The clinical presentation of severe and sustained muscle spasm is produced by a neurotoxic protein which causes the release of acetylcholine and norepinephrine at the presynaptic junction. The initial bite is mild to moderately painful and is often missed (Fig. 16.38). Within approximately 1 h, local erythema and muscle cramping begin, followed by generalized cramping involving large muscle groups such as the thighs, shoulders, abdomen, and back. Associated clinical features can include fasciculations, weakness, fever, salivation, vomiting, diaphoresis, and a characteristic pattern of facial swelling called *Latrodectus* facies (Fig. 16.39). Rare cases of seizure, uncontrolled hypertension, and respiratory arrest have occurred.

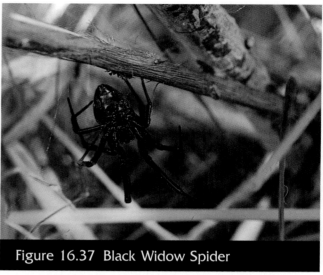

Figure 16.37 Black Widow Spider

Latrodectus mactans with characteristic hourglass marking on its abdomen. (Courtesy of Alan B. Storrow, MD.)

Differential Diagnosis

The black widow spider is relatively aggressive and will defend her web, which is often found in woodpiles, basements, and garages. Most envenomation occurs between April and October and is located on the hand and forearm. In cases where no history of spider bite can be elicited, a wide differential diagnosis—including causes of acute abdominal pain, muscle spasm, or possible toxic ingestion—must be entertained.

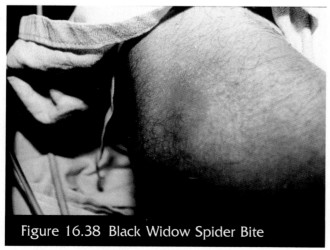

Figure 16.38 Black Widow Spider Bite

The bite of the black widow spider is clinically subtle. Local reaction is usually trivial, as in this confirmed bite with a small patch of mild erythema. (Courtesy of Gerald O'Malley, DO.)

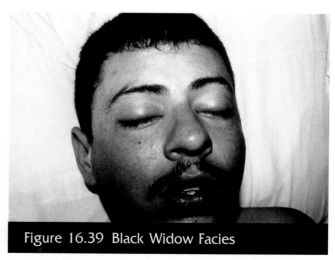

Figure 16.39 Black Widow Facies

A pattern of facial swelling, known as *Latrodectus* facies, may occur several hours after envenomation. (Courtesy of Gerald O'Malley, DO.)

Emergency Department Treatment and Disposition

Treatment of the local wound should include cleansing and tetanus prophylaxis. Severe pain and spasm may require intravenous benzodiazepines and narcotics. Calcium gluconate infusion has long been recommended to reduce symptoms, although evidence for its efficacy is lacking or contradictory. Antivenin exists and carries the same risk as all horse serum products. Antivenin should be strongly considered in cases of respiratory arrest, seizures, uncontrolled hypertension, and pregnancy.

Clinical Pearls

1. Of the five *Latrodectus* species indigenous to the United States, only three are black and only one has the orange-red hourglass marking (Fig. 16.37).
2. Calcium gluconate infusion is controversial for the treatment of muscle spasm. Benzodiazepines have replaced it as the drugs of choice.
3. Envenomation by *L. mactans* can mimic an acute abdomen.

Associated Clinical Features

The order Hymenoptera includes wasps (Fig. 16.40), bees, and ants. Envenomation usually results in local pain, mild erythema, swelling, and pruritus. However, the possibility of more severe reactions makes this subgroup the most important in terms of human envenomation. A systemic or toxic reaction may occur from one or multiple stings. This may manifest as gastrointestinal symptoms, headache, pyrexia, muscle spasms, or seizure. Anaphylaxis may occur within minutes and may cause death. A serum sickness–type reaction may occur 7 to 14 days after envenomation.

Solenopsis invicta was imported from South America and is the most prominent fire ant in the United States. It is primarily found in the South and builds mound nests in open grass settings, commonly in urban yards (Fig. 16.41). Disturbing the nests may result in severe swarming attacks. Bites are painful and produce sterile pustules that crust over in a few days (Fig. 16.42).

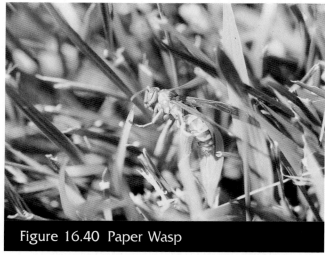

Figure 16.40 Paper Wasp

Paper wasps are found throughout the world and often establish nests close to or within human dwellings. (Courtesy of Sean P. Bush, MD.)

Differential Diagnosis

Other arthropod envenomations or plant exposures must be considered.

Emergency Department Treatment and Disposition

Anaphylaxis is treated with conventional therapy. Local reactions may be treated with ice packs, steroid cream, and oral antihistamines.

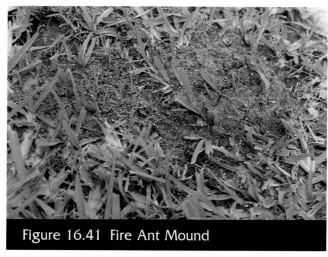

Figure 16.41 Fire Ant Mound

This typical fire ant mound is a raised area of dirt in an urban yard. (Courtesy of Alan B. Storrow, MD.)

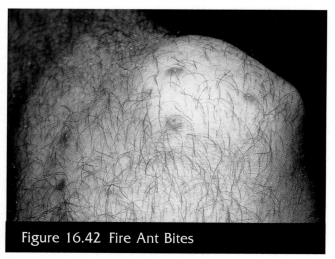

Figure 16.42 Fire Ant Bites

These fire ant bites on the anterior knee occurred after this patient knelt on a mound. These bites are 3 days old; the initial sterile pustules have begun to crust over. (Courtesy of Alan B. Storrow, MD.)

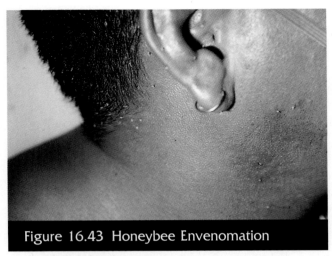

Figure 16.43 Honeybee Envenomation

Many honeybee stingers (barbs and venom sacs) are seen on this patient's cheek and ear and along the hairline. (Courtesy of Alan B. Storrow, MD.)

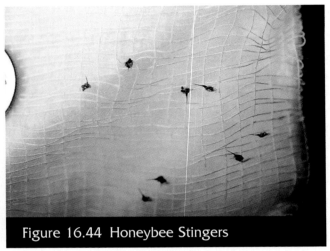

Figure 16.44 Honeybee Stingers

The barbs and attached venom sacs (stinger apparatus) after removal from the patient. (Courtesy of Alan B. Storrow, MD.)

Clinical Pearls

1. Honeybee stings are usually apparent since the stinger apparatus, including barb and venom sac, is often detached and present on the patient's skin (Figs. 16.43 and 16.44).
2. "Brazilian killer" or "Africanized" bees are now present in Texas, Arizona, and California. Their venom is not known to be more toxic; however, their aggressiveness, tendency to swarm in large numbers, and ability to travel long distances make them potentially more dangerous to humans.

Associated Clinical Features

The order Lepidoptera contains several families of caterpillars that are venomous to humans. The venom apparatus typically consists of barbed spines arranged in clumps or scattered about the dorsal surface of the insect (Fig. 16.45). They may contain venom or serve as a mechanical irritant. The venoms, about which little is known, are purely defensive in nature. Patients who are stung are often gardening or outdoors when they come in contact with the caterpillar. The typical envenomation presents with acute pain followed by erythema and mild swelling (Fig. 16.46). Caterpillars with a less sophisticated venom apparatus or less toxic venom may cause simple pruritus or urticaria. Systemic symptoms have been reported but are very rare.

The puss caterpillar or woolly slug (*Megalopyge opercularis*) is perhaps the most famous and important venomous U.S. caterpillar (Fig. 16.47). Found throughout the United States, it is very hairy and flat and may reach a length of 4 cm. It lives in shade trees and feeds on their vegetation.

Chiggers are the larvae of trombiculid mites and inflict intensely pruritic bites on their victims (Fig. 16.48). They are parasitic only as larvae and infest humans by crawling onto them (usually up the socks) and latching on. The mites secrete a salivary fluid containing digestive enzymes onto the victim's skin. Clothing precautions and repellents are usually effective in reducing unpleasant chigger infestations.

Centipedes are venomous arthropods that have one pair of legs per body segment, with the number of segments being variable. The first segment contains hollow curved "fangs" (really modified legs and not truly mouth parts) (Fig. 16.49) capable of penetrating human skin. These

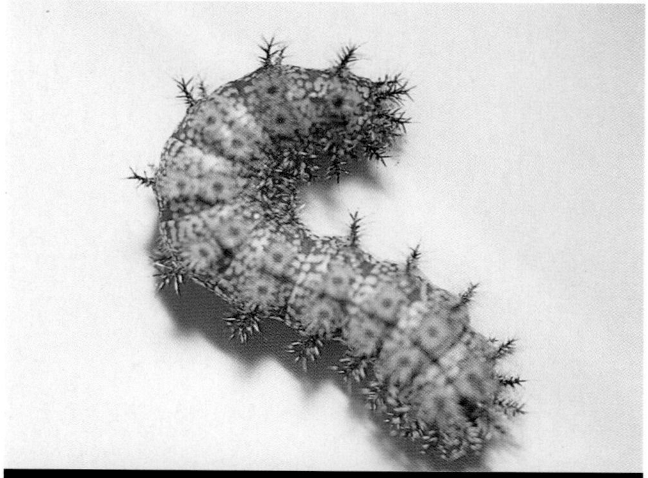

Figure 16.45 Caterpillar with Barbed Spines

Typical garden caterpillar with barbed spines arranged in clumps. (Courtesy of Alan B. Storrow, MD.)

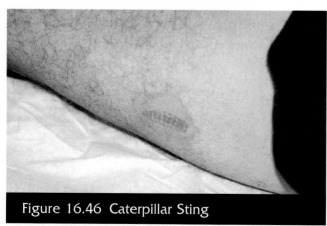

Figure 16.46 Caterpillar Sting

Appearance of a caterpillar sting at 2 h. The patient presented with moderate pain and severe itching. Note how the erythema follows the pattern of the caterpillar. (Courtesy of Alan B. Storrow, MD.)

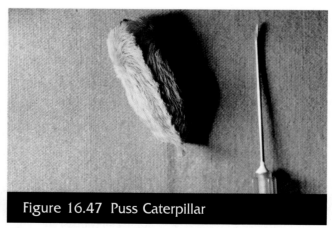

Figure 16.47 Puss Caterpillar

The "puss caterpillar" or "woolly slug" is likely the most important venomous caterpillar in the United States. The hairy appearance and small hair tail is characteristic. (Courtesy of Alan B. Storrow, MD.)

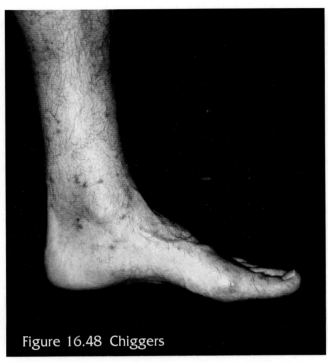

Figure 16.48 Chiggers

Chigger bites on a leg appear as puncta surrounded by erythema. (Courtesy of Kevin J. Knoop, MD.)

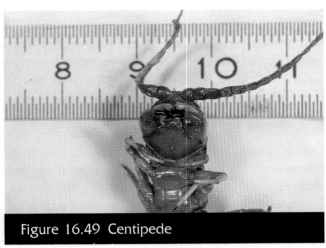

Figure 16.49 Centipede

Note the curved "fangs" (actually modified legs) on the first segment of this centipede from Texas. (Courtesy of Alan B. Storrow, MD.)

bear venom glands at the bases. Centipedes largely use their venom to kill their prey. When provoked, however, they may sting humans and produce local burning pain, erythema, and swelling. Severe systemic reactions may occur but are uncommon.

Differential Diagnosis

Other arthropod envenomations or plant exposures must be considered.

Emergency Department Treatment and Disposition

Treatment of envenomations from caterpillars, mites, and centipedes is purely symptomatic and consists of appropriate pain control, oral antihistamines (such as cyproheptadine or diphenhydramine), topical antipruritic creams, and basic wound care.

Clinical Pearls

1. The caudal appendages of centipedes are not associated with a venom apparatus.
2. Infiltration with local anesthetics may be useful in markedly painful centipede envenomations or for the removal of retained "fang" fragments.
3. Envenomations by the order Lepidoptera are usually from a caterpillar, not from a cocoon or adult stage.
4. Some caterpillars are capable of producing a very painful sting requiring opiate pain control.
5. Attached caterpillar spines may be removed with adhesive tape.

Associated Clinical Features

Scorpions are venomous nocturnal arthropods and a worldwide health concern. The most significant morbidity and mortality is attributable to the Buthidae family, which is characterized by a triangular central sternal plate (Figs. 16.50, 16.51). This family includes, among others, the venomous *Androctonus* genus in northern Africa, *Leiurus* in the Middle East, *Tityus* in South America, and *Centruroides* in North America.

Centruroides (Fig. 16.52) is found primarily in the southwestern United States and northern Mexico. It is characterized by a variable subaculear tooth beneath the stinger (Figs. 16.53, 16.54), may be striped, and is yellow to brown in color. These spiders prefer darkness and thus tend to hide in crevices, woodpiles, bedding, clothing, and shoes during the day. Envenomation produces a mild local reaction of pain, swelling, burning, and ecchymosis (Fig. 16.55).

However, envenomation with the species *Centruroides exilicauda,* the bark scorpion, can lead to progressive symptoms and death. The venom of *C. exilicauda* initially produces local paresthesias and pain (grade 1), which may be accentuated by tapping the involved area, also known

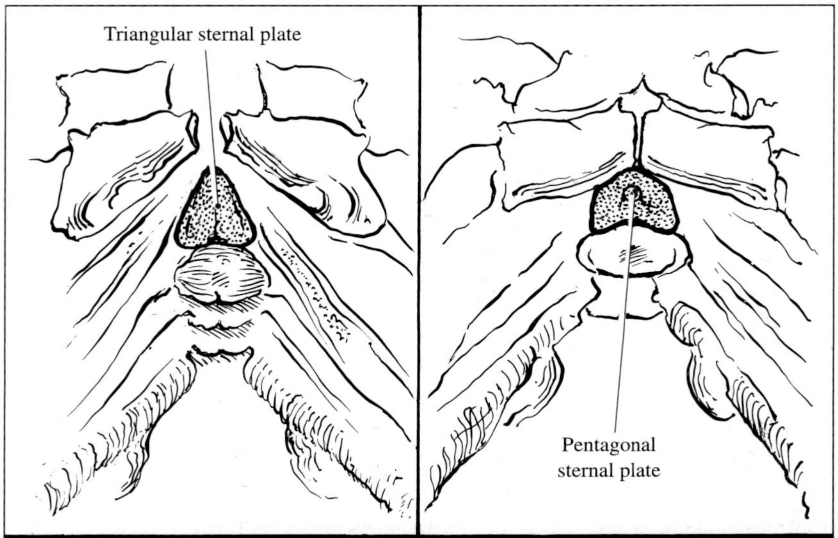

Triangular sternal plate

Pentagonal sternal plate

Figure 16.50 Buthidae Sternal Plate

The Buthidae family is associated with the most significant envenomations and is characterized by triangular sternal plates (left). Members of the other scorpion families have pentagonal sternal plates (right).

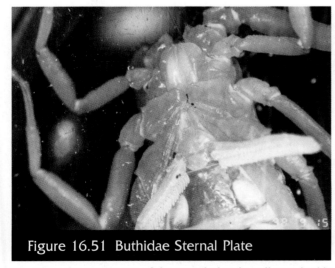

Figure 16.51 Buthidae Sternal Plate

The triangular appearance of the sternal plate is well seen in this scorpion, a member of the Buthidae family. (Courtesy of Sean P. Bush, MD.)

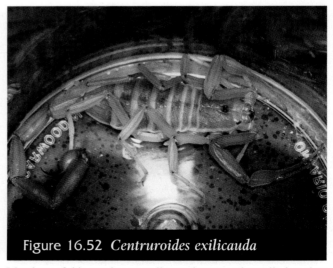

Figure 16.52 *Centruroides exilicauda*

Members of this species are yellow to brown and usually less than 5 cm long. Below the stinger is the telson, within which are two glands containing venom. (Courtesy of Sean P. Bush, MD.)

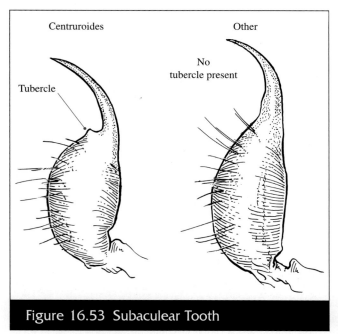

Figure 16.53 Subaculear Tooth

The barb noted at the base of the stinger is variably present in *Centruroides* (left) and absent in other species (right)

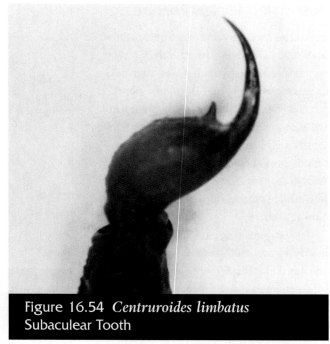

Figure 16.54 *Centruroides limbatus* Subaculear Tooth

A variable subaculear tooth is characteristic of *Centruroides*. This is an example of a large subaculear tooth on the telson from *C. limbatus*. *C. exilicauda* typically has a smaller, sometimes subtle "tooth." (Courtesy of Sean P. Bush, MD.)

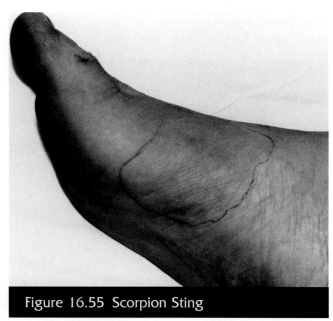

Figure 16.55 Scorpion Sting

Most scorpion envenomations are mild and produce local pain, swelling, paresthesias, and mild ecchymosis. (Courtesy of Stephen Corbett, MD.)

as the "tap" test. More severe envenomations may produce remote paresthesias (grade II) and either somatic or autonomic nerve dysfunction (grade III). Proteins in the toxin are thought to cause repetitive firing of neurons by binding to sodium channels. These symptoms may include tachycardia, nausea, wandering eye movements, blurred vision, difficulty breathing, trouble swallowing, restlessness, and involuntary shaking. Both somatic and autonomic dysfunction may be present (grade IV). These systemic reactions tend to be more severe in younger patients and may result in death, usually from respiratory arrest, if not treated properly.

Differential Diagnosis

The differential diagnosis of mild scorpion stings includes any insect bite or sting. Major envenomations produce a broad spectrum of neuromuscular symptoms, which may mimic severe black widow spider envenomation, toxic ingestions, or neuromuscular disorders.

Emergency Department Treatment and Disposition

Treatment depends on the severity of envenomation. Grade I or II envenomations are treated with supportive care (ice, oral analgesia) and tetanus immunization. There is no known role for the use of barbiturates, benzodiazepines, steroids, calcium, or epinephrine. The past use of large doses of barbiturates has been suggested to be a major contributor to reported deaths.

Envenomations that progress to grade III or IV must be treated aggressively and may require paralysis and intubation for severe spasms. Goat serum antivenin is available in Arizona (Samaritan Regional Poison Center in Phoenix, 602-253-3334) and can be considered. It does carry a risk of hypersensitivity reactions. Pain and paresthesias from a scorpion sting may persist for up to 2 weeks, but most systemic symptoms improve within 9 to 30 h without antivenin treatment and usually peak at approximately 5 h.

Clinical Pearls

1. Antivenin should be used cautiously, as hypersensitivity reactions are common.
2. If the scorpion is brought in, examine it for a triangular plate and subaculear tooth.
3. Almost all scorpions, including *Centruroides exilicauda,* fluoresce with intense brightness under cobalt light.

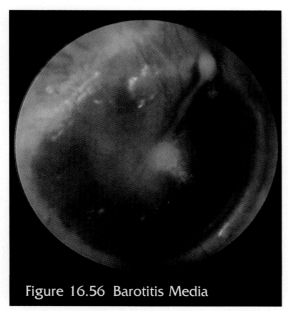

Figure 16.56 Barotitis Media

Tympanic membrane erythema and mild hemorrhage consistent with barotitis media. (Courtesy of Richard A. Chole, MD, PhD.)

Associated Clinical Features

Middle ear squeeze (barotitis media) results from a relative decrease in middle ear pressure produced as a diver descends. It can occur in as little as 2 to 3 ft of water. The tympanic membrane (TM) bulges inward, causing discomfort. At a depth of approximately 4 ft, the pressure difference is great enough to collapse the eustachian tube and cause obstruction. If attempts to equalize the pressure (e.g., Valsalva or Frenzel maneuver) fail, ascent is necessary. If a diver continues to descend, TM rupture may occur. The influx of water into the middle ear may cause extreme vertigo and lead to a diving disaster.

Barotitis media may present with pain only (grade 0), TM erythema (grade 1), erythema and mild TM hemorrhage (grade 2, Fig. 16.56), gross TM hemorrhage (grade 3), free middle ear blood (grade 4), or free blood with TM perforation (grade 5).

Differential Diagnosis

The differential diagnosis of diving-related ear pain includes otitis externa, otitis media, and ear canal squeeze.

Emergency Department Treatment and Disposition

Treatment includes ascent, decongestants, and analgesia. Antihistamines may be of use for allergy-related eustachian tube dysfunction. Antibiotics are recommended for preexisting infections or for TM rupture. Most cases resolve spontaneously within hours to days. The patient should not resume diving until the condition has resolved or the TM is completely healed.

Clinical Pearls

1. Barotitis media is the most common medical problem associated with diving.
2. Associated barotrauma should be investigated in cases of barotitis media.

Associated Clinical Features

Mask squeeze results when a diver fails to maintain the balance between the air pressure within his or her mask and the external water pressure during descent. Repeated nasal exhalations into the scuba mask while diving normally accomplish this. When this is not performed properly, extreme negative air pressure can build up inside the mask and may result in the rupture of capillary beds, leading to conjunctival hemorrhage and skin ecchymosis (Fig. 16.57).

Differential Diagnosis

Given a recent history of diving, the differential is limited but would include traumatic causes of facial ecchymosis and conjunctival hemorrhage.

Emergency Department Treatment and Disposition

Treatment consists of ascent and essentially supportive care. A history of recent eye surgery should be sought; if discovered, thorough eye examination should be performed and ophthalmologic consultation considered.

Clinical Pearls

1. Diver education and proper diving technique minimize the risk of mask squeeze.
2. Special consideration should be given to patients with recent keratotomy, as corneal incisions heal relatively slowly.

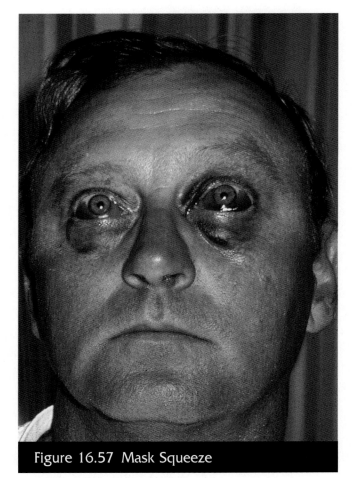

Figure 16.57 Mask Squeeze

Mask squeeze in a diver who descended to 45 FSW without exhaling into his mask. (Courtesy of Kenneth W. Kizer, MD; reprinted with permission from Auerbach PS (ed): *Wilderness Medicine: Management of Wilderness and Environmental Emergencies,* 3rd ed. St. Louis: Mosby–Year Book; 1995.)

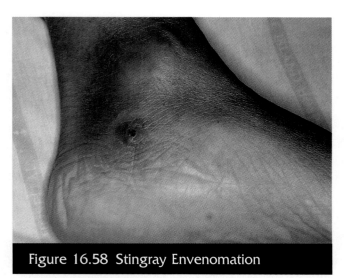

Figure 16.58 Stingray Envenomation

Puncture wound from stingray envenomation in a lower extremity. (Courtesy of Daniel L. Savitt, MD.)

Associated Clinical Features

Stingray envenomation involves a forceful thrust of the caudal spine or spines of the animal producing a puncture wound (Fig. 16.58) or laceration. Since the animals commonly burrow in sand, they may be accidently stepped on. The stingray has a barbed tail that reflexively impacts the victim, usually in the lower extremity. The force of injection causes the integumentary sheath covering the spine to rupture, potentially releasing venom, mucus, pieces of the sheath, and spine fragments. The wound usually produces immediate intense pain, edema, and bleeding. The initially dusky or cyanotic wound may progress to erythema, with rapid fat and muscle hemorrhage. Systemic symptoms may include nausea, vomiting, diarrhea, diaphoresis, muscle cramps, fasciculations, weakness, headache, vertigo, paralysis, seizures, hypotension, syncope, arrhythmias, and death.

Differential Diagnosis

All marine envenomations, specific to the particular environment, must be considered, since visualization of the offending creature is rare. Nonvenomous stings and simple trauma with infection must also be considered.

Emergency Department Treatment and Disposition

Rapid attention to a stingray envenomation is the key to successful treatment. The wound should be irrigated immediately and primary exploration accomplished to remove visible debris. Local suction and proximal constriction bands may be useful but are controversial. Irrigation should be promptly followed by immersion in hot water, to tolerance, for 30 to 90 min. Wounds should be further explored and debrided during soaking. Pain relief should be initiated early, and narcotics may be needed. After soaking, wounds should be formally explored, debrided, and dressed for delayed primary closure or primary closure with drainage. Prophylactic antibiotics are recommended. Patients can usually be discharged home after a 3- to 4-h observation period if no systemic symptoms arise. Tetanus prophylaxis should be given if indicated.

Clinical Pearls

1. Application of cryotherapy to stingray envenomations may prove disastrous.
2. Retained foreign bodies are a common problem in stingray wounds.
3. Bacteria cultured from marine envenomations are extremely diverse. Antibiotics chosen should include coverage of *Vibrio* species.

Associated Clinical Features

Sea urchins belong to the phylum Echinodermata and are nonaggressive, slow-moving creatures. Envenomation usually occurs after intentional or accidental handling. Long, brittle, venom-filled spines or the three-jawed globiferous pedicellariae are responsible for the injury. The spines frequently break and pedicellariae can remain attached and active for several hours. They may advance into muscle or joint spaces and cause infection (Fig. 16.59). The usual presentation is burning pain progressing to localized muscle aches. Erythema and edema may be present. Multiple envenomations may produce systemic symptoms including nausea, vomiting, abdominal pain, paresthesia, numbness, paralysis, hypotension, syncope, or respiratory distress. While the envenomation causes a reaction that may be quite painful, it is rarely life-threatening.

Differential Diagnosis

The differential diagnosis of sea urchin envenomation includes other marine envenomations and local trauma. Delayed presentations can mimic a host of local inflammatory reactions. A careful history of exposure is critical.

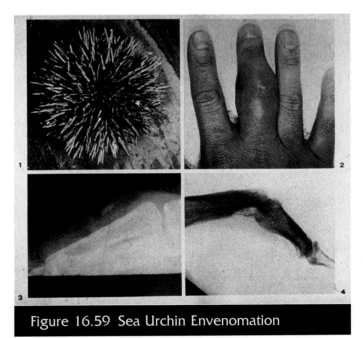

Figure 16.59 Sea Urchin Envenomation

Four images representing (1) a living sea urchin with characteristic spines; (2) puncture wound of the right middle finger revealing swelling during the chronic phase; (3) radiograph taken shortly after sea urchin injury, revealing the calcified sea urchin spine; and (4) osteolytic process of the right middle phalanx caused by an embedded sea urchin spine. (From Halstead BH: *Venomous Marine Animals of the World.* Washington, DC: US Government Printing Office, 1965.)

Emergency Department Treatment and Disposition

Following envenomation, the affected area should be submersed in nonscalding hot water for 30 to 90 min. Pedicellariae may be removed by applying shaving cream and gently scraping with a razor. Obvious embedded spines should be removed. Hand wounds often require surgical debridement. Retained spines often dissolve spontaneously; however, granulomas may form, producing locally destructive inflammation.

Clinical Pearls

1. Sea urchin envenomation involving a joint may produce severe synovitis.
2. Some species of sea urchin contain dye, which may give the false impression of a retained spine.
3. Sea urchins known to be hazardous to humans are generally found in the Indian Ocean, Pacific Ocean, and Red sea.

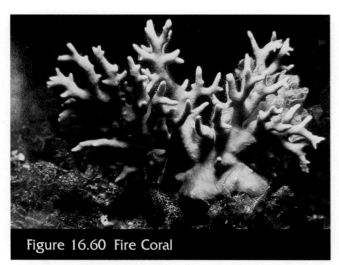

Figure 16.60 Fire Coral

After contact, fire coral most commonly causes immediate local burning pain, followed by erythematous papules or urticarial eruptions. Pruritus may last for several days. (Courtesy of Edward J. Otten, MD.)

Associated Clinical Features

The phylum Coelenterata contains approximately 10,000 different species, of which several hundred are a danger to humans. This diverse group includes hydrozoans (e.g., Portuguese man-of-war and fire coral, Fig. 16.60), scyphozoans (i.e., "true" jellyfish), and anthozoans (i.e., soft corals, stony corals, and anemones). They account for more marine envenomations than any other phylum. The important species involved in human injuries share sharp stinging cells called nematocysts. Nematocysts are enclosed in venom sacs and are present in tentacles that hang from air-filled structures. After external contact, the nematocysts are discharged from their sacs, often penetrate the skin, and release their venom. Nematocyst venom is an extremely complex substance containing numerous proteins and enzymes. Clinical presentation following envenomation ranges from the mild dermatitis to cardiovascular and pulmonary collapse. Mild envenomations usually result in a self-limited papular inflammatory eruption associated with burning and limited to areas of contact. Moderate to severe envenomations produce a spectrum of neurologic, cardiovascular, respiratory, and gastrointestinal symptoms. Anaphylactoid reactions—including hypotension, dysrhythmias, bronchospasm, and cardiovascular collapse—may play a role.

Differential Diagnosis

Coelenterate stings often produce a telltale linear pattern corresponding to the shape of tentacles (Figs. 16.61, 16.62). Sea anemones have tentacles loaded with nematocyst variations. Contact may cause painful urticarial lesions, paresthesias, edema, erythema (Fig. 16.63), and, if severe, ulceration, necrosis, and secondary infection. Coelenterate envenomation must also be considered as a potential contributing cause in unexplained cases of collapse resulting from swimming, diving, or near-drowning incidents.

Emergency Department Treatment and Disposition

Concurrently with primary resuscitation, nematocyst decontamination should be accomplished beginning with seawater flushing. The hypotonic nature of fresh water, as well as isopropyl alcohol, may cause additional nematocysts to fire and should be avoided. A 5% solution of acetic acid (vinegar) applied for at least 30 min is the most widely accepted detoxicant. It has been suggested to remove tentacles with the application of shaving cream, followed in 5 min by a careful scraping with a firm, dull object (e.g., tongue blade, credit card). Pruritus may be treated with antihistamines. Pain may be addressed with immersion in hot water or with systemic analgesics. Any victim with systemic symptoms requires at least 6 to 8 h of observation because rebound phenomena are common.

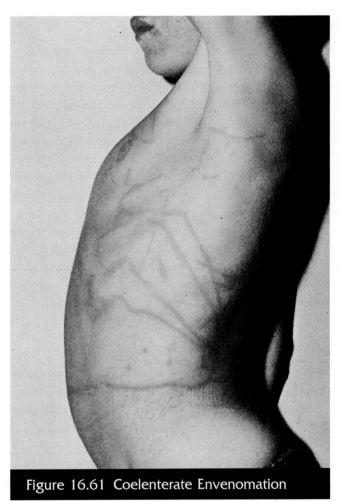

Figure 16.61 Coelenterate Envenomation

The sharp angulations and undulations characteristic of jellyfish envenomation. (From Halstead BH: *Venomous Marine Animals of the World*. Washington, DC: US Government Printing Office, 1965.)

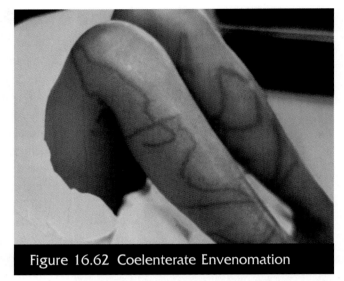

Figure 16.62 Coelenterate Envenomation

Jellyfish envenomation on the lower extremities. (Courtesy of the Department of Dermatology, Naval Medical Center, Portsmouth, VA.)

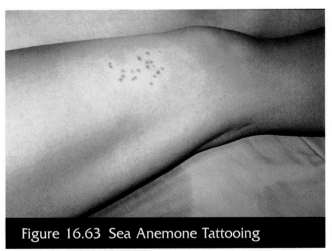

Figure 16.63 Sea Anemone Tattooing

Contact with sea anemones results mainly in local skin irritation, initially manifest as pruritus, burning, throbbing, and, sometimes radiation of pain to other areas. The area involved may reveal blistering, local edema, and violaceous petechial hemorrhages. The skin papules are confined to the areas of contact and may persist for 7 to 10 days. (Courtesy of Gerald O'Malley, DO.)

Clinical Pearls

1. The box jellyfish (*Chironex fleckeri*) is generally considered the most deadly of marine animals and is most predominant in Australian and Southeast Asian waters. It may produce severe systemic symptoms hours after exposure. A sheep-derived antivenin (Commonwealth Serum Laboratory, Australia) is available.

2. The detached tentacles of some species may contain active nematocysts for months, even when fragmented on the beach or floating in water.

3. The Portuguese man-of-war is present in the Floridian Atlantic coast and the Gulf of Mexico. It is known to have a neurotoxin that may cause severe pain and death.

4. There is considerable overlap in degrees of envenomation, from annoying dermatitis to multisystem involvement and death.

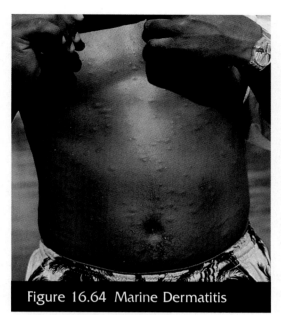

Figure 16.64 Marine Dermatitis

Typical appearance of marine dermatitis. (Courtesy of Richard A. Clinchy III, PhD.)

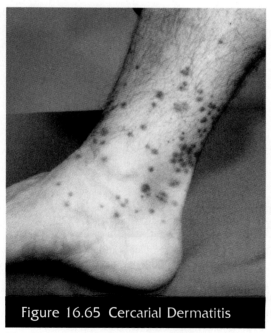

Figure 16.65 Cercarial Dermatitis

The discrete and highly pruritic papules of cercarial dermatitis commonly occur on exposed body areas. (Courtesy of David O. Parrish, MD. Used with permission from Parrish DO. Seabather's eruption or diver's dermatitis. *JAMA* 1993;270:2300–2301.)

Associated Clinical Features

Marine dermatitis, also known as "sea bather's eruption," is a pruritic condition commonly mislabeled *sea lice*. Symptoms usually occur a few minutes to 12 h after exposure. The offending organisms are probably numerous and include the larval form of the thimble jellyfish and the planula form of the sea anemone *Edwardsiella lineata*. The rash consists of erythematous wheals and papules, which may be extremely pruritic (Fig. 16.64). Systemic manifestations include fever, malaise, headache, conjunctivitis, and urethritis. Unlike cercarial dermatitis, marine dermatitis primarily affects areas of the body covered by caps, fins, and bathing suits.

Cercarial dermatitis, or "swimmer's itch," occurs when humans become accidental hosts of nonhuman schistosomes. This causes an immune response that results in itching, erythema, and mild edema. After 60 min, the classic signs are red macules that become pruritic papules 3 to 5 cm in diameter and surrounded by erythema (Fig. 16.65).

Differential Diagnosis.

A marine dermatitis should be considered when pruritic lesions follow seawater exposure. The incidence increases significantly during the late summer and fall off Long Island and in the late spring and early summer in south Florida. Contact dermatitis and some fungal skin disorders may present in a similar fashion.

Emergency Department Treatment and Disposition

Marine dermatitis is self-limited, rarely persisting beyond 10 days to 2 weeks. The dermatitis may be partially prevented by a vigorous soap-and-water scrub after saltwater bathing. Treatment is symptomatic, and calamine lotion with 1% menthol may bring relief. Topical steroids may provide additional relief. In severe cases, oral antihistamines and corticosteroids may be necessary.

Cercarial dermatitis is treated with isopropyl alcohol or calamine lotion. Severe cases may require systemic corticosteroids, whereas bacterial infection may require topical or oral antibiotics.

Clinical Pearls

1. Marine dermatitis primarily affects areas covered by caps, fins, and bathing suits.
2. Individual lesions may look like insect bites.

Associated Clinical Features

Scorpion fish are colorful venomous marine animals found primarily in tropical waters. Their exotic, beautiful appearance has made them increasingly popular among marine aquarists in the United States, and many envenomations have resulted from mishandling. They are well camouflaged in the wild and stings are usually caused by accidentally stepping on them. Scorpion fish are grouped into the genera Pterois (lion fish) (Fig. 16.66), Scorpaena (scorpion fish proper), and Synanceja (stone fish), with the severity of envenomation progressing respectively. All scorpion fish have multiple spines in association with venom glands; envenomation results from skin puncture followed by venom release into the tissues. Immediately following a scorpion fish sting, the victim experiences intense pain that, untreated, lasts for hours. The site may become warm, erythematous, and edematous and vesicles may arise. Lion fish stings are painful but relatively mild, usually limited to localized pain and tissue responses. Severe systemic effects are more common with stone fish envenomation and may produce a constellation of cardiovascular, pulmonary, neurologic, and gastrointestinal sequelae.

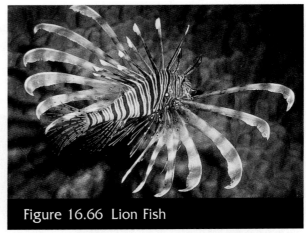

Figure 16.66 Lion Fish

The *Pterois* genus of the Scorpaenidae family includes the lion fish. Envenomations occur by erectile spines on the dorsal, pelvic, and anal fins of these fish. Its clinical manifestations are relatively mild and include intense, sharp, throbbing pain, with possible progression of pain radiation, erythema, ecchymosis, systemic symptoms, and necrosis. (Courtesy of Edward J. Otten, MD.)

Differential Diagnosis

History raises a high suspicion for scorpion fish stings in the wild and diagnosis is usually obvious domestically. The differential includes coelenterate, stingray, echinoderm, and sea snake envenomation. As with coelenterates, scorpion fish envenomation should be considered in the event of unexplained near drowning and swimmer collapse.

Emergency Department Treatment and Disposition

Hot water immersion for 30 to 90 min should be initiated as soon as possible. Rebound pain is common and should be treated with repeated hot water immersion. During immersion, the wound should be carefully inspected for pieces of spine and sheath, which may have broken off in the skin. Thorough warm saline irrigation should also be performed along with wound exploration. Severe pain should be treated with local injection of lidocaine without epinephrine and with narcotic analgesia. Antibiotic prophylaxis should be considered in high-risk wounds. Tetanus status should be addressed.

Clinical Pearls

1. Stone fish envenomations are by far the most dangerous of the scorpion fish stings and severe systemic reactions may occur. Stone fish antivenin (Commonwealth Serum Laboratories, Australia) is available.
2. Scorpion fish venom is heat-labile and hot water immersion therapy is effective in treating pain and inactivating venom.

Associated Clinical Features

Erysipeloid, also known as "fish handler's disease," is a bacterial skin infection caused by *Erysipelothrix rhusiopathiae.* This condition is frequently seen in those who handle raw meat, fish, and shellfish. The offending organism enters the body through a break in the skin and causes a local infection within 2 to 7 days. Lesions are characterized by an edematous central purplish-red area, surrounded first by central clearing and then circumscribed by an advancing raised, erythematous ring (Fig. 16.67). The area is usually pruritic and painful and may be associated with fever, malaise, and regional lymphadenopathy.

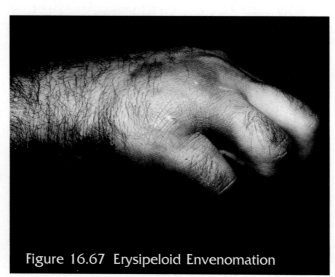

Figure 16.67 Erysipeloid Envenomation

Typical appearance of *Erysipelothrix rhusiopathiae* skin infection. [Courtesy of Paul S. Auerbach, MD; reprinted with permission from Auerbach PS (ed): *Wilderness Medicine: Management of Wilderness and Environmental Emergencies,* 3rd ed. St. Louis: Mosby–Year Book; 1995.]

Differential Diagnosis

History aids greatly in the diagnosis, but erysipeloid may be confused with contact or rhus dermatitis, insect bites, and fungal or other cutaneous infections.

Emergency Department Treatment and Disposition

If left untreated, erysipeloid will usually resolve spontaneously in about 3 weeks. Skin infections may be treated with penicillin VK, cephalexin, or erythromycin. If severe infection occurs in association with septicemia, endocarditis, or arthritis, penicillin G 2 to 4 million U IV q4 h for 4 to 6 weeks should be administered. Tetanus status must be addressed.

Clinical Pearls

1. A history of occupational or recreational exposure to fish or shellfish is the key to diagnosis.
2. *E. rhusiopathiae* is usually resistant to aminoglycoside antibiotics, and these should be avoided.

Associated Clinical Features

Poison ivy, oak, and sumac (Figs. 16.68, 16.69, and 16.70) cause more cases of allergic contact dermatitis than all other allergens combined. At least 70% of the U.S. population is sensitive to the *Toxicodendron* species.

The dermatitis begins as pruritus and redness usually within 2 days of exposure in susceptible persons. The degree of dermatitis depends on the patient's degree of sensitivity, amount of allergen exposure, and the reactivity of the skin at the exposed body location. The dermatitis may vary from erythema to erythema with papules to erythema with vesicles and bullae (Figs. 16.71 and 16.72). A linear distribution of the cutaneous lesions is strongly suggestive of *toxicodendron* dermatitis (Fig. 16.73). This distribution occurs after contaminated fingernails have scratched the skin or plant parts rubbed against it.

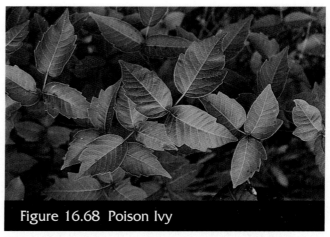

Figure 16.68 Poison Ivy

Toxicodendron radicans (poison ivy—shrub or climbing vine). Note that the leaves of poison ivy have three leaflets and the stems are commonly reddish orange. Poison ivy occurs throughout the United States. (Courtesy of Lawrence B. Stack, MD.)

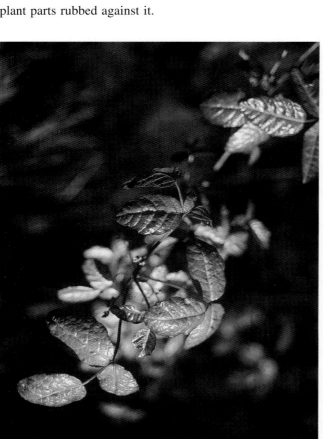

Figure 16.69 Poison Oak

Toxicodendron diversiloba (poison oak). Like poison ivy, the terminal part of the branch has a cluster of three shiny leaves. It grows as a tree or woody shrub and occurs west of the Rocky Mountains. (Courtesy of Ken Zafren, MD.)

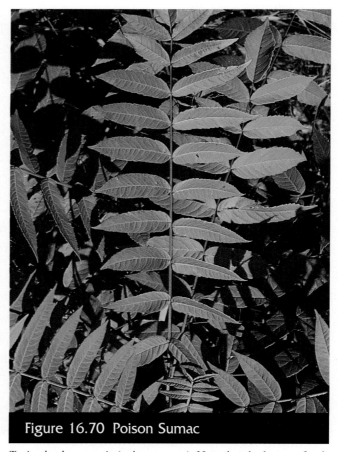

Figure 16.70 Poison Sumac

Toxicodendron vernix (poison sumac). Note that the leaves of poison sumac have 7 to 13 leaflets. It grows as a tree or woody coarse shrub. Only one species of poison sumac is found in the United States. (Courtesy of Lawrence B. Stack, MD.)

551

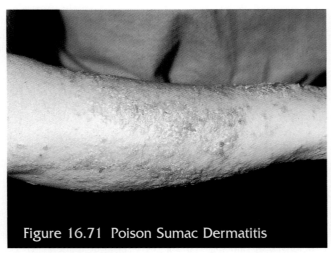

Figure 16.71 Poison Sumac Dermatitis

A moderately severe local reaction to poison sumac. Note the vesicles, bullae, and exudates characteristic of a contact dermatitis. (Courtesy of Alan B. Storrow, MD.)

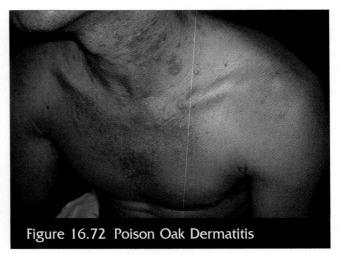

Figure 16.72 Poison Oak Dermatitis

Erythematous papules and vesicles. This firefighter was exposed to urushiol, the allergen of poison oak, ivy, and sumac, in smoke from burning poison oak. (Courtesy of Ken Zafren, MD.)

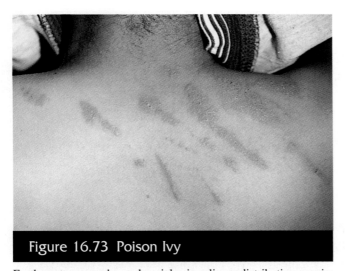

Figure 16.73 Poison Ivy

Erythematous papules and vesicles in a linear distribution consistent with *Toxicodendron* dermatitis. (Courtesy of Alan B. Storrow, MD.)

Differential Diagnosis

Medical problems that may appear like a *Toxicodendron* rash include photodermatitis, cellulitis, thermal burns, and other causes of contact dermatitis.

Emergency Department Treatment and Disposition

An immediate rinse or shower with warm water and soap may minimize the reaction. If symptoms are limited to erythema and papules and a small surface area, calamine lotion or topical steroid sprays may provide adequate symptomatic relief. Pruritus may be decreased with oral antihistamines (e.g., diphenhydramine or cyproheptadine) and oatmeal baths. Vesicles and bullae require Domeboro compresses (for 60 min three times daily) to help dry these lesions and relieve pruritus. Systemic corticosteroids tapered over 3 weeks are used in severe reactions. Secondary infection should be treated with systemic antibiotics against staphylococcal and streptococcal species.

Clinical Pearls

1. Fluid from the vesicles or bullae does not contain any allergen.
2. Removal of the allergen from the skin within 30 min of exposure may prevent dermatitis.
3. Deliberate removal of allergen from under the fingernails may prevent spreading.
4. Treatment with systemic steroids for less than 2 or 3 weeks may result in rebound exacerbations of the dermatitis.

Associated Clinical Features

Sporotrichosis is a fungal skin infection caused by *Sporothrix schenckii,* an organism primarily found on plants and flowers and in soil; the problem is common among gardeners and florists. It also affects those who handle animals, since the fungus may inhabit animals' claws. Infection arises as contaminated thorns, spines, or claws penetrate the victim's skin. After an average incubation period of 3 weeks, localized infections become apparent. "Fixed" cutaneous infections are localized to the inoculation site and are manifest as 2- to 4-mm papules or nodules. They may ulcerate, become surrounded by raised erythema, and are typically painless (Fig. 16.74). Progression to lymphocutaneous infections occurs in about 70% of cases. Patients present with a nodule at the site of penetration, with later appearance of subcutaneous nodules and skip areas along lymphatic tracks (Fig. 16.75). The lesions may wax and wane over months to years. Patients with cutaneous sporotrichosis typically lack systemic symptoms and, if laboratory profiles are performed, have unremarkable results.

Differential Diagnosis

Cellulitis, syphilis, anthrax, brown recluse spider envenomation, and other cutaneous mycoses may be confused with sporotrichosis. Other less common infections such as cat-scratch disease, nocardiosis, and tuberculosis may be considered. A straightforward history of injury is often helpful to pinpoint the diagnosis.

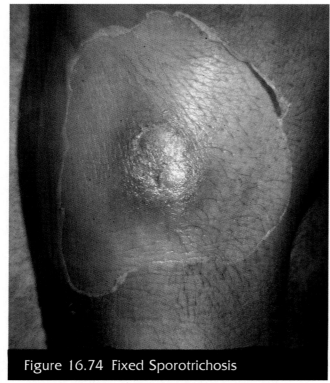

Figure 16.74 Fixed Sporotrichosis

The ulcer and surrounding erythema of fixed cutaneous sporotrichosis could be confused with a brown recluse spider bite. (Courtesy of Edward J. Otten, MD.)

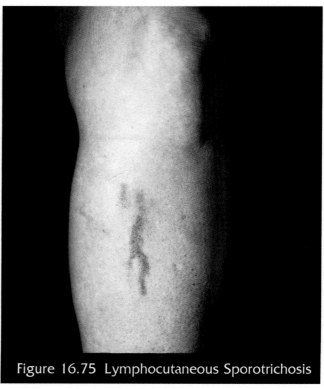

Figure 16.75 Lymphocutaneous Sporotrichosis

Lymphatic spread is common in cutaneous sporotrichosis. (Courtesy of Kevin J. Knoop, MD.)

Emergency Department Treatment and Disposition

Sporotrichosis may be successfully treated with oral potassium iodide for one month after clinical manifestations have resolved. Alternative therapy includes oral ketoconazole, while disseminated infections may require intravenous amphotericin B. Outpatient therapy is appropriate for nondisseminated infections. Tetanus status should be addressed.

Clinical Pearls

1. Fungal cultures and tissue biopsy cultures are somewhat useful to confirm the diagnosis.
2. Treatment must be continued for 1 month following clinical resolution to eradicate *S. schenckii.*
3. Although rare, a pulmonary form of sporotrichosis after inhalation exposure has been reported.

Associated Clinical Features

Peyote (*Liphophora williamsii*) is a cactus plant (Fig. 16.76) found primarily in the southwestern United States. The cactus contains a significant amount of mescaline, a potent hallucinogen with structural similarities to norepinephrine. Peyote buttons and seeds are frequently ingested for recreational use but are also used in the religious ceremonies of some Native American groups (peyotism). Toxicity of peyote is generally mild and self-limited. Mescaline induces some sympathomimetic effects due to its similarity to norepinephrine, and marked visual hallucinations and a sense of depersonalization follow. These effects are sometimes accompanied by unpleasant GI symptoms such as severe nausea and vomiting. Full recovery from these symptoms usually occurs within a few hours.

Differential Diagnosis

The differential diagnosis of peyote ingestion includes any hallucinogen poisoning. The timing of clinical effects makes mescaline similar to lysergic acid diethylamide (LSD).

Emergency Department Treatment and Disposition

Treatment of peyote ingestion is largely supportive; severe toxic effects are uncommon. Marked agitation may be managed with benzodiazepines.

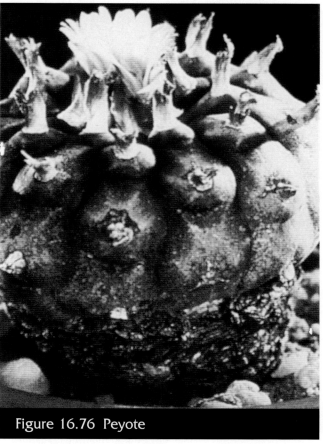

Figure 16.76 Peyote

Typical appearance of peyote cactus. Note the individual fleshy "buttons," which may be sliced and dried for storage. (Courtesy of Edward J. Otten, MD.)

Clinical Pearls

1. An individual peyote button contains about 45 mg of mescaline; a mescaline dose of 5 mg/kg produces psychic effects.
2. The emotional lability and anxiety produced by mescaline may predispose patients to accidental or self-inflicted trauma.

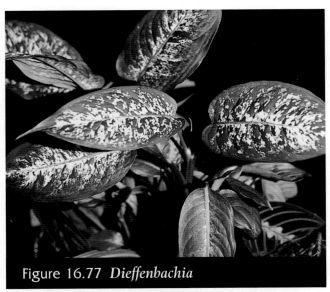

Figure 16.77 *Dieffenbachia*

Dieffenbachia is a common houseplant because of its colorful appearance and ease of indoor growth. (Courtesy of Kevin J. Knoop, MD.)

Associated Clinical Features

Dieffenbachia (dumbcane) is a common houseplant (Fig. 16.77) that causes toxic effects when ingested owing to large amounts of insoluble oxalate crystals in its leaves. The oxalate crystals are highly corrosive, and those who ingest the leaves experience painful burning of the lips, tongue, mouth, and esophagus. Marked swelling of the tongue, lips, and oropharynx can occur, and airway patency may become a major issue in managing these patients. Fortunately, calcium oxalate crystals are not absorbed and the profound hypocalcemia associated with soluble oxalates is not seen with *Dieffenbachia* poisoning.

Differential Diagnosis

The differential diagnosis of *Dieffenbachia* ingestion includes exposure to any caustic substances that may cause a similar pattern of burning when ingested.

Emergency Department Treatment and Disposition

Topical anesthetics are helpful in controlling severe pain from burning mucous membranes. Management is largely supportive, as the painful oral burns experienced with *Dieffenbachia* exposure usually limit ingestion. As with any oropharyngeal burn, airway issues must be addressed. A period of observation is appropriate to make sure that airway compromise does not occur with continued swelling. If leaves are swallowed, GI consultation should be considered to assess the extent of esophageal injury. Decontamination is usually not necessary, as the plant is rarely swallowed in significant amounts.

Clinical Pearls

1. Performance of nasopharyngoscopy may be helpful in assessment of airway patency for more posterior burns.
2. Patients should be instructed not to swallow topical anesthetics, as toxicity may result with extensive use.

Associated Clinical Features

Jimsonweed (*Datura stramonium*) is a toxic plant that contains tropane alkaloids consisting of atropine, scopolamine, and cocaine compounds. Ingestion may occur through the drinking of tea made from the leaves or flowers of jimsonweed or from eating the plant's seeds or leaves (Fig. 16.78). Poisoned victims demonstrate an anticholinergic toxidrome resulting from the antimuscarinic receptor effects of atropine and scopolamine. Clinically patients may exhibit altered mental status, xerostomia, xeroderma, xerophthalmia, blurred vision, mydriasis, tachycardia, decreased bowel and bladder motility, and hyperthermia.

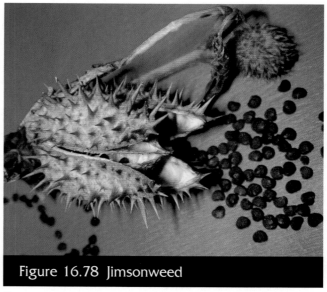

Figure 16.78 Jimsonweed

Jimsonweed plant with seeds. (Courtesy of Matthew D. Sztajnkrycer, MD, PhD.)

Differential Diagnosis

Jimsonweed poisoning carries a broad differential that comprises any toxin producing an anticholinergic toxidrome, including but not limited to antihistamines, antipsychotics, skeletal muscle relaxants, and tricyclic antidepressants.

Emergency Department Treatment and Disposition

Treatment initially consists of securing the ABCs (airway, breathing, circulation) and stabilization measures. Hypotension resulting from tropane alkaloid ingestion usually responds to fluid boluses, but vasopressor agents may be necessary. Once hemodynamic stability is achieved, the patient's detoxification must be addressed. Gastric lavage followed by activated charcoal is recommended but may be of little use, as toxins are absorbed rapidly. Whole-bowel irrigation is contraindicated with intestinal ileus and must be considered with great caution in jimsonweed ingestion owing decreased bowel motility. Physostigmine may be of benefit to treat severe anticholinergic toxicity, but extreme caution along with toxicology consultation is advisable, as the drug may induce AV block, asystole, seizures, hypotension, and bronchospasm.

Clinical Pearls

1. Examination of the axilla for xeroderma is very helpful to detect peripheral anticholinergic syndrome and distinguish between anticholinergic and sympathomimetic toxidromes.
2. Administering 1% pilocarpine drops does not reverse anticholinergic mydriasis.

Associated Clinical Features

Cardiac glycosides (CG) are found in the leaves of the *Nerium oleander* (Fig. 16.79), *Digitalis purpurea* (foxglove, Fig. 16.80), and *Convallaria majalis* (lily of the valley); if ingested, they produce clinical findings similar to digoxin toxicity. Toxicity can also occur if smoke from burning plants is inhaled. Foxglove and oleander tea may be a cause of CG toxicity. Therapeutic effects occur from inhibition of the cardiac cell membrane sodium-potassium adenosine triphosphate pump. These effects result in increased automaticity, improved conduction, and improved inotropy.

Toxic effects are an exaggeration of therapeutic effects. Bradydysrhythmias may result from impaired pacemaker function. Tachydysrhythmias may occur from increased automaticity. Nausea, vomiting, confusion, depression, and fatigue may be present. Headaches, paresthesias, weakness, scotomas, and color disturbance (yellow vision) may also be seen.

Differential Diagnosis

Conditions that may mimic CG ingestion include cardiac medication overdose, cardiac ischemia, myocardial infarction, pulmonary embolus, and any condition associated with cardiac disturbances.

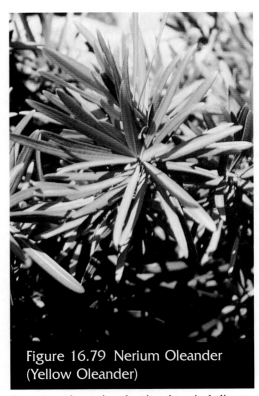

Figure 16.79 Nerium Oleander (Yellow Oleander)

A common decorative plant in subtropical climates often seen lining roads and highways. Flowers may be white, yellow, red, or purple. Plants may grow to a height of 15 ft. (Courtesy of Lawrence B. Stack, MD.)

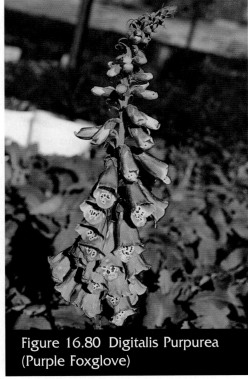

Figure 16.80 Digitalis Purpurea (Purple Foxglove)

The ornamental plant. (Courtesy of Lawrence B. Stack, MD.)

Emergency Department Treatment and Disposition

Atropine should be initially given for bradydysrhythmias. Refractory bradydysrhythmias require pacing. Ventricular tachydysrhythmias usually respond to phenytoin or lidocaine. Activated charcoal is the preferred method of decontamination. Cardioversion should be avoided in CG toxicity. Digoxin-specific Fab fragments are the treatment of choice for life-threatening dysrhythmias that fail conventional therapy.

Clinical Pearls

1. Treat CG overdose from plant exposure in the same way as an acute digoxin overdose.
2. Fab fragments have been used successfully to treat CG overdose from plant ingestion.
3. Calcium should be avoided in treating CG-associated hypokalemia, as it may worsen ventricular arrhythmias.

Associated Clinical Features

Mushrooms are the fruits of certain fungi. *Amanita phalloides* (the "death cap," Fig. 16.81) and *Amanita virosa* (the "destroying angel") species produce amantoxins and account for most fatalities due to mushroom ingestion. Mushroom poisoning commonly occurs in the early fall, when wild mushrooms are abundant and amateur foragers mistake poisonous mushrooms for edible ones.

Amantoxin poisoning results in an abrupt onset of nausea, vomiting, diarrhea, and abdominal pain 6 to 24 h after ingestion. Hematemesis, hematochezia, and severe dehydration resulting in hypotension may occur. Metabolic acidosis and electrolyte loss may be found on laboratory evaluation in severe poisoning. Gastrointestinal symptoms may last 12 to 24 h and are followed by a latent period of apparent improvement. This period is followed by a rise in liver enzymes and bilirubin and elevations in the PT and PTT. Liver and renal failure may become apparent.

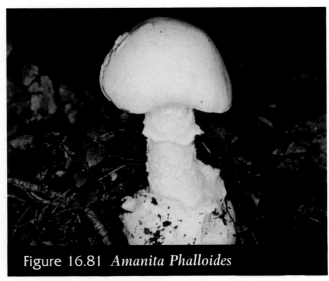

Figure 16.81 *Amanita Phalloides*

The "death cap" produces amatoxins and accounts for most of the fatalities due to mushroom ingestion. (Courtesy of Edward J. Otten, MD.)

Differential Diagnosis

The large differential surrounding acute abdominal pain and gastrointestinal bleeding should be entertained. Acute viral hepatitis may present similarly to mushroom ingestion.

Emergency Department Treatment and Disposition

Once the ABCs have been stabilized, gastric decontamination and activated charcoal administration are recommended. Specific interventions that may be helpful but are yet unproved include forced diuresis, charcoal hemoperfusion, high-dose cimetidine, high-dose penicillin, high-dose ascorbic acid, *N*-acetylcysteine, and hyperbaric oxygen therapy.

Clinical Pearls

1. A history of the ingestion of wild mushrooms by anyone not expert in their identification should prompt suspicion of this problem.
2. A single "death cap" may contain enough toxin to kill an adult.
3. Cooking these mushrooms does not substantially alter their toxicity.

Associated Clinical Features

The jequirty pea (*Abrus precatorius*), also known as the rosary pea, belongs to a family of poisonous plants that contain toxalbumins. The chief toxin of the jequirty pea is abrin, which is structurally very similar to the toxin ricin of the castor bean. Ingestion of jequirty peas rarely results in toxicity, as a majority of the abrin lies within the hard shell of the pea. However, when the peas are chewed or the shell is digested, gastroenteritis usually occurs. Nausea, vomiting, abdominal pain, and diarrhea are common but in severe cases may be accompanied by hemorrhagic gastritis, seizures, arrhythmias, marked dehydration, CNS depression, and even death. Unfortunately, because of the colorful, attractive nature of the jequirty pea (Fig. 16.82), most cases of severe toxicity occur in the pediatric age group.

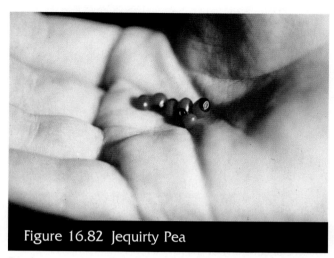

Figure 16.82 Jequirty Pea

Jequirty peas are also known as rosary peas, Indian beans, Buddhist's beads, crab's eyes, and prayer beads. They are about 5 mm in diameter and have a colorful glossy shell, usually red with a black center, although black and white may also be seen. (Courtesy of Kevin J. Knoop, MD.)

Differential Diagnosis

The differential diagnosis of jequirty pea ingestion includes any infectious or toxicologic cause of acute gastroenteritis.

Emergency Department Treatment and Disposition

Treatment of jequirty pea ingestion is largely supportive, as there is no specific antidote for abrin. In all cases, gastric decontamination is indicated and should include activated charcoal, gastric lavage, and whole bowel irrigation. In asymptomatic patients, decontamination, careful observation, and close follow-up is acceptable. With symptoms of toxicity, however, admission is recommended, as the potential for marked clinical worsening is present.

Clinical Pearls

1. Most jequirty pea ingestions are benign, as the vast majority of abrin toxin resides within the undigested shell of the plant.
2. Both toxalbumins, abrin in the jequirty pea and ricin in the castor bean, are structurally similar to botulinum toxin, cholera toxin, diphtheria toxin, and insulin.
3. The jequirty pea is found on a green vine native to India, but it can also be found in other tropical and subtropical areas such as the Caribbean and Florida.

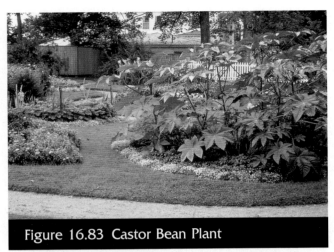

Figure 16.83 Castor Bean Plant

The castor bean plant is large and leafy; it may reach a height of 10 to 12 ft. (Courtesy of Alex Wilson.)

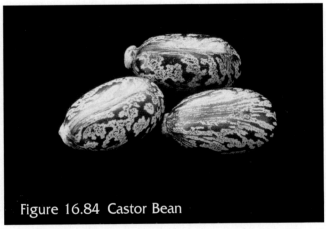

Figure 16.84 Castor Bean

Typical appearance of the castor bean. (Courtesy of Alex Wilson.)

Associated Clinical Features

Ricinus communis (castor bean) shares many similarities with its close neighbor the jequirty pea. Both are toxalbumin-containing plants; the chief toxin of the castor bean is ricin. As in the jequirty pea, most ingestions are not fatal because the toxin in the castor bean is located within the hard coats of the seeds (Figs 16.83 and 16.84). Three seeds are contained in each of the plant's brown capsules. Unless the shell is digested or chewed, ricin is not released and toxicity does not ensue.

When a toxic ingestion does occur, the clinical picture is very similar to that of jequirty pea ingestions, with nausea, vomiting, abdominal pain, and diarrhea developing in 1 to 3 h. Marked dehydration and hemorrhagic gastritis may occur in severe ingestions, but progression to death is uncommon, as ricin is poorly absorbed from the GI tract. Allergic reactions with anaphylaxis have been reported with handling of the seeds and are also seen among workers in factories where castor oil is produced.

Differential Diagnosis

The differential diagnosis of castor bean ingestion includes any infectious or toxicologic cause of acute gastroenteritis.

Emergency Department Treatment and Disposition

Treatment of castor bean ingestion is largely supportive, as there is no specific antidote for ricin. Gastric decontamination should be performed, including activated charcoal, gastric lavage, and whole bowel irrigation. In asymptomatic patients, decontamination, careful observation, and close follow-up is acceptable. With symptoms of toxicity, admission is recommended for further observation, as there is potential for marked clinical worsening.

Clinical Pearls

1. Like jequirty pea ingestions, castor bean ingestions are usually benign, as a vast majority of the toxin resides within the undigested shell of the plant.
2. The plant is commercially cultivated as a source of castor oil. Such oil has been used for centuries as a purgative and as a lubricant for machines.

Associated Clinical Features

Ascaris lumbricoides is a helminth that may cause crampy abdominal pain (Fig. 16.85). Exposure occurs through fecal contamination of food and water. Ascarides are commonly found in tropical climates such as Central America, South America, and Southeast Asia, although they are also endemic in the southeastern United States.

Presenting symptoms may include nonspecific abdominal pain and diarrhea. Migration into the biliary system through the ampulla of Vater or into the pulmonary tree may produce biliary colic and respiratory problems, respectively. Examination of the patient is often nonspecific, although an acute abdomen may occur if there is complete biliary or small bowel obstruction from a massive worm burden.

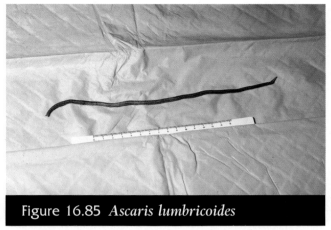

Figure 16.85 *Ascaris lumbricoides*

The helminth *Ascaris* after passage from the anus. (Courtesy of Bret T. Ackerman, DO.)

Differential Diagnosis

Other parasites that may cause diseases of the GI tract include *Giardia lamblia, Entamoeba histolytica,* and *Cryptosporidium. Strongyloides stercoralis* and the hookworms *Necator americanus* and *Ancylostoma duodenale* may produce similar abdominal symptoms.

Emergency Department Treatment and Disposition

The medications of choice for *Ascaris* include mebendazole, pyrantel pamoate, and albendazole.

Clinical Pearls

1. Microscopic examination of the stool often reveals the ova of *Ascaris.*
2. Pulmonary involvement of *Ascaris* is known as Loeffler syndrome.

CHAPTER 17

FORENSIC MEDICINE

William S. Smock
Lawrence B. Stack

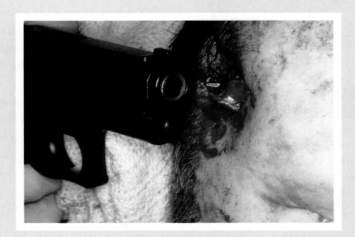

Associated Clinical Features

Gunshot injuries are classified as either entrance or exit wounds. Atypical wounds (grazing) may also be present. Physical findings in and around these wounds may offer evidence as to the actual mechanism, supporting or refuting the initial history given to the provider. As these findings may be transient, the emergency physician must be diligent in recognizing and documenting them at the time of presentation.

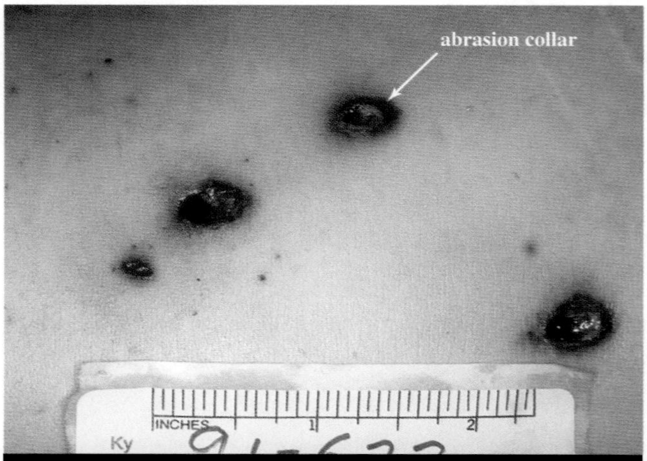

Entrance Wounds

Gunshot wounds of entrance are divided into four categories based on their range of fire: distant, intermediate, close, and contact. Range-of-fire is the distance from the gun's muzzle to the victim.

The size of the entrance wound bears no relation to the caliber of the inflicting bullet. Entrance wounds over elastic tissue will contract around the tissue defect and have a diameter much less than the caliber of the bullet.

Distant Wounds: The distant wound is inflicted from a range sufficiently distant that the bullet is the only projectile expelled from the muzzle that reaches the skin. There is no tattooing or soot deposition associated with a distant entrance wound. As the bullet penetrates the skin, friction between it and the epithelium results in the creation of an "abrasion collar" (Fig. 17.1). The width of the abrasion collar will vary with the angle of impact. Most entrance wounds will have an abrasion collar; however, gunshot wounds to the palms and soles are exceptions—there entrance wounds appear slit-like.

Intermediate-Range Wounds: Tattooing is pathognomonic for an intermediate-range gunshot wound and presents as punctate abrasions from contact with partially burned or unburned grains of gunpowder (Fig. 17.2). This tattooing cannot be wiped away. Clothing and hair, as intermediate objects, may prevent the gunpowder grains from making contact with the skin. Tattooing can, but rarely does, occur on the palms and soles owing to the thickness of their epithelium.

Tattooing has been reported with a range of fire as close as 1 cm and as far away as 4 ft. The density of the abrasions and the associated pattern will depend on the barrel length, muzzle-to-skin distance, type of gunpowder (ball, flattened ball, or flake), presence of intermediate objects, and caliber

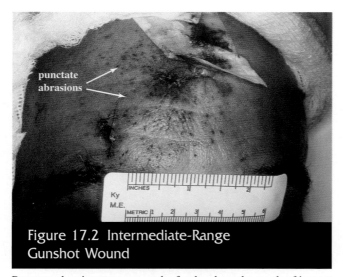

Figure 17.1 Distant Gunshot Wound

The elliptical abrasion collars associated with these gunshot wounds of entrance indicate that the projectile passed from right to left. The range of fire is classified as distant or indeterminate based on the lack of carbonaceous material or gunpowder tattooing. (Courtesy of William S. Smock, MD.)

Figure 17.2 Intermediate-Range Gunshot Wound

Punctate abrasions present on the forehead are the result of impact with unburned or partially burned gunpowder. This phenomenon is termed *tattooing.* Tattooing is pathognomonic for intermediate-range gunshot wounds. (Courtesy of William S. Smock, MD.)

of the weapon. Spherical powder travels farther and has greater penetration than flattened ball or flake powder.

Close-Range (Near Contact) Wounds: "Close range" is defined as the maximum range at which soot is deposited on the wound or clothing (Fig. 17.3) and typically is a muzzle-to-victim distance of 6 in. or less. On rare occasions, however, soot has been found on victims as far as 12 in. from the offending weapon. The concentration of soot will vary inversely with the muzzle-to-victim distance and its appearance will be affected by the type of gunpowder and ammunition used, the barrel length, the caliber, and the type of weapon.

Contact Wounds: A contact wound occurs when the barrel or muzzle is in contact with the skin or clothing as the weapon is discharged. Contact wounds can be described as tight, where the muzzle is pushed hard against the skin, or loose, where the muzzle is incompletely or loosely in contact with the skin or clothing. Wounds sustained from tight contact with the barrel can vary in appearance from a small hole with seared, blackened edges (from the discharge of hot gases and an actual flame) (Fig. 17.4), to a gaping, stellate wound (from the expansion of the skin from gases). Large stellate wounds are often misinterpreted as exit wounds based solely upon their size and without adequate examination of the wound.

In a tight contact wound, all materials—the bullet, gases, soot, incompletely combusted gunpowder, and metal fragments—are driven into the wound. If the wound is over thin or bony tissue, the hot gases will cause the skin to expand to such an extent that it stretches and tears. These tears typically have a triangular shape, with the base of the tear overlying the entrance wound. Larger tears are associated with ammunition of .32 caliber or greater or magnum loads.

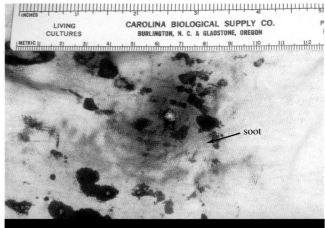

Figure 17.3 Near-Contact Gunshot Wound

The deposition of carbonaceous material or soot is seen on a T-shirt from a close-range gunshot wound. Clothing should be collected and placed in separate paper bags for transport to the crime laboratory. (Courtesy of William S. Smock, MD.)

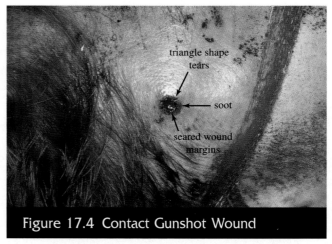

Figure 17.4 Contact Gunshot Wound

A contact gunshot wound from a 22-caliber handgun. (Courtesy of William S. Smock, MD.)

Stellate tears are not pathognomonic for contact wounds. Tangential wounds, ricochet or tumbling bullets, and some exit wounds may also be stellate in appearance. These wounds are distinguished from tight contact wounds by the absence of soot and powder within the wound. In some tight contact wounds, expanding skin is forced back against the muzzle of the gun, causing a characteristic pattern contusion called a *muzzle contusion* (Fig. 17.5). These patterns are helpful in determining the type of weapon (revolver or semiautomatic) used to inflict the injury and should be documented prior to wound debridement or surgery.

With a loose contact wound, where the muzzle is angled or held loosely against the skin, soot and gunpowder residue will be present in and around the wound (Fig. 17.6). The angle between

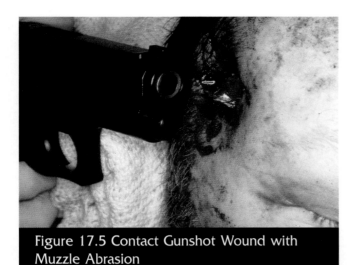

Figure 17.5 Contact Gunshot Wound with Muzzle Abrasion

A contact gunshot wound to the right temple with stellate tears, seared skin, soot deposition, and muzzle imprint. A muzzle abrasion or muzzle imprint on the patient's right temple was the result of the injection of gases into the skin, causing a rapid and forceful expansion of the skin against the barrel of this 9-mm semiautomatic pistol. (Courtesy of William S. Smock, MD.)

the muzzle and skin will determine the soot pattern. A perpendicular loose contact or near contact injury results in searing of the skin and deposition of the soot evenly around the wound. A tangential loose or near contact injury produces an elongated searing pattern and deposit of soot around the wound.

"Bullet wipe" is soot residue, soft lead, or lubricant, which may leave a gray rim or streak on the skin or clothing overlying an entrance wound (Fig. 17.7). This gray discoloration may also be found around the abrasion collar but is usually more prominent on clothing.

Exit Wounds

Determining whether a wound is an entrance or an exit wound should be based on the physical characteristics and physical evidence associated with the wound and *never upon the size* of the wound. Exit wounds are the result of a bullet pushing and stretching the skin from inside outward. The skin edges are generally everted, with sharp but irregular margins (Fig. 17.8). Abrasion collars, soot, searing, and tattooing are not associated with exit wounds. Soot can be seen at an atypical exit wound site if the entrance wound is close to the associated exit wound. Soot is propelled through the short wound tract and appears faintly on the exit wound surface.

Exit wounds assume a variety of shapes and appearances and are *not* consistently larger than their corresponding entrance wounds. The size of an exit wound is determined primarily by the amount of energy possessed by the bullet as it exits the skin and by the bullet's size, shape, and attitude. A bullet's usual nose-first attitude will change upon entering the skin to a tumbling and

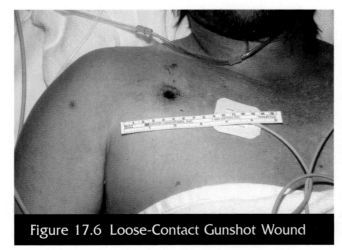

Figure 17.6 Loose-Contact Gunshot Wound

Self-inflicted contact wound to the right upper chest with a 9-mm handgun. The wound margins display searing and soot deposition. (Courtesy of William S. Smock, MD.)

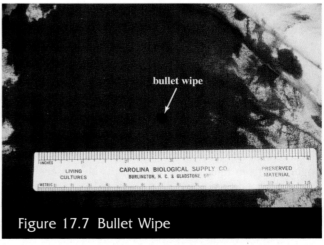

Figure 17.7 Bullet Wipe

"Bullet wipe" is residue and lead deposited on clothing or skin. The presence of this residue on clothing may help to determine whether the wound is an entrance wound. (Courtesy of William S. Smock, MD.)

yawing one. A bullet with sufficient energy to exit the skin in a sideways attitude or one that has increased its surface area by mushrooming may produce an exit wound larger than its entrance wound. Energy transferred to bone, with resultant ballistic fracture, may also result in a exit wound larger than the entrance wound (Fig. 17.9). A "false abrasion collar" or "shored exit" wound may mimic an entrance wound. This occurs when the epithelium is pressed against a supporting surface such as a floor, wall, chair, or firm mattress (Fig. 17.10).

Graze Wounds

Graze wounds are considered atypical and result from tangential contact with a passing bullet. The direction of the bullet's path is determined by careful wound examination. The bullet produces a trough with formation of skin tags on the lateral wound margins (Fig. 17.11). The base of these tags point toward the weapon and away from the direction of bullet travel.

Forensic Pearls

1. Distant-range gunshot wounds are inflicted from a distance greater than 4 ft and typically there is no tattooing, soot, or searing associated with the wound.
2. Intermediate-range gunshot wounds are inflicted at a distance from 1 cm to 4 ft and characteristically are associated with tattooing from burned and unburned gunpowder imbedded in the skin.

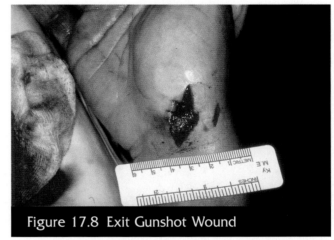

Figure 17.8 Exit Gunshot Wound

A stellate exit wound. Exit wounds may take on a variety of appearances. Stellate exit wounds should not be confused with contact wounds. The lack of soot and seared skin tells the physician that this is an exit wound. (Courtesy of William S. Smock, MD.)

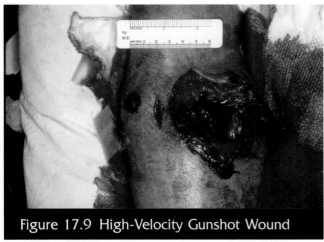

Figure 17.9 High-Velocity Gunshot Wound

A perforating high-velocity gunshot wound to a lower extremity. The gaping exit wound resulted from the transfer of energy from the projectile to the tibia. The impact propelled multiple bony fragments through the skin. (Courtesy of William S. Smock, MD.)

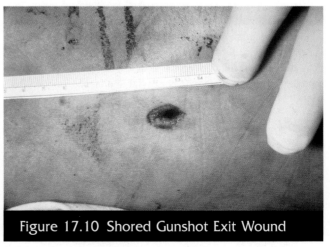

Figure 17.10 Shored Gunshot Exit Wound

A "shored exit" or "false abrasion collar" associated with a gunshot wound of exit. The false abrasion collar results when the skin is supported by a firm surface as the bullet exits. Shored exits occur when epithelium is pressed against a supporting surface (i.e., floor, wall, chair, or firm mattress). (Courtesy of William S. Smock, MD.)

3. Near or close-contact gunshot wounds are defined as the maximum range at which soot is deposited on the wound or clothing and typically occur at a distance of 6 in. or less.

4. Contact gunshot wounds (barrel is in contact with the skin or clothing at time of discharge) vary in appearance but frequently include triangular tears, searing, and gunpowder within the wound.

5. Abrasion collars, soot, searing, and tattooing are not associated with exit wounds.

6. Determination of whether a wound is an entrance or exit wound should be based on the physical characteristics of the wound and clothing and not on the size of the wound.

7. Emergency physicians should attempt to recognize, preserve, and collect short-lived evidence whenever the clinical situation allows.

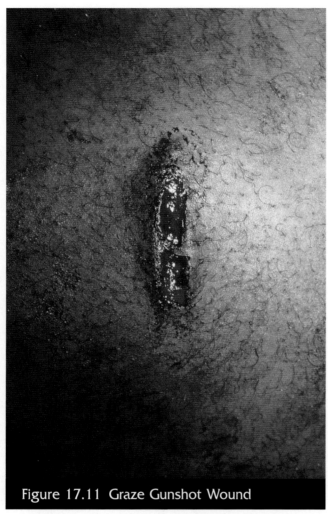

Figure 17.11 Graze Gunshot Wound

A superficial graze wound from a 9-mm projectile. Determining the directionality of a graze wound is difficult. The dark wound margins are the result of drying artifact and should not be confused with the deposition of soot. (Courtesy of William S. Smock, MD.)

Pattern Injuries of Domestic Violence, Assault, and Abuse

Every "weapon" (hand, belt, hot iron, knife, electrical cord, baseball bat, tire iron) leaves a mark, design, or pattern stamped or imprinted upon or just below the level of the epithelium. The imprints of these weapons are called *pattern injuries,* which are considerably reproducible. These injuries can be categorized into three major classifications according to their source: blunt force, sharp force, and thermal pattern injuries.

SHARP-FORCE-PATTERN INJURIES · DIAGNOSIS

Associated Clinical Features

There are two types of sharp-force injuries: incised and stabbed. The incised wound is longer than it is deep. The stab wound is defined as a puncture wound that is deeper than it is wide. The wound margins of sharp-force injuries are clean and lack the abraded edges of injuries from blunt forces. Forensic information can be gathered during the examination of a stab wound. Some characteristics of a knife blade, single- or double-edged, can be determined by visual inspection (Figs. 17.12 to 17.14). Characteristics such as serrated versus sharp can be determined if the blade was drawn across the skin during insertion or withdrawal from the victim. Serrated blades do not always leave these characteristic marks.

Forensic Pearls

1. Incised wounds are longer than they are deep.
2. Stab wounds are puncture wounds that are deeper than they are long.
3. Knife-blade characteristics (single or dual edged, serrated or smooth) can frequently be determined by visual inspection of the wound.

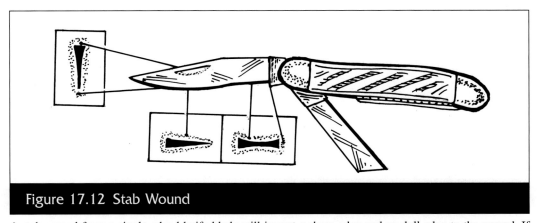

Figure 17.12 Stab Wound

A stab wound from a single-edged knife blade will impart a sharp edge and an dull edge to the wound. If the blade penetrates to the proximal portion of the blade, a contusion may result from contact with the hilt of the knife.

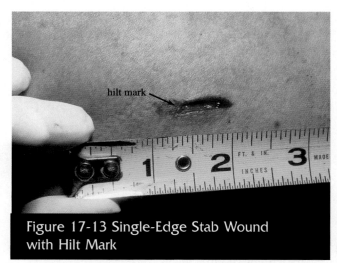

Figure 17-13 Single-Edge Stab Wound with Hilt Mark

A single-edged stab wound with a small hilt mark associated with the dull edge of the blade. (Courtesy of William S. Smock, MD.)

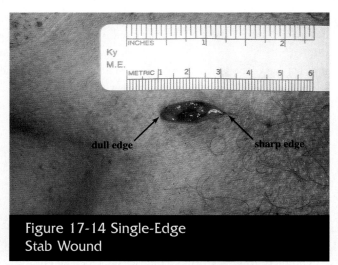

Figure 17-14 Single-Edge Stab Wound

A stab wound from a single-edged knife blade. The left side of the wound corresponds with the dull edge of the blade and the right side with the sharp edge of the blade. (Courtesy of William S. Smock, MD.)

Associated Clinical Features

The most common blunt force is the contusion (Fig. 17.15). The *pattern contusion* is a common injury that helps identify the causative weapon. A blow from a linear object leaves a contusion that is characterized by a set of parallel lines separated by an area of central clearing. The blood underlying the striking object is forcibly displaced to the sides, which accounts for the pattern's appearance. Pattern injuries that an emergency physician should recognize include those caused by the hand (slap marks, fingertip contusions, grab marks, choke holds, fingernail abrasions), solid objects (baseball bat, tire iron, 2 by 4, belt, shoe, comb), and bite marks (Figs. 17.16 to 17.18).

Other manifestations of blunt force trauma to the skin are the abrasion and the laceration. A weapon with a unique shape or configuration may stamp a mirror image of itself

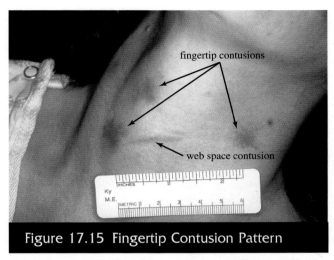

Figure 17.15 Fingertip Contusion Pattern

This patient exhibits fingertip contusions as well as a web-space contusion. These injuries are the result of being choked by her assailant's left hand. (Courtesy of William S. Smock, MD.)

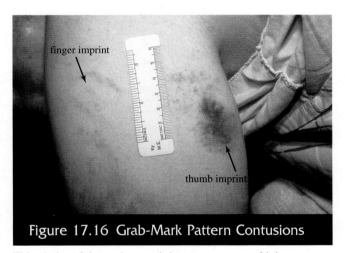

Figure 17.16 Grab-Mark Pattern Contusions

This victim of domestic assault has two patterns of injury present over the outer aspect of her upper arm. The contusion on the left reveals a central clearing bordered by two parallel lines, which is the result of forceful contact with an extended finger. The contusion on the right is the result of fingertip pressure applied by the thumb of her assailant. (Courtesy of William S. Smock, MD.)

This victim of assault presents with two pattern injuries. Diagonally oriented across both buttocks are pattern contusions with central clearing as well as parallel contusions. The vertically oriented contusions are the result of forceful contact as a blow was delivered with an open hand. The presence of these vertical contusions is virtually pathognomonic of inflicted injury. (Courtesy of William S. Smock, MD.)

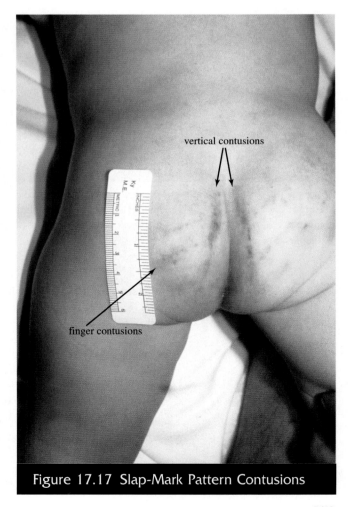

Figure 17.17 Slap-Mark Pattern Contusions

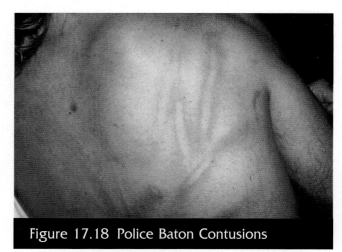

Figure 17.18 Police Baton Contusions

This patient sustained multiple blows from a police baton during his arrest. The central clearing bordered by two parallel contusions is indicative of impact with a rounded linear object. (Courtesy of William S. Smock, MD.)

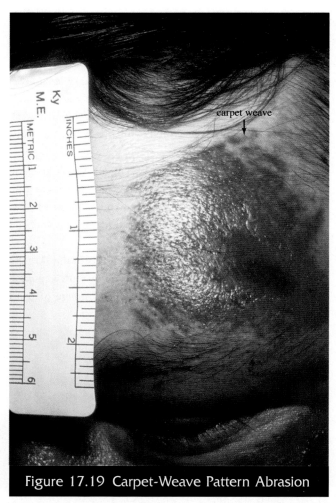

Figure 17.19 Carpet-Weave Pattern Abrasion

A pattern abrasion of the forehead from a domestic assault. The weave of the carpet is appreciated on the outer margins of the abrasions. This injury occurred when the patient's forehead was slammed into the carpet. (Courtesy of William S. Smock, MD.)

on the skin (Fig. 17.19). The presence of a subconjunctival hemorrhage may be suggestive of choking, strangulation, or suffocation.

Forensic Pearls

1. A contusion is the most common blunt-force injury pattern.
2. Blood underlying the force of the contusion is displaced to either side of the object, causing a *pattern contusion* in the shape of that object.
3. Emergency physicians must be able to recognize the pattern injuries caused by the hand, solid objects, and bites.

Associated Clinical Features

A thermal-pattern injury is a common form of abuse or assault, especially in children and the elderly. The detailed history of the incident should include the position of the patient relative to the thermal source. This will help determine whether the injury was inflicted or accidental. Pattern thermal injuries commonly encountered in the ED include *flat-iron burns, curling-iron burns, immersion burns,* and *splash burns* (Figs. 17.20 to 17.22). Immersion or dipping burns are characterized by a sharp or clear line of demarcation between burned and unburned tissue. In contrast, splash burns are characterized by an irregular or undulating line or by isolated areas of thermal injury, usually round or oval in shape, caused by droplets of hot liquid. The severity of the scald injury depends upon the length of the time the skin

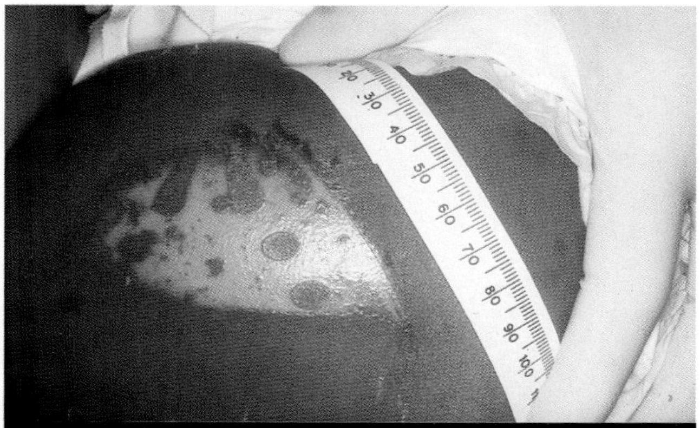

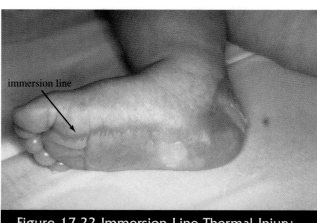

Figure 17.20 Clothes-Iron Thermal Injury Pattern

A thermal injury inflicted by an iron. The areas of sparing are associated with the iron's steam holes. (Courtesy of William S. Smock, MD.)

◄——— Superficial and partial-thickness burns were noted on the patient's anterior surface only. The areas of abdominal sparing indicate that the victim was flexed and curled at the time of injury. The child's caretaker, the mother's boyfriend, admitted to holding the child under a running hot-water tap. Partial-thickness burns on the penis and medial thighs are indicative of pooling of the liquid in those areas, resulting in a time-dependent injury. (Courtesy of William S. Smock, MD.)

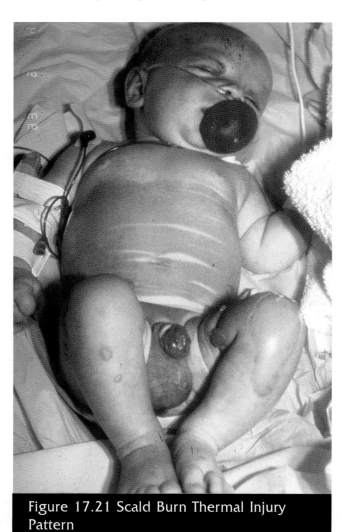

Figure 17.21 Scald Burn Thermal Injury Pattern

immersion line

Figure 17.22 Immersion-Line Thermal Injury Pattern

A classic "immersion line" is seen in a thermal-pattern injury. The line of demarcation is associated with the depth of the immersion. (Courtesy of William S. Smock, MD.)

was in contact with the offending substance and the temperature of the substance itself. Tap or faucet water causes full-thickness thermal damage in 1 s at 70°C, and 180 s at 48.9°C. Law enforcement agents routinely measure the household's or institution's water temperature in any investigation involving a scald injury of a child, a developmentally delayed person, or an elderly patient.

Forensic Pearls

1. A thermal-pattern injury is a common form of abuse seen in infants, institutionalized patients, and the elderly.
2. Emergency physicians must recognize thermal-pattern injuries of abuse.

CHAPTER 18

WOUNDS AND SOFT TISSUE INJURIES

Matthew D. Sztajnkrycer
Alexander T. Trott

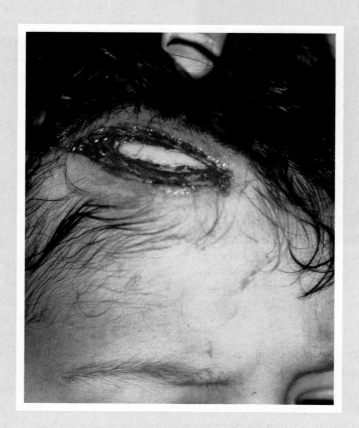

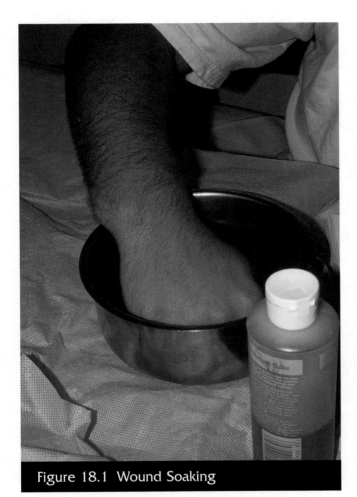

Figure 18.1 Wound Soaking

Soaking is an appropriate method for loosening debris and coagulated blood. While freeing the physician to perform other duties, soaking should never be used as a substitute for careful, thorough cleaning and irrigation. (Courtesy of Matthew D. Sztajnkrycer, MD, PhD.)

Associated Clinical Features

Wound cleaning and thorough irrigation are the most important steps in wound care in terms of reducing bacterial contamination and the subsequent risk for wound infection. Although they are time-consuming, failure to go through these procedures can result in infection or a cosmetically unacceptable scar.

Wound soaking (Fig. 18.1) is commonly used to loosen debris and coagulated blood. While soaking can assist in removing gross contaminants, it is not a substitute for irrigation. Irrigation is the most effective way to cleanse a wound of debris and contaminants as well as to reduce the bacteria count. Normal saline is the irrigation fluid of choice. An acceptable alternative is 10% povidone-iodine (Betadine) solution. When diluted to a 1% concentration (1 part per 10 parts saline), it can be safely applied to wounds while retaining its bactericidal activity.

Emergency Department Treatment and Disposition

Prior to wound cleansing and irrigation, the patient is made comfortable and given adequate anesthesia. It is prudent to have the patient lie supine so as to avoid possible vagally mediated responses to pain or the sight of wound manipulation. Gauze sponges soaked in 10% povidone-iodine solution diluted 1:10 to 1:20 may be used for cleansing the wound periphery. The sponges can be used for gentle mechanical scrubbing of a grossly contaminated wound. Cleansing continues until the area is visibly free from contaminants. Hair can be cleansed like skin and need not be removed unless it impedes the placement of sutures or staples. Removal of eyebrow hair is discouraged because of its slow or absent regrowth.

High-pressure irrigation is more effective than low-pressure irrigation in cleaning wounds. An 18- or 19-gauge intravenous catheter sheath or a commercially available splash shield, either attached to a 20- or 30-mL syringe, will generate a pressure stream of 5 to 8 psi (Figs. 18.2, 18.3). A typical bulb system's pressure stream is only 0.5 to 1 psi. The higher-pressure systems have been shown to decrease the risk of infection. Pulsatile irrigation systems, which can generate pressures of 50 to 70 psi, are effective in lowering bacteria counts and infection rates in large, grossly contaminated wounds, but they may cause trauma to wound margins. They offer no advantage for routine wounds cared for in the ED. Pulsatile irrigation is reserved for mutilating injuries, such as those caused by a lawn mower. Sustained high-pressure irrigation systems are associated with an increased incidence of wound infection.

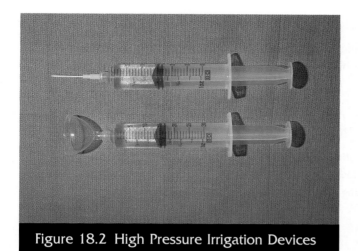

Figure 18.2 High Pressure Irrigation Devices

The ideal pressure for routine wound irrigation is 5–8 psi. This can be easily achieved through the use of a 20 to 30 cc syringe attached to a commercially available device with splash shield (top: Zerowet Splashshield, Zerowet, Inc, Palos Verdes Peninsula, CA), or an 18 or 19 gauge intravenous catheter sheath (bottom). (Courtesy of Matthew D. Sztajnkrycer, MD, PhD.)

It has been suggested that 500 to 1000 mL of irrigation fluid, or 60 mL/cm of wound length, should be used for most uncomplicated wounds. Debris that cannot be irrigated from the wound is either scrubbed or sharply debrided using iris scissors or a scalpel with a number 15 blade. The tissue should appear pink and viable, with a scant amount of fresh bleeding indicating good vascular supply.

Clinical Pearls

1. No matter how small the wound, universal blood and body fluid precautions, including gloves and face shield, should always be observed.
2. Antibiotics are no substitute for thorough wound cleansing and irrigation.
3. Povidone-iodine combined with an ionic detergent (Betadine scrub) is toxic to components of an open wound and is not recommended for wound irrigation or cleansing.
4. Shaving the eyebrow for wound repair is contraindicated, since hair in this area may not regrow.

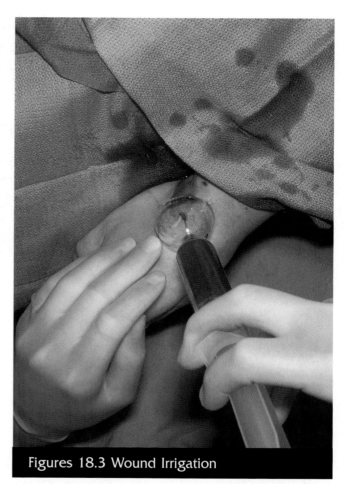

Figures 18.3 Wound Irrigation

After adequate anesthesia, an infected animal bite is opened and thoroughly irrigated using a 30 cc syringe and commercial splash shield. Note that even with the attached splash shield, there can be significant splatter and potential for body fluid exposure. Universal precautions should be followed at all times. (Courtesy of Matthew D. Sztajnkrycer, MD, PhD.)

Associated Clinical Features

All wounds require a thorough examination, including direct inspection and exploration. This can determine the presence of foreign bodies as well as injuries to nerves, tendons, blood vessels, joints, and other structures.

Emergency Department Treatment and Disposition

The patient must be comfortable for adequate wound exploration. Local or regional anesthesia is used, and the area is thoroughly cleaned and irrigated. Assess nerve function prior to anesthesia. The simplest way to control bleeding is by direct pressure. Should this fail, gauze moistened with 1:10000 epinephrine or tourniquets (Fig. 18.4) may be used for short periods. If epinephrine is used, the gauze should not be applied for longer than 5 min, and its use is contraindicated on fingers, toes, ears, the penis, and the nose tip.

Adequate exposure of the wound can be achieved with hemostats used to separate wound edges (Fig. 18.5). The hemostats are applied to the superficial fascia, not the dermis, as that might injure and further devitalize tissue. Small self-restraining devices, such as Wheatlanders retractors, can further assist in exposure. If exposure is still not ade-

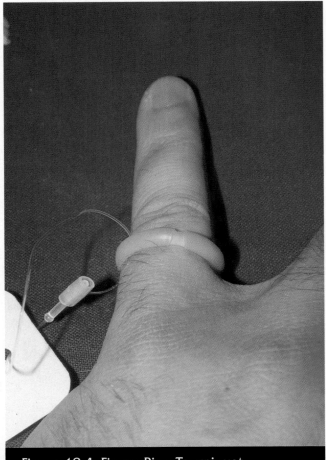

Figure 18.4 Finger Ring Tourniquet

The key to proper wound exploration is adequate hemostasis and subsequent exposure. The ring tourniquet is an effective means of hemostasis. Removal after the procedure is important to prevent finger ischemia and necrosis. Another effective method of hemostasis involves using a Penrose drain tightened with hemostats. (Courtesy of Matthew D. Sztajnkrycer, MD, PhD.)

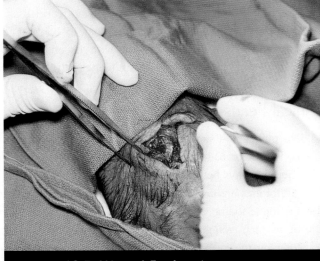

Figure 18.5 Wound Exploration

Once hemostasis has been obtained, in this case through the use of an inflated blood pressure cuff, the wound can be exposed and properly explored. Exploration reveals the two severed ends of an extensor tendon. (Courtesy of Matthew D. Sztajnkrycer, MD, PhD.)

quate despite hemostasis and separation, the wound margins may be slightly extended to allow better visualization. Extension is performed by using a scalpel with a number 15 blade or fine iris scissors. The wound is extended from one end, through the epidermis and dermis only, to avoid further injury to underlying structures. Once the superficial fascia has been exposed, it may be carefully and bluntly dissected using forceps or scissors.

Clinical Pearls

1. Scalp lacerations should be explored digitally to palpate for depressed skull fractures.
2. After functional testing, all wounds over tendons should be explored to determine tendon integrity. This examination should include visualization of the tendon through its range of motion, with particular attention to limb position at the time of injury. In the neutral hand position, a tendon laceration may be remote from the wound site.
3. Never probe a wound blindly or blindly attempt to control bleeding with hemostats.

Associated Clinical Features

Every foreign body has the potential to act as a nidus for infection and to impair wound healing. The majority of wound debris may be removed through meticulous, copious irrigation. However, direct visualization and removal with instruments may be required. Objects can either be inert (nonreactive) or organic (reactive). Examples of inert objects include bullets, needles, and metal objects. While these may cause chronic pain, they do not provoke an inflammatory response. Organic materials—such as wood, bone, stone, rubber, and soil—may cause infection and must be completely removed. The most common objects retained in hand wounds are, in decreasing order of frequency, wood splinters, glass fragments, metallic objects, and needles. Plain radiographs may be used to identify tooth fragments, metals, and most glass (Fig. 18.6). Ultrasound may play a minor role in wound foreign body identification, although it is not routinely practical. Direct inspection is the preferred method.

Differential Diagnosis

Apparent foreign bodies in wounds may represent open fractures, blood or fibrin coagulum, or neurovascular structures.

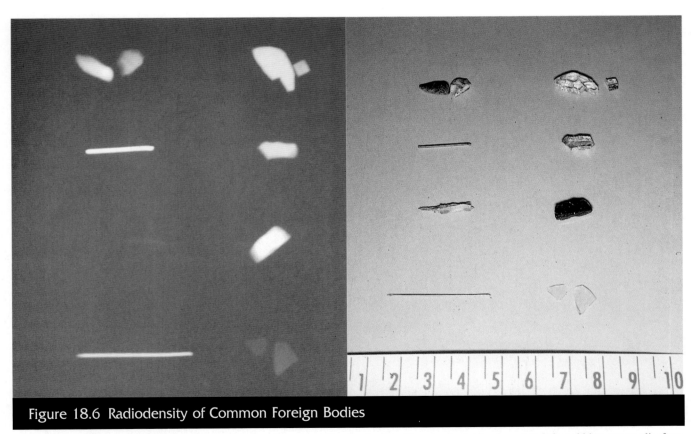

Figure 18.6 Radiodensity of Common Foreign Bodies

The plain radiograph demonstrates the radiodensity of common foreign bodies. Counterclockwise from top left: pebbles, paper clip fragment, wood splinter, hollow needle, lightbulb glass, dark ("beer bottle") glass, transparent glass, and automobile windshield glass. Note that, although faint, the wood splinter is visible on the plain radiograph. Ruler markings are in centimeters. (Courtesy of Matthew D. Sztajnkrycer, MD, PhD.)

Emergency Department Treatment and Disposition

Patient reliability in determining the presence of a foreign body is inaccurate in approximately half of all cases. Certain clinical situations should raise the suspicion of retained foreign bodies. These include lacerations caused by broken glass, perioral injuries in association with traumatic loss of dentition, and injuries to the hands and feet with needles, nails, or splinters. Prior to anesthesia, one may elicit a foreign-body sensation by gently running gloved fingers over the wound. After adequate hemostasis and anesthesia have been implemented, gentle probing of the wound with a hemostat will generate a distinct "grating" sensation in the presence of some foreign bodies. However, aggressive probing is discouraged. Good hemostasis cannot be overemphasized. Even small amounts of blood can impair exploration.

Suspicion of a retained foreign body mandates local wound exploration and the consideration of radiographic (Fig. 18.7) or ultrasound evaluation. Nearly 80% of objects can be identified on plain radiographs. More specifically, 95% of glass fragments greater than 2 mm in size can be identified through the use of plain radiographs; fragments as small as 0.5 mm can be identified in 50 to 60% of cases. Nonradiodense objects, including wood, chicken bones, and some plastics, may still be identified as filling defects or outlined by air drawn into the wound at the time of injury.

The decision to remove inert objects is based upon location and potential for subsequent tissue damage and functional limitation. Inert objects need not be removed and will frequently be encapsulated within soft tissue, causing no sequelae. While biologically inert, glass foreign bodies are frequently symptomatic and all but the smallest fragments should be removed. All organic objects have to be removed. Localization and retrieval of identified foreign bodies can be complicated, and time-consuming; consultation may be required.

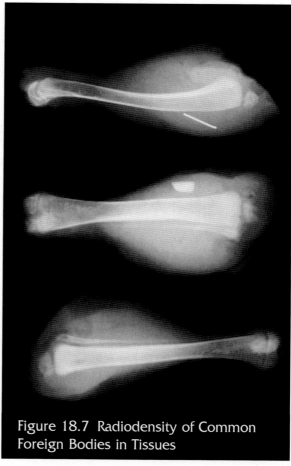

Figure 18.7 Radiodensity of Common Foreign Bodies in Tissues

The paper clip, dark glass, and wood splinter (*top to bottom*) described above were inserted into chicken legs and radiographs taken. The wooden splinter is no longer clearly visible within the soft tissue of the chicken. For purposes of foreign-body localization, a minimum of two radiographic views at 90 degrees to one another are obtained and the site of the foreign body entry clearly marked. (Courtesy of Matthew D. Sztajnkrycer, MD, PhD.)

Clinical Pearls

1. A thorough history of wound mechanism can alert the treating health care worker to the potential for a retained foreign body.
2. An alert patient often may be able to report a foreign-body sensation in the wound. This "feeling" should prompt thorough wound exploration and consideration of radiographs or ultrasound.
3. In attempting to locate an object with radiographs, the laceration is marked and two views of the area, at 90 degrees to one another, are obtained for proper spatial orientation. A paper clip taped to the wound edge is often used.
4. Missed retained foreign bodies are a very common source of litigation in emergency medicine.

Associated Clinical Features

Traumatic surface wounds are usually caused by one of three mechanisms: shearing, tension, or compression. Such a division helps to guide management decisions, predict the chance of infection, and determine the extent of eventual scar formation.

Shearing Injuries

These are caused by sharp objects, such as glass shards or knives; they generate a simple division of tissues (Figs. 18.8, 18.9). They are low-energy injuries, with minimal tissue destruction. The majority of uncomplicated shearing injuries (i.e., those not involving a neurovascular or other anatomically important structure) can be repaired primarily in the ED. They have a low incidence of wound infection; scar formation is usually minimal and cosmetically acceptable.

Puncture wounds are typically due to sharp, elongated objects that pierce the skin and penetrate into deeper tissues (Fig. 18.10). Such wounds have a higher potential for infection, foreign-body retention, or underlying structure injury.

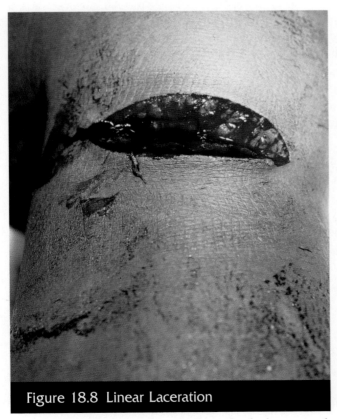

Figure 18.8 Linear Laceration

A large but uncomplicated linear leg laceration is demonstrated. Given the depth and gaping nature of the wound, it can be closed using a layered closure to remove surface tension at the wound edges and promote a more cosmetically acceptable outcome. (Courtesy of Alan B. Storrow, MD.)

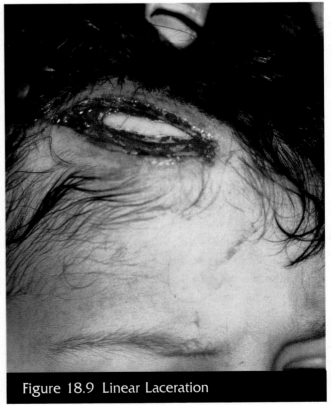

Figure 18.9 Linear Laceration

A long linear laceration involving the forehead and scalp, with exposed galea. The wound is explored and palpated for evidence of a depressed or open linear skull fracture. Closure of large galeal lacerations is recommended to prevent spread of infection. Large frontal galeal lacerations are also repaired to prevent a cosmetic deformity of the frontalis muscle. (Courtesy of Kevin J. Knoop, MD, MS.)

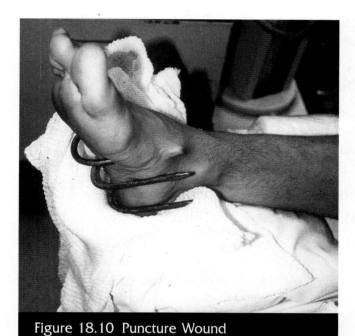

Figure 18.10 Puncture Wound

A puncture wound to the foot with a contaminated garden instrument. Tetanus status must be carefully addressed in such an injury. A radiograph of the foot demonstrated no associated bony injuries. (Courtesy of Matthew D. Sztajnkrycer, MD, PhD.)

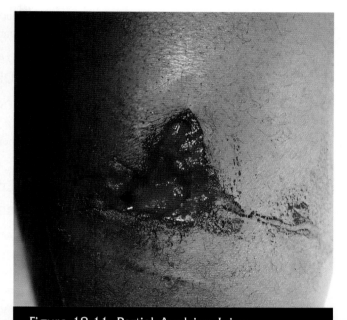

Figure 18.11 Partial Avulsion Injury

This patient has sustained a typical partial avulsion laceration from a fall onto the edge of a staircase. Note the triangular "flap" in the upper left quadrant of the wound. Closure of partial avulsion injuries must be particularly meticulous to reduce any further compromise of the flap tip's vascular supply. (Courtesy of Alan B. Storrow, MD.)

Tension or Partial Avulsion Injuries

These occur when objects strike the skin at a sharp angle, commonly generating a triangular flap (Fig. 18.11). A flap of this type results in vascular disruption to the two sides of the wound and thus is at risk for further compromise, ischemia, and necrosis. The energy required to generate such an injury is greater than that needed for shearing injuries; the result is greater tissue destruction and an increased potential for ischemia (Fig. 18.12). These two factors place the partial avulsion injury at increased risk for wound infection and scar formation. Care must be taken during examination and repair to preserve the remaining vascular supply to the flap; otherwise the flap may become ischemic. In addition, distal-based partial avulsion injuries are at an even greater risk for vascular compromise.

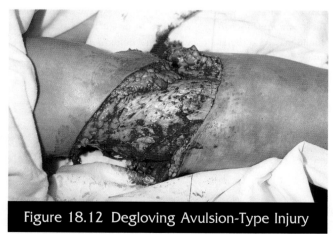

Figure 18.12 Degloving Avulsion-Type Injury

The patient sustained a complex degloving injury after her lower extremity became tangled in a rope while she was water-skiing. (Courtesy of Alan B. Storrow, MD.)

Crush or Compression Injuries

These occur when a blunt object strikes tissue at a right angle, imparting a high degree of kinetic energy. This force results in significant underlying tissue destruction of the skin and underlying supportive fascial layers. Crush injuries are typically ragged, with irregular wound edges and a complex

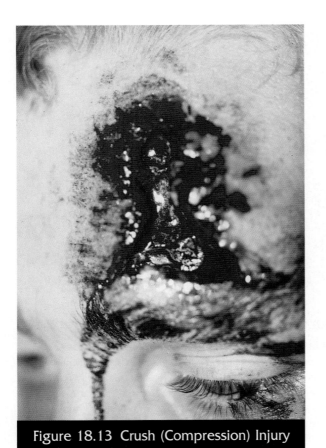

Figure 18.13 Crush (Compression) Injury

A fall from a bicycle has resulted in a complex stellate laceration, characterized by ragged, irregular wound edges. The potentially high forces involved in producing a crush wound may be sufficient to cause deeper damage. Computed tomography of the head unfortunately demonstrated a left frontal hemorrhagic contusion. (Courtesy of Matthew D. Sztajnkrycer, MD, PhD.)

laceration pattern (Fig. 18.13). Despite meticulous wound care and careful primary closure, the resulting scars may be cosmetically poor.

Differential Diagnosis

The differential for a traumatic wound includes other mechanisms of laceration: avulsion, partial or complete amputation, abrasion, hematoma, or contusion.

Emergency Department Treatment and Disposition

All patients with traumatic wounds, regardless of mechanism, should have their tetanus immunization status addressed (Table 18.1). The physical examination is directed to functional and neurovascular status. To obtain optimal wound healing, adequate hemostasis, thorough irrigation, removal of devitalized and contaminated tissues, and appropriate closure tension must be achieved. All wounds must be thoroughly inspected for the presence of foreign bodies and underlying injuries. Plain radiographs are appropriate to help rule out open fractures and may be useful in the identification of certain foreign bodies. If open fractures are suspected or confirmed, intravenous antibiotics are administered and an orthopedic surgeon is consulted. Repair of traumatic wounds depends on the depth, complexity, and location of the wound. Deep wounds are closed in layers or by using a vertical mattress technique to remove dead space and take tension off the wound. Superficial wounds may be repaired with staples, simple interrupted sutures, or running sutures. In certain circumstances, Steri-Strips or adhesive glues may be warranted.

Table 18.1

RECOMMENDATIONS FOR TETANUS PROPHYLAXIS

Tetanus Immunization Status	Clean, Minor Wounds		All Other Wounds[a]	
	Td	TIG	Td	TIG
Unknown or < 3 doses	Yes	No	Yes	Yes
> 3 Doses				
Last dose < 5 years	No	No	No	No
Last dose 5–10 years	No	No	Yes	No
Last dose > 10 years	Yes	No	Yes	No

Key: Td, tetanus-diphtheria toxoid; TIG, tetanus immune globulin (250 U).
[a] Defined as contaminated wounds, puncture wounds, avulsion injuries, burns, crush injuries.
Source: Adapted from Hollander JE, Singer AJ: State of the art: laceration management. *Ann Emerg Med* 1999; 34:356–367.

Clinical Pearls

1. Shearing injury is the most common wound mechanism seen in the ED.
2. The vascular supply to the flap is tenuous and improper closure may further compromise the tissue, especially at the tip. A repair using a corner stitch will help minimize further ischemia.
3. Crush injuries have an increased susceptibility to infection. Thorough cleansing, copious irrigation, and judicious debridement are required.

Associated Clinical Features

The ear is composed of a poorly vascularized cartilaginous skeleton covered by tightly adherent skin. There is little subcutaneous tissue, and an injury to the ear that results in hematoma formation can cause pressure necrosis of the cartilage, infection, loss of shape and stability, and a poor cosmetic outcome. The goal of repair in ear lacerations is complete coverage of exposed cartilage (Fig. 18.14) and evacuation or prevention of hematoma.

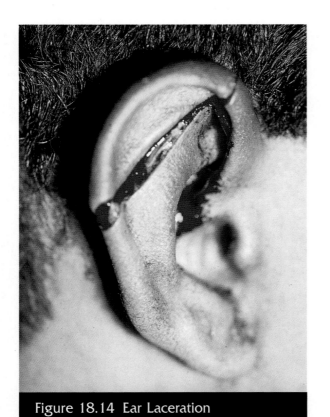

Figure 18.14 Ear Laceration

This patient has presented after sustaining an uncomplicated, linear laceration to the pinna. Closure must cover all exposed cartilage. (Courtesy of Alan B. Storrow, MD.)

Differential Diagnosis

In addition to simple lacerations of the ear, trauma to the ear may include abrasions, partial avulsions, soft tissue swelling, and perichondral hematomas.

Emergency Department Treatment and Disposition

Prior to laceration repair, the area is examined for signs of acute hematoma formation or other associated traumatic injuries. Hemotympanum or Battle's sign suggests the presence of a more serious closed head injury, especially basilar skull fracture. Blunt trauma may result in barotrauma to the eardrum, including perforation. Examination can be facilitated by local anesthesia infiltration or, in the case of larger or more complex lacerations, a field block.

Simple lacerations through the earlobe or involving the helix but that do not expose cartilage can be repaired with interrupted 6-0 nonabsorbable monofilament sutures. Simple lacerations that involve the cartilage are primarily repaired by ensuring complete coverage of the exposed cartilage by careful apposition of overlying skin. The skin generally provides sufficient support that no sutures are required for the cartilage itself. If the wound is irregular and cartilage debridement is required to avoid undue wound tension, the debridement is kept to a minimum. No more than 5 mm of cartilage can be removed or the cartilaginous skeleton may be deformed.

A perichondral hematoma must be drained within 72 h to prevent potential pressure necrosis and development of a "cauliflower" ear (see Figs. 1.26 and 1.27). Drainage is accomplished through a small incision directly over the hematoma and expression of coagulum. Ear wounds are best dressed with a mastoid pressure dressing either primarily or after later hematoma drainage. Such a dressing reduces the chances for future hematoma formation and its complications.

Ear sutures are removed in 3 to 5 days in children, 4 to 5 days in adults.

Clinical Pearls

1. Epinephrine-containing anesthetic agents are not to be used for ear lacerations.
2. Hematomas are rechecked in 24 h to evaluate for reaccumulation.

3. If cartilage has been exposed or a hematoma drained, antistaphylococcal antibiotic coverage is recommended.

4. Complex lacerations and hematomas of the ear are best cared for in conjunction with a consultant. (Fig. 18.15)

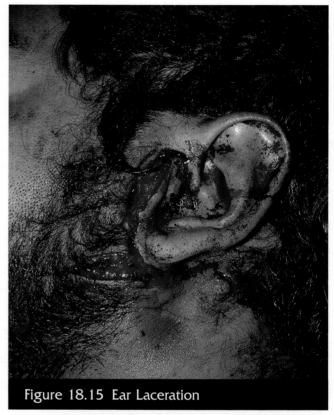

Figure 18.15 Ear Laceration

After being assaulted with a glass bottle, a patient presents to the emergency department with a complex ear laceration, involving the tragus and peri-auricular area. Care must be taken to evaluate important structures in the area, including the parotid duct and seventh cranial nerve. (Courtesy of Matthew D. Sztajnkrycer, MD, PhD.)

Associated Clinical Features

Lip lacerations may result in significant cosmetic defects if not properly repaired. The lip has two significant anatomic landmarks: the mucosal border, which divides intraoral and external portions of the lip, and the vermilion border, which separates the mucosa of the lip from the skin of the face. Another important anatomic structure of the lip is the underlying orbicularis oris muscle. Meticulous alignment of the vermilion border and its associated "white line" is the cornerstone of cosmetic repair. Lip anatomy may be distorted by the kinetic energy of the impact as well as the resultant edema surrounding the wound. Lacerations of the lip's vermilion border may be partial- or full-thickness, compromising the orbicularis oris.

Differential Diagnosis

Lacerations to the lip may not involve the vermilion border but may be limited to the mucosa or the intraoral portion. Facial lacerations in close proximity to the vermilion border may mimic a laceration that crosses the border. Other injuries—including abrasions, hematomas, and soft-tissue swelling—may initially mimic a vermilion border laceration.

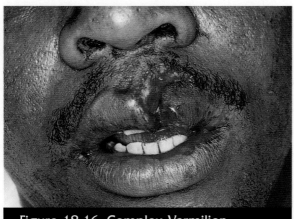

Figure 18.16 Complex Vermilion Border Laceration

After being assaulted, this patient sustained a large laceration through the vermilion border and the orbicularis oris muscle. Examination of the wound demonstrated an underlying fracture of the alveolar ridge with subluxation of the number 10 tooth. (Courtesy of Matthew D. Sztajnkrycer, MD, PhD.)

Emergency Department Treatment and Disposition

Given the high bacterial content of the oral cavity, lip lacerations will not remain clean during the repair. The goal of irrigation is to remove gross contaminants such as tooth fragments or dirt. If tooth fractures are noted, the wound must be explored for fragments. A radiograph may also prove useful for foreign-body evaluation. Anesthesia for laceration repair is best performed using either an infraorbital (upper lip) or mental (lower lip) nerve block. Local infiltration may further distort tissues and obscure the alignment of the vermilion border.

If the vermilion border is violated by a superficial laceration, then the first suture, typically 6-0 in size, is placed at the vermilion border to reestablish anatomic relationships (see Fig. 6.13). Once alignment is judged adequate, simple interrupted sutures are used for completion. If the laceration extends within the oral cavity, absorbable 5-0 sutures are used to close the intraoral component.

With deep or "through and through" lacerations involving the orbicularis oris (Fig. 18.16), the muscle layers are initially approximated with deep, usually 5-0, absorbable sutures. Once the muscle is approximated, the first skin suture is again placed at the level of the vermilion border and the repair is completed as described above.

Sutures are removed in 3 to 5 days in children, 4 to 5 days in adults. The patient is advised to eat soft foods, not to apply excessive force to the suture line, and to rinse after eating to prevent the accumulation of food particles.

Clinical Pearls

1. Misalignment of the vermilion border by as little as 1 mm may result in a cosmetically noticeable defect. Any repair of vermilion border lacerations should begin with alignment and suturing of this structure.
2. Regional anesthesia rather than local infiltration is optimal for repair, as it causes less distortion of the anatomic structures.
3. A marking pen may be used to identify landmarks prior to placing the sutures, as suturing itself causes some tissue edema, bleeding, and distortion.
4. Any patient with a lip laceration requires a thorough inspection of the oral cavity for associated trauma, including dental fractures, oral lacerations, and mandibular injuries.

Associated Clinical Features

Tendon injuries are often associated with lacerations to the hand or wrist. These injuries should be suspected either by the anatomic location of the laceration or when patients report an inability to flex or extend a digit or digits. A thorough neurovascular examination is critical to evaluate for associated injuries. Accurate assessment of motor function is necessary in any hand injury, although partial tendon injuries, including near complete (90%) tendon lacerations, may still result in normal mechanical function. Testing for strength might show diminished tendon function (Fig. 18.17), although function may be difficult to evaluate in the setting of an acute, painful injury. Any wound suspected of harboring a tendon laceration must be carefully explored in spite of normal testing.

Differential Diagnosis

In addition to tendon lacerations, trauma may generate partial tendon lacerations, trauma to the tendon sheath, or bony injuries including avulsion fractures. In cases of remote injury, the differential diagnosis also includes bony injury, tenosynovitis, and arthritis.

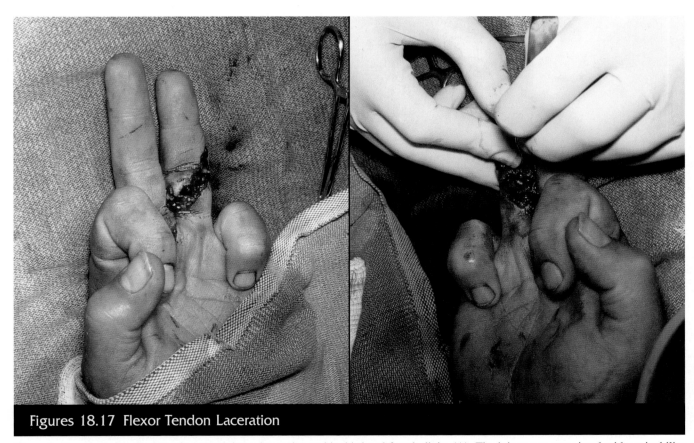

Figures 18.17 Flexor Tendon Laceration

The patient presented to the ED after sustaining a laceration to his third and fourth digits (A). The injury was associated with an inability to flex these two digits. Wound exploration revealed the distal segment of the transected flexor tendon apparatus (B). (Courtesy of Matthew D. Sztajnkrycer, MD, PhD.)

Emergency Department Treatment and Disposition

Prior to wound examination, a thorough examination of the extremity is performed to assess neurovascular and motor function. All individual flexor and extensor tendons are assessed, including deep and superficial flexor digitorum tendons. Abnormal resting posture of the involved extremity can indicate tendon injury. Tendons are taken through a full range of motion, including re-creation of limb position at the time of injury, in order to detect injuries along the length of the tendon. Adequate tendon exploration requires excellent hemostasis, which can be achieved through direct pressure or the brief use of a blood pressure cuff or other tourniquet.

Initial wound care should include irrigation, exploration for foreign bodies, debridement, antibiotics, and tetanus prophylaxis if indicated.

Partial tendon lacerations are treated conservatively, with splinting in neutral position and appropriate follow-up. Extensor tendon lacerations (Fig. 18.18) can be repaired primarily in the ED under limited conditions and in consultation with a specialist. Flexor tendon lacerations require consultation (Fig. 18.19).

Clinical Pearls

1. Tendon function may remain unaffected despite a near complete tendon laceration.
2. All wounds with potential tendon lacerations are carefully explored through a full range of motion in order to detect lacerations along the course of the tendon.
3. Flexor tendon lacerations are immediately referred to a hand specialist.

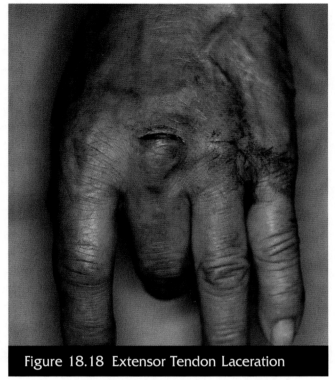

Figure 18.18 Extensor Tendon Laceration

Note the laceration over the third metacarpal head. Inability to extend the long finger is strong clinical evidence of complete disruption of the extensor tendon. (Courtesy of Kevin J. Knoop, MD, MS.)

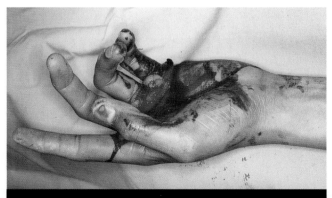

Figure 18.19 Flexor Tendon Laceration

This patient with a palmar laceration is unable to flex his index finger secondary to complete disruption of the flexor tendon. (Courtesy of Daniel L. Savitt, MD.)

Associated Clinical Features

Bites account for approximately 6% of all ED patients with traumatic wounds. Dog bites predominate (Fig. 18.20), at 60 to 80%, with cat bites accounting for another 5 to 15%. The frequency of human bites varies by institution but has been reported to range from 3.6 to 23%. Bite injuries are most likely to occur in children between age 5 and 14. The microbiology of bite wounds is frequently polymicrobial, but clinically relevant bacterial species include *Pasteurella* (*P. multocida, P. canis, P. dagmatis*), *Streptococcus, Staphylococcus, Moraxella,* and *Enterococcus.* The microbiology of human bites is more complex than that of cat and dog bites. *Eikenella corrodens* has been recovered from nearly 30% of all human bites, including 25% of all clenched-fist injuries. All mammalian bites are at risk for infection by anaerobic organisms such as *Fusobacterium, Bacteroides, Porphyromonas, Prevotella,* and *Peptostreptococcus*; human bites demonstrate the greatest risk of anaerobic infection.

A number of risk factors are predictive of bite wound complications and influence wound management strategies. Three quarters of these wounds in adults occur on the extremities, but the majority of wounds in children occur on the face and head. The hand is at highest risk for developing infection (30%), while the most resistant anatomic location is the face (1.4 to 5.8%).

Wounds caused by fangs, especially cat fangs that penetrate deeply into tissues, are associated with a high risk of infection. Large open wounds caused by shearing, as seen in the bites of dogs or larger animals (Fig. 18.21), are less likely to become infected. Superficial lacerations with minimal tissue disruption are associated with a low risk of infection regardless of species.

Emergency Department Treatment and Disposition

The management of bite wounds depends on location, wound type, severity, and signs of infection. Contusions and superficial abrasions may be treated with thorough cleansing, while larger

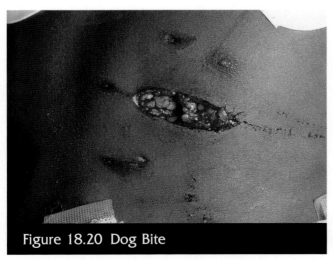

Figure 18.20 Dog Bite

An 8-year-old girl presented to the ED after being attacked by several dogs. She sustained multiple shearing lacerations to her chest and back. (Courtesy of Matthew D. Sztajnkrycer, MD, PhD.)

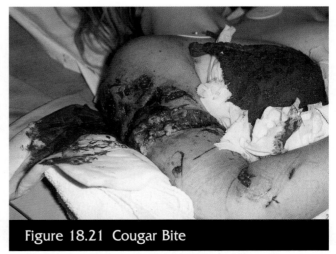

Figure 18.21 Cougar Bite

This patient has sustained large wounds as a result of a cougar attack. In contrast to the small penetrating injuries seen with house cat and small dog bites, the weight and force of large animals often results in shearing injuries. (Courtesy of Alan B. Storrow, MD.)

wounds that violate the epidermis and dermis require standard wound care protocols. All devitalized tissue must be thoroughly debrided to reduce the possibility of wound infection. Copious pressure irrigation after debridement is recommended. Radiographs are obtained to exclude bony injury or retained dentition. Appropriate cultures can be obtained in purulent wounds, although the polymicrobial results usually do not affect management.

Closure of dog bites is not recommended for wounds more than 8 to 12 h old, puncture wounds, hand lacerations, or high-risk wounds. Because of the excellent blood supply, bite wounds on the face may be considered for closure after 8 to 12 h. Cat bites and scratch wounds are best left open and treated with thorough irrigation and debridement. Large, easily irrigated human bites less than 12 h old on the trunk or a proximal extremity may be sutured with a single layer of nonabsorbable suture material. Facial bites without evidence of infection and less than 12 h old may likewise be closed. Other human bites should generally be left open and considered for delayed primary closure. Clenched-fist injuries are left open and managed in consultation with a hand specialist.

For established infections caused by cat and dog bites, empiric antibiotic therapy is started with broad-spectrum antibiotics such as ampicillin-sulbactam, cefoxitin, or ceftriaxone, alternatively, ciprofloxacin and clindamycin can be used. In children, trimethoprim-sulfamethoxazole may be substituted for ciprofloxacin. Infection by *P. multocida* classically starts within 24 h of the bite, is marked by prominent pain and swelling, and is associated with a serosanguineous gray exudate. The antibiotic of choice for *Pasteurella* is penicillin; doxycycline is an alternative. Antibiotics are used for nearly all bite wounds, although the efficacy of this approach has not been substantiated. Amoxicillin-clavulanate or dicloxacillin plus penicillin are suggested regimens to cover typical skin flora and *Pasteurella* species.

Clinical Pearls

1. Fang puncture wounds may be carefully widened using a number 15 scalpel blade to improve irrigation. The incised wound is left open to close by secondary intention.
2. All patients with bite wounds from susceptible animals are assessed for rabies exposure as well as tetanus status.
3. Given cosmetic concerns and low infection risk, dog bites to the face can be sutured even after 8 to 12 h.
4. Although rare, a potentially fatal cause of dog-bite infection is *Capnocytophaga canimorsus* (CDC group DF-2), a gram-negative rod. Patients with this infection are often immunocompromised or asplenic and may present with sepsis and disseminated intravascular coagulation. The recommended antibiotic for treatment is amoxicillin-clavulanate.

Associated Clinical Features

Because of their design and nature, accidental impalement with fishhooks poses problems with removal. Often, the hook cannot be removed by the patient because of the barbs. Several different methods have been described to remove fishhooks (Fig. 18.22).

Emergency Department Treatment and Disposition

The wound is thoroughly cleaned and irrigated. Tetanus status is determined. After adequate anesthesia has been obtained, several different removal methods may be employed depending upon the location and type of hook.

Superficially embedded hooks or hooks with small barbs may be removed in a retrograde fashion, by backing the hook out through the original site of penetration. A small incision is frequently required in line with the concavity of the fishhook. A technique utilizing string has also been described. The string should have good tensile strength, such as 0-silk or umbilical tape. The string is looped around the curved portion of the hook and then carefully and gently pulled in a direction parallel to and away from the shaft of hook. At the same time, the shaft and eye-

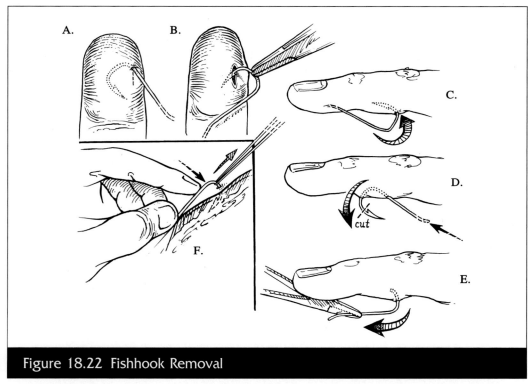

Figure 18.22 Fishhook Removal

Hooks with small barbs that are only superficially embedded may be carefully backed out through the original puncture site (A and B). This may require a small incision, made in line with the concavity of the curve of the hook. The push-through technique is useful for hooks with large barbs or those more deeply embedded. The hook is pushed out through the skin, the barb removed, and the remainder of the hook subsequently removed through the original penetration site (C, D, and E). The traction (string) technique provides an alternative for removing hooks with small barbs. While pressing down on the shaft of the hook, traction is applied with 0 silk or umbilical tape. A swift yank of the cord in the direction opposite the barb will dislodge the hook (F). Care is taken to warn bystanders of the potential for the fishhook to fly across the room.

let are depressed against the skin and slightly rotated to disengage the barbs. The string is then sharply pulled, releasing the hook. This technique has the advantage of not requiring anesthesia.

The most common and successful removal technique is the "push-through and cut" technique. This is recommended for deeply embedded hooks or hooks with large barbs. Basic skin preparation and local wound infiltration are performed in the standard manner. The hook shaft is manipulated with a hemostat in order to push the hook and barbs through the dermis (Fig. 18.23). The end of the hook and barb is removed with wire cutters and the shaft is backed out through the wound.

Clinical Pearls

1. Thorough irrigation and debridement of devitalized tissue is necessary after removal of the fishhook.
2. Hooks embedded in cartilaginous structures, such as the ear or nose, are best managed with the push-through methods.
3. Hooks that penetrate joint spaces are removed with the push-through technique, as fine barbs may break off with the retrograde technique. These wounds should be managed in consultation with an orthopedic surgeon.
4. Fishhooks that penetrate the globe of the eye are left in place and emergent ophthalmologic consultation obtained. The patient is placed in the semirecumbent position to decrease intraocular pressure and the globe is protected with an eye shield. Pressure patches are contraindicated, as they may extrude intraocular contents.

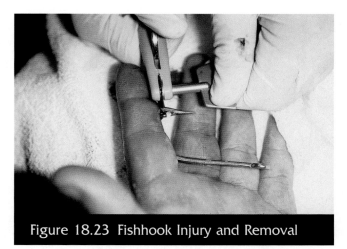

Figure 18.23 Fishhook Injury and Removal

A patient presented to the ED with a fishhook embedded in his finger. The push-through technique was used to remove the hook. Use of a ring cutter proved unsuccessful; a bolt cutter was eventually required to remove the distal portion of this large hook. (Courtesy of Alan B. Storrow, MD.)

Associated Clinical Features

The majority of wounds seen in the ED are uncomplicated lacerations generated from shearing or flap injuries and are readily amenable to primary wound closure. Each wound will have different technical factors that influence the repair. The cornerstones of wound closure are layer matching, wound edge eversion, and prevention of excessive wound edge tension.

In repairing any laceration, it is important to suture individual layers to their counterparts (e.g., superficial fascia to superficial fascia). Failure to do so may result in improper healing and poor cosmetic results. Wound edge eversion is equally important in the initial repair, as scars have a tendency to contract over time. Everted wounds flatten with scar maturation, while noneverted wounds contract into linear pits, with resultant poor cosmetic results (Figs. 18.24, 18.25).

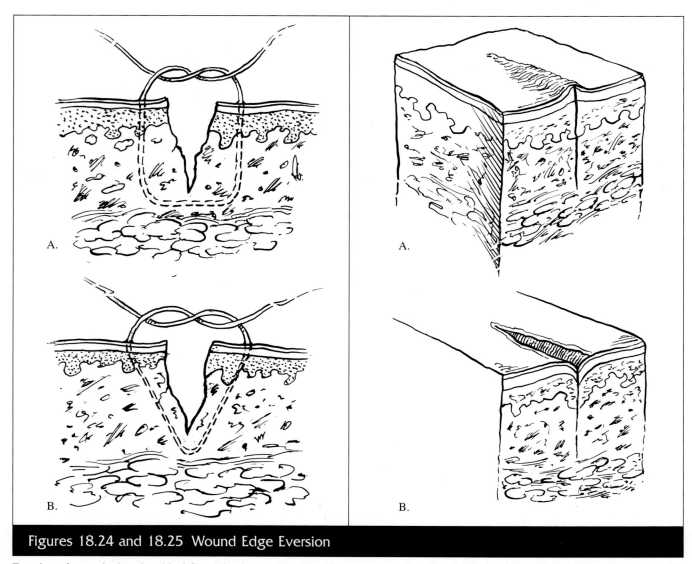

Figures 18.24 and 18.25 Wound Edge Eversion

Eversion of wound edges is critical for optimal wound healing. For proper eversion, the needle point should enter the epidermis at a 90-degree angle, generating a square or bottle-shaped suture configuration 18.24A. This results in a slight rise of the skin edges above the skin plane 18.25A. Such eversion will flatten at the level of the skin plane during healing. Entry at a shallower angle 18.24B often leads to wound edge inversion, eventual contraction of the wound edges below the skin plane, and subsequent scar formation 18.25B.

The repair of any wound will place a degree of tension upon the wound. Excessive wound tension by the sutures may result in impaired capillary blood flow to the healing wound, with possible necrosis and a cosmetically unacceptable scar. The first suture throw is critical in determining the amount of tension on the wound. When brought together, wound edges should just touch and be slightly everted, as wound edges tend to become slightly edematous after repair.

Emergency Department Treatment and Disposition

All laceration repairs should begin with a thorough evaluation. Tetanus status is addressed. Different wound closure techniques include simple interrupted sutures, staples, running sutures, dermal sutures, tissue adhesives, and tape (Steri-Strips). Suture material, size, and duration before removal are determined by the anatomic site of the wound (Table 18.2). Use of deep, absorbable sutures may be necessary to reduce wound tension before superficial repair (Fig. 18.26).

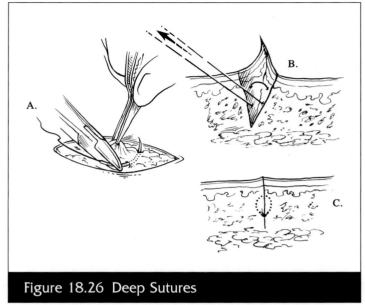

Figure 18.26 Deep Sutures

Judicious placement of deep sutures allows approximation of the dermis, reduces tension on the wound edges, and may facilitate final superficial closure. The needle is driven from deep within the wound to a superficial level (A). On the opposite side of the wound, the needle is driven from superficial to deep (B). By having the leading and trailing suture come out on the deep side *and* on the same side of the superficial cross suture (B). The resultant knot is buried within the wound (C).

Table 18.2

SUTURE MATERIALS, SIZE, AND DURATION BY ANATOMIC SITE

Anatomic Site	Skin	Deep	Duration
Scalp	5-0, 4-0 Monofilament	4-0 Absorbable	6–8 days
Ear	6-0 Monofilament	N/A	4–5 days
Eyelid	7-0, 6-0 Monofilament	N/A	4–5 days
Eyebrow	6-0, 5-0 Monofilament	5-0 Absorbable	4–5 days
Nose	6-0 Monofilament	5-0 Absorbable	4–5 days
Lip	6-0 Monofilament	5-0 Absorbable	4–5 days
Oral mucosa	N/A[a]	5-0 Absorbable	N/A
Face/forehead	6-0 Monofilament	5-0 Absorbable	4–5 days
Chest/abdomen	5-0, 4-0 Monofilament	3-0 Absorbable	8–10 days
Back	5-0, 4-0 Monofilament	3-0 Absorbable	12–14 days
Arm/leg	5-0, 4-0 Monofilament	4-0 Absorbable	8–10 days
Hand	5-0 Monofilament	5-0 Absorbable	8–10 days[b]
Extensor tendon	4-0 Monofilament	N/A	N/A
Foot/sole	4-0, 3-0 Monofilament	4-0 Absorbable	12–14 days

[a] Not applicable.
[b] Add 2 to 3 days for joint extensor surfaces.
Source: Adapted from Trott AT: *Wounds and Lacerations: Emergency Care and Closure,* 2d ed. St. Louis, MO: Mosby–Year Book, 1997.

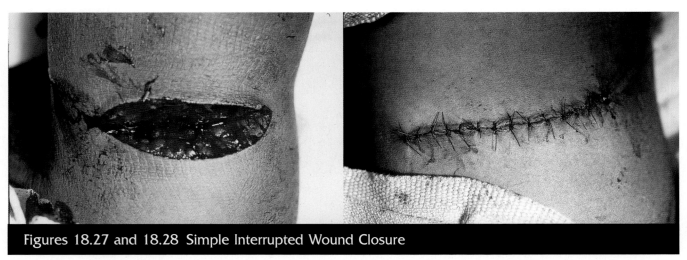

Figures 18.27 and 18.28 Simple Interrupted Wound Closure

An uncomplicated linear laceration generated by a sharp object. For anesthesia and hemostasis, the wound edges are infiltrated with lidocaine containing epinephrine. The wound is subsequently closed with simple interrupted sutures. Attention is paid to obtaining a degree of wound edge eversion. (Courtesy of Alan B. Storrow, MD.)

Simple Interrupted Closures

This closure involves single nonabsorbable sutures, each independently tied (Figs. 18.27, 18.28). They can provide excellent wound edge approximation and are the most common type of wound closure used in the ED.

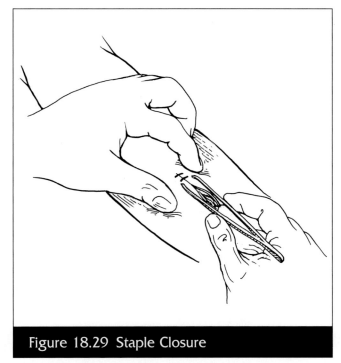

Figure 18.29 Staple Closure

Meticulous care must be taken when using staples to properly approximate and evert wound edges. This can be facilitated through the use of forceps during staple closure.

Staples

Studies have demonstrated that staples, a rapid means of closing linear wounds, engender less inflammatory response, resist infection more effectively, and generate greater wound tensile strength than sutures. Staples are best utilized in repairing linear, sharp lacerations of the scalp, trunk, and extremities (Fig. 18.29). Staples are not used on the face, over joints, or on the hands or feet.

Running Closure

This rapid closure technique involves taking several bites along the length of a wound without tying individual knots. Knots are tied only at the beginning and end. This method is most useful for superficial linear lacerations greater than 5 cm in length. Particular care must be taken to achieve equal wound tensions with each bite. Proper wound eversion may be difficult.

Dermal Closures

Also known as the subcuticular closure, this technique involves the use of absorbable sutures placed in the superficial fascia and dermis, with the knot buried in the wound.

The dermal closure may be achieved using either simple interrupted or running techniques. When properly performed, it provides excellent cosmetic results and avoids the need for suture removal.

Wound Adhesives

Cyanoacrylate adhesives have advantages in wound closure because of speed of closure, reported low infection rate, lack of repeat visit for suture removal, and no anesthesia requirement. Wounds closed using adhesives are at increased risk of immediate dehiscence, but no difference in tensile strength has been reported at 7 days. The wound edges must be approximated during application; thus two operators may be required for optimal closure. Proper application requires considerable practice in technique.

Clinical Pearls

1. In order to obtain proper wound edge eversion, the point of the needle should generally enter the epidermis and dermis at a 90-degree angle before it is brought around through the tissue.
2. The bites on both sides of a wound should be equidistant for both optimum wound healing and cosmetic outcome.
3. In gaping wounds, surface tension may be reduced with the use of deep sutures. The minimum number of such sutures is used because they may act as a foreign body and a potential nidus for infection. Deep sutures also stimulate a greater healing response and may therefore generate a larger final scar.
4. Use of cyanoacrylate wound adhesives does not obviate the need for good wound care, including thorough irrigation and exploration. Local or regional anesthesia may still be required.

Associated Clinical Features

Although the majority of lacerations can be managed by using simple wound closure techniques, certain lacerations require more advanced techniques. These include the horizontal and vertical mattress stitch and the corner stitch.

Emergency Department Treatment and Disposition

The *vertical mattress suture* is a useful technique for generating wound edge eversion, particularly in deep wounds (Fig. 18.30). The suture is performed by first taking a large tissue bite through the fascial layer approximately 1 to 1.5 cm from the wound edge and crossing equidistant to the other wound edge. The needle is then reversed and a second small bite through the epidermal-dermal junction 1 to 2 mm from the wound edge is taken. This suture has several additional advantages. It acts as both a deep and superficial closure, thereby reducing wound tension. It is particularly useful in areas of marked skin laxity, such as the dorsum of the hand.

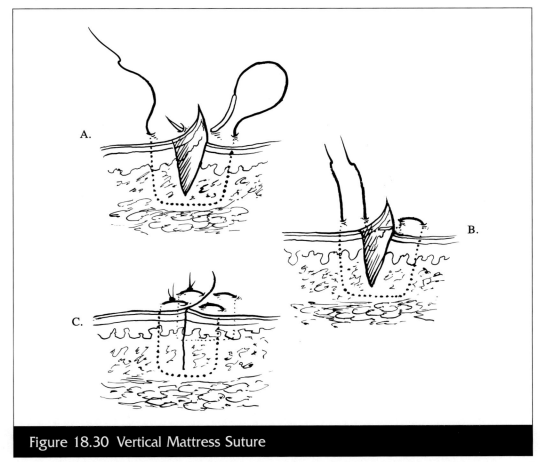

Figure 18.30 Vertical Mattress Suture

The suture is placed by first taking a large deep bite of tissue approximately 1 cm away from the wound edge and exiting at the same location on the other side of the wound. A second small superficial bite is then performed in the reverse direction (A). When the bites are complete (B), tying results in nice apposition of the wound edges (C). This technique is especially useful in areas of lax skin, such as the elbow or dorsum of the hand.

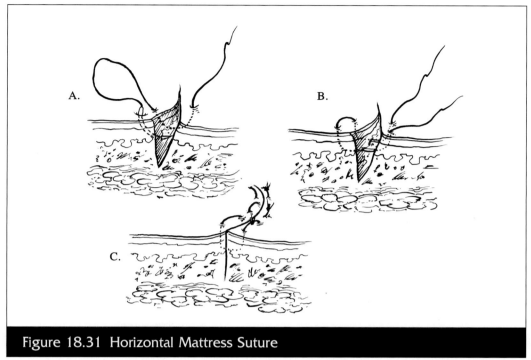

Figure 18.31 Horizontal Mattress Suture

Useful in achieving wound edge eversion, the horizontal mattress suture begins with a standard suture throw. A second bite is taken approximately half a centimeter from the first exit (A) and brought through at the original starting edge, half a centimeter from the original entry point (B and C).

The *horizontal mattress suture* may also be used to optimize wound edge eversion (Fig. 18.31). With this suture, the needle is introduced through the skin in the standard manner for a simple interrupted stitch. Rather than tie the knot at this point, a second bite is taken approximately 5 mm from the first. The knot is subsequently tied on the side of the initial bite. As well as causing wound edge eversion, this technique is particularly useful in areas under significant tension, such as the knee.

Many wounds result in the generation of jagged irregular wound margins, with triangular corners or small flaps. These wounds have tenuous vascular supplies, and improper suturing may further compromise the viability of the tissue. A common technique for securing the triangular corner of a wound without further compromising the small capillary beds is the *corner stitch* (Figs. 18.32, 18.33, 18.34). The technique is effectively a half-buried mattress suture, where the needle is initially introduced through the skin in the noncorner area of the wound. The needle is brought out through the dermis and then passed horizontally through the dermis of the triangular portion of the wound. It is then

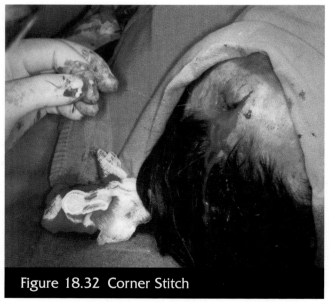

Figure 18.32 Corner Stitch

Flaps generated by partial avulsion injuries must be repaired with care to avoid compromising the tenuous blood supply of the flap. A corner stitch is an excellent technique that can solve many tricky wound problems. (Courtesy of Matthew D. Sztajnkrycer, MD, PhD.)

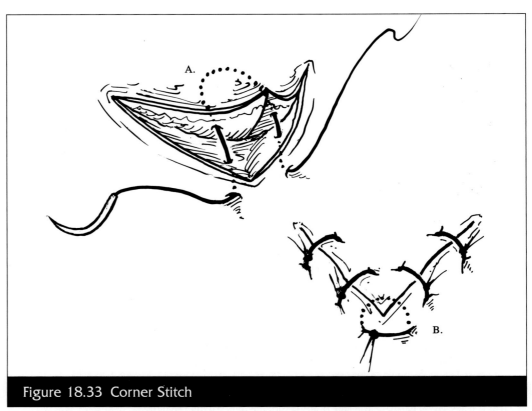

Figure 18.33 Corner Stitch

The corner stitch is performed through the use of a half-buried horizontal mattress suture. The suture begins percutaneously away from the corner of the wound. The suture needle is then brought horizontally through the corner at the level of the dermis and back out through the epidermis at the opposite noncorner portion of the wound (A). This technique avoids placing suture material near the apex of the flap (B).

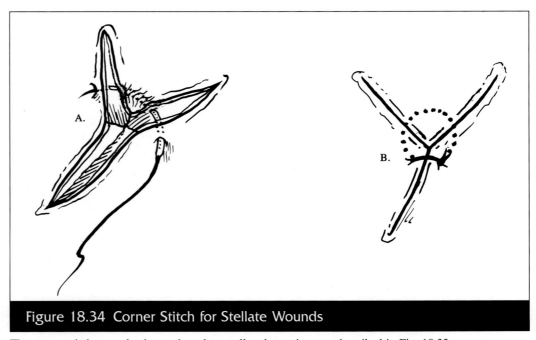

Figure 18.34 Corner Stitch for Stellate Wounds

The corner stitch may also be used to close stellate lacerations, as described in Fig. 18.33.

brought through the dermis on the other portion of the wound and out through the opposite non-corner area, where the knot is tied. Once the corner is secured, simple sutures are used to repair the rest of the wound, with care taken to place the sutures far enough from the tip to optimize circulation.

Clinical Pearls

1. Utilization of a mattress suture can aid in wound edge eversion, dead space removal, and tension reduction.
2. A single corner stitch may be used to close several corners of a stellate wound. The corner stitch is one of the most useful techniques in the ED management of complex wounds.

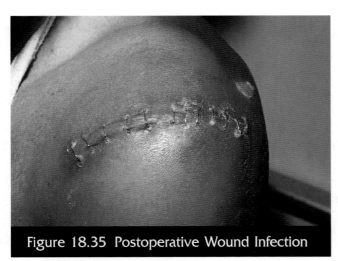

Figure 18.35 Postoperative Wound Infection

The patient presented to the ED with increasing pain and redness at the site of his staple closure. The area was erythematous, tender, and warm and had scant purulent drainage around some of the staples. (Courtesy of Matthew D. Sztajnkrycer, MD, PhD.)

Associated Clinical Features

Despite appropriate and meticulous care, all wounds are subject to three main complications: infection, dehiscence, and hypertrophic scar formation. Nearly all wounds evaluated in the ED have occurred under nonsterile conditions and should be considered contaminated. Disruption of the epidermis allows a portal of entry for skin flora, while contaminants may harbor microorganisms. Bacterial concentrations vary depending upon the anatomic location; the highest epidermal bacterial concentrations are found on the scalp, axillae, mouth, feet, nail folds, and perineum. A key factor in determining bacterial concentration in the wound is time elapsed until presentation. Wounds should therefore be thoroughly cleaned and irrigated in a timely manner following presentation. Wound infection is suggested by pain, warmth, erythema, edema, and purulent drainage from the wound site (Fig. 18.35).

Wound healing occurs via a structured process of epithelialization, neovascularization, collagen synthesis, wound contraction, and remodeling. New collagen fibril synthesis occurs by day 2, and peak synthesis occurs by day 5 to 7. Damaged collagen is subsequently degraded by proteolytic enzymes and replaced with the newly synthesized collagen. A nadir in wound strength occurs between days 7 and 10; during this weakest point, which frequently coincides with suture removal, the wound is at risk for dehiscence (Fig. 18.36) or breakdown. Factors that may contribute to wound dehiscence by impairing wound healing include infection, drugs (especially corticosteroids), foreign bodies, advanced age, poor nutritional status, diabetes mellitus, and peripheral vascular disease.

At the opposite extreme to wound dehiscence, wound healing may occur in an exaggerated manner, resulting in hypertrophic scars and keloid formation (Fig. 18.37). Hypertrophic scars are the result of excessive collagen deposition within the borders of the original wound, generating excessive scar bulk. These wounds occur at areas of increased tissue stress. Keloids represent inappropriate scarring that extends beyond the boundaries of the original wound. While keloids are most commonly described in the African-American population, they may occur in any darkly pigmented skin areas.

Emergency Department Treatment and Disposition

Sutures and staples represent foreign bodies within the wound and generate varying degrees of inflammatory reaction. Local wound infections are treated with suture removal and thorough irrigation and drainage as well as possible radiographic and visual exploration of the wound for missed foreign bodies. A 7-day course of a first-generation cephalosporin or antistaphylococcal penicillin is appropriate for most infections. For animal bites, other antibiotics may be more appropriate. More advanced wound infections, including those with evidence of lymphangitic streaking and systemic toxicity, should be managed with parenteral antibiotics.

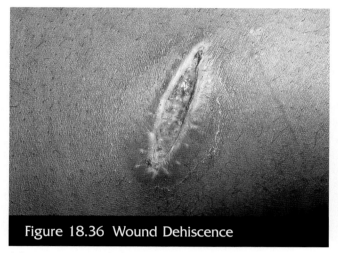

Figure 18.36 Wound Dehiscence

After suture removal, the patient returned to the ED. The wound had dehisced but had a clean base of granulation tissue. The wound was allowed to close by secondary intention. (Courtesy of Alan B. Storrow, MD.)

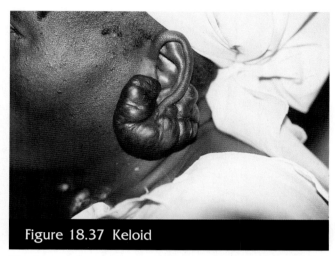

Figure 18.37 Keloid

The degree of excessive scar bulk extending beyond the original wound margins may be dramatic and cosmetically significant. (Courtesy of Thea James, MD.)

Wound dehiscence is treated conservatively by treating the underlying causes and allowing healing via secondary intention. Dehiscence of wounds in cosmetically sensitive areas is best managed in conjunction with a consultant.

Hypertrophic scars and keloids are managed in conjunction with a consultant. Treatment modalities include corticosteroids, compressive dressings, surgical excision, and radiation therapy.

Clinical Pearls

1. All accidental wounds are considered contaminated and treated as such. Thorough irrigation and cleansing is of paramount importance in preventing wound infection.
2. Expedient ED wound care is important, since bacterial contamination increases over time.
3. The tensile strength of the wound reaches its nadir between 7 to 10 days.
4. All patients with wounds in areas of increased tissue stress and a history of hypertrophic scarring are treated with splinting and physical therapy to minimize the risk of excessive scarring.

CHAPTER 19

EMERGENCY ULTRASOUND

Paul R. Sierzenski
Michael J. Lambert
Theodore J. Nielsen

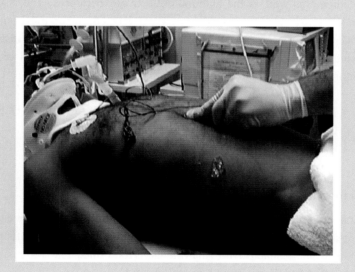

Emergency medicine ultrasound has the basic goal of improving patient care. This chapter strives to provide a "visual blueprint" for the reader who uses emergency medicine ultrasonography in his or her practice. It is intended to serve as a practical imaging reference when an emergency screening ultrasound examination is being performed and assumes a basic knowledge and experiential base in ultrasound examinations. For practitioners without this prerequisite body of knowledge, it may provide useful information about the scope of the emergency screening ultrasound examination (ESUE).

Success in performing an ESUE is dependent on the physician's goal-directed approach to each examination. This demands that the physician use ultrasound to identify, confirm, or exclude specific sonographic findings that are consistent with specific disease states or life-threatening conditions.

Basic ultrasound information—including transducer recommendations, scanning protocols, anatomic schematics, and ultrasound images—are presented throughout the chapter. Applicable protocols are patterned after imaging guidelines of the American Institute of Ultrasound in Medicine as well as the authors' collective experiences. The issues of the efficacy, accuracy, and/or sensitivity of this modality are not debated; rather, a "visual blueprint" for ESUEs is provided. Once again, this chapter is not presented as a primary instructional tool, but rather as a rapid visual review for the physician trained in ESUE applications.

Information is presented about the following ESUE protocols:

1. Trauma: focused assessment with sonography for trauma (FAST)
2. Cardiac: echocardiography (ECHO)
3. Abdominal (gallbladder, aorta, and kidney)
4. Pelvic/endovaginal

Transducers

Sonography is performed using transducers of varying frequencies. Lower or higher frequencies are selected for more or less depth of penetration. Many manufacturers produce multifrequency transducers available with small or large footprints. The various transducers recommended for use in the ESUE are listed below (Fig. 19.1).

- *Microconvex*: This transducer has the advantage of a tight curvature and small footprint that allows for easy access between ribs and for subxiphoid imaging. This is an excellent transducer for the FAST, especially for the beginner, who may have difficulty scanning or interpreting with rib shadowing present. This probe is also helpful in the thin patients with a high-positioned gallbladder requiring intercostal windows for optimal imaging. These transducers are generally more expensive than the standard curve-linear transducer.
- *Convex Array*: Considered a standard abdominal transducer, it is used by many sonographers and provides wide near and far fields of view (ideal in evaluating the aorta). The long curved footprint of this type of transducer may make subxiphoid cardiac imaging difficult, as will the noted presence of "rib shadowing," which is inevitable with this transducer in scanning the right/left upper quadrants in the coronal plane. This is the transducer of choice for imaging the gallbladder at a frequency of 3.5 MHz; it is used by many vascular laboratories in evaluating the abdominal aorta. It is also the preferred transducer for renal ultrasound.

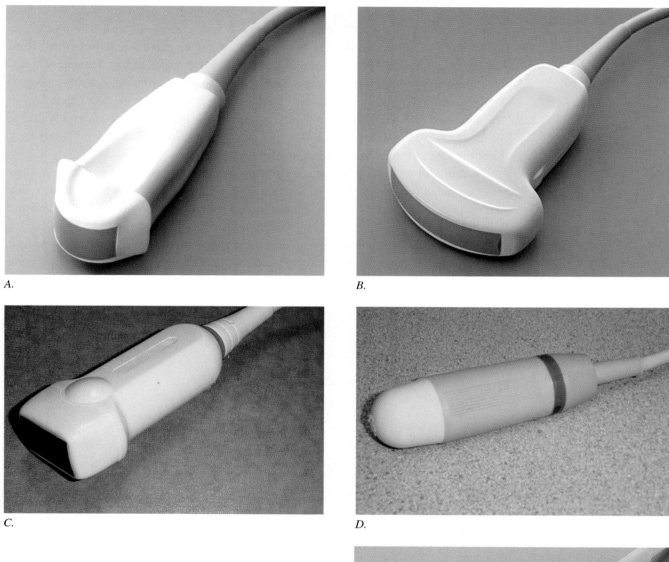

A.

B.

C.

D.

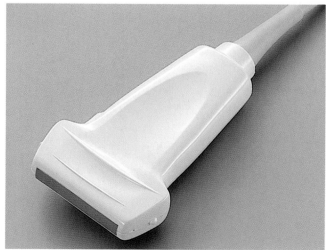

E.

Figure 19.1 Transducers

Various transducers recommended for use in the emergency screening ultrasound exam (ESUE). *A.* Microconvex. *B.* Convex array. *C.* Phased array. *D.* Mechanical sector. *E.* Linear. (*A*, *B*, and *E*, Courtesy of SonoSite, Inc.; *C* and *D*, Courtesy of Windy City Ultrasound, Inc..)

- *Phased Array*: This transducer is the transducer of choice for cardiac ultrasound. It results in a narrow near field of view. The image obtained is a true "pie-shaped" image. As a result, the phased array often has a small, flat footprint and is easy to maneuver between ribs. These transducers are frequently marketed in the 2.0- to 4.0-MHz ranges and will yield less resolution than the curved array transducers of higher frequencies. The advantage of this transducer is in scanning the obese patient who may be difficult to image during the FAST examination. The disadvantage is that the image quality is slightly less than that of geometrically steered (linear and curved array) transducers of the same frequency. This is not the preferred transducer for transabdominal pelvic sonography.
- *Mechanical Sector*: Many manufacturers still produce mechanical sector transducers. These provide a small footprint with a pie-shaped image and are usually much less expensive than phased-array transducers. Mechanical transducers are more likely to wear over time and tend to be less tolerant to incidental impacts (a common occurrence in the ED).
- *Linear*: This transducer is frequently used for superficial structures and vascular ultrasound. It usually is available in frequencies ranging from 5.0 MHz upward. It can be helpful in the very thin patient or the patient with an extremely superficial gallbladder.

The focused assessment with sonography for trauma (FAST) is an organized series of sonographic windows or views that attempts to identify the presence or absence of fluid in anatomic potential spaces (e.g., pericardium or Morison's pouch) or anatomically dependent areas (e.g., pelvis, posteroinferior thorax, and splenorenal recess). It is, in fact, a cardiac and thoracoabdominal survey that allows the physician to identify or exclude immediate or potential life threats in the trauma patient. Though intended for the evaluation of the traumatized patient, the FAST examination and its components are also extremely valuable in the evaluation of several emergent complaints and clinical conditions.

Clinical Indications for the FAST Examination

- Blunt abdominal trauma
- Penetrating thoracic/abdominal trauma
- Unexplained hypotension (trauma and nontrauma)
- Evaluation of the pregnant trauma patient
- Acute dyspnea with suspected pleural/pericardial effusion or tamponade

In its simplest form, the FAST examination uses four primary sonographic windows to evaluate the patient. It is recommended that these windows be scanned in sequence, but isolated views may be obtained when indicated (e.g., suspected pleural effusions in the dyspneic patient).

Required Views for the FAST Examination

1. Subxiphoid-cardiac window (subcostal view)
2. Right upper quadrant (Morison's pouch)
3. Left upper quadrant (splenorenal view)
4. Suprapubic window (pelvic view)

Recommended Transducers for the FAST Examination

- *Microconvex*
- *Convex array*
- *Phased array*

Most abdominal sonography is performed using transducers of 3.5 to 5.0 MHz. The FAST examination is an echocardiographic and thoracoabdominal examination. This presents the dilemma of using a transducer that can image all three of these areas but only with some sonographic compromise.

FAST Window 1: Subxiphoid-Cardiac (Subcostal View)

Technique

- The patient is supine.
- The transducer is directed under the xiphoid process toward the left shoulder in a horizontal plane (Fig. 19.2).
- Direct the transducer indicator to the patient's right.

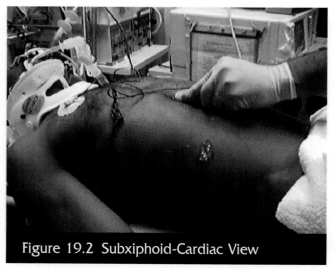

Figure 19.2 Subxiphoid-Cardiac View

The transducer is directed under the xiphoid process toward the left shoulder in a horizontal plane. (Courtesy of Michael J. Lambert, MD, RDMS.)

- Pivot, sweep, and tilt the transducer to view of all four cardiac chambers.
- Identify the heart, four cardiac chambers, and surrounding pericardium (Fig. 19.3).

Abnormal Findings

- Hemopericardium (pericardial effusion): Dark black, anechoic region noted between the bright pericardium and the walls of the heart (occasionally internal echoes representing fibrin, clot, or cardiac tissue may be present) (Fig. 19.4).

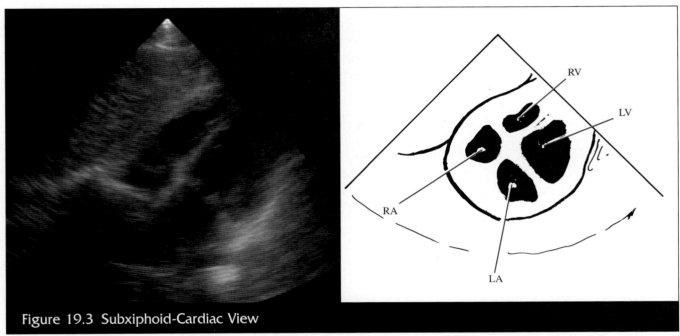

Figure 19.3 Subxiphoid-Cardiac View

The heart, four cardiac chambers, and surrounding pericardium are seen in this view. (Courtesy of Michael J. Lambert, MD, RDMS.)

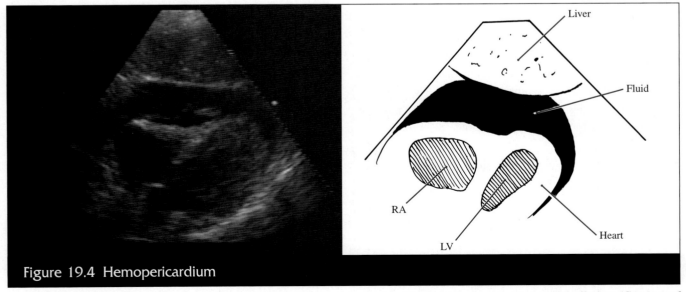

Figure 19.4 Hemopericardium

The dark black, anechoic region between the bright pericardium and the walls of the heart represents a pericardial effusion. (Courtesy of Paul R. Sierzenski, MD, RDMS, FAAEM.)

- Asystole: No cardiac activity present.
- Hyperdynamic cardiac activity: Extensive cardiac contraction with maximal collapse of the cardiac chambers, often associated with tachycardia and hypovolemia.

FAST Window 2: Right Upper Quadrant (Morison's Pouch)

Technique

- The patient is supine.
- The transducer indicator is aimed toward the axilla in a coronal plane.
- The transducer is directed as a coronal section through the body in the midaxillary line, extending from the 9th through 12th ribs. Start between the 11th and 12th ribs initially, then move cephalad or caudal to complete the evaluation (Fig. 19.5).
- Identify the liver and right kidney interface. This region is the potential space known as Morison's pouch. Normally, these organs' surrounding tissues are in direct contact with one another (Fig. 19.6).
- Evaluate the right diaphragmatic recess and the subdiaphragmatic recess.

Abnormal Findings

- Hemoperitoneum: Dark black, anechoic region between the liver and right kidney or in the subdiaphragmatic recess (Fig. 19.7). May be positive with a ruptured ectopic pregnancy.

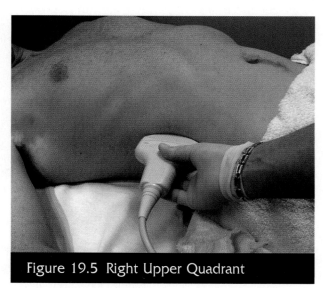

Figure 19.5 Right Upper Quadrant

The transducer is directed as a coronal section through the body in the midaxillary line extending from the 9th through 12th ribs. (Courtesy of Windy City Ultrasound, Inc.)

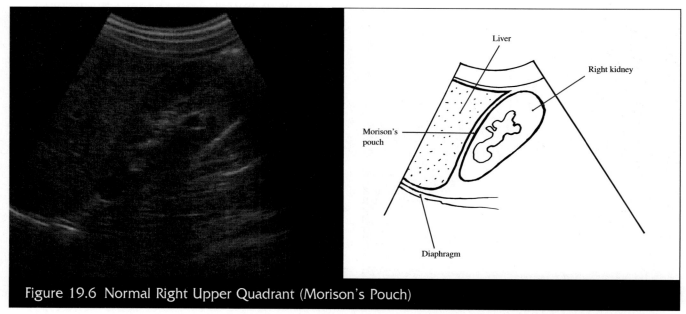

Figure 19.6 Normal Right Upper Quadrant (Morison's Pouch)

At the liver and right kidney interface is the potential space known as "Morison's pouch." Normally the surrounding tissues of these organs are in direct contact with one another. (Courtesy of Windy City Ultrasound, Inc.)

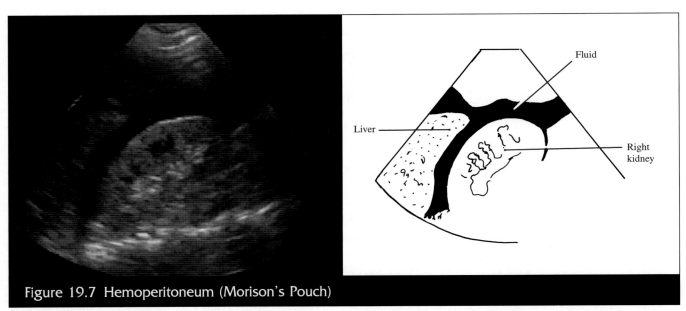

Figure 19.7 Hemoperitoneum (Morison's Pouch)

The dark black, anechoic region between the liver and right kidney or in the subdiaphragmatic recess represents fluid in Morison's pouch. (Courtesy of Michael J. Lambert, MD, RDMS.)

- Right hemothorax: Anechoic (dark) region above the level of the diaphragm.
- Solid organ injury: Solid organ injury such as hepatic and renal lacerations as well as organ rupture have been described but are beyond the scope of this chapter.
- Hydronephrosis: Dilatation of the renal sinus with dark, anechoic fluid within the bright renal sinus (see "Renal Ultrasound," below).

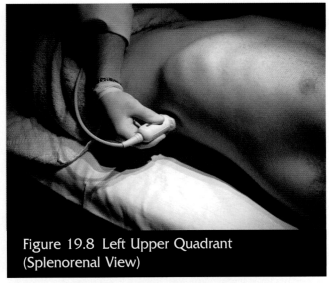

Figure 19.8 Left Upper Quadrant (Splenorenal View)

The transducer is directed as a coronal section through the body in the midaxillary line extending from the 9th through 12th ribs. (Courtesy of Windy City Ultrasound, Inc.)

FAST Window 3: Left Upper Quadrant (Splenorenal View)

Technique

- The patient is supine.
- The transducer indicator is directed toward the axilla in a coronal plane.
- The transducer is directed as a coronal section through the body in the midaxillary to posterior axillary line extending from the 9th through 12th ribs. Start between the 11th and 12th ribs initially, then move cephalad or caudal to complete the evaluation (Fig. 19.8).
- Identify the spleen and left kidney interface. This region is a physiologic potential space. Normally the surrounding tissues of these organs are in direct contact with one another (Fig. 19.9).
- Evaluate the left diaphragmatic recess and the left subdiaphragmatic recess.

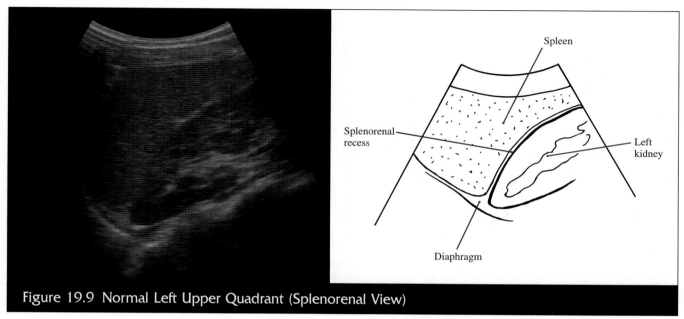

Figure 19.9 Normal Left Upper Quadrant (Splenorenal View)

The spleen and left kidney interface is a physiologic potential space (splenorenal recess). Normally the surrounding tissues of these organs are in direct contact with one another. (Courtesy of Paul R. Sierzenski, MD, RDMS, FAAEM.)

Abnormal Findings

- Hemoperitoneum: Anechoic (dark) region between the spleen and left kidney or between the spleen and the diaphragm (Fig. 19.10).
- Left hemothorax: Dark black, anechoic region above the level of the diaphragm (Fig. 19.11).

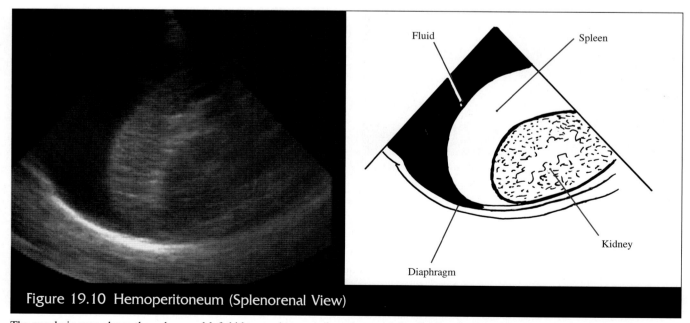

Figure 19.10 Hemoperitoneum (Splenorenal View)

The anechoic area above the spleen and left kidney or between the spleen and the diaphragm represents fluid in the potential space. This image represents fluid above the spleen but below the level of the diaphragm. (Courtesy of Michael J. Lambert, MD, RDMS.)

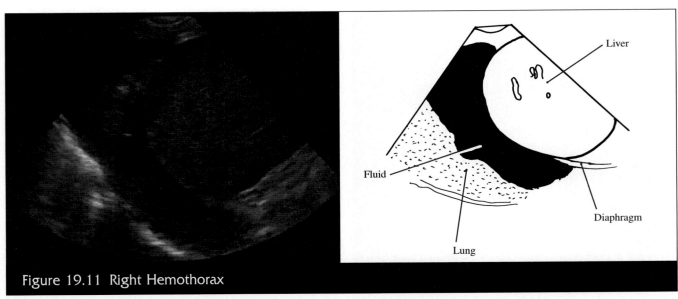

Figure 19.11 Right Hemothorax

Fluid *above* the level of the diaphragm represents a hemothorax. (Courtesy of Michael J. Lambert, MD, RDMS.)

- Solid organ injury: Solid organ injury such as splenic and renal lacerations as well as organ rupture have been described but are beyond the scope of this chapter.

- Hydronephrosis: Dilatation of the renal sinus with dark black, anechoic fluid within the bright renal sinus (see "Renal Ultrasound," below).

FAST Window 4: Suprapubic

Technique

Sagittal View (Longitudinal)

- The patient is supine.
- The transducer is placed just above the symphysis pubis.
- The transducer is directed into the pelvis with the transducer indicator oriented toward the patient's head (Fig. 19.12).
- Identify the bladder (triangular in this view when fully distended), uterus (pear-shaped if present), and rectum (Fig. 19.13).

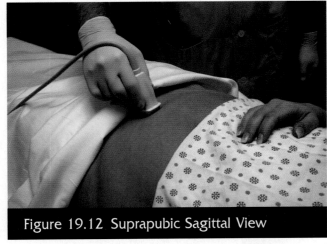

Figure 19.12 Suprapubic Sagittal View

The transducer is directed with the transducer indicator oriented toward the patient's head and placed just superior to the symphysis pubis. (Courtesy of Windy City Ultrasound, Inc.)

Transverse View

- The patient is supine.
- The transducer is placed about 1 to 2 cm above the symphysis pubis.
- The transducer is directed with the transducer indicator oriented toward the patient's right, with the beam angled caudally into the pelvis (Fig. 19.14).
- Identify the bladder (rectangular in this view when fully distended), uterus (oval hyperechoic structure if present) and rectum (Fig. 19.15).

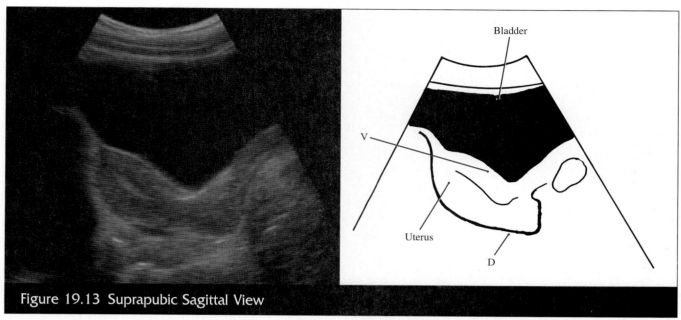

Figure 19.13 Suprapubic Sagittal View

In this view, when fully distended, the bladder is triangular in shape. If present, the uterus is pear-shaped. Fluid may collect in the vesi-couterine (V) (potential space seen between the bladder and uterus in this view) and/or rectouterine (D) (pouch of Douglas) (space seen posterior to the border of the uterus and rectum) pouches. (Courtesy of Windy City Ultrasound, Inc.)

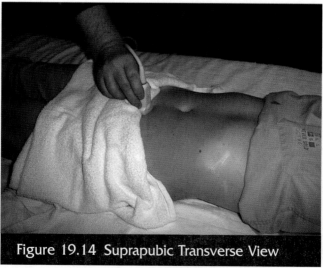

Figure 19.14 Suprapubic Transverse View

The transducer indicator is oriented toward the patient's right and the beam angled caudally into the pelvis. (Courtesy of Windy City Ultrasound, Inc.)

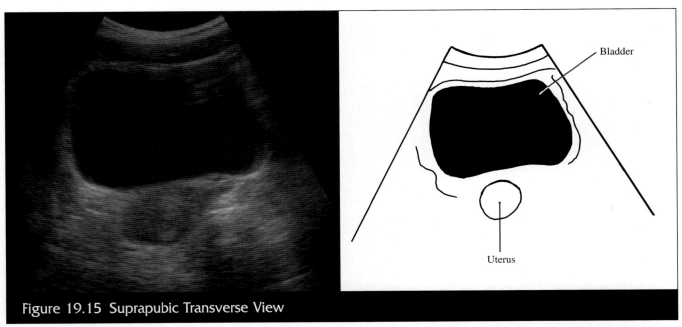

Figure 19.15 Suprapubic Transverse View

In this view, the bladder assumes a rectangular shape when fully distended. If present, the uterus is an oval hyperechoic structure. (Courtesy of Windy City Ultrasound, Inc.)

Abnormal Findings

- Hemoperitoneum: Anechoic (dark) regions between the bladder and uterus or the uterus and rectum or as loops of bowel floating lateral to the bladder in the transverse view and lateral or superior to the bladder in the sagittal view (Fig. 19.16).

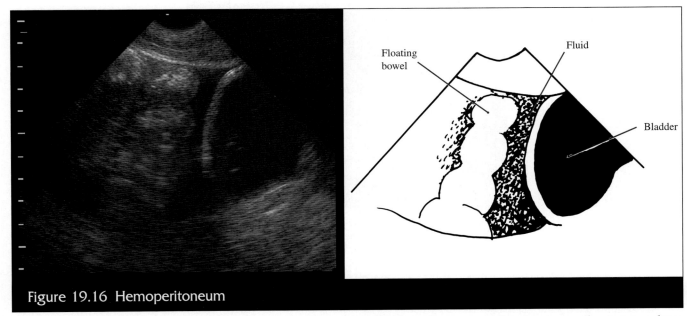

Figure 19.16 Hemoperitoneum

Hemoperitoneum can be seen as dark black, anechoic regions between the bladder and uterus, as well as the uterus and rectum or as loops of bowel floating lateral to the bladder in the transverse view and lateral or posterior to the bladder in the sagittal view. (Courtesy of Paul R. Sierzenski, MD, RDMS, FAAEM.)

Scan Pearls for the FAST Examination

Subxiphoid-Cardiac

1. When your view is obscured by gas, slide the transducer slightly to the patient's right subcostal region, using the liver as an echogenic window.

2. If you are unable to view the heart in the true subxiphoid or subcostal window, move to a parasternal long axis view (see "Cardiac Ultrasound (ECHO)," below).

3. A frequent mistake in imaging is to direct the transducer toward the spine rather than coronally to the shoulder. You will often require less than a 30 degree angle between the transducer and the skin.

4. Start imaging with the depth/scale setting at its maximum (e.g., 20 to 24 cm). This should allow you to image the anterior and posterior pericardium in your initial view. Gradually decrease the depth/scale (e.g., 14 to 18 cm) to fill the entire sector image with the heart as you continue to optimize your image.

RUQ and LUQ

1. The diaphragmatic recess includes a *superior region,* which is the inferior border of the right thorax, and an *inferior region (subdiaphragmatic recess),* which is the superior border of the abdomen. Fluid in the diaphragmatic recess can represent a hemothorax when located superior/cephalad to the diaphragm or a hemoperitoneum or subphrenic hematoma (inferior to the diaphragm) in the setting of trauma.

2. Identify the kidneys from the superior to the inferior poles in the coronal plane. It may seem easier at first to perform a short axis view; however, the sonographer risks missing early small fluid collections if only a middle renal transverse section is imaged.

3. If you are uncertain whether a finding is actually present, evaluate it in a second plane. To do this, turn the transducer 90 degrees from your initial transducer position and see if the finding is still noted on the image.

4. It is important to note that the LUQ is not synonymous to the RUQ; the spleen is not tethered to the diaphragm as the liver is by the coronary ligament. Sonographically we tend to see fluid collect in the left subdiaphragmatic area more than the right. This area should be evaluated.

Suprapubic

1. It is important to remember that the bladder is within the pelvis; therefore the transducer must be directed posteriorly and inferiorly to image the bladder and its neighboring structures.

2. When in the sagittal plane, simply rotate the transducer 90 degrees counterclockwise with the transducer indicator oriented to the patient's right, and you will transition to a transverse view.

Two-dimensional echocardiography (2D ECHO) can yield significant diagnostic information for the patient presenting with cardiac arrest, shock, shortness of breath, and a host of other complaints or physical findings. Although the physician can easily become intimidated by all the diagnostic possibilities that can be identified or potentially missed in performing echocardiography, one can, with experience, incorporate ED ECHO into the diagnostic armamentarium without becoming overextended.

It is important to note that, unlike abdominal sonography, cardiac ultrasound is by convention oriented with the transducer indicator for the display screen to the right of the screen (which will effectively be the patient's left). This may be a significant cause of initial confusion for many who have not performed echocardiography before. Most ultrasound systems today include cardiac presets that automatically reverse the orientation to the right of the display screen. The following section describes a sonographic approach for a correctly oriented image using standard cardiac windows.

Clinical Indications for ED Cardiac Ultrasound (ECHO)

- Cardiac arrest, PEA
- Penetrating thoracic/abdominal trauma
- Unexplained hypotension or shock
- Dyspnea
- Acute myocardial infarction
- Suspected aortic dissection

Specific pathologic states confirmed or excluded with ED ECHO include asystole (confirmation), cardiac activity (confirmation), pericardial effusion, and aortic root dilatation/dissection.

The sonographic windows for ED ECHO act as an extension of the subxiphoid view presented within the trauma/FAST examination. The ED ECHO utilizes cardiac windows that are familiar to cardiologists and sonographers alike. The four ED ECHO windows will allow the emergency physician to evaluate asystole, pericardial effusions, and the aortic root.

Required Views for Emergency Department ECHO

1. Subxiphoid (subcostal) (see "FAST Examination," above)
2. Parasternal long-axis view (PSLAx)
3. Parasternal short-axis view (PSSAx)
4. Apical four-chamber view (A4C)

Recommended Transducers for ECHO

- *Phased array*
- *Microconvex*
- *Mechanical sector*

ECHO Window 1: Subxiphoid-Cardiac (Subcostal View)

Technique

- The patient is supine.
- The transducer is placed inferior to the xiphoid process and directed toward the left shoulder

in a horizontal plane. (The transducer indicator should be directed in the same orientation as the indicator mark of the screen; this is frequently to the patient's right in an abdominal preset, but it is toward the left in a cardiac preset) (see Fig. 19.2).

- Pivot, sweep, and tilt the transducer to view all four cardiac chambers.
- Identify the heart, four cardiac chambers, and surrounding pericardium (see Fig. 19.3).

Abnormal Findings

- Hemopericardium (pericardial effusion): Anechoic (dark) region noted between the bright pericardium and the walls of the heart (occasionally internal echoes representing, fibrin, clot, or cardiac tissue may be present) (see Fig. 19.4).
- Asystole: No cardiac activity present.
- Hyperdynamic cardiac activity: Extensive cardiac contraction with maximal collapse of the cardiac chambers, often associated with tachycardia.

Scan Pearls for Subxiphoid-Cardiac

- See "Scan Pearls for the FAST Examination," above.

ECHO Window 2: Parasternal Long-Axis View (PSLAx)

Technique

This assumes a leftward image orientation—e.g., transducer indicator to the right of the screen. This will effectively be toward the patient's head.

- The patient is supine or in the left lateral decubitus (LLD) position with the left arm extended above the head for easier transducer access.
- The transducer is placed in the fourth or fifth left parasternal intercostal space with the transducer indicator directed at the right clavicle or shoulder (Fig. 19.17).
- Identify the right ventricle, left atrium, left ventricle, aortic valve, aortic root, aortic outflow tract, and surrounding pericardium (Fig. 19.18).

Abnormal Findings

- Hemopericardium: Anechoic (dark) region noted between the hyperechoic (bright) pericardium and the walls of the heart (see Fig. 19.4).
- Aortic root dilatation: An aortic root measurement greater than 3.8 cm is abnormal and should suggest either aortic dissection or aneurysm in the emergency patient with chest pain or back pain or in the appropriate clinical setting. Further evaluation is recommended.
- Dilated descending aorta: The descending thoracic aorta can be seen in the far field in this view posterior to the left atrium. A descending thoracic aorta greater than 3.8 cm is suspicious for aneurysm or dissection and requires further evaluation.

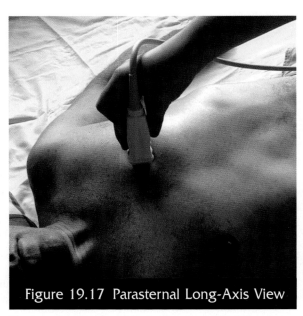

Figure 19.17 Parasternal Long-Axis View

The transducer is placed in the fourth or fifth left parasternal intercostal space with the transducer indicator oriented toward the right clavicle or shoulder. (Courtesy of Windy City Ultrasound, Inc.)

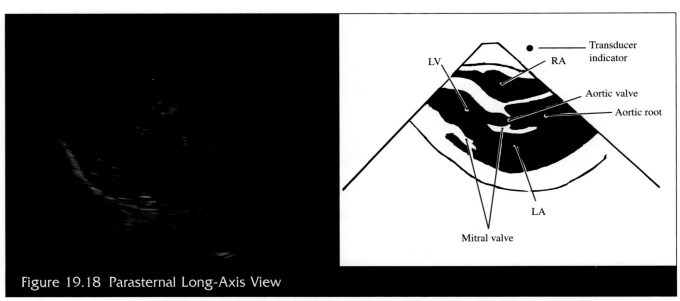

Figure 19.18 Parasternal Long-Axis View

The left atrium, left ventricle, aortic valve, aortic root, aortic outflow tract, and surrounding pericardium can be visualized. (Courtesy of Michael J. Lambert, MD, RDMS.)

Scan Pearls for the Parasternal Long-Axis View

1. A true parasternal long-axis view (a sagittal image through the heart) will visualize the aortic root within the image. If the aortic root is not present, you are likely in an oblique plane and will need to gently angle the transducer in either direction to optimize the image.

2. It is critical to make deliberate, slow, small adjustments of the transducer in imaging the heart, since even small movements at the skin surface can translate into large changes in beam angle at just 5 to 10 cm deep from the surface.

3. Normal spontaneous respiration is usually fine for cardiac imaging. Patients who are tachypneic can be very challenging, and verbally coaching the patient's breathing patterns is best. If you note a great deal of artifact due to lung interposition, place the patient in the left lateral decubitus position; have him or her inhale and slowly exhale while you scan. When you have an acceptable window, ask the patient to stop exhaling and hold his or her breath while you capture your images.

4. Remember that the parasternal long axis is approximated by a line running from the right acromioclavicular joint and the left antecubital fossa (when the arm is lying by the patient's side).

ECHO Window 3: Parasternal Short-Axis View (PSSAx)

Technique

This assumes a leftward image orientation—e.g., transducer indicator to the right of the screen. This will effectively be toward the patient's head.

- The patient is supine or in the left lateral decubitus position.
- From the parasternal long-axis position, rotate the transducer 90 degrees clockwise (to the pa-

tient's left) or place the transducer in the fourth or fifth left parasternal intercostal space in a line connecting the left clavicle/shoulder and the right hip (Fig. 19.19).

• Identify the left ventricle (circular), right ventricle (crescent-shaped), and surrounding pericardium (Fig. 19.20).

Abnormal Findings

• Hemopericardium: Dark black, anechoic region noted between the bright pericardium and the walls of the heart (see Fig. 19.4).

• Dilated right ventricle: The right ventricle is normally a crescent-shaped structure; if this is a rounded, dilated structure, it suggests elevated right-sided pressures, as seen with pulmonary emboli and severe pulmonary hypertension.

Scan Pearls for the Parasternal Short-Axis View

1. The standard parasternal short-axis view is obtained with the image plane at the level of the papillary muscles. Visualization of the papillary muscles should ensure a true transverse section through the left ventricle and provides a prime location for the evaluation of left ventricular contraction and motion.

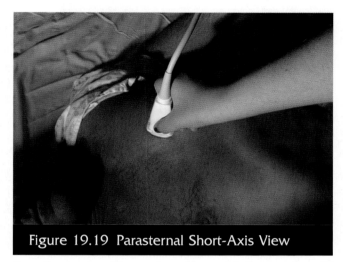

Figure 19.19 Parasternal Short-Axis View

From the parasternal long-axis position, rotate the transducer 90 degrees clockwise (to the patient's left) or place the transducer in the fourth or fifth left parasternal intercostal space in a line connecting the left clavicle/shoulder and the right hip. (Courtesy of Windy City Ultrasound, Inc.

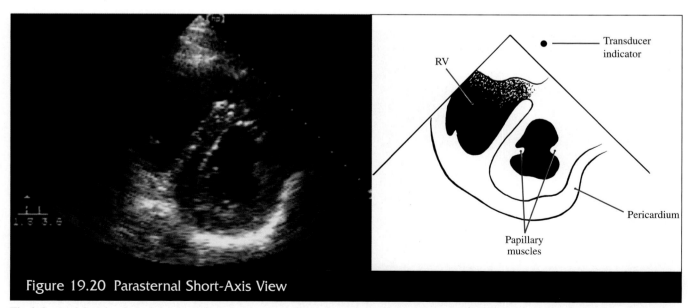

Figure 19.20 Parasternal Short-Axis View

The left ventricle (circular), right ventricle (crescent-shaped), aortic valve, and surrounding pericardium can be identified. (Courtesy of Paul R. Sierzenski, MD, RDMS, FAAEM.)

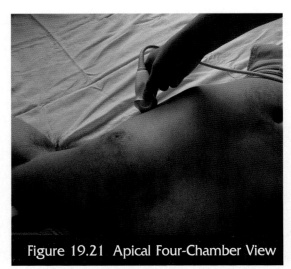

Figure 19.21 Apical Four-Chamber View

The transducer is placed over the cardiac apex or the point of maximal intensity, with the beam directed toward the right clavicle/shoulder in a plane coronal to the heart. The transducer indicator is directed toward the left axilla. (Courtesy of Windy City Ultrasound, Inc

ECHO Window 4: Apical Four-Chamber View (A4C)

Technique

This assumes that a leftward image orientation is the standard sonographic approach.

- The patient is supine or in the left lateral decubitus position.
- The transducer is placed over the cardiac apex or the point of maximal intensity (PMI) with the beam directed toward the right clavicle/shoulder in a plane coronal to the heart. The transducer indicator is directed toward the left axilla (Fig. 19.21).
- Identify the left ventricle, right ventricle, left atrium, right atrium, and surrounding pericardium (Fig. 19.22).

Abnormal Findings

- Hemopericardium: Anechoic (dark) region noted between the hyperechoic pericardium and the walls of the heart (see Fig. 19.4).
- Dilated right atria/ventricle: If the right atria/ventricle are rounded or appear rigid and poorly contracting, this may suggest elevated right-sided pressures as seen with pulmonary emboli and severe pulmonary hypertension.

Scan Pearls for Apical Four-Chamber View

1. See "Scan Pearls for the FAST Examination, Subxiphoid-Cardiac," item 4, above.
2. It is critical to realize the variance in the resting position of the heart. It is evident, using this view, that there can be relatively significant differences and acoustic windows from patient to patient with the four-chamber apical view.

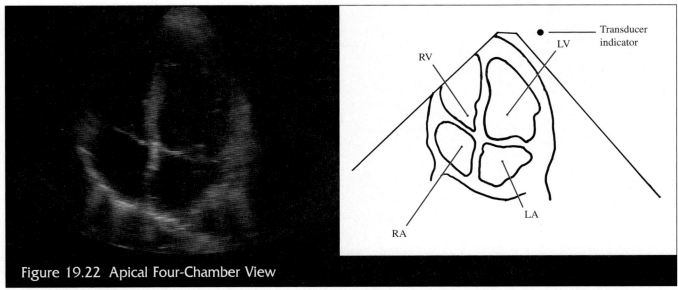

Figure 19.22 Apical Four-Chamber View

The right ventricle (RV), left ventricle (LV), right atrium (RA), left atrium (LA), and surrounding pericardium are visualized in this view. (Courtesy of Paul R. Sierzenski, MD, RDMS, FAAEM.)

The application of abdominal ultrasound in emergency medicine seems, for many physicians, self-evident. Abdominal aortic aneurysm (AAA), gallbladder disease, and renal colic are all common diagnoses in patients presenting to the ED. The ability to rapidly diagnose or exclude these disease states can decrease patient morbidity and mortality. The abdominal emergency screening ultrasound examination (ESUE) can aid in this diagnostic process.

The clinical indications for an abdominal ESUE may vary with each ED and ED physician. There are three specific pathologic states that we believe the proficient emergency physician should be able to identify: AAA, gallstones, and hydronephrosis. This series on abdominal ESUE presents the applications of gallbladder, aortic and renal ultrasound.

Required Views for Abdominal Ultrasound

1. Gallbladder (sagittal, transverse, oblique views)
2. Aorta (transverse, sagittal views)
3. Renal (coronal, sagittal views)

Gallbladder Ultrasound

Ultrasound of the gallbladder can be among the most rewarding ESUEs to perform. Patients can receive a rapid focused ultrasound to determine if gallstones or gallbladder pathology is the etiology of their pain or presenting symptoms, and they are often relieved to be given a visual presentation of their illness. No ESUE calls for more careful positioning of the patient than the gallbladder and biliary ultrasound. Position the patient to minimize bowel gas from your view, accentuate possible pathology, and verify suspected findings. This can be a technically difficult ultrasound to perform.

Clinical Indications for Gallbladder Ultrasound

- Right-upper-quadrant pain
- Jaundice/icterus
- Epigastric pain

It is important to recognize the limited nature of gallbladder ultrasounds performed by emergency physicians. Thorough evaluation of the biliary tract is a routine component of a standard radiology abdominal ultrasound but can be technically and diagnostically difficult, especially in the patient with acute pain. For this reason, measurement of the hepatic and common bile ducts is not included as an initial key component to the basic gallbladder ESUE. Techniques for measurement of the common bile duct are reviewed below; these should be performed by an emergency physician proficient in abdominal ultrasound. Although the sonographic identification of gallstones may seem straightforward, the sonographic findings for cholecystitis can frequently be subtle.

Recommended Transducers for Gallbladder Ultrasound

- *Convex array*
- *Microconvex*
- *Phased array*
- *Mechanical sector*

Most abdominal sonography is performed using transducer frequencies of 3.5 to 5.0 MHz. In rare instances, lower or higher frequencies are needed for more or less depth of penetration.

Gallbladder Ultrasound Window 1: Sagittal View

Technique

- The patient is supine or in the left lateral decubitus position. Other positions—including prone, right lateral decubitus, semierect, and standing—may be helpful in scanning the gallbladder.
- The transducer is placed in the subxiphoid region with the orientation indicator directed toward the patient's head and swept below the right costal margin to approximately the midclavicular line (Figs. 19.23, 19.24).
- Identify the liver, portal vein, common bile duct, hepatic artery, gallbladder, and main lobar

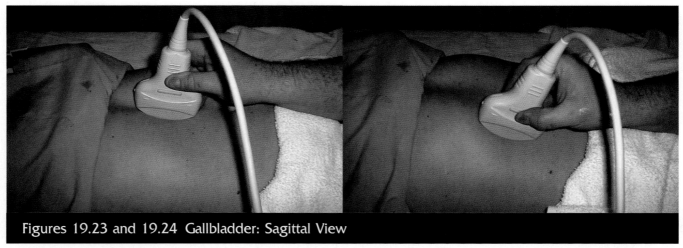

Figures 19.23 and 19.24 Gallbladder: Sagittal View

The transducer is placed in the subxiphoid region with the orientation indicator directed toward the patient's head and moved along the right costal margin approximately to the midclavicular line. (Courtesy of Windy City Ultrasound, Inc.)

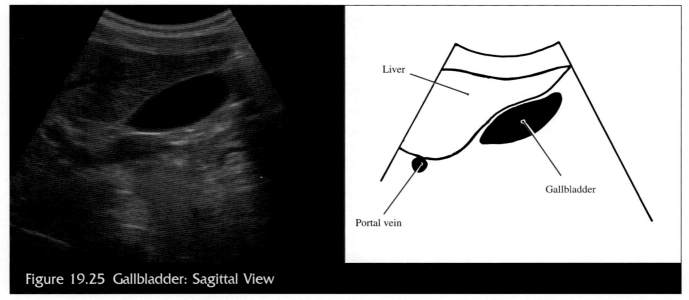

Figure 19.25 Gallbladder: Sagittal View

Various structures can be seen in this sagittal view. Although not apparent in the drawing, the gallbladder and portal vein are within the liver. Moving the patient to the left lateral decubitus position may improve this view. (Courtesy of Windy City Ultrasound, Inc.)

fissure (spanning these two structures). Measure the thickness of the common bile duct when able (Fig. 19.25).

- Scan through the gallbladder completely from the medial to lateral borders of the gallbladder.

Gallbladder Ultrasound Window 2: Transverse View

Technique

- The patient is supine or in the left lateral decubitus position.
- From the sagittal position, rotate the transducer 90 degrees counterclockwise to the patient's right and move along the right costal margin (Fig. 19.26).
- Identify the liver, gallbladder, inferior vena cava, right kidney (if visualized), and common bile duct (if visualized) (Figs. 19.27 to 19.29).

Abnormal Findings

- Gallstones: Bright oval to round hyperechoic structure(s) within the gallbladder, often with a posterior shadow on ultrasound (Fig. 19.30).
- Pericholecystic fluid: An anechoic stripe that borders the outer gallbladder wall and should be visualized in two views. This fluid is often but not necessarily circumferential (Fig. 19.31).

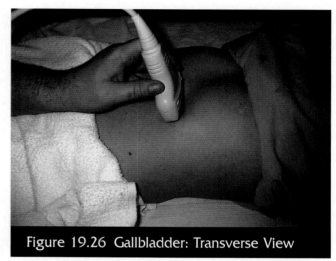

Figure 19.26 Gallbladder: Transverse View

The transducer is rotated 90 degrees counterclockwise from the sagittal position and moved along the right costal margin. (Courtesy of Windy City Ultrasound, Inc.)

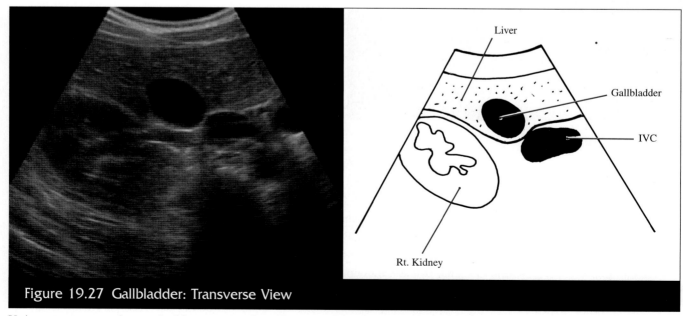

Figure 19.27 Gallbladder: Transverse View

Various structures can be seen in this transverse view. (Courtesy of Windy City Ultrasound, Inc.)

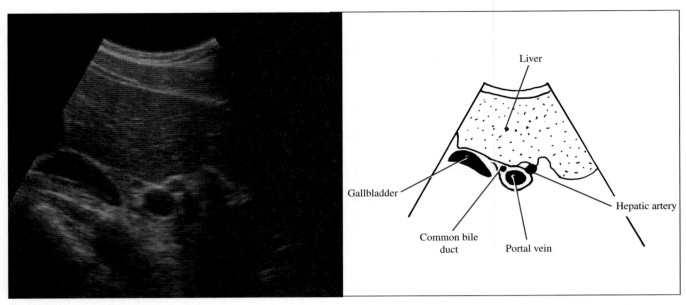

A.

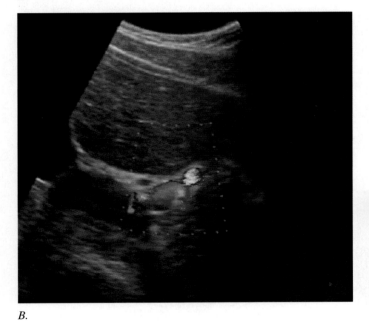

B.

Figure 19.28 Gallbladder: Portal Triad

The portal triad (portal vein, common bile duct, and hepatic artery) is readily seen in this transverse view. Although not apparent in the drawing, these structures are within the liver. (*A*). Color-flow Doppler (*B*) facilitates identification of these structures. (Courtesy of Windy City Ultrasound, Inc.)

- Thickened gallbladder wall: A gallbladder wall that measures 4 mm or more is considered abnormal.
- Sonographic Murphy's sign: Tenderness of the gallbladder when compressed under direct visualization with the ultrasound transducer.
- Dilated common bile duct (CBD): A CBD with an internal diameter greater than 4.0 mm is dilated; however, documented measurements up to 8.0 mm can be normal in the elderly. One rule of thumb is that 4 mm up to age 40 and thereafter an increase of 1 mm per decade represents the normal range.

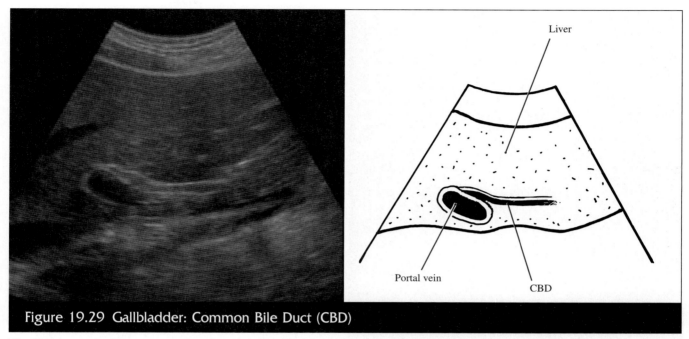

Figure 19.29 Gallbladder: Common Bile Duct (CBD)

The CBD is seen in this transverse view. Once it is identified, its thickness should be measured. (Courtesy of Windy City Ultrasound, Inc.)

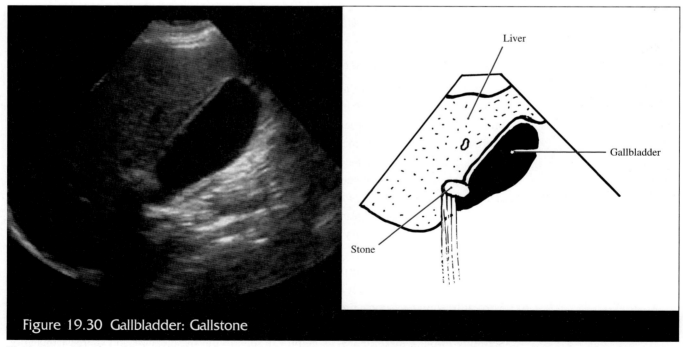

Figure 19.30 Gallbladder: Gallstone

The bright oval-to-round hyperechoic structure within the gallbladder with a posterior shadow is the classic gallstone presentation seen on ultrasound. (Courtesy of Michael J. Lambert, MD, RDMS.)

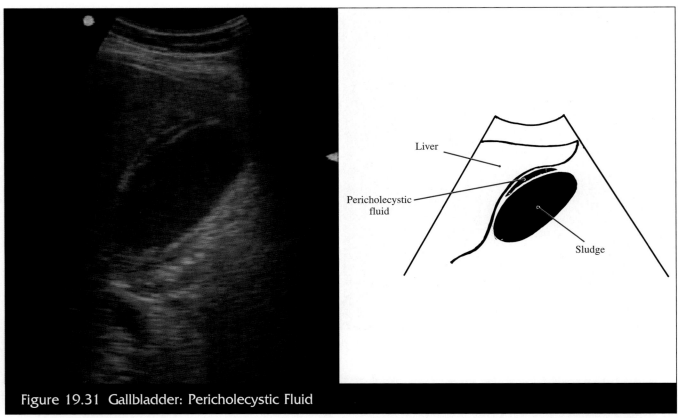

Figure 19.31 Gallbladder: Pericholecystic Fluid

A circumferential anechoic stripe that borders the outer gallbladder wall is consistent with pericholecystic fluid. A small gallstone with posterior shadowing is also seen. (Courtesy of Windy City Ultrasound, Inc.)

Scan Pearls for Gallbladder Ultrasound

1. It is frequently necessary to have the patient take a deep breath and hold it to allow the gallbladder to descend into sonographic view.
2. Measure the anterior wall when evaluating wall thickness. The thickness of the posterior wall is often affected by "posterior enhancement"; therefore it may falsely appear thickened.
3. The duodenum is located medially to the gallbladder. It may be interpreted as a gallstone even by proficient sonographers if care is not taken to evaluate the gallbladder completely and to observe for peristalsis on areas suspected to be bowel.
4. If you suspect gallstones but do not visualize "shadowing," confirm that your focal point is at the area of interest and try changing the transducer frequency if possible (e.g., increase from 3.5 to 5.0 MHz).
5. If pericholecystic fluid is suspected but difficult to determine, it may be helpful to increase the frequency or convert to a linear transducer.
6. Most ultrasound systems provide a cinematic loop, or "cineloop," that will allow the sonographer to recall on average 20 to 40 images that occurred before the image was frozen. Scrolling through these images is helpful in identifying the cleanest and sharpest image of the CBD to measure.
7. The gallbladder tends to migrate inferiorly in elderly patients, so that it may lie significantly below the costal margin.

Ultrasound of the abdominal aorta is used to diagnose or exclude an abdominal aortic aneurysm (AAA). As the general population ages, the diagnosis of AAA should occur with more frequency, and the use of ultrasound of the abdominal aorta in the ED for patients with abdominal, back, or flank pain should also increase.

Clinical Indications for Abdominal Aorta Ultrasound

- Abdominal, back, or flank pain
- Pulsatile abdominal mass
- Hypotensive patient with abdominal pain or distention

Early diagnosis of AAA can improve patient survival. When a patient is in shock, there is no bedside test superior to an ESUE of the aorta to diagnose an AAA. Since aortic aneurysms occur as both fusiform (most common) and saccular types, it is essential that the ESUE of the aorta include both sagittal and transverse components. It is generally accepted that an aortic measurement of greater than 3.0 cm in diameter is abnormal, with a significant risk of aortic rupture starting with measurements greater than 5.0 cm. This section illustrates the abdominal vasculature, which will aid in identification of the abdominal aorta and evaluation of AAAs.

Required Views for Abdominal Aorta Ultrasound

- Transverse view
- Sagittal view

Recommended Transducers for Abdominal Aorta Ultrasound

- *Convex array*
- *Microconvex*
- *Phased array*
- *Mechanical sector*

Abdominal Aorta Window 1: Transverse View

Technique

- The patient is supine.
- Place the transducer in the epigastrium with the transducer indicator oriented to the patient's right. Move down the abdominal aorta to the bifurcation (about the level of the umbilicus) (Fig. 19.32).

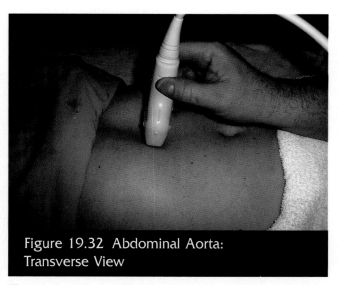

Figure 19.32 Abdominal Aorta: Transverse View

The transducer is placed in the epigastrium with the transducer indicator oriented to the patient's right; it is then moved down the abdominal aorta to the bifurcation. (Courtesy of Windy City Ultrasound, Inc.)

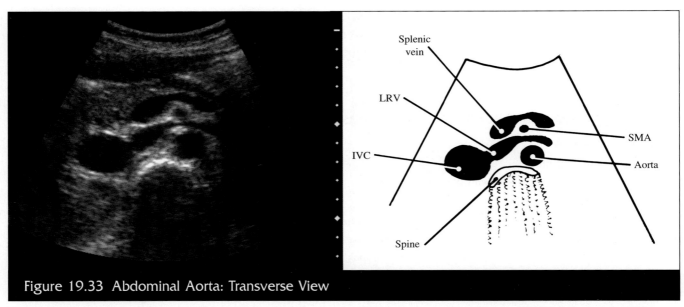

Figure 19.33 Abdominal Aorta: Transverse View

Various structures are identified, including the liver, inferior vena cava (IVC), superior mesenteric artery (SMA), splenic vein (SV), aorta, and "spinal stripe." (Courtesy of Windy City Ultrasound, Inc.)

- Identify the liver, aorta, inferior vena cava (IVC), superior mesenteric artery (SMA), splenic vein (SV), and "spinal stripe" at the level of the proximal aorta (Fig. 19.33).
- Identify the IVC, aorta, and spinal stripe at the mid- and distal aorta.

Abnormal Findings

- AAA: Anteroposterior measurements of more than 3.0 cm are suspicious for an aneurysm (Fig. 19.34).

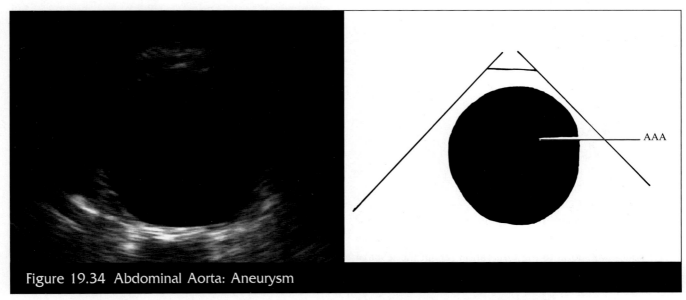

Figure 19.34 Abdominal Aorta: Aneurysm

A large abdominal aortic aneurysm (AAA) is seen in this view. (Courtesy of Michael J. Lambert, MD, RDMS.)

Abdominal Aorta Window 2: Sagittal View

Technique

- The patient is supine.
- Place the transducer in the epigastrium with the transducer indicator oriented toward the patient's head. Move down the abdominal aorta to the bifurcation (about the region of the umbilicus) (Fig. 19.35).
- Identify the liver, aorta, inferior vena cava (IVC), celiac trunk, and superior mesenteric artery (SMA) (Fig. 19.36).

Abnormal Findings

- AAA: Anteroposterior measurements of more than 3.0 cm are suspicious for an aneurysm.

Scan Pearls for Abdominal Aorta Ultrasound

1. The ESUE of the abdominal aorta should begin in the transverse view, since this view provides the greatest amount of information and is essential for the diagnosis of a saccular aneurysm.
2. Measure the entire diameter of the aorta or aneurysm and not just the lumen or false lumen. Include measurements of the proximal, mid-, and distal aorta.
3. If a significant amount of bowel gas is present, sit the patient at 45 degrees and apply constant gentle pressure.

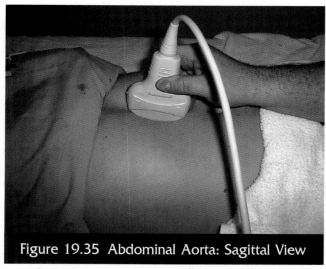

Figure 19.35 Abdominal Aorta: Sagittal View

The transducer is placed in the epigastrium with the transducer indicator oriented toward the patient's head; it is then moved down the abdominal aorta to the bifurcation. (Courtesy of Windy City Ultrasound, Inc.)

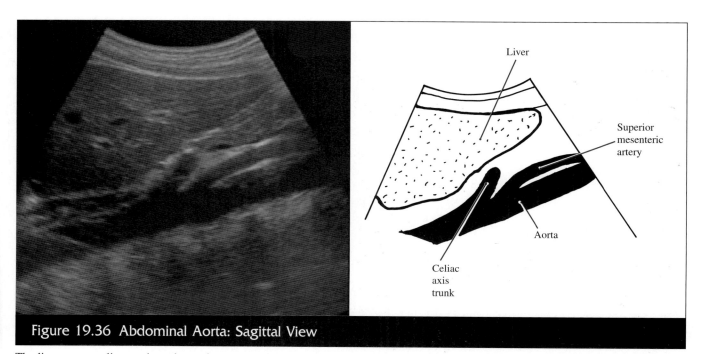

Figure 19.36 Abdominal Aorta: Sagittal View

The liver, aorta, celiac trunk, and superior mesenteric artery (SMA) are identified in this view. (Courtesy of Windy City Ultrasound, Inc.)

4. The IVC will generally collapse when you have the patient abruptly "sniff"—a result of the negative pressure transmitted to the venous system by this maneuver.

5. If pulsed Doppler is available, it may be used to discriminate between the highly pulsatile flow of the aorta and the low-amplitude rumble of the IVC.

Renal ultrasound can yield helpful diagnostic information for the patient presenting with abdominal or flank pain consistent with renal colic. Obstructive uropathy due to kidney stones is the principal pathology identified with renal ultrasound. However, it is not standard practice for emergency physicians to perform renal ultrasound to identify renal or ureteral calculi; rather, the kidneys are evaluated for hydronephrosis. The presence of hydronephrosis in the patient with renal colic is presumed to be a direct result of ureteral obstruction. There is no accurate means of determining the degree of obstruction by the presence of hydronephrosis.

Clinical Indications for Renal Ultrasound

- Flank pain
- Renal colic
- Abdominal pain in the elderly
- Hematuria
- Costovertebral angle (CVA) tenderness

The diagnostic dilemma for many emergency physicians is how to effectively utilize the renal ESUE in the patient with suspected renal colic. Although hydronephrosis is the primary sonographic finding in renal ESUE, renal cysts, calculi, and renal masses may also be identified.

The recommended sonographic approach to the kidney is identical to that for the RUQ and LUQ windows in the trauma/FAST examination previously discussed. The coronal view allows the sonographer to visualize the right or left kidney from the superior to inferior poles. The renal ESUE is best interpreted when comparative images are obtained between the right and left kidneys. It is important to realize that many approaches to the renal system, described in other texts, may be useful at times; however, the coronal view is familiar to the emergency physician. For that reason it is our primary window for evaluating the kidneys on the renal ESUE.

Required Views for Renal Ultrasound

- Coronal views (right and left)

Renal Ultrasound Window 1: Right and Left Coronal Views

Recommended Transducers for Renal Ultrasound

- *Convex array*
- *Microconvex*
- *Phased array*
- *Mechanical sector*

Technique

- The patient is supine.
- The transducer indicator is oriented toward the patient's head.
- The transducer is directed as a coronal section through the body in the midaxillary to posterior axillary lines (Fig. 19.37). Begin scanning between the 9th to 11th ribs on the right and the 8th to 11th ribs on the left.

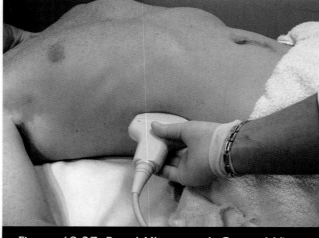

Figure 19.37 Renal Ultrasound: Coronal View

The transducer is directed in the midaxillary to posterior axillary lines for scanning between the 9th to 11th ribs on the right and the 8th to 11th ribs on the left. (Courtesy of Windy City Ultrasound, Inc.)

- Identify the liver, right kidney, renal cortex (with pyramids), and central renal sinus (Fig. 19.38).
- Identify the spleen, left kidney, renal cortex (with pyramids), and central renal sinus (Fig. 19.39).

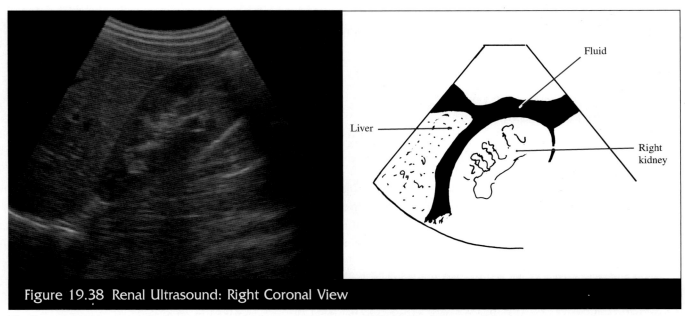

Figure 19.38 Renal Ultrasound: Right Coronal View

The liver, right kidney, and diaphragm are seen in this view. (Courtesy of Windy City Ultrasound, Inc.)

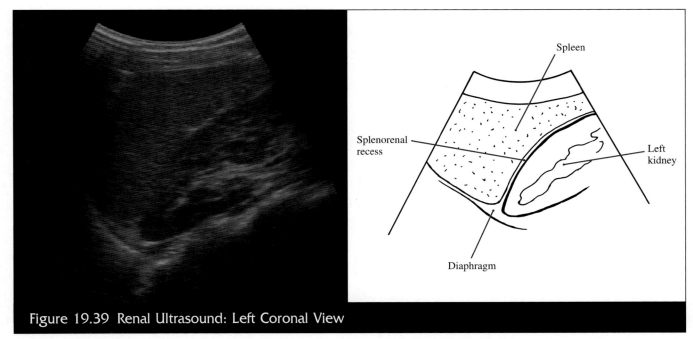

Figure 19.39 Renal Ultrasound: Left Coronal View

The spleen, left kidney, and diaphragm are seen in this view. (Courtesy of Windy City Ultrasound, Inc.)

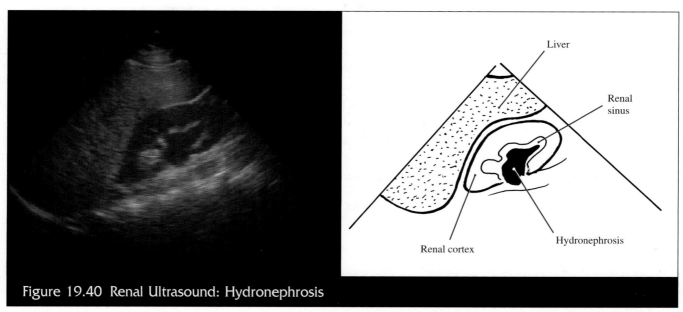

Figure 19.40 Renal Ultrasound: Hydronephrosis

Dilatation of the renal sinus with dark black, anechoic fluid within the bright renal sinus is consistent with hydronephrosis. (Courtesy of Paul R. Sierzenski, MD, RDMS, FAAEM.)

Abnormal Findings

- Hydronephrosis: Dilatation of the renal sinus with dark black, anechoic fluid within the bright renal sinus (Fig. 19.40).
- Renal calculi: Bright hyperechoic oval/round structures within the cortex or renal sinus (posterior shadowing is often present).
- Renal cyst: Anechoic structure often at the periphery of the renal cortex with a thin wall, and posterior acoustic enhancement.

Scan Pearls for Renal Ultrasound

1. If your machine has "dual" or "multi-image" modes, selecting this feature will allow you to make an on-screen side-by-side comparison of both kidneys.
2. Rib shadows will be evident with this coronal view. Have the patient hold his or her breath in inspiration and move the transducer a rib space higher or lower to visualize the kidney from the superior to the inferior pole.

Pelvic ultrasound is frequently used to evaluate the patient presenting with pelvic pain and/or vaginal bleeding, who may have a host of underlying clinical conditions. Among these are ovarian cyst, tuboovarian abscess, ovarian torsion, fetal demise, urinary retention, incomplete or threatened abortion, molar pregnancy, appendicitis, urinary tract infection, ureteral calculi, or pelvic inflammatory disease. However, the primary goal of the pelvic emergency screening ultrasound examination (ESUE) is to exclude an ectopic pregnancy. Pelvic ultrasound is accomplished with two different scanning techniques: transabdominal and endovaginal.

Pregnant patients presenting with abdominal pain or vaginal bleeding during the first trimester must have an ectopic pregnancy excluded. This is commonly accomplished in the ED setting by identifying an intrauterine pregnancy.

Clinical Indications for Pelvic Ultrasound

- Pelvic/abdominal pain
- Vaginal bleeding (pregnant or nonpregnant patient)
- Suspected pregnancy

Scan Requirements for Pelvic Ultrasound

1. Transabdominal ultrasound (uses the bladder as an acoustic window): sagittal and transverse views
2. Endovaginal ultrasound (provides a wider field of view, with better definition of anatomy): sagittal and coronal views

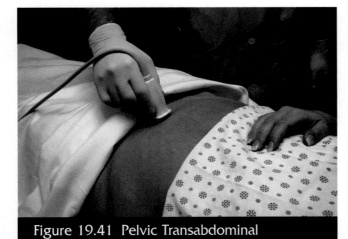

Figure 19.41 Pelvic Transabdominal Ultrasound: Sagittal View

The transducer is placed superior to symphysis pubis, with the transducer indicator directed in a line through the umbilicus (H = head, F = foot). (Courtesy of Windy City Ultrasound, Inc.)

Pelvic Transabdominal Sonography (TAS) Window 1: Sagittal View

Recommended Transducers for Pelvic TAS

- *Convex array*
- *Microconvex*
- *Phased array*
- *Mechanical sector*

Technique

- The patient is supine.
- Place transducer superior to symphysis pubis, with the transducer indicator directed toward the umbilicus (Fig. 19.41).
- Identify the bladder (triangular), uterus, rectum, ovaries, and the vesicouterine and rectouterine pouches (pouch of Douglas) (Fig. 19.42).

Abnormal Findings

- Free intraperitoneal fluid: Anechoic (dark) bands of fluid located in the vesicouterine and/or rectouterine pouch.

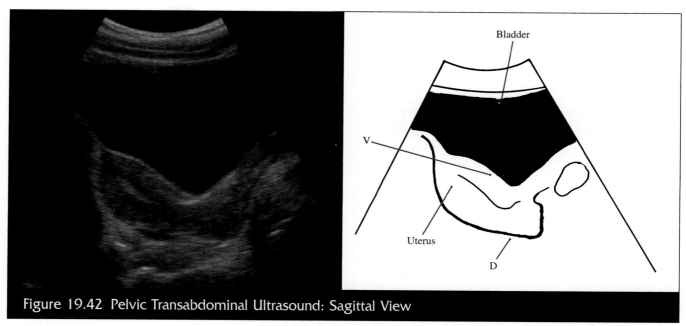

Figure 19.42 Pelvic Transabdominal Ultrasound: Sagittal View

The bladder (triangular in this view) and uterus are seen. The rectum, ovaries, and vesicouterine (V) and rectouterine (pouch of Douglas) (D) pouches may be seen with movement of the probe. (Courtesy of Windy City Ultrasound, Inc.)

Pelvic Transabdominal Sonography (TAS) Window 2: Transverse View

Technique

- The patient is supine.
- From the TAS sagittal view, rotate the transducer 90 degrees counterclockwise or place it superior to symphysis pubis, directed in a line connecting the anterior superior iliac crests (gradually angle caudally) (Fig. 19.43).
- Identify the bladder (rectangular), uterus (if present), rectum, ovaries, and the vesicouterine and rectouterine pouches (pouch of Douglas) (Fig. 19.44).

Abnormal Findings

- Free intraperitoneal fluid: Dark anechoic bands of fluid located in the vesicouterine and/or rectouterine pouch.

Scan Pearls for Transabdominal Ultrasound

1. A full bladder allows better visualization of structures posterior to the bladder in transabdominal ultrasound. An empty/minimally filled bladder is preferred for endovaginal ultrasound.
2. A *small* amount of free fluid found in the posterior cul-de-sac of the pelvis can be physiologic.

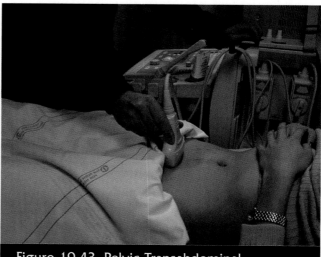

Figure 19.43 Pelvic Transabdominal Ultrasound: Transverse View

The transducer is rotated 90 degrees counterclockwise from the sagittal view and directed in a line connecting the anterior superior iliac crests. The transducer is angled caudally to complete the view. (Courtesy of Windy City Ultrasound, Inc.)

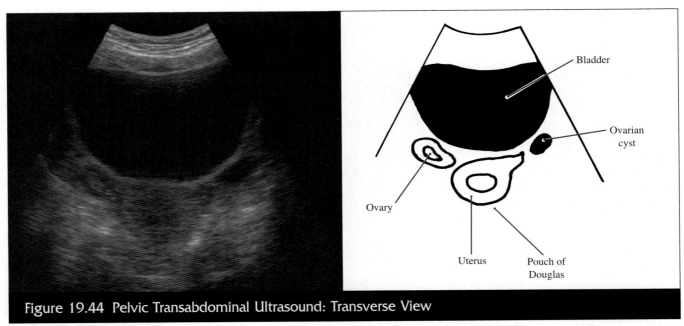

Figure 19.44 Pelvic Transabdominal Ultrasound: Transverse View

The bladder (rectangular in this view) uterus, and ovary are seen. The rectum and the vesicouterine and rectouterine pouches (pouch of Douglas) may be seen with movement of the probe. (Courtesy of Windy City Ultrasound, Inc.)

Endovaginal Sonography (EVS) Window 1: Sagittal View

Technique

- The patient is supine (lithotomy position).
- With a latex condom/shield covering the transducer, place it into the vagina, directed toward the anterior fornix in a line through the umbilicus (Fig. 19.45).
- The transducer indicator is directed up.
- Identify the bladder (sliver), uterus, rectum, ovaries, and the vesicouterine (anterior) and rectouterine (posterior) cul-de-sacs (Fig. 19.46).

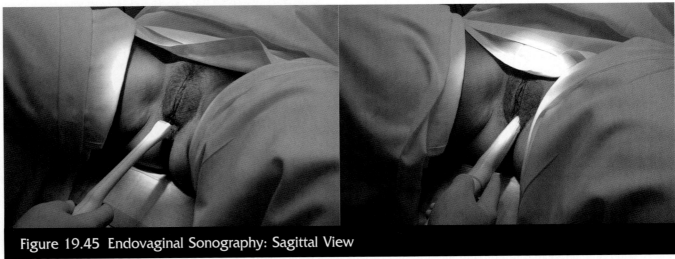

Figure 19.45 Endovaginal Sonography: Sagittal View

The transducer is directed toward the anterior fornix in a line through the umbilicus (A); it is then placed into the vagina (B). The probe is advanced gradually. (Courtesy of Windy City Ultrasound, Inc.)

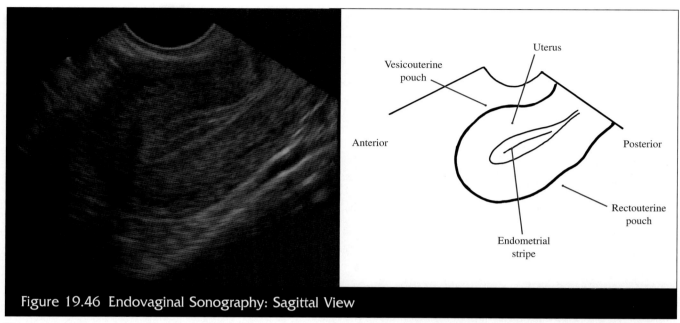

Figure 19.46 Endovaginal Sonography: Sagittal View

The uterus with an endometrial stripe is seen in this view. Other structures to be identified include the bladder, rectum, ovaries, and vesicouterine and rectouterine pouches. (Courtesy of Windy City Ultrasound, Inc.)

Abnormal Findings

- Free intraperitoneal fluid: Anechoic (dark) bands of fluid located in the vesicouterine and/or rectouterine pouch.
- Ectopic pregnancy: Extrauterine gestation may have an accompanying "pseudosac" (an anechoic fluid collection within the endometrial echo of the uterus) in the uterus (Fig. 19.47).

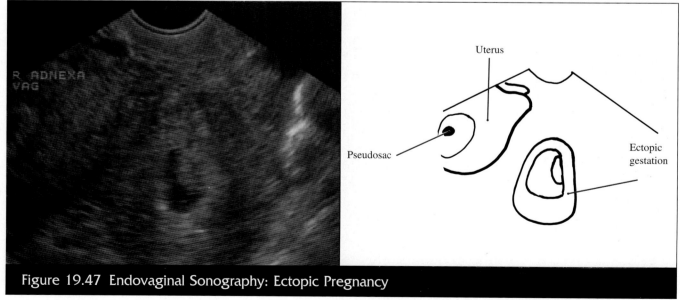

Figure 19.47 Endovaginal Sonography: Ectopic Pregnancy

An extrauterine gestation with an accompanying "pseudosac" (an anechoic fluid collection without a clear double decidual reaction) in the uterus is seen. (Courtesy of Michael J. Lambert, MD, RDMS.)

Endovaginal Sonography (EVS) Window 2: Coronal View

Technique

- The patient is supine (ideally in the lithotomy position).
- From the EVS sagittal view, rotate the transducer counterclockwise 90 degrees or, with a latex condom/shield covering the transducer, place the transducer into the vagina directed toward the posterior fornix in a line through the umbilicus (Fig. 19.48).

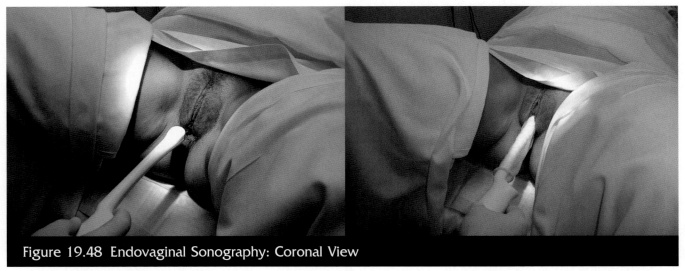

Figure 19.48 Endovaginal Sonography: Coronal View

From the sagittal view, the transducer is rotated counterclockwise 90 degrees (*A*) and directed toward the posterior fornix in a line through the umbilicus. (Courtesy of Windy City Ultrasound, Inc.)

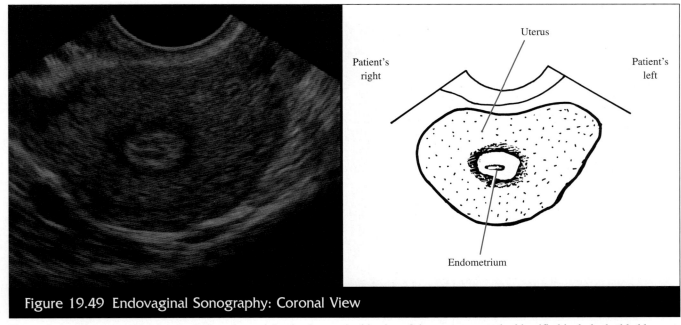

Figure 19.49 Endovaginal Sonography: Coronal View

The oval-shaped uterus with a hyperechoic endometrial stripe is seen in this view. Other structures to be identified include the bladder, rectum, ovaries, and the vesicouterine and rectouterine pouches. (Courtesy of Windy City Ultrasound, Inc.)

- Identify the bladder (sliver), uterus (ovoid) (Fig. 19.49), rectum, ovaries (Fig. 19.50), and the vesicouterine and rectouterine pouches (pouch of Douglas).
- Identify an intrauterine pregnancy if present (Fig. 19.51).

Abnormal or Positive Findings

- Free intraperitoneal fluid: Anechoic (dark) bands of fluid located in the vesicouterine (anterior) or rectouterine (posterior) cul-de-sac.

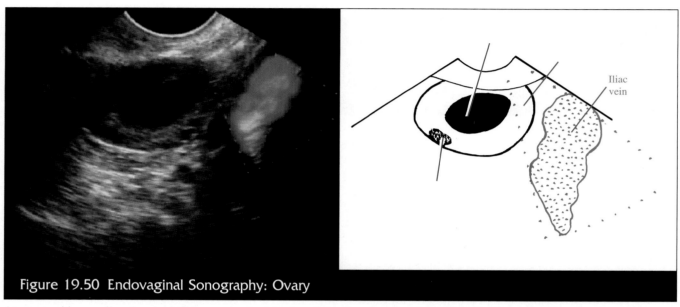

Figure 19.50 Endovaginal Sonography: Ovary

An ovary with a small cyst and a follicle are seen in this view. Color-flow Doppler, if available, facilitates identification of vascular structures. The iliac vein is seen in this view. (Courtesy of Michael J. Lambert, MD, RDMS.)

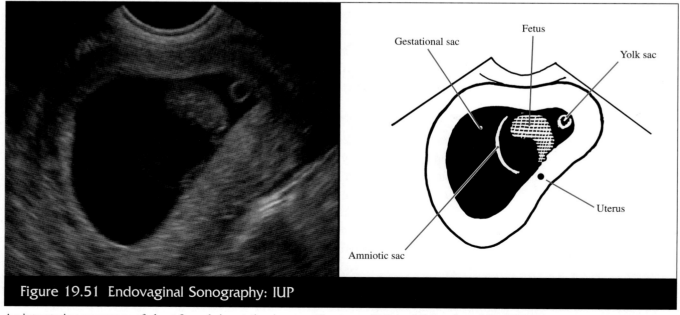

Figure 19.51 Endovaginal Sonography: IUP

An intrauterine pregnancy of about 9 weeks' gestation is seen. (Courtesy of Michael J. Lambert, MD, RDMS.)

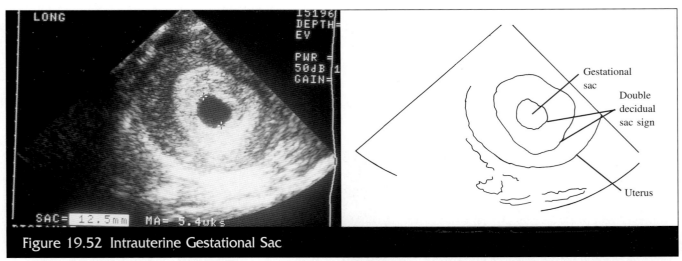

Figure 19.52 Intrauterine Gestational Sac

Discrete ring of an intrauterine gestational sac seen on transvaginal ultrasound. No yolk sac is visualized. A double decidual sac sign is seen, however, lending evidence of a true gestational sac versus a pseudogestational sac formed from a decidual cast in ectopic pregnancy. A thorough look in the adnexa is important in diagnosing ectopic pregnancy when a gestational sac is the only finding. (Courtesy of Janice Underwood, RDMS.)

- Live intrauterine pregnancy: Greater than 5-mm gestational sac with a thick, concentric echogenic ring within the endometrial echo of the uterus and both of the following: fetal pole with cardiac activity.
- Intrauterine pregnancy (IUP): Greater than 5-mm gestational sac with a thick, concentric echogenic ring within the endometrial echo of the uterus and one of the following: yolk sac, fetal pole, or double decidual sign (the decidua capsularis and decidua vera seen as two distinct hypoechoic layers surrounding the early gestational sac) (Fig. 19.52).
- Abnormal IUP: Gestational sac greater than 10 to 12 mm without yolk sac, gestational sac greater than 16 mm without fetal pole, or definitive fetal pole without cardiac pulsation.
- No definitive IUP: The uterus appears empty and no definitive ectopic pregnancy is visualized. Possible diagnosis includes early IUP, abortion, ectopic pregnancy.
- Ectopic pregnancy: Greater than 5-mm gestational sac and thick, concentric echogenic ring *outside* the endometrial echo of the uterus and one of the following: definitive yolk sac, obvious fetal pole, cardiac activity.

Scan Pearls for Endovaginal Ultrasound

1. On insertion of the transducer, identify the bladder.
2. In the sagittal view, identify the endometrial stripe from the fundus of the uterus to the cervix. This is accomplished by tilting the probe (anteriorly to posteriorly) while maintaining a sagittal plane of the uterus.
3. Return to the fundus of the uterus in a sagittal view and slowly evaluate the right and then left borders of the uterus in the longitudinal axis.
4. Turn the transducer counterclockwise 90 degrees to enter the coronal plane. The uterus should appear oval in this view. Scan posteriorly to the cervix and then superiorly to the fundus of the uterus to exclude the presence of a bicornuate uterus.

5. If a pregnancy or intrauterine sac is identified, further evaluate with measurements and an assessment of fetal cardiac activity.

6. To evaluate the ovaries, begin with the patient's right ovary and scan initially in the longitudinal (sagittal) plane, then rotate the transducer counterclockwise 90 degrees and evaluate the ovary in the coronal plane. The ovaries ideally will be located anteromedially to the external iliac vessels. This is often only a guide to their location, and a methodical approach is often required to visualize both ovaries.

7. If the uterus is difficult to identify, withdraw the transducer slightly. A common error in EVS is inserting the transducer too far, thus bypassing the uterus and imaging only bowel.

CHAPTER 20
HIV CONDITIONS

Shane Cline
Michael Krentz

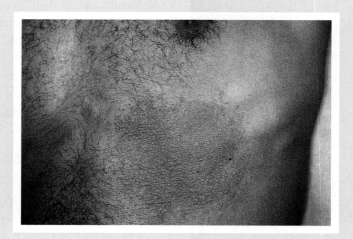

Associated Clinical Features

Clinical illness accompanies primary HIV infection in approximately two-thirds of patients, usually within several days to several weeks of exposure. Acute HIV infection is often undiagnosed or underdiagnosed in the ED setting. The most common symptoms after seroconversion include fever, malaise, headache, photophobia, sore throat, enlarged lymph nodes, arthralgias, abdominal pain, diarrhea, and a typically maculopapular rash with lesions on the face, neck, and trunk (Fig. 20.1). This rash is seen in over half of persons with symptomatic acute HIV infection and can have many presentations. The lesions are usually 5 to 10 mm in diameter and are erythematous, nonpruritic, and nontender. Mucocutaneous inflammation and ulceration of the buccal mucosa is also a common finding and distinctive feature. Less frequently, patients will demonstrate neurologic signs and symptoms consistent with meningoencephalitis, myelopathy, peripheral neuropathy, or Guillain-Barré syndrome. Therefore HIV infection should be considered in the differential diagnosis of aseptic meningitis. The acute illness usually lasts from a few days to two weeks. Laboratory studies may show lymphopenia and thrombocytopenia.

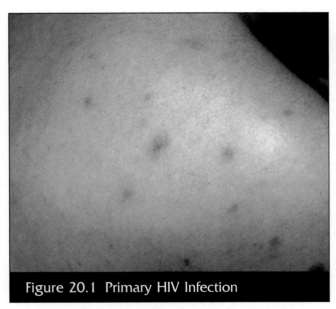

Figure 20.1 Primary HIV Infection

A maculopapular rash is seen in over half of persons with symptomatic acute HIV infection. This less typical papular/vesicular rash was present in a patient with primary HIV infection. (Courtesy of Gregory K. Robbins, MD, MPH.)

Differential Diagnosis

Formerly considered to be similar to a mononucleosis-like viral syndrome, primary HIV infection does present with some unique features. Perhaps the most distinctive physical manifestation is the skin rash, which is rarely found in primary presentations of mononucleosis, toxoplasmosis, and cytomegalovirus infection. The rashes of rubella and roseola do not affect palms and soles. Other considerations in the differential diagnosis include hepatitis A or B, disseminated gonococcal infection, drug reactions, and secondary syphilis.

Emergency Department Treatment and Disposition

HIV testing is rarely performed in the ED owing to the difficulty of obtaining informed consent, lack of time for thorough counseling, and uncertain follow-up. Moreover, the diagnosis of acute HIV infection is difficult to make with standard serologic tests. Emergency physicians should take a careful history for HIV risk factors and should be cautious but honest in entertaining this diagnosis. Patients should be educated about safe sex and referred for further outpatient testing and evaluation. Prompt follow-up is critical, since immediate antiviral therapy is indicated for persons with acute HIV infection.

Clinical Pearls

1. Although historically HIV infection has been seen predominately in patients who belong to high-risk groups, the epidemiology is changing. When any sexually active patient presents to the ED with an acute, severe febrile illness, acute HIV infection should be included in the differential diagnosis.

2. Consider acute HIV infection as a potential etiology in patients with aseptic meningitis, pharyngitis, or a maculopapular rash.

3. Ensure proper follow-up for patients in whom the diagnosis of acute HIV infection is entertained.

Associated Clinical Features

Oral infections are seen in over half of all HIV patients. Oral candidiasis can occur at all stages of HIV disease. The severity of the infection depends on the degree of immunosuppression. The most common species is *Candida albicans. Candida tropicalis* can cause severe infections. Another 150 different species of *Candida* have become increasingly resistant because of the chronic use of systemic antifungal therapy.

Oral thrush is classified as pseudomembranous, angular, or erythematous. Pseudomembranous candidiasis involves removable whitish plaques on the tongue and buccal mucosa (Fig. 20.2). Patients with angular cheilitis demonstrate erythema and fissures at the angles of the mouth. Erythematous thrush appears as smooth red patches along the soft and hard palate. Oral candidiasis can be diagnosed clinically and by microscopic observation of hyphae with 10% KOH preparation.

Esophageal candidiasis frequently accompanies oral candidiasis. The most common symptoms are dysphagia and odynophagia. Barium swallow and endoscopy aid in making the diagnosis. Typical findings observed with an air-contrast barium swallow are ulcerative plaques, causing filling defects along the long axis of the esophagus and producing the classic "shaggy" mucosal appearance. Endoscopy provides for the definitive diagnosis (Fig. 20.3), and allows the examiner to obtain biopsies and viral, bacterial, and fungal cultures.

Like other conditions in immunocompromised patients, vaginal candidiasis can be severe, causing a whitish discharge and vulvar erythema. Women will commonly present to the ED for evaluation of vaginal candidiasis as their first clinical manifestation of the HIV infection.

Differential Diagnosis

HIV-related candidal infections must be differentiated from a variety of other entities, depending on the site of infection:

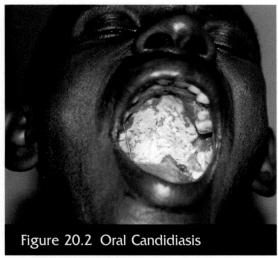

Figure 20.2 Oral Candidiasis

Removable whitish plaques on the palate are seen in this HIV patient with pseudomembranous candidiasis. (Courtesy of Thea James, MD.)

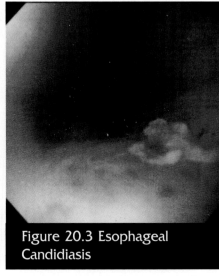

Figure 20.3 Esophageal Candidiasis

Endoscopy demonstrating esophageal candidiasis in this HIV patient. (Courtesy of Edward C. Oldfield III, MD.)

Oral	Esophageal	Vaginal
Cytomegalovirus	Cytomegalovirus	Chlamydial
Herpes simplex	Herpes simplex	Gonococcal
Hairy tongue	HIV esophagitis	Bacterial
HIV stomatitis	Medication-related ("pill esophagitis")	
Kaposi's sarcoma	*Mycobacterium avium intracellulare*	

Emergency Department Treatment and Disposition

Poor oral intake secondary to pain associated with severe oral or esophageal candidiasis can cause dehydration and malnutrition, sometimes requiring intravenous hydration and admission. Empiric treatment is appropriate in patients suspected of having esophageal candidiasis. Endoscopy should be performed in those patients whose symptoms do not improve in 3 to 5 days. There is no "standard" treatment for candidiasis in the HIV patient. Both oral and vaginal candidiasis can be treated with standard nystatin or clotrimazole troches. Alternatively, systemic treatment with either ketoconazole or fluconazole is usually effective for oral, vaginal, and esophageal candidiasis. For severe or refractory cases of candidiasis, amphotericin B is the drug of choice.

Clinical Pearls

1. Popular one-dose oral treatments for oral or vaginal candidiasis are associated with a high rate of relapse in HIV patients.
2. Consider possible drug interactions when prescribing antifungal medications. For example, the absorption of ketoconazole is impaired by the simultaneous administration of antacids and cimetidine. Ketoconazole levels are also decreased in patients taking rifampin or isoniazid. Because of these drug interactions, many clinicians favor the use of fluconazole, since lack of gastric acid or the presence of food does not affect its absorption. Fluconazole does raise the serum levels of warfarin, rifabutin, or sulfonylureas.
3. Ensure follow-up in 3 to 5 days when treating empirically for presumptive esophageal candidiasis.
4. Oral candidiasis is a poor prognostic sign, predictive of progression to AIDS in the HIV-positive patient.

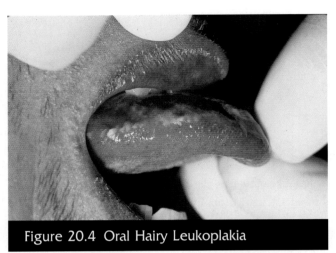

Figure 20.4 Oral Hairy Leukoplakia

Filiform projections and whitish plaques along the side of the tongue are characteristic. (Courtesy of Briana Hill, MD.)

Associated Clinical Features

Caused by the Epstein-Barr virus, oral hairy leukoplakia is frequently encountered in HIV patients who present to the ED with unrelated symptoms. The patient may demonstrate characteristic filiform projections and whitish plaques along the side of the tongue (Fig. 20.4). The buccal mucosa may also be affected. Most often oral hairy leukoplakia is asymptomatic, although occasionally this condition can cause pain. The diagnosis is usually made clinically. However, definitive diagnosis can be made by biopsy, which characteristically reveals acanthosis and parakeratosis.

Differential Diagnosis

Commonly seen in HIV patients are numerous conditions that can be confused with hairy leukoplakia. These include oral candidiasis, geographic tongue, oral herpes simplex virus, cytomegalovirus, Kaposi's sarcoma, and idiopathic aphthous ulcerations.

Emergency Department Treatment and Disposition

Patients known to be HIV-positive can be educated and reassured. If the patient is symptomatic, zidovudine, oral acyclovir, or topical tretinoin may be prescribed in consultation with an infectious disease specialist.

Clinical Pearls

1. The presence of hairy tongue in a patient who is not known to have HIV requires follow-up and serologic testing and may expand the emergency physician's workup.
2. Hairy leukoplakia is rarely associated with conditions other than HIV.
3. Oral candidiasis can be distinguished by utilizing a swab in an attempt to remove the exudate characteristic of thrush and by observing pseudohyphal elements microscopically.

Associated Clinical Features

Prior to the emergence of HIV, Kaposi's sarcoma (KS) was known only as a rare endothelial tumor found in older patients of European/Mediterranean descent. In HIV patients, KS most often affects male homosexual or bisexual patients. The etiologic agent, human herpesvirus 8, is strongly implicated as the viral cofactor that plays an important role in the development of KS.

Kaposi's sarcoma is usually multicentric, involving the skin and visceral organs. In lighter-skinned individuals, cutaneous KS is usually violaceous (Fig. 20.5), whereas it is black in those who are darker-skinned (Fig. 20.6). Visual presentations vary. Early lesions are usually less than 0.5 cm in diameter, nontender, and flat. Later they become larger and nodular. Any area of the skin can become involved, especially the soles of the feet and the mucous membranes. The palms are rarely affected.

Differential Diagnosis

Other conditions that can present similarly to Kaposi's sarcoma include drug reactions, melanomas, opportunistic infections, bacillary angiomatosis, and thrombotic thrombocytopenic purpura.

Emergency Department Treatment and Disposition

Since the diagnosis of cutaneous KS requires biopsy, the patient should be referred to dermatology and infectious disease for follow-up. Early KS can be treated with immunomodulators and antiviral agents, whereas late KS or rapidly progressive KS is treated with systemic chemotherapy or radiation therapy.

Clinical Pearls

1. HIV patients who present with persistent raised purple lesions warrant biopsy.
2. Perform a careful skin and oral examination in HIV patients.
3. Note that half of patients with oral involvement have other GI tract involvement as well.
4. KS can be an early manifestation of HIV infection in patients with normal CD4 cell counts.

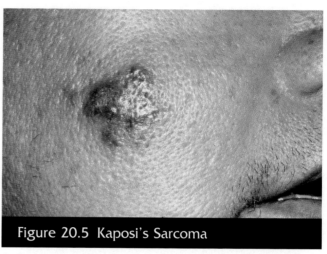

Figure 20.5 Kaposi's Sarcoma

A single violaceous patch is seen on the face of an HIV-positive patient. (Courtesy of George Turiansky, MD.)

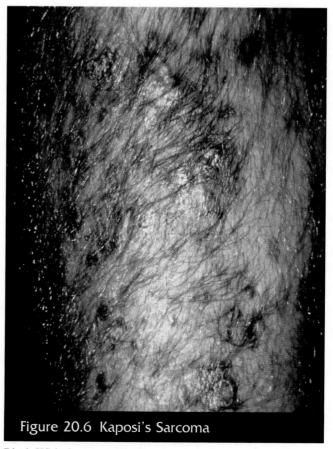

Figure 20.6 Kaposi's Sarcoma

Black KS lesions, as typically seen in darker-skinned individuals. (Courtesy of the Department of Dermatology, National Naval Medical Center, Bethesda, MD.)

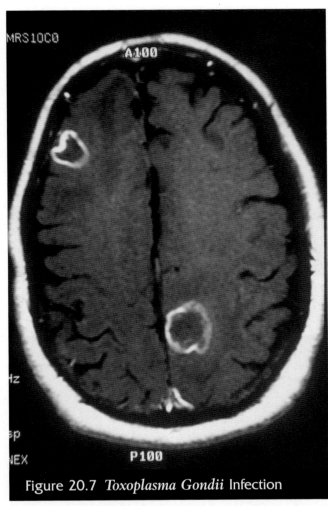

Figure 20.7 *Toxoplasma Gondii* Infection

Contrast head CT showing typical multiple ring-enhancing lesions seen in *T. gondii* CNS infection. (Courtesy of Edward C. Oldfield III, MD.)

Associated Clinical Features

Toxoplasmosis is a common opportunistic infection affecting HIV patients with less than 100 CD4 cells/μL. It can present as encephalitis, chorioretinitis, pneumonia, or a disseminated disease. The most common cause is reactivation of a latent infection.

Central nervous system (CNS) toxoplasmosis most often presents with symptoms consistent with a mass lesion (headache, focal neurologic deficit, seizure), or as encephalitis (fever and altered mental status). Diagnosis can be difficult. Contrast computed tomography (CT) of the head most typically reveals multiple ring-enhancing lesions with a predilection for the basal ganglia or corticomedullary junction (Fig. 20.7). Magnetic resonance imaging (MRI) of the head is a better test for the diagnosis. Serum serologic tests have no role in the diagnosis; however, cerebrospinal fluid (CSF) antibodies to *T. gondii* can be helpful. Often the diagnosis is based on response to empiric treatment, as evidenced by an improvement in symptoms and reduction in the size of the lesions.

Ocular toxoplasmosis is a common complication of HIV disease. Patients typically present with a visual disturbance such as decreased vision, floaters, or visual field deficits. Eye pain or swelling is rare. Retinitis is typically diagnosed by indirect ophthalmoscopic evaluation revealing exudates and hemorrhage (Fig. 20.8). Toxoplasmosis retinitis appears different than cytomegalovirus (CMV) retinitis because it involves deeper strata of the retina, resulting in less edema and hemorrhage.

Differential Diagnosis

Other pathologic CNS conditions to consider may be classified as either infectious (bacterial meningitis, tuberculous meningitis, herpes encephalitis, progressive multifocal leukoencephalopathy, syphilis, fungal infections, etc.) or noninfectious (lymphoma, metastasis, drug reaction).

Ocular toxoplasmosis can appear similar to cytomegalovirus, varicella zoster, herpes simplex virus, *Pneumocystis* infection, fungal infection, ischemic retinopathy, ocular syphilis, and drug reactions.

Emergency Department Treatment and Disposition

Stabilization of the patient is the initial intervention for CNS toxoplasmosis. Subsequently, analgesics and antipyretics should be administered if indicated. If the patient presented with a seizure, the emergency physician should consider loading with intravenous phenytoin or fosphenytoin.

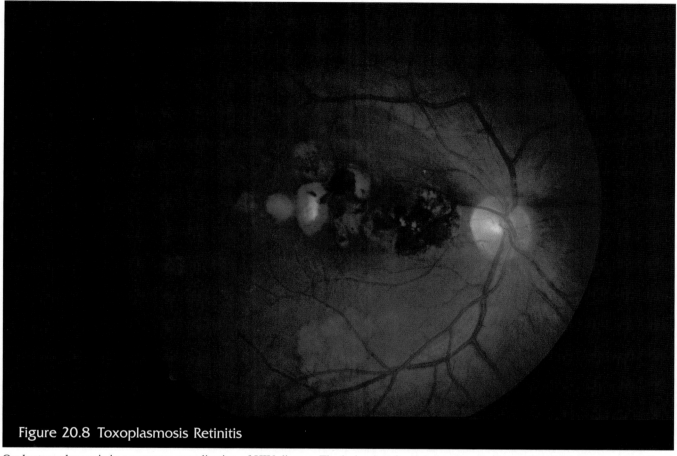

Figure 20.8 Toxoplasmosis Retinitis

Ocular toxoplasmosis is a common complication of HIV disease. The lesion is a focal destructive chorioretinitis which leaves well-defined, heavily pigmented scars, especially in the macular area. (Courtesy of Department of Ophthalmology; Naval Medical Center, San Diego, CA.)

The workup should include a noncontrast head CT followed by a contrast head CT and a lumbar puncture. Infectious disease consultation should then be obtained. When the diagnosis of CNS toxoplasmosis is made, treatment includes pyrimethamine and sulfadoxine for 6 weeks or until symptoms or neuroimaging findings have resolved. As in the case of *Cryptococcus* infections in HIV patients, chronic suppressive treatment is required. The dose of trimethoprim-sulfamethoxazole used for prophylaxis against *Pneumocystis carinii* pneumonia is sufficient.

For ocular toxoplasmosis, a thorough slit-lamp examination, including fluorescein staining and measurements of intraocular pressure, should be done before consulting ophthalmology.

Clinical Pearls

1. Space-occupying lesions, which are common in HIV patients, can cause increased intracranial pressure. Under most circumstances, perform a head CT before attempting a lumbar puncture in order to prevent iatrogenic herniation.
2. Consider steroids and seizure prophylaxis for patients with severe cerebral edema as evidenced by severe confusion, lethargy, coma, or even papilledema.
3. Educate patients with HIV to cook their meat thoroughly and to be compulsive about hand washing. Cat owners should be instructed to wear gloves while cleaning the litter box.

Associated Clinical Features

Cytomegalovirus (CMV) infects over three-quarters of HIV patients, usually resulting from reactivation of a latent infection. Most patients have progressive disease with a CD4 cell count of less than 100/μL. CMV infection can present as chorioretinitis, central nervous system disease, GI disease, or pulmonary disease.

Patients with ocular CMV typically complain of unilateral vision loss. If untreated, the condition progresses to bilateral blindness. The funduscopic examination usually reveals exudates, hemorrhages, edema, and dense opaque lesions, giving it the typical "cottage cheese and ketchup" appearance (Fig. 20.9).

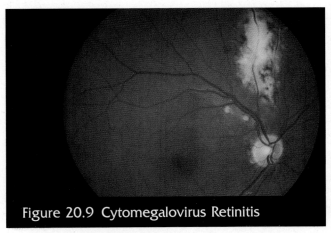

Figure 20.9 Cytomegalovirus Retinitis

Funduscopic examination shows exudates and hemorrhages ("cottage cheese and ketchup" appearance) seen with CMV retinitis. (Courtesy of Edward C. Oldfield III, MD.)

Differential Diagnosis

Although many opportunistic infections (fungal, toxoplasmal, herpetic) can mimic cytomegalovirus infections, the differential diagnosis should include ischemic retinopathy and drug reactions.

Emergency Department Treatment and Disposition

First-line therapy consists of either ganciclovir or foscarnet given intravenously. Intraocular ganciclovir implants can be combined with either. Relapse or progression of CMV retinitis is common, thus requiring chronic suppressive maintenance therapy.

Clinical Pearls

1. Because the diagnosis can be difficult, ocular complaints in HIV patients require a complete ophthalmologic examination and possible ophthalmology referral.
2. Unlike patients with candidal esophagitis, whose chief complaint is dysphagia, patients with CMV esophagitis typically complain of odynophagia or substernal chest pain and very infrequently of dysphagia.
3. Bone marrow suppression is a major toxic effect of ganciclovir.

Associated Clinical Features

HIV patients infected with *Cryptococcus neoformans* can present with the disseminated form (Fig. 20.10) or with primary central nervous system (CNS) or pulmonary manifestations. Cryptococcal meningitis is a common opportunistic infection of the CNS, usually occurring in patients with advanced HIV infection whose CD4 cell counts are less than $50/\mu L$. Presenting symptoms are often nonspecific. Most commonly, patients with cryptococcal meningitis complain of headache, fever, and malaise that may be anywhere from 1 day to 4 months in duration. Diagnosis is made by lumbar puncture. Cerebrospinal fluid (CSF) findings usually reveal a normal CSF glucose concentration, a mildly elevated CSF protein concentration, and a CSF leukocyte count of less than $20/\mu L$. Although the sensitivity is not extremely high, an india ink stain in the ED can be beneficial (see Fig. 21.22). A CSF cryptococcal latex antigen test can also be obtained and has a sensitivity of 90%, as compared with 50% for an india ink stain. Definitive diagnosis is by culture.

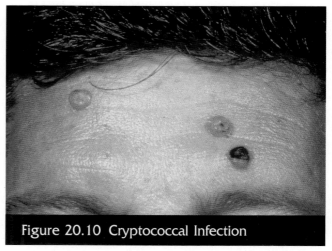

Figure 20.10 Cryptococcal Infection

Cryptococcal skin lesions in disseminated form. Note that the umbilicated centers give a similar appearance to that of molluscum contagiosum. (Courtesy of Briana Hill, MD.)

Differential Diagnosis

Diseases that might mimic cryptococcal meningitis include other fungal infections (*Histoplasma* and *Nocardia*), bacterial infections (bacterial meningitis, tuberculous meningitis, brain abscess), viral encephalitis (herpes simplex virus, herpes zoster, progressive multifocal leukoencephalopathy), protozoal infections (toxoplasmosis), and space-occupying lesions (lymphomas, Kaposi's sarcoma).

Emergency Department Treatment and Disposition

As with all patients, the most critical first step in the ED is stabilization. In general, HIV patients with fever and headache should receive an antipyretic and have blood for two cultures drawn. Empiric antibiotics (ceftriaxone, 2g IV) should be administered if the patient appears "sick" or has unstable vital signs. Empiric administration of antivirals or antifungals should be discussed with an infectious disease specialist. Most often the workup should include noncontrast computed tomography (CT) followed by contrast CT of the head and lumbar puncture (LP). If the lumbar puncture reveals cryptococcus, the standard treatment consists of amphotericin B with flucytosine for a period of 6 weeks. High cerebrospinal fluid (CSF) pressure can cause many of the symptoms of cryptococcal meningitis. Serial spinal taps, an indwelling lumbar drain, or ventriculoperitoneal shunting may be indicated. Fluconazole is the maintenance treatment of choice for cryptococcal meningitis.

Clinical Pearls

1. Perform the LP after the CT, and do so with the patient in a lateral position so as to obtain a proper opening pressure.

2. Obtain a fourth tube of CSF for special studies such as directogens (*Haemophilus influenzae type B, C. neoformans, Neisseria meningitides, Streptococcus pneumonia, Streptococcus agalactiae*), acid-fast stains and cultures, VDRL, cytology, PCR (varicella zoster, enteroviruses, herpes simplex virus, parvovirus B19, JC 19 virus).

3. "False-positive" india ink stains can occur with other encapsulated organisms such as *Klebsiella pneumoniae, Rhodotorula, Candida,* and *Proteus.*

4. Blood cultures are positive in more than three-quarters of patients with cryptococcal meningitis.

Associated Clinical Features

In primary varicella infection, the virus migrates from the skin to the sensory nerves, where it becomes latent. This primary phase can be much more severe in HIV patients, sometimes causing central nervous system involvement, pneumonitis, and hepatitis. Contrary to patterns seen in immune-competent patients, primary varicella in HIV patients is more extensive, with deep-seated, slow-healing, and often recurrent lesions that may last for months.

Reactivation of the varicella virus (rarely HSV) characterizes herpes zoster, with acute inflammation of one or more of the dorsal root ganglia. A prodrome of lancinating pain and hyperalgesias over the skin surface for 3 to 4 days is followed by the appearance of a herpetic eruption of painful vesicles with red bases in a dermatomal distribution (Fig. 20.11). Reactivation herpes zoster is seen in 10 to 20% of HIV patients and is often the first clinical indication of an immune deficiency. Approximately 5% of patients will develop "zoster paresis," with a motor weakness following the rash.

HIV patients with herpes zoster are at risk for dissemination of the virus (Fig. 20.12), possibly leading to meningoencephalitis, retinitis, and pneumonitis. Cerebral angiitis is a complication of herpes zoster involving the ipsilateral carotid or middle cerebral artery, with subsequent contralateral aphasia or focal deficits. Reactivation of the virus in the ophthalmic division of the trigeminal nerve (Fig. 20.13) can cause conjunctivitis, keratitis, ocular muscle palsies, ptosis, and mydriasis.

The diagnosis of herpes zoster in the ED is usually made clinically. Culture, serologic testing, or PCR confirms unequivocally. A Tzanck smear can be obtained by scraping the base of a lesion in an attempt to demonstrate multinucleated giant cells (see Fig. 13.15).

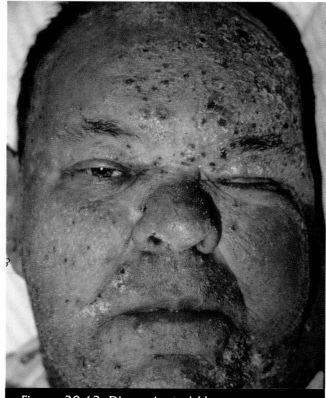

Figure 20.12 Disseminated Herpes Zoster Infection

Vesicles are seen over the entire face, representing disseminated HZV infection (multiple dermatomal distributions). (Courtesy of the Department of Dermatology, National Naval Medical Center, Bethesda, MD.)

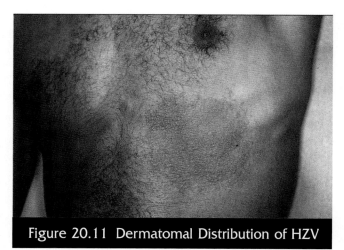

Figure 20.11 Dermatomal Distribution of HZV

Many tiny vesicles on an erythematous base are grouped in a dermatomal distribution in this HIV patient. (Courtesy of Jeffery Gibson, MD.)

661

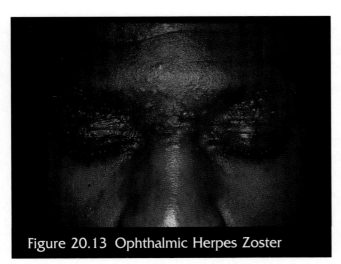

Figure 20.13 Ophthalmic Herpes Zoster

This patient has vesicles in the ophthalmic division of cranial nerve V bilaterally. (Courtesy of Daniel Savitt, MD.)

Differential Diagnosis

Etiologies for other vesicular lesions commonly encountered in HIV patients include herpes simplex virus, enterovirus, insect bites, contact dermatitis, and opportunistic infections.

Emergency Department Treatment and Disposition

Patients with disseminated disease or ophthalmic zoster should receive intravenous acyclovir (10 to 12.5 mg/kg IV q 8 h). Moreover, treatment of zoster ophthalmicus should include topical antibiotics and an immediate ophthalmology referral. For uncomplicated mild cases of herpes zoster, acyclovir (800 mg five times a day for 10 days) or famciclovir (500 mg tid for 7 days) is recommended. [Valacyclovir should be used with caution in HIV patients, since it is associated with thrombotic thrombocytopenic purpura (TTP).] Acyclovir or famciclovir cause a more rapid resolution of cutaneous lesions if started within 72 h of their appearance, but they do not change the incidence of postherpetic neuralgia. Valacyclovir may be more effective than acyclovir or famciclovir. In the absence of response to one of the oral regimens, the patient should be switched to intravenous acyclovir or foscarnet (if resistance is suspected). Immunocompromised patients should not be placed on steroids. Narcotics, capsaicin cream, and tricyclic antidepressants can be used for pain control.

From a preventive standpoint, the Centers for Disease Control (CDC) recommends that immunocompromised patients receive postexposure prophylaxis with varicella zoster immune globulin if they present within 96 h of exposure. Furthermore, susceptible patients should be vaccinated.

Clinical Pearls

1. Avoid prescribing oral antivirals and discharging patients home without close follow-up.
2. Worsening cases of herpes zoster, complicated herpes zoster, or ophthalmic zoster all require intravenous acyclovir and admission.
3. Herpes zoster encephalitis can occur months after the cutaneous phase and can be difficult to diagnose. Common presenting symptoms include mental status changes, headache, fever, photophobia, and vomiting. Ensure follow-up for patients diagnosed with shingles who are less than 50 years old, since they may require workup of a potential underlying immunodeficiency.

Associated Clinical Features

Eosinophilic folliculitis is a common dermatologic condition that usually involves the face, neck, trunk, and extremities (Figs. 20.14, 20.15). Patients complain of severe pruritus. The skin lesions usually start as small groups of pustules and vesicles. These can later coalesce to create irregular lakes of erosions and polycyclic plaques with central hyperpigmentation. Most patients with this condition will demonstrate CD4 cell counts of less than 250/μL. Approximately half of these patients will have moderate eosinophilia and moderate leukocytosis.

Differential Diagnosis

HIV patients have a high incidence of seborrheic dermatitis, which can be confused with this condition. Inquiry about concurrent medications or environmental exposures may suggest either a drug reaction or insect bites. Kaposi's sarcoma and lymphomas can present similarly to this condition. Other dermatologic conditions to be considered are scabies, staphylococcal folliculitis, photodermatitis, pruritus nodularis, xerostomia, and ichthyosis.

Emergency Department Treatment and Disposition

The diagnosis requires dermatology referral for biopsy. Antihistamines, topical steroids, itraconazole, and ultraviolet B phototherapy are effective.

Clinical Pearls

1. The severe pruritus associated with this condition helps distinguish it from bacterial folliculitis.
2. Patients with eosinophilic folliculitis may present with prurigo nodularis and lichen simplex chronicus as a consequence of severe itching and rubbing.

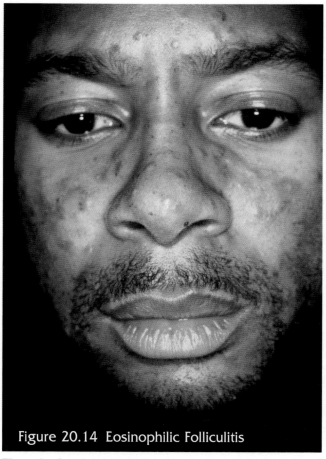

Figure 20.14 Eosinophilic Folliculitis

The rash of eosinophilic folliculitis consists of small groups of pustules and vesicles, as seen on the face of this patient. (Courtesy of the Department of Dermatology, National Naval Medical Center, Bethesda, MD.)

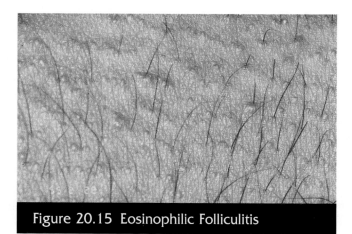

Figure 20.15 Eosinophilic Folliculitis

A magnified view showing pustules at the base of each hair follicle. (Courtesy of the Department of Dermatology, National Naval Medical Center, Bethesda, MD.)

663

Associated Clinical Features

As HIV infection progresses and the CD4 cell count declines, HSV infections become more frequent and severe, with delayed healing and prolonged shedding. The lesions can be oral, labial, esophageal, genital, or rectal (Fig. 20.16). These ulcerations are often associated with regional adenopathy. HSV esophagitis is often associated with oral or labial HSV. In contrast to cytomegalovirus (CMV) where there is a large solitary esophageal ulcer, multiple small ulcers characterize HSV esophagitis. Perirectal lesions are often beefy red and extremely tender, with a predilection for the gluteal cleft. Perirectal HSV may also be associated with proctitis and anal fissures.

Ocular HSV may be demonstrated by observing dendritic lesions after fluorescein staining (see Figs. 2.30 to 2.32). HSV is associated with a syndrome of acute retinal necrosis characterized by pain, keratitis, and iritis that may lead to retinal detachment. Recurrent herpetic whitlow in HIV patients can be severe, with extensive cutaneous erosions on the fingers. Dissemination can cause encephalitis, pneumonitis, hepatitis, and colitis. The diagnosis is usually made clinically but can be confirmed a Tzanck preparation, biopsy, or culture.

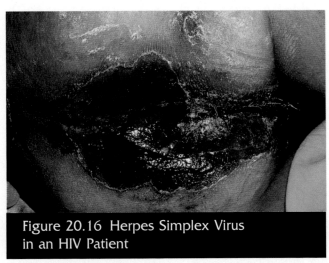

Figure 20.16 Herpes Simplex Virus in an HIV Patient

Severe, recurrent perirectal HSV lesions in an HIV patient. (Courtesy of Briana Hill, MD.)

Differential Diagnosis

Vesicular lesions such as those caused by contact dermatitis, herpes zoster, eosinophilic folliculitis, molluscum contagiosum, and drug reactions can resemble herpes simplex virus.

Emergency Department Treatment and Disposition

Acyclovir (200 mg five times a day for 10 days) or famciclovir (500 mg tid for 7 days) are standard treatments. Valacyclovir should be used with caution in patients with HIV since it is associated with TTP. Ocular HSV requires prompt ophthalmology referral. Severe, refractory, or disseminated HSV is an indication for admission and intravenous acyclovir. Intravenous acyclovir should be used with caution in dehydrated patients because it can crystallize in the renal tubules. For frequent recurrent oral or genital outbreaks, suppressive regimens (acyclovir 600 to 800 mg qd) are indicated.

Clinical Pearls

1. Anticipate disseminated disease in HIV patients.
2. Presentations of HSV may be atypical compared to HSV in immunocompetent individuals.
3. Suspect HSV in any HIV patient with a poorly healing, painful perirectal lesion.
4. Resistance to acyclovir and cross-resistance to ganciclovir are relatively common. Foscarnet may be considered as an alternative.

Associated Clinical Features

Molluscum contagiosum, usually an asymptomatic, benign disease, may be severe in HIV patients. The disease is caused by a poxvirus. HIV patients have a predilection for facial rash, sometimes with ocular involvement (Fig. 20.17). The rash can also involve the groin or become generalized. Typical presentations consist of groups of 2 to 20 small, discrete, "waxy" lesions with central umbilication. The incubation period for the virus ranges from 2 weeks to 6 months. Diagnosis is usually clinical but can also be made with a "squash" preparation—i.e., a Wright stain demonstrating intracytoplasmic inclusions.

Differential Diagnosis

Other dermatologic lesions that are often mistaken for molluscum contagiosum are cutaneous *Cryptococcus*, basal cell cancer, keratoacanthoma, and condyloma accuminata.

Emergency Department Treatment and Disposition

If the diagnosis is suspected in the ED, the patient should be reassured and referred to a dermatologist. The latter may utilize one of the following treatments: trichloroacetic peels, mechanical removal, cryosurgery, or the drug cidofovir. The recurrence rate is high.

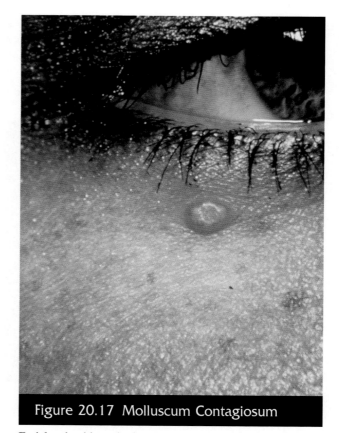

Figure 20.17 Molluscum Contagiosum

Facial rash with ocular involvement is a common site of infection in HIV patients. Note the central umbilication. (Courtesy of the Department of Dermatology, National Naval Medical Center, Bethesda, MD.)

Clinical Pearls

1. Although these lesions can regress spontaneously, removal is advisable to prevent autoinoculation.
2. Clinically, it may be difficult to distinguish between cutaneous *Cryptococcus* and molluscum contagiosum. Dermatology or infectious disease consultation and biopsy may be required.

Associated Clinical Features

Suspect *Pneumocystis carinii* pneumonia (PCP) in any HIV patient who presents with complaints of dyspnea and nonproductive cough. Presentations can be indolent, acute, or subacute. Associated symptoms include fever, fatigue, anorexia, weight loss, and chest pain. The CBC is usually normal except for lymphopenia. The LDH is often elevated. Arterial blood gases most often reveal a respiratory alkalosis and an increased A-a gradient. Findings on chest radiographs can be variable; however, the most common manifestation is diffuse interstitial alveolar infiltrates (Fig. 20.18). Previous recommendations that HIV patients with CD4 counts less than $200/\mu L$ should receive lifelong prophylaxis are changing. Therefore emergency physicians may encounter this condition more frequently in the future. Definitive diagnosis requires observing organisms in lung tissue. The most sensitive method is by open-lung or transbronchial biopsy. However, the more common diagnostic method is bronchoscopy and bronchoalveolar lavage revealing organisms on methenamine-silver stain.

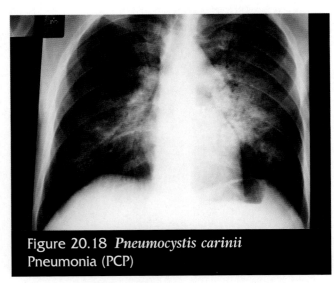

Figure 20.18 *Pneumocystis carinii* Pneumonia (PCP)

Chest radiograph showing diffuse interstitial alveolar infiltrates of PCP. (Courtesy of Edward C. Oldfield III, MD.)

Differential Diagnosis

The differential diagnosis of an HIV patient presenting to the ED with a pulmonary complaint is broad. In terms of frequency, community-acquired bacterial pneumonias are at the top of the list. Inquiry about previous purified protein derivative (PPD) status, travel, and ill contacts are important. This history might lead the examiner to suspect tuberculous pneumonia, histoplasmosis, cryptococcosis, coccidioidomycosis, or aspergillosis.

Another important question is the CD4 nadir, which might lead to suspicion of cytomegalovirus or toxoplasmal infection. Sometimes the findings on the chest radiograph can help in making the diagnosis.

Emergency Department Treatment and Disposition

The first priority in treating PCP is general supportive care. Trimethoprim-sulfamethoxazole, orally or intravenously, is the standard treatment. Pentamidine, atovaquone, and clindamycin are also effective. A 5-day course of prednisone should be added if the P_{O_2} is less than 70 or the A-a gradient is greater than 35. This has been shown to reduce the rates of intubation and death. Formerly, HIV patients received prophylaxis for the following indications: CD4 cell count less than $200/\mu L$, unexplained fever for more than 2 weeks, or an episode of oral candidiasis. However, if the viral load and CD4 counts are under good control, many infectious disease specialists are now stopping PCP prophylaxis.

Clinical Pearls

1. Include PCP in the differential diagnosis of any HIV patient who presents with a persistent fever or respiratory complaint.
2. PCP can also affect the bone marrow, spleen, liver, GI tract, pancreas, palate, pericardium, thymus, central nervous system, or eyes.

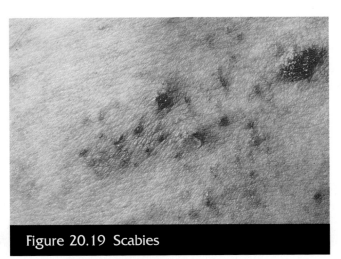

Figure 20.19 Scabies

Typical scabies rash showing unroofed papules secondary to scratching. Several small burrows are also seen. (Courtesy of George Turiansky, MD.)

Associated Clinical Features

Human scabies is one of the most common contagious dermatoses; it is caused by the mite *Sarcoptes scabiei.* In HIV patients, this organism can cause "crusted scabies," also known as Norwegian scabies (see Fig. 13.61), which denotes an overwhelming scabies infestation. In typical scabies, the mites cause extremely pruritic burrows, vesicles, and papules (Fig. 20.19) in a characteristic distribution involving the finger webs, sides of the hands and feet, breasts, waist, and groin. In contrast, crusted scabies typically affects the hands and the feet with asymptomatic crusting. Norwegian scabies typically does not cause significant pruritus. Typical scabies involves approximately 15 mites per infected individual, whereas Norwegian scabies involves a hyperinfestation with thousands to millions of mites per individual. Scabies is spread by direct physical contact, and it can occur in epidemic form. Risk factors include poor hygiene, crowding, and exposure to pets.

Differential Diagnosis

Often, Norwegian scabies will not be included in the differential due to lack of pruritus. Other conditions to consider are drug reactions, which are extremely common in HIV patients, and pediculosis in sexually promiscuous patients and prostitutes. Dermatoses such as psoriasis and Kaposi's sarcoma should also be included in the differential diagnosis.

Emergency Department Treatment and Disposition

Most often the diagnosis of scabies is made clinically, with evidence of burrows and severe pruritus in a characteristic distribution. Definitive diagnosis is made from examination of shavings from the lesions. Placing mineral oil over a suspected lesion and then shaving it with a number 15 blade can demonstrate the mites, which are usually 0.3 to 0.4 mm in length. Sometimes eggs, egg casings, or feces can be seen. Norwegian scabies is diagnosed similarly, with demonstration of the mites on a mineral oil or potassium hydroxide microscopic examination.

Permethrin cream has a low toxicity and is the treatment of choice for scabies. Patients are instructed to apply the cream from the neck down and leave it on for 8 h before removal. The patient's clothes and bedding should be washed in hot water. Antihistamines alleviate the pruritus.

For HIV patients with Norwegian scabies, permethrin should be applied to the face, scalp, behind the ears, and from the neck downward. Repeat treatments may be needed. Sometimes 6% salicylic acid, a keratolytic agent, should be prescribed to improve penetration of the scabicide. For severe or refractory cases, oral ivermectin (200 μg/kg for one dose) can be tried.

Clinical Pearls

1. *Wear gloves*!
2. Oral antibiotics are often indicated for Norwegian scabies because of skin breakdown.
3. Treat close contacts.
4. Tell patients that although the scabicide will kill the mites, the itching may last for weeks. Patients often seek repeat treatments and inappropriately receive additional scabicides, which can cause contact dermatitis.

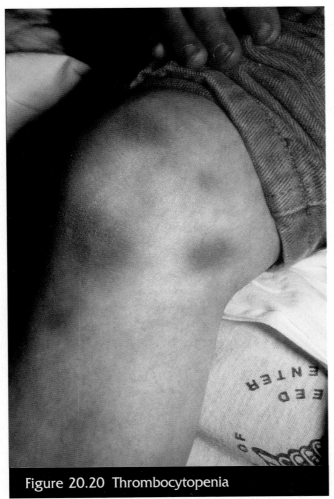

Figure 20.20 Thrombocytopenia

Ecchymosis in an HIV patient with thrombocytopenia. (Courtesy of Edward C. Oldfield III, MD.)

Associated Clinical Features

Thrombocytopenia occurs in 30 to 60% of all HIV patients. It can occur independently at all stages of HIV infection and by itself does not have significant prognostic value. This is different from HIV-associated anemia and granulocytopenia, which occur concomitantly with the severity of the course of the HIV infection. The etiology of HIV-associated thrombocytopenia is usually multifactorial, with decreased bone marrow production and increased platelet destruction, which can be either immune- or nonimmune-mediated. Immune destruction occurs secondary to molecular mimicry between the HIV 120 antigen and the platelet GpIIb/IIIa receptor. Infections and fevers can decrease the life span of platelets in HIV patients, contributing to the thrombocytopenia. HIV patients with thrombocytopenia can present to the ED with bleeding (especially from the oral mucosa), ecchymosis (Fig. 20.20), and petechiae.

Differential Diagnosis

The skin findings of thrombocytopenia can be confused with manifestations of opportunistic infections or Kaposi's sarcoma. If laboratory findings indicate a thrombocytopenia, the clinician should exclude pseudothrombocytopenia by assuring that the smear does not contain clumped megakaryocytes. Aside from primary thrombocytopenia associated with HIV, the emergency physician should consider drug toxicity, idiopathic thrombocytopenic purpura (ITP), thrombotic thrombocytopenic purpura (TTP), hemolytic uremic syndrome (HUS), and infections.

Emergency Department Treatment and Disposition

The emergency physician's efforts are initially focused on stabilization of the patient with two large intravenous lines, type and cross-match, and crystalloid infusion if significant bleeding has occurred. Because of the complexity of the differential diagnosis and potentially complicated treatment of HIV thrombocytopenia, an infectious disease specialist should be consulted early. In most cases, HIV patients with platelet count greater than 50,000 can be managed conservatively. Zidovudine can increase platelet counts in over 50% of patients. If the platelet count is less than 20,000 many infectious disease specialists recommend gamma globulin infusion and parenteral steroids. Other possible treatments include dapsone, vincristine, and, as a last resort, splenecotomy. Even if the patient is to be managed conservatively, bone marrow analysis should be arranged on an outpatient basis to rule out other causes of thrombocytopenia.

Clinical Pearls

1. Observe universal precautions!
2. Perform thorough skin and oral examinations in all patients with HIV looking for evidence of thrombocytopenia.
3. Take a careful drug history and consider other infectious etiologies before assuming the thrombocytopenia is directly secondary to HIV infection.
4. Spontaneous bleeding is rare unless the platelet count is less than 10,000.

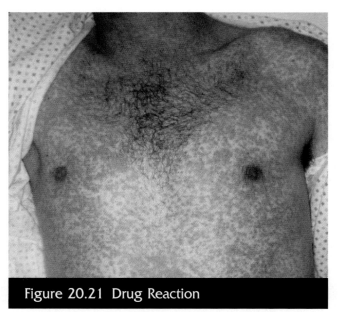

Figure 20.21 Drug Reaction

Exanthematous drug reaction in an HIV patient. (Courtesy of Kenneth Skahan, MD.)

Associated Clinical Features

For unknown reasons, HIV patients have a 5 to 20 times higher rate of drug reactions than non-HIV patients. Up to 5% of ED visits by HIV patients are due to complications of pharmacologic therapy. Many of these reactions are manifest dermatologically, in order of decreasing frequency: (1) exanthems (Fig. 20.21), (2) urticaria/angioedema, (3) fixed drug reactions (see Fig. 13.46), (4) erythema multiforme (see Fig. 13.1), and (5) photosensitivity reactions (see Fig. 13.58). The most common classes of medications associated with rashes are antivirals, antibiotics, and antifungals.

Differential Diagnosis

In addition to cutaneous drug reactions, the emergency physician should consider other primary dermatologic conditions. Often the timing of drug initiation can be helpful. Most drug reactions occur within 1 to 2 weeks of the initiation of the drug, but they can also occur months or years later. Another consideration is that the skin findings may be a manifestation of opportunistic infection or neoplasm, such as Kaposi's sarcoma or lymphoma.

Emergency Department Treatment and Disposition

The emergency physician may need to consult an infectious disease specialist, a pharmacist, or a dermatologist to help clarify the existence of a drug reaction. Clues besides recent initiation of a new drug are eosinophilia greater than 1000 or elevated liver function tests. Individual treatment varies depending on the situation. The offending agent should be discontinued. Antihistamines and steroids are indicated in certain situations.

Clinical Pearls

1. Do not forget to ask about alternative medicines and nonprescription medications.
2. One-half of all HIV patients will react adversely to sulfa drugs.
3. Be aware of Stevens-Johnson syndrome and toxic epidermal necrolysis (TEN).
4. Notify Medwatch or a similar hospital agency regarding serious or unusual reactions.

Associated Clinical Features

Acute necrotizing ulcerative gingivitis (ANUG), also known as Vincent's angina or trench mouth, is commonly seen in HIV patients (Fig. 20.22). The triad associated with ANUG is oral pain, halitosis, and ulcerations along the interdental papillae. Other signs and symptoms include "metallic taste," "wooden teeth" sensation, tooth mobility, fever, adenopathy, and malnutrition. The cause of this aggressive, destructive process is infection by oral anaerobes (*Treponema, Selenomonas, Fusobacterium, Prevotella*).

ANUG represents a spectrum of disease from mild ulcerations to severe cellulitis and spread of the infection to the soft tissues, cheeks, lips, and bones.

Differential Diagnosis

The differential diagnosis includes typical gingivitis, pharyngitis, HIV-associated idiopathic ulcerations, herpes simplex virus, and oral candidiasis. Emergency physicians should always consider Ludwig's angina. Noma (cancrum oris, gangrenous stomatitis), a rare disease of childhood associated with malnutrition, is characterized by an anaerobic destructive infectious process of the orofacial tissues that can resemble ANUG.

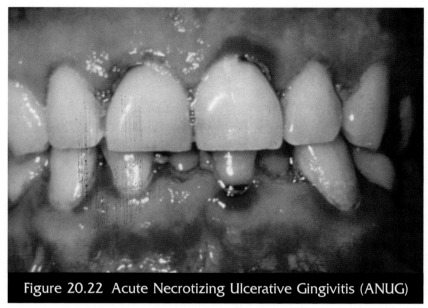

Figure 20.22 Acute Necrotizing Ulcerative Gingivitis (ANUG)

ANUG (Vincent's angina or "trench mouth") caused by spirochetal and fusiform bacteria in an HIV patient. Note the punched-out ulcerations of the interdental papillae, which are pathognomonic. (Courtesy of the Department of Dermatology, National Naval Medical Center, Bethesda, MD.)

Emergency Department Treatment and Disposition

ANUG is most frequently seen in three population groups: (1) HIV patients, (2) malnourished children, and (3) young adults who are under a great deal of stress. The first steps for the emergency physician are to eliminate other, potentially more serious life-threatening infections and to address hydration status. Treatment includes (1) eliminating contributing factors (stress, poor nutrition, poor sleep, alcohol and tobacco use), (2) chlorhexidine rinses twice a day, (3) surgical debridement by an oral surgeon, and (4) oral pencillin and metronidazole.

Clinical Pearls

1. Do not miss Ludwig's angina (brawny submandibular induration and tongue elevation—see Fig. 6.23) or noma.
2. ANUG is most frequently confused with herpes simplex virus.

CHAPTER 21

MICROSCOPIC FINDINGS

Diane M. Birnbaumer

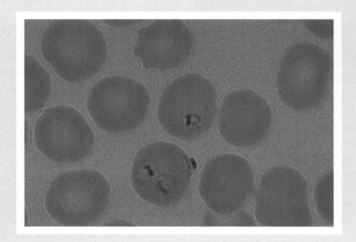

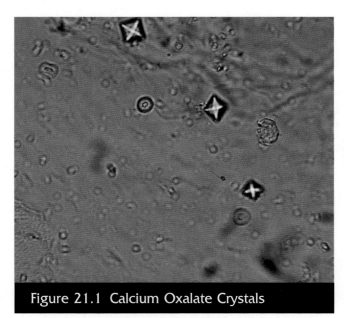

Figure 21.1 Calcium Oxalate Crystals

Calcium oxalate crystals come in two shapes. The classically described octahedral, or envelope-shaped, crystals are made of calcium oxalate dihydrate. Calcium oxalate monohydrate crystals are needle-shaped. They are seen in acid or neutral urine. They may be found in the urine of patients with ethylene glycol ingestion. In addition, the urine of patients with ethylene glycol ingestion may also fluoresce under a Wood's lamp. (From Susan K. Strasinger: *Urinalysis and Body Fluids,* 3d ed. Philadelphia: Davis; 1994.)

Uses

To evaluate for the presence of cells, casts, and crystals. See Figs. 21.1 to 21.5.

Materials

Freshly collected urine specimen, centrifuge, graduated centrifuge tubes, glass microscope slide, coverslip.

Method

1. Pour 10 mL of freshly collected urine into a graduated centrifuge tube.
2. Centrifuge at ×400 to ×450 gravity for 5 min.
3. Decant 9 mL of supernatant, leaving 1 mL in the tube.
4. Resuspend the centrifuged pellet in the remaining 1 mL of urine by stirring with a pipet.
5. Place one drop of resuspended urine on a glass microscope slide.
6. Overlay with a coverslip.
7. Examine initially using scanning ×10 power, emphasizing the periphery of the coverslip, since urinary elements tend to gather at the edges.
8. Switch to ×40 power to focus on specific urinary elements such as cells, casts, and crystals. Use ×100 power as needed for specific identification.

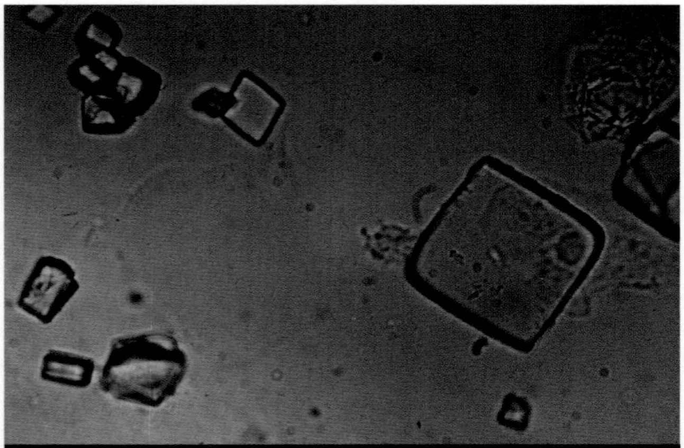

Figure 21.2 Uric Acid Crystals

Uric acid crystals often have a yellow hue and a variety of sizes and shapes. They are found in acidic urine. (From Susan K. Strasinger: *Urinalysis and Body Fluids,* 3d ed. Philadelphia: Davis; 1994.)

676

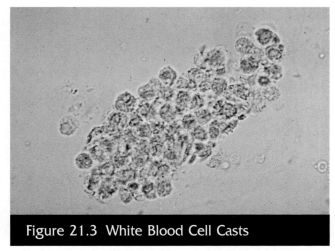

Figure 21.3 White Blood Cell Casts

Usually two to three cells in width, white blood cell casts are indicative of upper urinary tract infection such as pyelonephritis. (Courtesy of the American Society of Clinical Pathologists.)

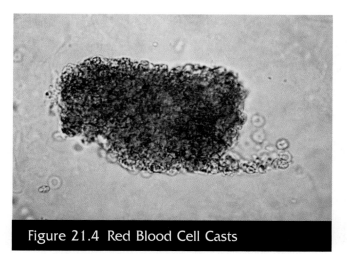

Figure 21.4 Red Blood Cell Casts

Red blood cells casts range from 3 to 10 cells in width and are seen in glomerulonephritis. (Courtesy of the American Society of Clinical Pathologists.)

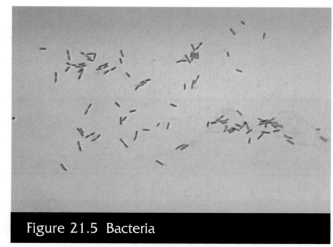

Figure 21.5 Bacteria

Bacteria are often seen in urine specimens and either can be consistent with infection or may result from local contamination from surrounding skin during specimen collection. (Courtesy of Roche Laboratories, Division of Hoffman-LaRoche Inc., Nutley, NJ.)

Uses

To determine the presence of uric acid crystals (in patients with gout) or calcium pyrophosphate crystals (in patients with pseudogout) in joint fluid. See Figs. 21.6 and 21.7.

Materials

Freshly collected joint fluid, glass microscope slide, coverslip, polarizer.

Method

1. To prevent interference from polarizing artifacts, clean the slide and coverslip with alcohol prior to using them.
2. Using freshly collected unspun joint fluid, place a drop of joint fluid on the glass microscope slide.
3. Overlay coverslip.
4. View the slide using the polarizer.
5. Scan at ×10 power; ×100 power is needed to see intracellular crystals.

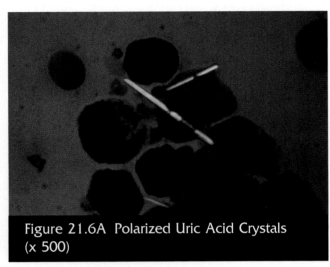

Figure 21.6A Polarized Uric Acid Crystals (x 500)

Intracellular needle-like uric acid crystals are seen within the polymorphonuclear cells from the joint fluid in a patient with gout using a direct polarizing light. (From Susan K. Strasinger: *Urinalysis and Body Fluids,* 3d ed. Philadelphia: Davis; 1994.)

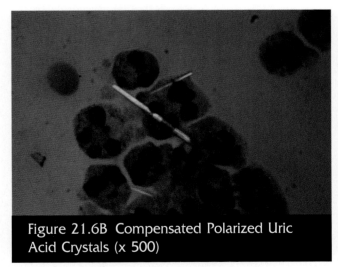

Figure 21.6B Compensated Polarized Uric Acid Crystals (x 500)

Once crystals are found with a direct polarizing light, identification is made by using a compensated polarized light. The yellow crystal is aligned parallel to the slow vibration component of the compensator (negatively birefringent). The blue crystal is perpendicular (Crossed Urate Blue). (From Susan K. Strasinger: *Urinalysis and Body Fluids,* 3d ed. Philadelphia: Davis; 1994.)

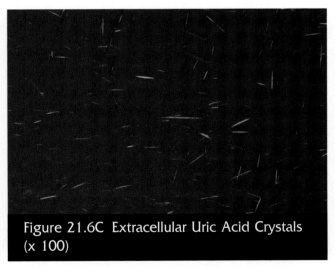

Figure 21.6C Extracellular Uric Acid Crystals (x 100)

Extracellular uric acid crystals are seen under compensated polarized light. Notice the change of color with crystal alignment. (From Susan K. Strasinger: *Urinalysis and Body Fluids,* 3d ed. Philadelphia: Davis; 1994.)

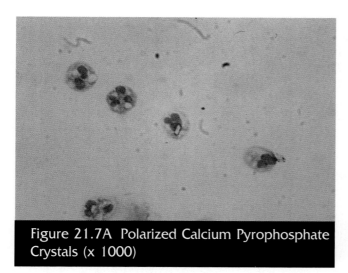

Figure 21.7A Polarized Calcium Pyrophosphate Crystals (x 1000)

Intracellular rhomboid crystals in the joint of a patient with pseudogout. They may also appear as rods. (From Susan K. Strasinger: *Urinalysis and Body Fluids,* 3d ed. Philadelphia: Davis; 1994.)

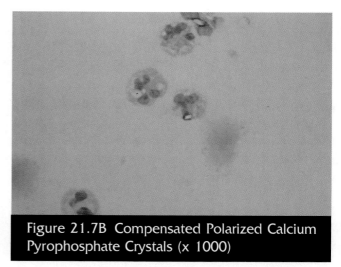

Figure 21.7B Compensated Polarized Calcium Pyrophosphate Crystals (x 1000)

The blue calcium pyrophosphate crystal is aligned parallel to the slow vibration component of the compensator (positively birefringent). (From Susan K. Strasinger: *Urinalysis and Body Fluids,* 3d ed. Philadelphia: Davis; 1994.)

Uses

To determine adequacy of specimen (e.g., sputum); to determine the morphology of predominant organisms in a specimen. See Figs. 21.8 to 21.11.

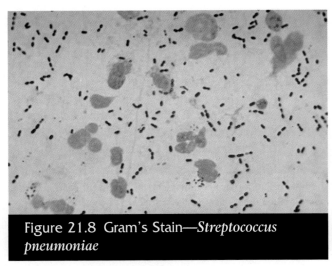

Figure 21.8 Gram's Stain—*Streptococcus pneumoniae*

Gram-positive, kidney-shaped diplococci of *S. pneumoniae*. (Courtesy of Roche Laboratories, Division of Hoffman-LaRoche Inc. Nutley, NJ.)

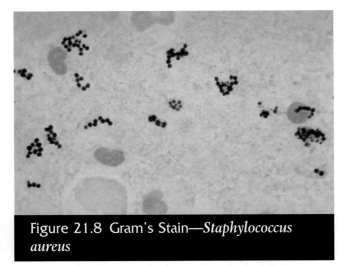

Figure 21.8 Gram's Stain—*Staphylococcus aureus*

Small clusters of gram-positive cocci seen in *S. aureus* infection. (Courtesy of Roche Laboratories, Division of Hoffman-LaRoche Inc. Nutley, NJ.)

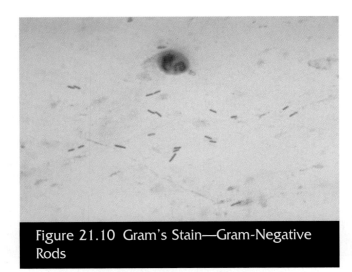

Figure 21.10 Gram's Stain—Gram-Negative Rods

Gram-negative rods of *Pseudomonas aeruginosa*. (Courtesy of Roche Laboratories, Division of Hoffman-LaRoche Inc. Nutley, NJ.)

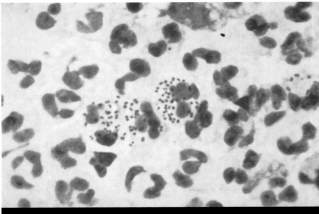

Figure 21.11 Gram's Stain—Neisseria gonorrhoeae

Multiple gram-negative, intracellular diplococci from a patient with *N. gonorrhoeae*. (Courtesy of Morse, Moreland, Thompson: *Atlas of Sexually Transmitted Diseases*. London: Mosby-Wolfe; 1990.)

Materials

Freshly collected specimen to be examined, glass microscope slide, crystal violet, Gram's iodine, acetone-alcohol (acetone, 30 mL, and 95% alcohol, 70 mL), safranin, Bunsen burner.

Method

1. Put specimen on dry, clean glass microscope slide and allow to air dry.
2. Heat-fix specimen by gently passing over flame.
3. Cover specimen with crystal violet for 1 min.
4. Rinse off completely with water; do not blot.
5. Cover specimen with Gram's iodine for 1 min.
6. Rinse off completely with water; do not blot.
7. Decolorize for 30 s with gentle agitation in acetone-alcohol.
8. Rinse off completely with water; do not blot.
9. Cover with safranin for 10 to 20 s.
10. Rinse off completely with water and let air-dry.

Uses

To examine lesions (chancres, mucous patches, condyloma lata, skin rash) for the presence of *Treponema pallidum* (Fig. 21.12).

Materials

Compound microscope with dark-field condenser (dark-field microscope), glass microscope slide, coverslip, physiologic saline.

Method for Obtaining and Viewing the Specimen

1. From chancre or condyloma lata:
   a. Gently abrade the lesion with a dry gauze.
   b. Dab away any bleeding.
   c. Touch slide to exudative fluid in base of lesion.
   d. Overlay coverslip and view immediately under dark-field microscope using ×40 and ×100 objectives.

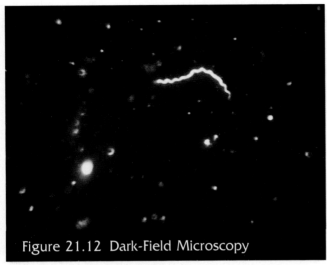

Figure 21.12 Dark-Field Microscopy

Examined under a dark-field microscope at ×40 or ×100 power, spirochetes appear as motile, bright corkscrews against a black background. (Courtesy of Morse, Moreland, Thompson: *Atlas of Sexually Transmitted Diseases*. London: Mosby-Wolfe; 1990.)

2. From mucous patch:
   a. Touch slide to mucous patch.
   b. Overlay coverslip and view immediately under dark-field microscope using ×40 and ×100 objectives.
3. From skin lesion:
   a. Gently scrape surface of skin lesion with edge of a number 15 scalpel blade.
   b. Dab away any bleeding.
   c. Touch slide to exudative fluid rising from skin lesion.
   d. Overlay coverslip and view immediately under dark-field microscope using ×40 and ×100 objectives.

Uses

To examine for clue cells, *Trichomonas,* and sperm. See Figs. 21.13 to 21.15.

Materials

Aqueous sodium chloride, glass microscope slide, coverslip.

Method

1. Place a drop of saline onto the middle of the glass slide. (Alternative method: Place several drops of saline in a small glass test tube and place the swab in the tube. The swab can then be wiped onto a slide at a later time.)
2. Mix a small amount of vaginal fluid to be examined into the saline drop.
3. Overlay a coverslip.
4. Examine directly through microscope at ×40 and ×100 (oil immersion).

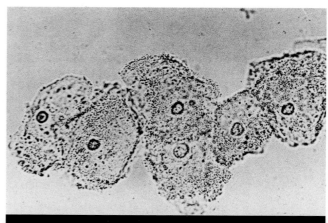

Figure 21.13 Clue Cells

"Glitter cell" or "clue cell": Epithelial cell covered with adherent bacteria in a wet mount of a vaginal specimen from a patient with *Gardnerella vaginalis* (also known as nonspecific vaginitis or bacterial vaginosis). Note the refractile appearance, indistinct borders, and ragged edges of the epithelial clue cell. (Courtesy of Curatek Pharmaceuticals.)

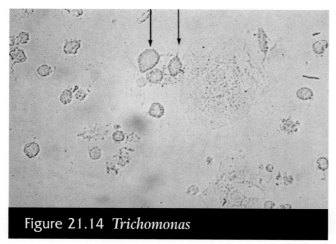

Figure 21.14 *Trichomonas*

Saline wet mount demonstrating oval-bodied, flagellated trichomonads. They are similar in size to leukocytes and can be distinguished from them by their motility and presence of flagella. (Courtesy of H. Hunter Hansfield: *Atlas of Sexually Transmitted Diseases.* New York: McGraw-Hill; 1992.)

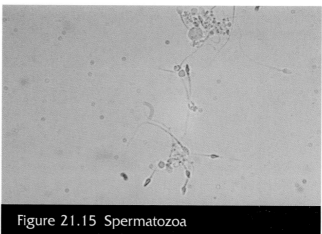

Figure 21.15 Spermatozoa

Spermatozoa may be motile or immotile. (From Susan K. Strasinger: *Urinalysis and Body Fluids,* 3d ed. Philadelphia: Davis; 1994.)

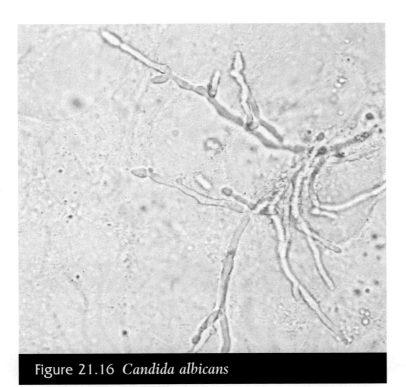

Figure 21.16 *Candida albicans*

Potassium hydroxide preparation of vaginal secretions from a patient with vaginal candidiasis due to *Candida albicans*. Note the pseudohyphae characteristic of this organism. (Courtesy of H. Hunter Hansfield: *Atlas of Sexually Transmitted Diseases*. New York: McGraw-Hill; 1992.)

Uses

To examine for yeast and fungus. See Fig. 21.16.

Materials

Aqueous potassium hydroxide (KOH) 10%, glass microscope slide, coverslip.

Method

1. Place a drop of KOH onto the middle of the glass slide.
2. Suspend a small amount of vaginal fluid into the drop of KOH.
3. Overlay a coverslip.
4. Let sit at room temperature for 30 min; as an alternative, gently heat the slide over a Bunsen burner but do not boil.
5. Examine under microscope for hyphae and spores.

Uses

To evaluate a patient for the presence of fecal leukocytes. See Fig. 21.17.

Materials

Freshly collected liquid stool specimen, glass microscope slide, coverslip, methylene blue.

Method

1. Place a drop of liquid stool onto the glass slide.
2. Add two drops of methylene blue to the stool specimen.
3. Mix thoroughly.
4. Overlay with a coverslip.
5. Place the edge of a piece of filter paper adjacent to the coverslip to absorb any excess methylene blue.
6. Examine using ×10 objective to scan specimen and ×40 and ×100 to identify specific leukocytes.

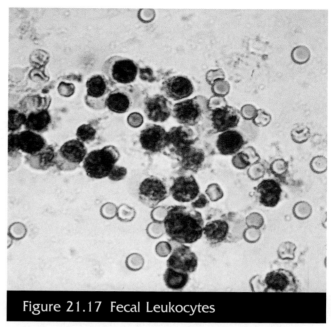

Figure 21.17 Fecal Leukocytes

Multiple white cells in the stool specimen from a patient with bacterial diarrhea. (Courtesy of Herbert L. DuPont, MD.)

Uses

To determine fungal dermatoses or skin infestations. See Figs. 21.18 to 21.21.

Materials

Fresh skin scraping, glass microscope slide, coverslip, 10% potassium hydroxide or mineral oil.

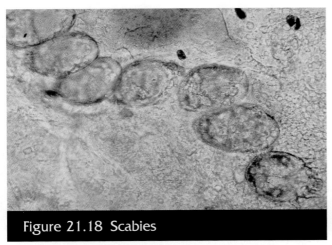

Figure 21.18 Scabies

Skin scraping from a patient with scabies. Note the intact mite at the lower right of the photograph, and the ova and fecal pellets. (Courtesy of the Department of Dermatology, Naval Medical Center, Portsmouth, VA.)

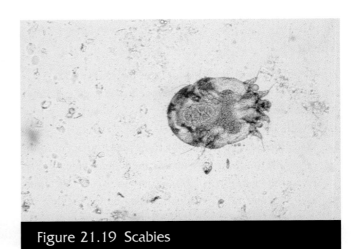

Figure 21.19 Scabies

Adult female scabies mite. (Courtesy of Morse, Moreland, Thompson: *Atlas of Sexually Transmitted Diseases.* London: Mosby-Wolfe; 1990.)

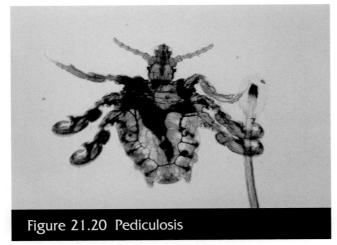

Figure 21.20 Pediculosis

Phthirus pubis, the crab louse. Note the short body and claw-like legs, which are ideally suited for clinging to the hair shaft. (Courtesy of the Department of Dermatology, Naval Medical Center, Portsmouth, VA.)

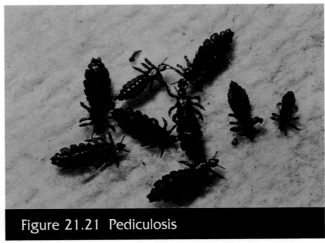

Figure 21.21 Pediculosis

Phthirus corporis, the body louse. Note the elongated body. (Courtesy of the Department of Dermatology, Naval Medical Center, Portsmouth, VA.)

Method

1. Specimen collection:
   a. Gently scrape skin lesion with edge of a number 15 scalpel.
2. Slide preparation:
   a. Pediculosis may be seen grossly clinging to individual hairs or under low power. Live nits may fluoresce with a Wood's lamp.
   b. For scabies, place a drop of KOH or mineral oil onto the slide.
   c. Suspend a small amount of the scraping onto the drop.
   d. Overlay a coverslip.
   e. Let sit at room temperature for 30 min; as an alternative, gently heat the slide over a Bunsen burner but do not boil.
   f. Examine under microscope for hyphae, spores, or infestations.

Cerebrospinal Fluid Examination

INDIA INK PREPARATION

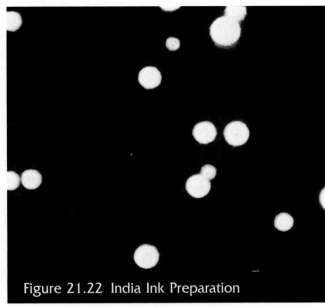

Figure 21.22 India Ink Preparation

Budding yeast with prominent capsule on india ink preparation from a patient with *C. neoformans* meningitis. (Courtesy of Morse, Moreland, Thompson: *Atlas of Sexually Transmitted Diseases.* London: Mosby-Wolfe; 1990.)

Uses

To examine cerebrospinal fluid for organisms with capsules, particularly *Cryptococcus neoformans.*

Materials

India ink, glass microscope slide, coverslip. See Fig. 21.22.

Method

1. Lightly centrifuge cerebrospinal fluid to concentrate cells at bottom of tube (1 to 2 min).
2. Pour off excess fluid (retain if further testing may be necessary).
3. Take a drop from the bottom of the centrifuge tube and place it in the middle of a glass microscope slide.
4. Place a drop of india ink into the specimen drop; gently mix.
5. Overlay a coverslip.
6. Examine at ×10 to screen specimen, use ×40 objective to confirm findings.

Uses

To evaluate for the presence of ring trophozoites. See Fig. 21.23.

Materials

Air-dried blood smear, Coplin jar of Wright's stain, slide rack, pH 7.2 buffer, blotting paper.

Method

1. Place a drop of blood on the middle of a slide.
2. Hold another slide evenly on top of the slide at a 45-degree angle and drag the slide over the drop of blood to the opposite edge to spread the blood evenly.
3. Allow the blood to dry for 5 to 10 min.
4. Stain air-dried smears in a closed Coplin jar of Wright's stain for 5 min.
5. Place the slide on a rack.
6. Rinse and treat with pH 7.2 buffer primed with 1 mL Wright's stain per 400 mL for 3 min.
7. Rinse in pH 7.2 buffer for 20 s.
8. Blot dry and mount on microscope at ×100 (oil immersion).

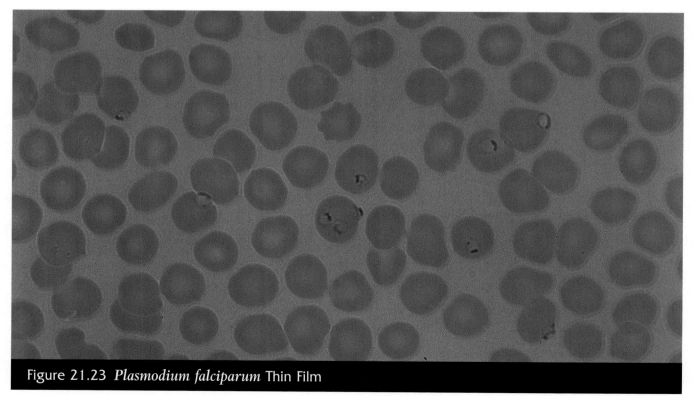

Figure 21.23 *Plasmodium falciparum* Thin Film

Ring forms (trophozoites) of *P. falciparum* are seen on the Wright's stain thin film in a patient with intermittent fever who had recently traveled to Africa. (Courtesy of James P. Elrod, MD, PhD.)

INDEX

Note: Page numbers followed by the letter *f* indicate figures; page numbers followed by the letter *t* indicate tables.